Textbook of Allergy for the Clinician

Second Edition

Editors

Pudupakkam K Vedanthan
Clinical Professor of Medicine
University of Colorado
Denver, Colorado
USA

Harold S Nelson
Professor of Medicine
National Jewish Health
Denver, Colorado
USA

Shripad N Agashe
University of Bangalore
Karnataka
India

PA Mahesh
Department of Respiratory Medicine
J S S University
Mysore, Karnataka
India

Rohit Katial
National Jewish Health
Denver, Colorado
USA

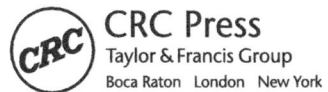

CRC Press
Taylor & Francis Group
Boca Raton London New York

CRC Press is an imprint of the
Taylor & Francis Group, an **informa** business

A SCIENCE PUBLISHERS BOOK

Cover credit:

Picture of Mast Cell: Reproduced by kind permission of Mariana Castells, M.D., Ph.D., Director Mastocytosis Center, Brigham and Women's Hospital, Professor of Medicine, Harvard Medical School, USA.

Alternaria mold picture: From the personal collection of Dr Shripad N Agashe, Co editor.

CT Skull picture: Personal collection of Pudupakkam K Vedanthan MD Lead editor.

Picture of Silk Worm Pupa: Personal collection of Pudupakkam K Vedanthan M.D. Lead editor.

Second edition published 2021
by CRC Press
6000 Broken Sound Parkway NW, Suite 300, Boca Raton, FL 33487-2742

and by CRC Press
2 Park Square, Milton Park, Abingdon, Oxon, OX14 4RN

© 2021 Taylor & Francis Group, LLC

First edition published by CRC Press 2014

CRC Press is an imprint of Taylor & Francis Group, LLC

Reasonable efforts have been made to publish reliable data and information, but the author and publisher cannot assume responsibility for the validity of all materials or the consequences of their use. The authors and publishers have attempted to trace the copyright holders of all material reproduced in this publication and apologize to copyright holders if permission to publish in this form has not been obtained. If any copyright material has not been acknowledged please write and let us know so we may rectify in any future reprint.

Except as permitted under U.S. Copyright Law, no part of this book may be reprinted, reproduced, transmitted, or utilized in any form by any electronic, mechanical, or other means, now known or hereafter invented, including photocopying, microfilming, and recording, or in any information storage or retrieval system, without written permission from the publishers.

For permission to photocopy or use material electronically from this work, access www.copyright.com or contact the Copyright Clearance Center, Inc. (CCC), 222 Rosewood Drive, Danvers, MA 01923, 978-750-8400. For works that are not available on CCC please contact mpkbookspermissions@tandf.co.uk

Trademark notice: Product or corporate names may be trademarks or registered trademarks and are used only for identification and explanation without intent to infringe.

Library of Congress Cataloging-in-Publication Data
```
Names: Vedanthan, P. K. (Pudupakkam K.), editor.
Title: Textbook of allergy for the clinician / Pudupakkam K. Vedanthan,
   Clinical Professor of Medicine, University of Colorado  Denver, Colorado
   [and four others].
Description: Second edition. | Boca Raton : CRC Press, 2021.
Identifiers: LCCN 2020041197 | ISBN 9780367405526 (hardcover)
Subjects: LCSH: Allergy.
Classification: LCC RC584 .T49 2021 | DDC 616.97/5--dc23
LC record available at https://lccn.loc.gov/2020041197
```

ISBN: 978-0-367-40552-6 (hbk)

Typeset in Times New Roman
by Radiant Productions

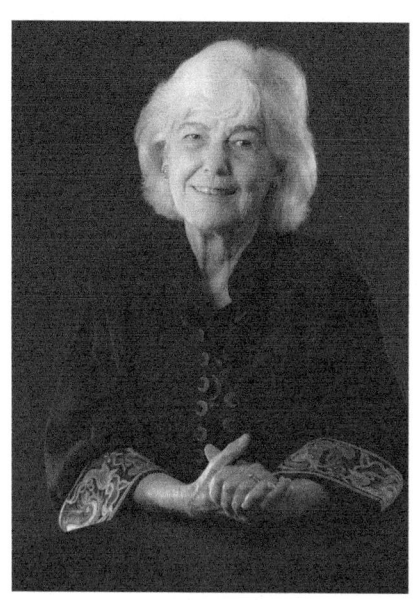

'In loving memory of Sarah Milledge Nelson Ph.D.
29 November 1931 to 27 April 2020'

Foreword

It is a pleasure to introduce this new edition of the 'Textbook of Allergy for the Clinician'. All the chapters have been updated, and new chapters have been added by authors from renowned institutions. Specifically, new chapters address topics that are particularly 'hot' in allergy and clinical immunology: Risk factors in asthma and allergies, office procedures and the updated chapter on food allergy. Separate chapters address asthma in pediatric and adult patients. The chapter on asthma has been expanded to include treatment with biologic medications. The scope of the content is comprehensive.

The audience is clinically 'targeted' and includes medical students, residents and fellows in training, nurses, physicians' assistants, nurse practitioners and others who contribute to recognition and treatment of patients with allergic and immunological diseases. The updated textbook will also have value in developing countries where the specialty of allergy and immunology is growing and where there is greater need for awareness of these illnesses and their management.

This is an international effort with contributions from educational centers in the United States, United Kingdom, Singapore and India.

Correspondence:
Charles H. Kirkpatrick, M.D.
Department of Medicine
University of Colorado Anschutz Medical Campus
B-164, R2
12700 East 19th Ave.
Aurora, CO 80045
charles.kirkpatrick@cuanschutz.edu

Preface

We are very pleased and eager to present the Textbook of Allergy for The Clinician, 2nd Edition. The first edition, published in 2014, was very well received especially by the training programs in India and served as the primary text as well as for ready references. There have been significant advances in the fields of allergy, asthma and immunology, especially in areas like food allergy, drug allergy, severe asthma, biological therapy, allergen immunotherapy, atopic dermatitis, latex allergy, as well as laboratory diagnostic techniques. An earnest attempt has been made to cover all these developments. The 2nd edition of our text book with 35 chapters has international impressions and variety, through the participation of 62 authors and co-authors from three different continents, namely America, Asia and Europe. Our senior colleague and co-editor Dr. Harold Nelson has been a constant pillar of support and has personally edited all the chapters in this edition. His support and guidance is highly appreciated by the editorial board. We want to sincerely thank all the authors, co-authors and their supporting staff and families for the cooperation and understanding in submitting the manuscripts in a timely manner. We want to thank the editorial staff at CRC Press (Taylor & Francis) for the expert guidance, cooperation and assistance. We thank International Asthma Services (IAS) Colorado USA for sponsoring this educational outreach. We sincerely thank our families for their understanding and continued support. We hope this edition will serve the purpose of updating and renewing the knowledge of all our students, colleagues and health professionals.

April 4th 2020

Dr Pudupakkam K Vedanthan
Dr Harold S Nelson
Dr Shripad N Agashe
Dr PA Mahesh
Dr Rohit Katial

Acknowledgements

Pudupakkam K Vedanthan

I feel privileged to be the Lead Editor for the Textbook of Allergy for the Clinician, 2nd edition. This textbook is truly international featuring 62 authors from four countries specifically India, Singapore, UK and the USA. As the main editor, it is of utmost importance that I encourage medical students, residents and fellows in training, and physicians in specialty courses to update their knowledge of allergy, asthma and immunology. My co-editor, mentor and teacher, Dr. Harold S. Nelson, has been a constant source of strength, support, and guidance through this process of planning, executing, and editing each of the chapters for this edition. The editorial board is highly appreciative of his support.

I dedicate this work to very important individuals in my personal and professional life, including: my father, late Dr. P. D. Krishnasawmi, a well-known and respected medical practitioner; my mother, late Mrs. P. D. Seethammal; my favorite teachers and mentors, Dr. K. G. Das, Retired Professor of Medicine, Mysore Medical College, India; late Dr. Henry Claman; late Dr. Elliott Middleton; late Dr. Hyman Chai and Dr. Harold S. Nelson. These people have instilled the value of hard work, dedication and sincerity. My special thanks to my wife Mrs. Kamala Vedanthan, to our daughter Ms. Ranjani Vedanthan who was especially helpful in editing, as well as our son Dr. Rajesh Vedanthan for his constant support and valuable suggestions. I owe a lot of gratitude to Mr. Mohan Murthy, my old friend, high school classmate from a family of publishers 'Shakthi Press' in the city of Mysuru, India for the invaluable help in making sure all the manuscript guidelines were satisfied. I sincerely thank the members of the editorial board for their suggestions, support, and overall teamwork. The publishers (CRC Press: Taylor and Francis) and their staff in the editorial department have been a constant source of guidance and assistance. I wholeheartedly thank and appreciate all the authors and co-authors for their sacrifice and the extra efforts to submit the manuscript in a timely manner. Everyone was very cooperative throughout the multiple steps involved in presenting the updated edition of this textbook.

PA Mahesh

At the outset, I would like to gratefully acknowledge Dr. Hal Nelson for taking on the brunt of the editing work. I would like to acknowledge my wife Dr. Amrutha D.H. and son Chirag for their patience. My parents Dr. Anand Rao P. and Neerada Rao P. for their encouragement, spirit of never giving up and positive inputs always. My father is a general practitioner and has been an important influence on me in understanding how to relate to patients and develop the important skill of patient communication. As a medical student, I was amazed at the dedication and commitment of my uncle, Dr. P. Laxminarayan Rao, Professor in Physiology and Former Dean Kasturba College, Manipal (only the second Indian to complete 50 years of teaching in physiology), who also instilled in me a desire to be a teacher. I am also greatly indebted to my mentor, Professor P. Ravindran, for helping me to develop both the attitude and aptitude in academics, clinical medicine and research. He remains my main role model and has guided my career decisions and has always led by example.

Shripad N Agashe

I wish to dedicate the chapter on aerobiology to my late wife D.R. Nirmala S. Agashe, retired Professor of Mathematics, Bangalore University who struggled so much and encouraged me to continue my academic pursuit. I am also thankful to my daughters Sandhya and Swapna who looked after me all these years, helped me and encouraged in all my academic work. I am thankful to Dr. Jacob N. Abraham, retired

Professor of Botany, St. Joseph College, Bangalore, India, for his assistance in the chapter on aerobiology. I am very grateful to Dr. Harold Nelson and Dr. Vedanthan for handling the lion's share in preparation of this edition

Rohit Katial

This textbook is being assembled in the midst of the COVID-19 pandemic and highlights the importance of caring and supporting each other. I am grateful to my parents for providing me the skills to be able to not only contribute to this textbook but assist society in a meaningful manner during such challenging times. I thank both my family for their support, and I thank my colleagues for the collaborative effort leading to the 2nd edition of such a widely used textbook which will educate generations to come.

About the Sponsor

INTERNATIONAL ASTHMA SERVICES (IAS) (www.globalchestintitatives.org) is proud to continue to support the educational outreach, by presenting the Text Book of Allergy For the Clinician, 2nd Edition published by the CRC Press. IAS is a 501 c3 charitable organization based in Colorado U S A. IAS was established in 1992 by Dr. P. K. Vedanthan and his group of volunteers for the purpose of: 1. Improving the care of allergic and asthma patients around the world. 2. Education of patients, their families and the public in general. 3. Transfer of technology as well as training of health professionals. 4. Charitable allergy asthma awareness camps for the needy.

IAS has been especially active in India serving as the hub for additional training and education of health professionals through the partnership with major medical institutions and universities. IAS has actively participated in educational and charitable activities in several developing countries like Nepal, Sri Lanka, Myanmar, Mauritius, Kenya and Russia. By supporting the publication of the text Book of Allergy for the Clinician, 2nd edition, IAS has taken a significant step forward towards education of medical students, residents and fellows in training, general and specialty physicians, nurses and other health professionals around the globe.

Contents

Dedication iii
Foreword v
Preface vii
Acknowledgements ix
About the Sponsor xi

1. **Basics of Allergy: Immunological and Clinical** 1
   Rafeul Alam, Dipa K Sheth and *Magdalena M Gorska*

2. **Immunology of Allergic Diseases** 10
   Mandakolathur R Murali

3. **History Taking: Evaluation of Allergic Disorders** 19
   Gabriel K Wong and *Mamidipudi Thirumala Krishna*

4. **Allergy Skin Testing** 32
   Pudupakkam K Vedanthan and *Harold Nelson*

5. ***In vitro* Laboratory Tests for the Diagnosis of Allergy** 43
   Vijaya Knight, Preveen Ramamoorthy and *Ronald J Harbeck*

6. **Aerobiology for the Clinician: Basic and Applied Aspects, Pollen Sources, Pollen Calendars** 49
   Shripad N Agashe

7. **Risk Factors for Allergies and Asthma** 69
   Harold Nelson

8. **Rhinitis: Allergic and Nonallergic** 78
   Vinay Mehta, Srinivasan Ramanuja and *Pramod S Kelkar*

9. **Chronic Rhinosinusitis, Nasal Polyps and Aspirin Exacerbated Respiratory Disease** 89
   Farshad N Chowdhury and *Todd T Kingdom*

10. **Allergic Diseases of the Eye** 99
    Andrew Braganza and *Alo Sen*

11. **Rhinolaryngoscopy for the Allergist** 108
    Jerald W Koepke and *William K Dolen*

12. **Pediatric Asthma** 125
    Michael Teik Chung Lim, Mahesh babu Ramamurthy and *Daniel Yam-Thiam Goh*

13. **Adult Asthma** 139
    Flavia CL Hoyte, Eugene M Choo and *Rohit K Katial*

14. **The Pharmacotherapy of Rhinitis and Asthma** 147
    Amanda Grippen Goddard, Harold S Nelson, Rohit Katial and *Flavia Hoyte*

15. **Allergen Immunotherapy** 165
    Harold S Nelson

16.	**Pulmonary Function Testing** *Ekta Kakkar, Flavia CL Hoyte, Devasahayam J Christopher* and *Rohit K Katial*	178
17.	**Common Office Tests and Procedures for the Allergist** *Vinay Mehta*	185
18.	**Environment and Lifestyle in Allergic Disease** *Anubha Tripathi* and *Thomas AE Platts-Mills*	207
19.	**Effects of Air Pollution on Allergy and Asthma** *Sundeep Salvi* and *Sneha Limaye*	219
20.	**Asthma and COPD—Similarities and Differences** *Balamugesh Thangakunam* and *Devasahayam J Christopher*	231
21.	**Occupational Asthma** *Bill Brashier* and *Amruta Wankhede*	241
22.	**Anaphylaxis** *Amanda Cox* and *Julie Wang*	255
23.	**Insect Venom Allergy** *William H Bermingham, Alex G Richter* and *Mamidipudi T Krishna*	271
24.	**Urticaria and Angioedema** *Jenny M Stitt* and *Stephen C Dreskin*	287
25.	**Atopic Dermatitis** *Luz Fonacier* and *Amanda Schneider*	303
26.	**Contact Dermatitis** *Luz Fonacier* and *Eleanor Feldman*	312
27.	**Food Allergy—Introduction, Epidemiology, Pathogenesis and Clinical Presentation** *PA Mahesh, Hugo Van Bever* and *Pudupakkam K Vedanthan*	321
28.	**Food Allergy—Diagnosis and Management** *Neha T Agnihotri, Jialing Jiang, Christopher M Warren* and *Ruchi S Gupta*	332
29.	**Immunodeficiency Diseases** *Mandakolathur R Murali*	347
30.	**Integrative Allergy and Asthma for Traditional Practice** *William S Silvers* and *Heidi Bailey*	366
31.	**Ayurveda and Yoga Therapy for Allergy and Asthma** *Satyam Tripathi, Kashinath G Metri, Purnandu Sharma, Amit Singh* and *Ahalya Sharma*	376
32.	**Yoga Breathing Techniques in Asthma** *Pudupakkam K Vedanthan* and *R Nagarathna*	381
33.	**Drug Allergyr** *Jay M Portnoy* and *Aarti Pandya*	387
34.	**Latex Allergy** *Ronald D DeGuzman* and *Pudupakkam K Vedanthan*	403
35.	**Allergy–Asthma Practice: East vs West** *Mark Holbreich, Pudupakkam K Vedanthan, PA Mahesh* and *Sitesh Roy*	410

Index 423
About the Editors 427

1

Basics of Allergy
Immunological and Clinical

Rafeul Alam,[1,*] *Dipa K Sheth*[2] *and Magdalena M Gorska*[1]

INTRODUCTION

The immune system is composed of an adaptive immune system and an innate immune system. The adaptive immune system distinguishes itself from the innate system by the following features: (a) **Specificity** of antigen recognition, (b) **Diversity** of the antigen receptor repertoire, (c) Rapid clonal **expansion**, (d) **Adaptiveness** to the changing environment and (e) Immunological **memory**. The innate system lacks fine specificity, has limited diversity and rudimentary memory but manifests rapid engagement. Lymphocytes are the primary cells of adaptive immunity; they include T cells, B cells and NK cells. Each individual cell type will be described in this chapter.

Lymphoid cell generation

Generation of Antigen-specific Receptors: The growth of B and T cells from pluripotent stem cells requires successive differentiation through a series of stages that starts in the bone marrow and ends in the thymus (T cells) or peripheral lymphoid tissue (B cells) (Marrack et al. 2000, Carding et al. 2002, Calame 2001). During differentiation lymphocytes are able to recognize self and non-self antigens through the expression of antigen-specific receptors known as T Cell Receptors (TCR) and B Cell Receptors (BCR) (Nemazee 2000). TCRs are comprised of ab or gd subunits whereas BCRs are composed of membrane-bound immunoglobulins (Fig. 1.1). Approximately 90% of peripheral blood T cells are $\alpha\beta$+ and the remainder cells are $\gamma\delta$+, although the proportion of the latter reaches 25–30% in the gastrointestinal mucosa and skin.[2] The generation of TCRs and BCRs creates an impressive repertoire in the order of > 10^{14} through combinatorial joining of V, D and J (b and d chains) or V and J (Fig. 1.2). Recombination is triggered by IL-7 and involves recombination-activating gene-1 and -2 (RAG-1 & -2) and a DNA repair enzyme (metallo-b-lactamase) encoded by the gene Artemis (Hesslein and Schatz 2001). *The deficiency of the RAG enzymes, IL-7 receptor- and the Artemis gene product causes Severe Combined Immunodeficiency (SCID). A partial deficiency of RAG-1 & -2 causes Omenn syndrome.* The BCR is capable of recognizing small and large peptides, in contrast, the TCR recognizes small stretches of linear peptides of 10–12 amino-acids in length.

---

[1] Division of Allergy and Immunology, National Jewish Health & University of Colorado, Denver. Colorado. USA. Email: gorskam@njhealth.org
[2] Division of Allergy and Immunology, National Jewish Health, Denver. Colorado USA, Email: dipa.sheth@gmail.com
* Corresponding author: alamr@njhealth.org

2 *Textbook of Allergy for the Clinician*

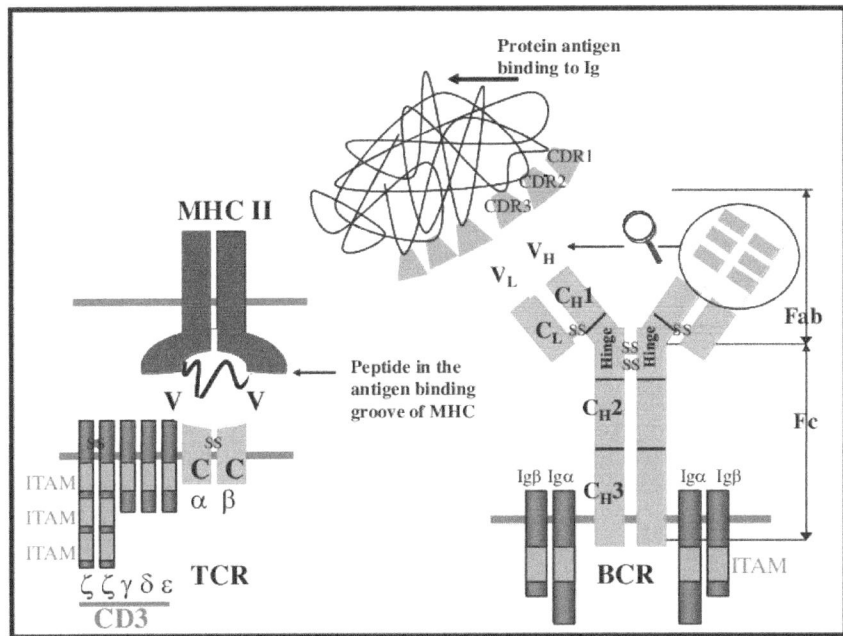

Figure 1.1. The composition of the T cell receptor (TCR) and the B cell receptor (BCR). TCR is composed of the CD3 complex and ab (or gd) subunits. ab (or gd) subunits bind the MHC-bound antigenic epitope, the CD3 complex transduces intracellular signaling. BCR is composed of the surface immunoglobulin and the Iga and Igb accessory molecules. MHC: Major histocompatibility complex; V: variable region of the receptor; C: constant region of the receptor; z z g d e are subunits of the CD3 complex; a and b are TCR subunits; Ig: membrane-bound immunoglobulin; Iga and Igb are BCR accessory BCR molecules; Hc and Lc are constant regions of the heavy (H) or light (L) chain of immunoglobulin; Hv and Lv are variable regions of the heavy (H) or light (L) chain of immunoglobulin; CDR: complementarity determining region.

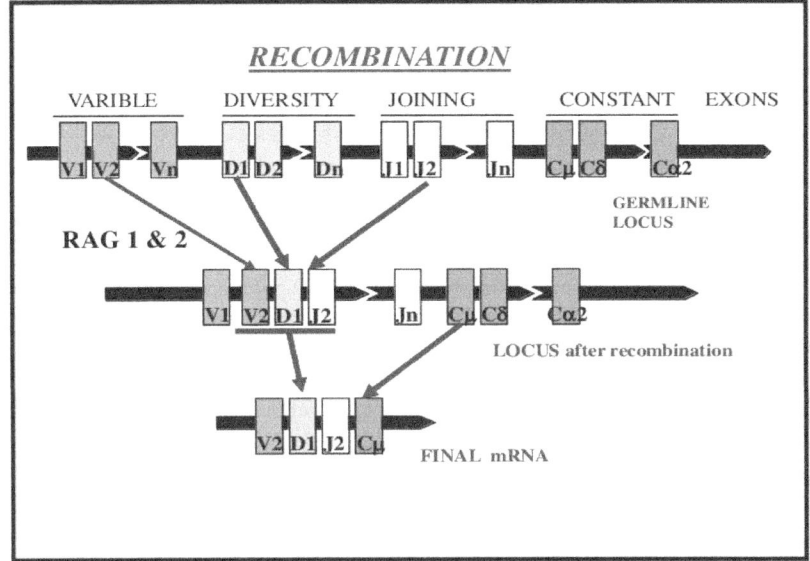

Figure 1.2. The immunoglobulin heavy chain locus as the example of genomic organization of antigen receptors. V, D, J exons encode the variable region of the immunoglobulin antigen-binding site and C exons encode the constant region.

Thymic Selection of T Cells: During the generation of antigen receptors, self MHC-reactive and non-reactive TCRs are generated (Hennecke and Wiley DC 2001).

T cells require signaling through the TCR for survival and proliferation; T cells that are unable to recognize self-MHC or have very low avidity TCRs for self-MHC die because of the lack of the TCR signal (death by neglect). T cells, which recognize self-MHC in conjunction with the self-peptide, are expanded (**positive selection**). Positively selected T cells with very high avidity for self-peptides (auto-reactive T cells) are killed (**negative selection**). Ninety-five percent of T cell precursors die due to negative selection/failing to express the appropriate TCR.

B cell precursors are not subjected to extensive deletions; self-reactive B cells undergo another round of receptor gene rearrangement (receptor editing) to replace an auto-reactive BCR with a normal BCR. In the early phase of differentiation, immature T cells express both CD4 and CD8 co-receptors (double-positive cells) (Sebzda et al. 1999, Germain 2002) CD4 T cells are selected through interaction with class II MHC molecules and CD8 T cells through interaction with class I MHC molecules.

Two tyrosine kinases—Lck (Lymphocyte-specific protein tyrosine kinase) and ZAP70 (zeta-associated protein 70) play a critical role in the selection of CD4 and CD8 T cells, respectively. *Patients with congenital deficiency of Lck have severe combined immunodeficiency because of the failure of CD4 differentiation; ZAP70 deficiency results in a severe defect of CD8 T cell differentiation.* A small fraction of T cells, mostly of gd subtype, is negative for both CD4 and CD8 (double negative) (Carding et al. 2002).

Immune surveillance—naïve lymphocyte

In order to increase the probability of antigen encounter, lymphocytes continuously circulate across various tissues. Naïve T and B cells preferentially migrate to lymph nodes due to homing receptors L-selectin and CCR7 (Moser and Loetscher 2001). Their ligands, CCL19 and CCL21 are expressed on High Endothelial Venules (HEV) of lymph nodes.

Events following an antigen encounter

Antigen Presentation: Professional Antigen Presenting Cells (APC) are those that express high levels of class II MHC molecules and possess the capacity to internalize, process and present foreign antigens in the MHC groove. APC cells include Dendritic Cells (DC), B cells, monocytes/macrophages and their tissue counterparts. Immature DCs, residing in the peripheral tissue, phagocytose and process foreign antigens (Table 1.1) (Guermonprez et al. 2002). Pathogen-derived molecules and cytokines from inflamed tissue, trigger DC maturation, enhance antigen processing and expression of foreign-peptide-loaded MHC proteins. Mature DCs secrete cytokines and upregulate different co-stimulators and CCR7.

Table 1.1. Major histocompatibility complex molecules.

	MHC I	**MHC II**
Genes	HLA-A, B, C	HLA-DP, DQ, DR
Structure	Transmembrane a chain bound to b2-microglobulin, only the a chain interacts with the peptide	Transmembrane a and b chain, both chains interact with the antigenic peptide
Presented peptide	Peptides derived from self/non-self intracellular proteins, e.g., viral peptides	Peptides derived from extracellular proteins, e.g., bacterial peptide
Mechanism of presentation	Intracellular proteins are degraded by the ubiquitin/proteasome pathway in the cytosol; transported by TAP to endoplastic reticulum and loaded onto MHC; the MHC/peptide complex translocates to the cell membrane	Extracellular proteins are endocytosed and degraded by lysosomal proteases; subsequently peptides-containing endosomes are fused to MHC-containing vesicles; peptides are loaded onto MHC and the complex translocates to the cell membrane
Presenting Cells	All nucleated cells, including APC	Antigen Presenting Cells (APC): dendritic cells, B cells, macrophages
Interacting T cell	CD8 T cell	CD4 T cell

Table 1.2. T Cell co-stimulatory molecules.

Receptor	Expression	Ligand	Role	Knock-out mice
CD28 family members					
CD28	C constitutive	B7.1 (CD80) I inducible (though CD40 stimulation), B7.2 (CD86) constitutive on APC	E essential for initiation of naïve T cell response, enhances IL-2 production, protects from apoptosis, lack of CD28 signaling results in T cell anergy	Di diminished IL-2 pr production, CD25 expression, immunoglobulin secretion and class switching, deficient Th2 response, CD8 response largely intact
CD152 (CTLA-4)	Inducible on activated cells	B7.1/B7.2	Inhibits activated T cell proliferation and IL-2 production, terminates T cell response	Massive lymphoproliferation and multiple organ destruction, T cells are skewed towards Th2
ICOS	Inducible on activated cells	B7RP-1, constitutive, mainly B cells and macrophages	Important for differentiation and effector function of Th1/Th2 cells, enhances IL-4, 10, 13 but not IL-2 production, promotes T cell memory generation	Impaired formation of germinal centers and class switching, low levels of immunoglobulins, T cells do not secrete IL-4 & IL-13. IFNg & IL-5 production unperturbed.
PD1	Inducible on activated cells	B7-H1/B7-DC, inducible on APC	Inhibits activated T cell proliferation and cytokine production	Lupus-like disorder, high titer of immunoglobulins
TNF family members					
CD134 (OX40)	Inducible, transiently expressed, within 24–120 h after T cell stimulation	OX40L, inducible on APC	Promotes clonal expansion of activated T cells during primary response and enhances memory generation	CD4 T cells can not sustain IL-2 production and clonal expansion during the primary response; reduced number of memory T cells, impaired Th2 response and lung inflammation in the asthma model, CD8 response largely normal
CD27	Inducible on activated T cells	CD27L	As above (OX40), particularly important for CD8 T cells	Reduced clonal expansion and memory formation; CD8 T cells much more affected
CD137 (4-1BB)	Inducible	4-1BBL	Enhances CD8 cell function	Increased T cell proliferation, reduced effector cell function
Light-R		Light	Enhances proliferation, cytokine production and cytotoxicity of CD8 cells after superantigen stimulation	Impairment of CD8 response to superantigens, normal response to classical antigen stimulation

Co-stimulators (Table 1.2) play a critical role in determining the nature of the immune response. The expression of CCR7 enables migration to the draining lymph nodes.

T cells

Mature DC present antigenic epitopes to a specific T cell through the formation of the 'immunological synapse' (Dustin 2002). TCR and co-stimulatory molecules (e.g., CD4/CD8, CD28) engage with their counter ligands on APCs in the immunological synapse. The TCR is associated with the CD3 complex (composed of a, b, g, d, e and two z subunits). Proper assembly of this receptor complex is important for TCR signaling. *The lack of the CD3g subunit causes severe immunodeficiency whereas that of the CD3e subunit induces a milder form of immunodeficiency.* The binding of the TCR to the peptide-MHC complex results in the activation of CD4- and CD3-associated tyrosine kinases—Lck: lymphocyte specific kinase and Src: Rouse sarcoma. These kinases phosphorylate CD3-associated z chains at ITAM (immunoreceptor tyrosine-based activation motif) sites, which allow docking of multiple signaling molecules and transduction of signals through downstream pathways (Hermiston et al. 2002).

B cells

Binding of a foreign multivalent antigen by the BCR triggers four processes: B cell proliferation, differentiation into antibody producing plasma cells, memory formation and antigen presentation to T cells. Proliferating B cells form the germinal center in the lymph node. The BCR engages Src: Rouse sarcoma-type kinases to initiate signal transduction (Gauld et al. 2002). Following binding of antigens to surface immunoglobulins, B cells internalize, process (Table 1.1), express the antigenic epitopes in the MHC groove and present to T cells. T cells modulate B cell functions in a number of ways. T cell-derived cytokines—IL-4, IL-5, IL-6, IL-2 and IFN-g enhance B cell proliferation and differentiation into antibody secreting plasma cells. The physical interaction of T cells with B cells allows signaling through the CD40L-CD40 co-receptors, which, in the presence of IL-4, plays an essential role in immunoglobulin class switching. Naïve B cells initially express IgM and IgD on the cell surface; with stimulation the B cell switches immunoglobulin classes and produces IgG, IgA or IgE. *Patients deficient in CD40L suffer from hyper IgM syndrome and are unable to class switch to IgG, IgA or IgE* CD40 signaling that involves the activation of the NF-kB pathway. *Patients deficient in NEMO, protein involved in NF-kB regulation, present with life-threatening infections due to low levels of IgG (accompanied by increased IgM levels).* CD40 engagement facilitates B cell proliferation, differentiation, memory, survival, somatic hypermutation and immunoglobulin secretion. *In patients deficient in CD40L, the activation of B cells and formation of germinal centers are abolished.* The description of T cell subsets and the role of immunoglobulins are provided Tables 1.3, 1.4, and 1.5.

Table 1.3. Mechanisms of CD8 cell cytotoxicity.

Group	Mediator	Function
Cytotoxic Granular Proteins	Perforin	Perforins insert themselves into the target cell membrane and form pores. CD8 T cells use these pores to inject the content of the granules directly into the cytosol of the target cell.
	Granzymes	Proteases inducing rapid target cell death through activation of pro-apoptotic molecules: caspases, BID, DFF45
Receptors	FasL	FasL associates with the Fas receptor on the target cell. Fas directly activates caspases and triggers apoptosis of the target cell.
	TWEAK TRAIL	TWEAK and TRAIL induce apoptosis through similar mechanisms.
Cytokines	TNFa	Activates caspases in target cells

Table 1.4. T helper cells.

Subset	Differentiation factors		Cytokines produced
	Cytokines	Transcriptional factors	
Th1	IL-12	T-bet, STAT-4, STAT-1	IFNg, IL-2, TNF-ß
Th2	IL-4	GATA-3, STAT-6, NF-ATc, JunB	IL-3, 4, 5, 9, 10, 13, IL-25
Th17	IL6/IL1 plus TGFb	RORgT, STAT3	IL17, IL21-23

Table 1.5. Functions of immunoglobulins.

Class	Immunoglobulin function
IgD	Forms BCR on B cells
IgM	Forms BCR on B cells, binds pathogens and toxins, activates complement
IgG (IgG$_{1-4}$)	Directly neutralizes toxins, blocks pathogen adhesion, activates complement, facilitates ADCC*, acts as an opsonin, i.e., activates phagocytes, inhibits lymphocyte function through FcRgII (CD32)
IgA (IgA$_{1-2}$)	Directly neutralizes toxins, blocks pathogen adhesion at mucosal sites, facilitates ADCC*
IgE	Induces mast cell and basophil degranulation, prolongs mast cell survival, facilitates eosinophil-mediated ADCC* against parasites

*ADCC-Antibody Dependent Cell mediated Cytotoxicity molecules to the cell surface for presentation to CD4 ab T cells and double-negative or CD8 gd T cells, respectively.

Effector phase

T cell phenotype: Activated T and B cells in the lymph node downregulate CCR7, begin to express receptors for chemokines that are preferentially expressed in the peripheral tissue and migrate to the site of pathogen entry. CD4 T cells (also called Th0) differentiate into T helper 1 cells (Th1), T helper 2 cells (Th2), and T helper 17 (Th17) cells, whereas CD8 T cells differentiate into cytotoxic T cells (Tables 1.3 and 1.4). Under specific circumstances cytotoxic CD8 T cells can differentiate into Tc1 and Tc2 cells, whose cytokine production profile is similar to that Th1 and Th2 cells. The differentiation of Th1, Th2 and Th17 cells is induced by IL-12, IL-4, and IL6, IL1 (in humans) and TGFb (in mice) respectively (Glimcher 2001). The foregoing cytokines are typically secreted by the antigen-presenting cell and/or other accessory cells. For Th1 differentiation IL-12 signaling via STAT-4 is essential, which activates the master Th1 regulator—T-bet, a transcription factor that induces sustained production of Th1 cytokines and also blocks Th2 differentiation. IL-4 signaling via STAT-6 and other signaling molecules, induces the master Th2 switch—GATA-3. GATA-3 stimulates Th2 cytokine production and inhibits Th1 differentiation (Table 1.4). IL6 stimulated STAT3 in the presence of TGFb induces RORgT, the master regulator of Th17. Th1 cells are primarily induced by and play a critical role in the defense against intracellular pathogens. Th2 cells are induced by extracellular pathogens/antigens. Th17 cells are induced by pathogens but are involved in autoimmunity in addition to defense against pathogens.

CD8 T cells have two distinct mechanisms of cytotoxicity: perforin and Fas ligand (Fig. 1.3) (Russell and Ley 2002). Perforin is a membrane pore-forming molecule, which allows release of granular enzymes directly into the cytosol of the target cell. Granzyme B induces rapid apoptosis of the target cell through caspase-dependent and caspase-independent manners.

Natural killer cells

Natural Killer (NK) cells do not possess the antigen receptor, making it a component of innate immunity (Moretta et al 2002). NK cells express receptors for MHC I molecules belonging to KIR family (Killer cell Inhibitory Receptor). NK cells are spontaneously active unless they are inhibited by self-MHC molecules, so they are well-suited to perform immunosurveillance for non-self MHC-bearing targets (e.g., transplanted cells, tumors, virally-modified cells, etc.). NK cells also mediate Antibody-Dependent Cell mediated Cytotoxicity (ADCC). NK cells release their toxic mediators upon binding to IgG-coated tumors or virally infected cells; the mechanism of cytotoxicity of NK cells is very similar to that of cytotoxic CD8 T cells (Table 1.3). A subset of T cells also expresses NK1.1; they are known as NK T cells and have a limited TCR repertoire (Godfrey et al. 2000). Following stimulation, NK T cells rapidly produce high levels of IL-4, IFNg and TNFa.

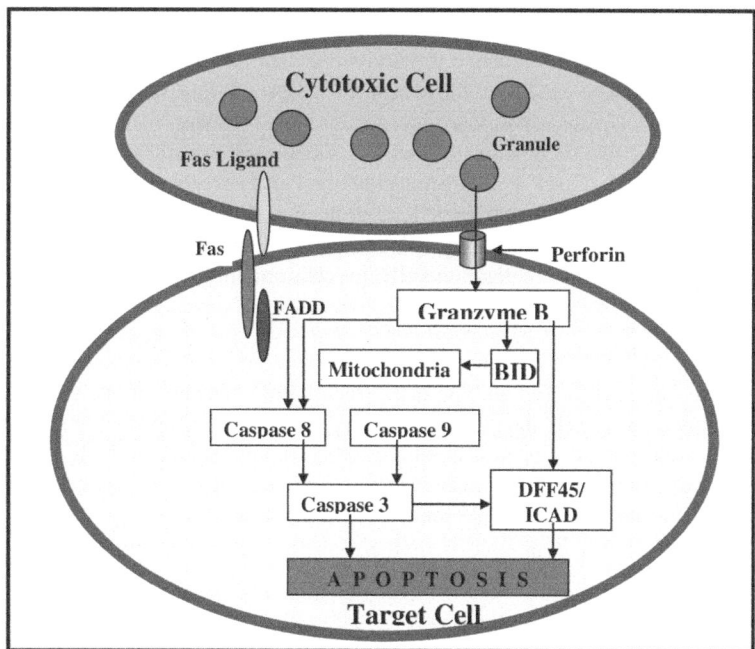

Figure 1.3. Antigen processing and presentation. Endogenously produced proteins (self proteins and viral proteins) are degraded in the proteasome, transported by TAP to endoplasmic reticulum, where they are combined with Class I molecules and transported to the cell surface for presentation to CD8 T cells. Unlike class I molecules, class II and CD1 molecules do not associate with endogenous proteins in the endoplasmic reticulum. Instead they associate with an invariant chain (Ii) and transported to the exosome. Extracellular proteins and lipids are endocytosed and degraded by lysosomal enzymes. Subsequently, they are combined with class II and CD1 molecules, respectively and the invariant chain is degraded. The exosome then transports the antigenic epitope-bound class II and CD1

Innate lymphoid cells (ILCs)

Recent studies have identified a distinct population of innate lymphoid cells (Klose and Artis 2016, Mjosberg et al. 2011). These ILCs are analogous to T helper cells in their function. ILC1, ILC2 and ILC3 have a cytokine profile that is similar to that of Th1, Th2 and Th17. Although their frequency is low compared to T helper cells, ILCs produce much higher quantities of effector cytokines (e.g., IL5 and IL13 production by ILC2s) and significantly contribute to the pathogenesis of inflammatory diseases and host defense.

Immunological tolerance

The elimination of auto-reactive T and B cells in the thymus and bone marrow, respectively, through negative selection is called central tolerance (Walker and Abbas 2002). There is evidence that some self-reactive T and B cells manage to escape the negative selection; their receptors may recognize MHC/self-peptide with an affinity that is not high enough to elicit negative selection. Despite the presence of auto-reactive cells, autoimmunity does not develop due to peripheral tolerance. DCs expressing self-peptides are not activated and therefore have very low levels of co-stimulatory molecules. They also secrete IL-10, so the majority of lymphocytes become anergic instead of being activated. Presentation of self-antigens in the absence of co-stimulation may also lead to clonal deletion through apoptosis. Auto-reactive cells as well as inflammatory cells in the peripheral organs are suppressed by a population of CD4+CD25+FoxP3+ cells, called regulatory T cells (Tregs) (Shevach et al. 2001). These cells secrete IL-10 and TGFb and block proliferation of lymphocytes.

Persistence of memory

Some antigen-specific lymphocytes manage to survive the 'shrinkage' phase of the immune response known as long-lived memory cells. In the event of a second attack, pathogen-specific memory lymphocytes mount an accelerated and more vigorous immune response, resulting in faster elimination of the invading target. The two populations of memory T cells are: effector memory T cells and central memory **T cells** (Kaech et al. 2002). The effector memory T cells do not express CCR7 and L-selectin, homes to peripheral tissues and conveys immediate protection against pathogens by rapidly producing cytokines. Central memory T cells home to lymph nodes due to the expression of CCR7 and L-selectin. Upon antigen stimulation they differentiate into effector cells and migrate to the peripheral tissue.

Conclusions

The immune system has evolved to combine many seemingly opposing virtues such as diversity and specificity, distinction between self and non-self and preparedness for acute emergency and maintenance of long-term memory. It has developed a unique genetic recombination mechanism that produces an unlimited repertoire utilizing a limited number of genes. For versatility, adaptivity and sophistication, the immune system remains unparalleled to all other biological systems.

Clinical pearls

1. *The deficiency of the RAG enzymes, IL-7 receptor- and the Artemis gene product causes severe combined immunodeficiency (SCID). A partial deficiency of RAG-1 & -2 causes Omenn syndrome.*
2. *Patients with congenital deficiency of Lck have severe combined immunodeficiency because of the failure of CD4 differentiation; ZAP70 deficiency results in the severe defect of CD8 T cell differentiation* (see Chapter 12).
3. *Patients deficient in CD40L suffer from the hyper IgM syndrome and are unable to class switch to IgG, IgA or IgE.*
4. *Patients deficient in NEMO, protein involved in NF-kB regulation, present with life-threatening infections due to low levels of IgG (accompanied by increased IgM levels).*
5. *In patients deficient in CD40L, the activation of B cells and formation of germinal centers are abolished.*
6. This chapter is in part based upon a review article that was previously published as "Lymphocytes". Alam, R. and Gorska, M. (authors); In the Primer on Allergic and Immunologic Diseases, 5th Edition, W. T. Shearer and James Li, editors, J. Allergy Clin. Immunol. 2003; 111(2 Suppl): S476–85.

References

Calame KL. Plasma cells: finding new light at the end of B cell development. Nat Immunol 2001; 2: 1103–8. 4.
Carding SR., Egan PJ. Gammadelta T cells: functional plasticity and heterogeneity. Nature Rev Immunol 2002; 2: 336–45.
Dustin ML. Membrane domains and the immunological synapse: keeping T cells resting and ready. J Clin Invest 2002; 109: 155–60.
Gauld SB, Dal Porto JM, Cambier JC. B cell antigen receptor signaling: roles in cell development and disease. Science 2002; 296: 1641–2.
Germain RN. T-cell development and the CD4-CD8 lineage decision. Nature Rev Immunol 2002; 2: 309–22.
Glimcher LH. Lineage commitment in lymphocytes: controlling the immune response. J Clin Invest 2001; 108: s25–s30.
Godfrey DI, Hammond KJ, Poulton LD, Smyth MJ, Baxter AG. NKT cells: facts, functions and fallacies. Immunol Today 2000; 21: 573–83.
Guermonprez P, Valladeau J, Zitvogel L, Thery C, Amigorena S. Antigen presentation and T cell stimulation by dendritic cells. Annu Rev Immunol 2002; 20: 621–67.
Hennecke J, Wiley DC. T cell receptor-MHC interactions up close. Cell 2001; 104: 1–4.
Hermiston ML, Xu Z, Majeti R, Weiss A. Reciprocal regulation of lymphocyte activation by tyrosine kinases and phosphatases. J Clin Invest 2002; 109: 9–14.
Hesslein DG, Schatz DG. Factors and forces controlling V(D) J recombination. Adv Immunol 2001; 78: 169–232.

Kaech SM, Wherry EJ, Ahmed R. Effector and memory T-cell differentiation: implications for vaccine development. Nature Rev Immunol 2002; 2: 251–62.

Klose, CS, Artis D. 2016. Innate lymphoid cells as regulators of immunity, inflammation and tissue homeostasis. Nat Immunol. 17: 765–74.

Marrack P, Bender J, Hildeman D, Jordan M, Mitchell T, Murakami M, et al. Homeostasis of alpha beta TCR+ T cells. Nat Immunol 2000; 1: 107–11.

Mjösberg, JM., Trifari S, Crellin NK, Peters CP, van Drunen CM, Piet B, et al. 2011. Human IL-25- and IL-33-responsive type 2 innate lymphoid cells are defined by expression of CRTH2 and CD161. Nat Immunol. 12: 1055–62.

Moretta L, Bottino C, Pende D, Mingari MC, Biassoni R, Moretta A. Human natural killer cells: their origin, receptors and function. Eur J Immunol 2002; 32: 1205–11.

Moser B, Loetscher P. Lymphocyte traffic control by chemokines. Nat Immunol 2001; 2: 123–8.

Nemazee D. Receptor selection in B and T lymphocytes. Annu Rev Immunol 2000; 18: 19–51.

Russell JH, Ley TJ. Lymphocyte-mediated cytotoxicity. Annu Rev Immunol 2002; 20: 323–70.

Sebzda E, Mariathasan S, Ohteki T, Jones R, Bachmann MF, Ohashi PS. Selection of the T cell repertoire. Annu Rev Immunol 1999; 17: 829–74.

Shevach EM, McHugh RS, Piccirillo CA, Thornton AM. Control of T-cell activation by CD4+ CD25+ suppressor T cells. Immunol Rev 2001; 182: 58–67.

Walker LS, Abbas AK. The enemy within: keeping self-reactive T cells at bay in the periphery. Nature Rev Immunol 2002; 2: 11–9.

2

Immunology of Allergic Diseases

Mandakolathur R Murali

INTRODUCTION

For centuries manifestations of allergic diseases such as asthma, anaphylaxis and food allergy were described eloquently but its mechanism remained a mystery. The discovery of IgE antibody, its relationship to mast cells and kinetics mediator release elucidated clinical phenotypes of allergic responses. Understanding Innate immune responses and adaptive CD4+TH2 responses ushered in the era of immune regulation. Therapeutic approaches evolved from modulating bronchoconstriction and bronchialreactivity to more targeted approaches. These include anti-IgE therapy, allergen immunotherapy, role of anti-cytokine receptor modulation. Understanding the role of microbiota and targeting aberrant adaptive immune responses to stop the atopic march are in progress and is the subject matter of this chapter.

Historic evolution of allergic disease

The earliest report of allergic diseases is that of King Menes of Egypt, who succumbed to the sting of a wasp at some point between 3640 and 3300 B.C. (Cohen and Samter 1979a). The astute Roman philosopher, Lucretius observed exaggerated responses in some humans to usually occurring substances but not in others and remarked "what is food for some may be fierce poisons for others" (Cohen and Samter 1979b). It should noted he brought into focus the concept that the clinical disease was due to the interaction of environmental agents (in this case food) with some (susceptible) humans and not all humans. However, the modern era of allergy started in 1819 with the classical description of hay fever (allergic rhinitis) by John Bostock (Bostock 1819). In 1869 Charles Blackley, investigated his own affliction with hay fever, by performing the first skin test by applying pollen through a small break in the skin and noting that in 20 minutes the site of the prick had a hive-like response. He also observed that a similar break in skin to which pollen was not applied, had no hive (Cohen and Samter 1979d). This was the birth of allergen skin testing and also highlighted the value of a negative control. Following the descriptions of the two Englishman, Bostock and Blackley, Morrill Wyman a physician in Boston challenged himself and eight others with pollen from wormwood (a member of the ragweed family, Ambrosia). He and some of his subjects were seized by features that resembled the autumnal catarrh. Later, he described in his own family consisting of his father, his siblings and his children, autumnal catarrh over three generations. Morrill thus added the familial nature of the disease as well as the role of *in vivo* provocative challenge—an observation that led to an oral food challenge in the diagnosis of food allergy. Thus, the sentinel elements of an allergic disease, that are generally harmless environmental

---

Harvard Medical School, Massachusetts General Hospital, Boston, MA, Email: Murali50@aol.com

stimuli cause adverse airway reaction in some but not all, often with a familial clustering, and which can be reproduced by skin tests or a provocative challenge (Cohen and Samter 1979c). One can thus state that these early observations set the stage for exploring the interaction of environmental stimuli (pollen, foods, wasp stings) with the genetic nature of the human subject (based on a familial nature). Thus, was born the gene by environmental reactions concept of allergic diseases.

Terminology and nomenclature of allergic diseases also evolved with better recognition of the clinical presentations as well as mechanisms. In 1902 Richet and Portier coined the word 'anaphylaxis' for the untoward and explosive systemic reaction with a detrimental outcome including death that they observed during their studies of immunization and differentiated anaphylaxis from the beneficial protective effect or 'prophylaxis' seen with a vaccine (Portier and Richet 1902). In 1906 Clemens Von Pirquet introduced the term 'allergy' to describe 'strange or untoward' reactions a few subjects experienced when immunized with vaccines or harmless substances (Von Pirquet 1906).

Based on the observations of successful immunization with diphtheria and tetanus toxoids in preventing these diseases, and hoping to achieve the same results with reactions to pollens such as in hay fever, Noon and Freeman established the basis of immunotherapy or 'allergy shots' in 1911(Noon 1911, Freeman 1911). They showed that immunotherapy involves injecting the allergy sufferer with small, incremental doses of the substance or allergen that caused the allergic disease. The idea was built on the premise that over time the immune system will become less sensitive to the allergen and the symptoms will mitigate.

In 1921 Prausnitz and Kustner showed that the serum from a sensitized individual can be introduced into the skin of a non-sensitized person (recipient) and the recipient will demonstrate at the transfer site an 'allergic hive' when challenged by the same specific antigen. This was called the P-K reaction and suggested that the allergic factor in the serum was transferrable (Prausnitz 1962). The serum factor responsible for allergic reaction was identified in 1967 by Kimishige and Teruko Ishizaka in USA, who along with Johannsen and Bennich showed it was the immunoglobulin IgE (Ishizaka and Ishizaka 1967) (Johansson et al. 1968). This was the beginning of the immunological basis of allergic diseases.

Sir William Osler, the father of modern medicine in the western world has a classic description of asthma in his textbook "Principles and Practice of Medicine" published in 1892 (Osler 1892). In it he described some of the cardinal clinical and pathological features of asthma. These included recognition of a familial occurrence, often beginning in childhood and lasting into old age, having many similarites to hay fever, and with paroxysms of symptoms on exposure to hay, dust, cat as well as changes in climate, atmosphere, colds and respiratory infections and at times triggered by fright, emotion or certain foods. He described spasm of the bronchial muscles, swelling of the bronchial mucous membrane and a special form of inflammation of the smaller bronchioles. The epithelium was denuded and could be found in sputum as 'Creola bodies' along with thick gelatinous masses obstructing the airway amidst Curshmann spirals and Charcot-Leyden crystals. Thus, early observations highlighted the role of the epithelium, inflammation, familial nature of the disease, factors that precipitate it and the association with hay fever and adverse reaction to foods. This taken with observations of Bostock, Blackley and Wyman and the discovery of IgE escalated studies on the immunology of allergic diseases.

Immunological understanding till the 70's

The discovery of IgE and assays for specific IgE (formerly called RAST tests, a term that should be relegated to history) coupled to clinical observations and skin test reactivity to specific allergens led to the concept that atopy is the genetic predisposition to produce specific IgE following exposure to allergens and that specific IgE contributes to allergic inflammation. Mast cells and basophils have high affinity receptors for IgE (FcεR1) and cross linking two contiguous molecules of IgE by specific antigen or the IgE receptor by anti-receptor antibody, resulted in IgE—dependent mast cell activation with secretion of a wide array of mediators (Soter and Austen 1976). These mediators such as histamine, leukotrienes, platelet activating factors, etc., had the biological properties to cause not only smooth muscle contraction (early reaction) but also the propensity to recruit eosinophils, basophils, mononuclear cells (late reaction) with the latter response being associated with enhanced airway reactivity (Bronchial Hyper Responsiveness or

BHR) to irritant stimuli, cold air, exercise, pollutants such as ozone, etc. That mast cells can be activated by allergic and non-allergic stimuli and that the resulting inflammation causes bronchial hyper reactivity along with exaggerated airway smooth muscle response to methacholine (cholinergic agonist) dominated the 1970's with initial therapeutic success in treating bronchospasm with a whole class of Beta 2 agonists. Overzealous use of bronchodilators is thought to underlie the epidemic of asthma deaths reported in the UK, New Zealand and Australia. In the 1960's it was related to isoprenaline and the epidemic of asthma deaths in New Zealand in the 1980's to a high dose fenoterol (Pearce 2009). It thus became clear that while bronchospasm may dominate the exacerbations, the underlying persistence of BHR is driven by the cellular immune inflammation that was clinically manifested as late phase response on skin tests as well as on bronchial provocation tests. This led to the investigation of the nature and mechanistic contribution of the mononuclear cells, chiefly lymphocytes, in allergic inflammation.

Immunological insights in the 80's

The next breakthrough came with the identification of a special subset of T cells capable of secreting cytokines that selectively interact with mast cells, basophils and eosinophils. These are T-cells positive for CD3 and CD4. They secreted IL-3, IL-4, IL-5, IL-9 and IL-13 as well as GM-CSF. While IL-3 and GM-CSF interact with basophils and mast cells, IL-4 and IL-13 promote B cell class switch to IgE production which can then bind to the FcεR1s on basophils and mast cells setting the stage for degranulation and acute exacerbation when they encounter a specific allergen (Robinson et al. 1992). IL-5 recruit's eosinophils and their degranulation releases Major Basic Protein (MBP) and Eosinophilic Cationic Protein (ECP), IL-9 enhances mast cell recruitment, increases expression of FcεR1 as well as augmenting mucous production. IL-13 contributes to bronchial hyper responsiveness. This subset of T cells is the TH2 type CD4 cells and its description in human airways validates the earlier observations of Mossman and Kaufman who had described the T cell functional dichotomy in murine model (Mossman et al. 1986). Th1 cells secrete IL-2, interferon-γ, IL-3 and contribute to macrophage activation as well as granuloma formation as seen in tuberculosis, sarcoidosis and implicated in Crohn's disease and rheumatoid arthritis. Th2 cells are incriminated in allergic diseases such as allergic, rhinitis, asthma, food allergy, eosinophilic esophagitis—atopic dermatitis, eosinophilic granulomatosis with polyangiitis (EGPA) formerly known as the allergic granulomatosis of Churg–Strauss, and in helminthiasis. Th1 and Th2 cells arise by differentiation from precursor naïve CD4 TH0 cells and this is dictated by direct interaction with antigen presenting cells, particularly the dendritic cells that are present at the epithelial surfaces of the skin, respiratory and gastrointestinal surfaces as well as the cytokine milieu. The genetic susceptibility dictates the emergence of the atopic state thus again emphasizing the gene by environment interaction of allergic diseases.

Immunological advances till early 2000's

Almost 15 years ago, Holgate suggested on the basis of observations in asthma corroborated with biopsies and culture bronchial Epithelial Cells (EC) that ECs are a major cause in the initiation of the immune injury (Holgate et al. 2000). The ECs control many aspects of allergic sensitization and plays a pivotal role in allergic inflammation, remodeling and bronchial hyperactivity. The significance of Creola bodies is thus emerging. The role of this Epithelial-Mesenchyme Tropic Unit (EMTU) in the perpetuation of the allergic inflammation sheds light on the clinical observation called 'atopic march'. The clinical constellation of Atopic Dermatitis (AD), allergic rhinitis and asthma often affect the same patient and develop in temporal succession. This progression from AD in infancy to allergic rhinitis and asthma in childhood and young adulthood and even persisting in adult life is called the atopic march (Spergel 2010). Nearly 80% of children with AD will subsequently develop allergic rhinitis or asthma (Leung et al. 2004). The complex genetic trait of asthma is due to a gene by environment interaction. The relationship between genetic and epigenetic influences as well as the risk and protective factors in the evolution of allergic diseases or atopic march are depicted in Fig. 2.1. Intertwined with the concept of atopic march and the increasing prevalence of allergic diseases in the western world as contrasted to the developing nations is

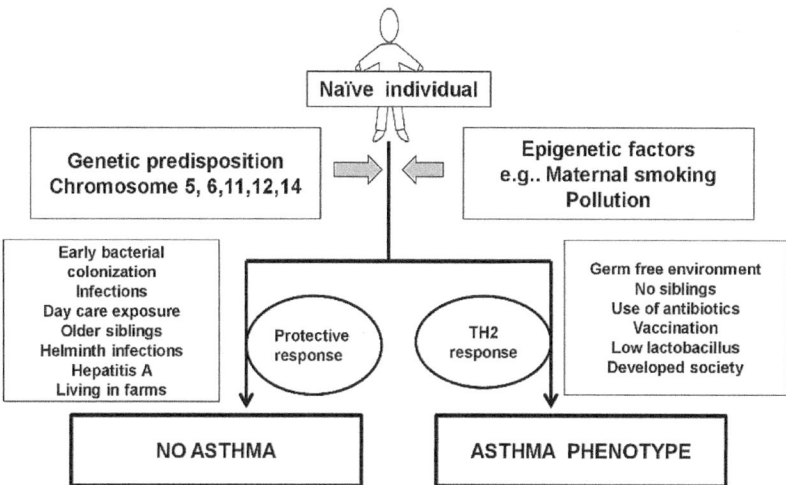

Figure 2.1. The complex genetic trait of asthma is due to gene by environmental interaction.

the 'hygiene hypothesis'. In 1989, David Strachan evaluated the associated risk between allergic rhinitis and 16 perinatal, social and environmental factors. He noted that family size had a significant inverse correlation with the development of allergy. Extrapolating that smaller family size may reduce individual exposure to respiratory infections; Strachan suggested that such infections might indeed be protective against the development of atopic disease (Strachan 1989). The inverse relationship between Hepatitis A infection and atopy has been explained on the basis that the cellular receptor for the hepatitis A virus in humans is a homolog of the TIM-1 on CD4 cells. Epidemiologically, HAV infection is associated with a reduced risk of developing atopy, and because the incidence of HAV infection has been significantly reduced in industrialized countries over the past 30 years, the discovery of a genetic interaction between HAV and TIM-1 provides the first molecular genetic evidence for the hygiene hypothesis (McIntire et al. 2001). Numerous epidemiological studies have shown that children who grow up on traditional farms are protected from asthma, hay fever and allergic sensitization. Early-life contact with livestock and their fodder, and consumption of unprocessed cow's milk have been identified as the most effective protective exposures. Studies on the immunobiology of farm living indicate activation and modulation of innate and adaptive immune responses by intense microbial exposures and possibly xenogeneic signals delivered before or soon after birth (Von Mutius 2000). Thus the hygiene hypothesis signals the role of microbiota as a possible modulator of allergic diathesis and this is an area of considerable research presently.

The airway Epithelial Cell (ECs) are interposed between the host's immune cells (both innate and adaptive) and the environment and represents the first line of defense against microorganisms, allergens, pollutants, atmospheric gases and irritant fumes. ECs express many Pattern Recognition Receptors (PRRs) to rapidly detect and respond to Pathogen-Associated Molecular Patterns (PAMPs) found on microbes or to Damage Associated Molecular Patterns (DAMPs) released on tissue damage, cell death or cellular stress. Microbial Associated Molecular Patterns (MAMP) of commensal as well symbiotic bacteria interact with epithelial and mucosal cells to regulate immune homeostasis. This forms the basis of microbiota and metabolome driven regulation of allergic inflammation. Activated ECs influence Dendritic Cell (DCs) via release of cytokines and thus the adaptive T cell response. It is to be noted the newly identified genes that increase asthma susceptibility are preferentially expressed in the epithelium. (e.g., SPINK5, MUC8, HLA-G, DPP10, chitinase 3 like-1, etc. (Cookson 2004). Further altered barrier function has been recently recognized as an important feature of atopic dermatitis (filaggrin mutations), food allergy and rhinosinusitis. In addition to innate defects in barrier function, environmental agents such as allergens (dust mites, pollens, fungi) have protease activity and break down tight junctions. Viruses also derange tight junctions as do protease containing detergents. Damage to ECs results in a decrease of the adhesion molecule E-cadherin. Decrease in E-cadherin results in loss of the tonic inhibitory control on DC function and facilitates allergen sensitization and production of TSLP and may therefore contribute to loss of inhalational tolerance to allergens in allergic airway disease. The epithelial to mesnchyme transformation is facilitated by loss of E-cadherin and also leads to increased Epidermal Growth Factor (EGF) mediated smooth muscle hyperplasia and airway remodeling. EC damage also results in a decrease in prostaglandin E2, which suppresses DC reactivity by acting on the EP4 receptor. Several other lipid mediators (lipoxin A4, resolvins, etc.) that suppress lung inflammation are also reduced in the airways of subjects with asthma (Holgate 2010).

Airway epithelium influences DC function and thus T cell differentiation. Airway ECs produce CCL2 and CCL20 in response to house dust mite inhalation and attract monocytes and immature DCs to the lung. Triggering of TLR 4 on ECs by dust mite also induces production of thymic stromal lymphopoietin (TSLP), GM-CSF, IL-25 and Il-33. These innate cytokines have pleiotropic effects. They share the propensity to activate DCs and prime TH2 responses, by inducing chemokines that attract TH2 cells or upregulating expression of surface molecules such as OX40L that facilitates TH2 development (Lambrecht and Hammad 2012). In addition, TSLP inhibits the production of the Th1 polarizing cytokine IL-12. The expression of TSLP is increased in bronchial biopsies and sputum from humans who have asthma, particularly in severe disease (Ying et al. 2005, Semlali et al. 2010). Further; genetic polymorphisms in the promoter region of TSLP are associated with increased risk of asthma. Diesel exhaust fumes, cigarette smoke and proteolytic allergens induce epithelial cells to produce TSLP. TSLP activates not only DCs but also other innate cells such as basophils, mast cells, eosinophils and innate non-T and non-B cells called innate lymphoid cells or nuocytes (Neil et al. 2010, Saenz et al. 2010). Basophils are an early source of IL-4 and enhance TH2 development initiated by DCs. Nuocytes are IL-25 and IL-33 responsive and produce IL-5 and IL-13 and thus contributes to eosinophilia, goblet cell metaplasia and airway hyper responsiveness (Chang et al. 2011).

Immunology of allergic diseases beyond 2000

Taking a page from Sir William Osler's observations that "asthma has many causes and physicians are to be well aware of the various causes that bring it about" studies in the last decade have focused on different phenotypes of asthma and immune pathways. The advent of Omalizumab and its impact on IgE dependent immune inflammation as well as the emerging pipeline of biologicals and small molecules that modulate immune networks, has resulted in an era of evidence based translational research that encompasses both the innate and adaptive immunity in the context of genetic heterogeneity and epigenetic influences. While some of these asthma phenotypes are well defined others may be an overlap of immune mechanisms. Sally Wenzel has proposed five different phenotypes with distinct immunopathological features (Wenzel 2012). These are depicted in Table 2.1.

The cytokines influencing the adaptive CD4+ T cell differentiation are featured in Fig. 2.2, it is to be noted that innate immune cells such as ECs and DCs also influence these pathways.

Besides TSLP there are two other EC derived cytokines that have a TH2 polarizing effect. They are the IL-1 and IL-18 family member IL-33 acting through its receptor, ST2 and IL-25 which is one of the six members of the IL-17 cytokine family. TSLP, IL-33 and IL-25 are generated by the airway epithelium in response to cytotoxic epithelial injury as well as by activation of PRRs such as TLR3 and

Table 2.1. Asthma phenotypes and immunopathological features.

Phenotype	Natural history	Immunopathology
Early-onset, allergic	Early onset, mild to severe	Specific IgE, TH2 cytokines, thickened sub epithelial basement membrane
Late-onset, eosinophilic	Adult-onset, often severe	Th2 with major role for IL-5, eosinophilia dominates
Exercise-induced	Mild, intermittent with exercise	Mast-cell activation, TH2 cytokines. Cysteinyl leukotrienes
Obesity-related	Adult onset	Lack of TH2 markers, oxidative stress, possible role for leptin
Neutrophilic	Variable, including sudden exacerbation and death	Sputum neutrophilia, TH 17 pathway, IL-8

Immunology of Allergic Diseases 15

TLR5. The ligand for TLR3 is a viral double-stranded RNA and for TLR5 the ligand is bacterial flagellin. IL-33 functions as an alarmin to alert the immune system to physical stress or infection. IL-25 and IL-33 activate the recently recognized, innate type-2 immune effector leukocyte, the nuocyte. The nuocyte functions as the connecting link between the innate and adaptive TH2 response, in that activated nuocytes secrete IL-4, IL-5, IL-9 and IL-13 all of which cause B cell activation, increased IgE production and eosinophilia as well as promoting goblet cell hypertrophy and increase airway hyper responsiveness—features that are an integral part of allergic inflammation (Holgate 2012).

Besides the nuocyte, TH9 cells are implicated in asthma. It remains to be established whether IL-9 secreting T cells are distinct from TH2 cells or whether TH2 cells differentiate into TH9 cells. TH9 cells do not express the well-defined transcription factors such as T-bet (for TH1), GATA-3 (for TH2) RORγ3 for TH17 and Foxp3 (for iTregs). TH9 cells secrete IL9 that not only promotes mucous production but

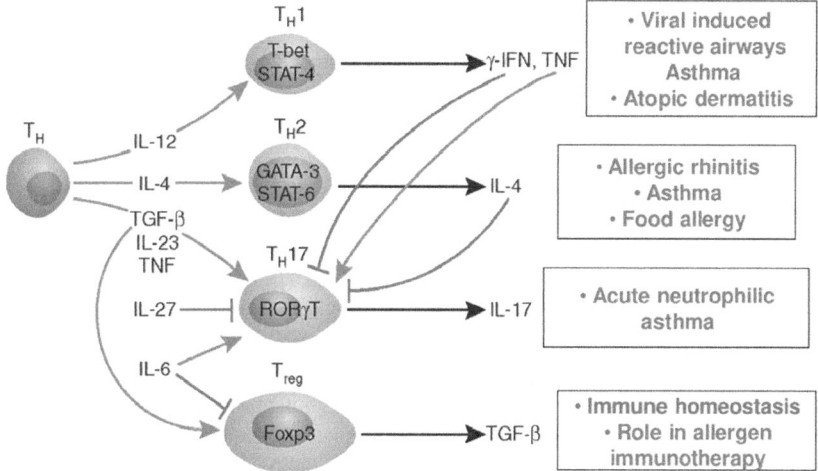

Figure 2.2. Cytokines CD 4+T cells and diseases.

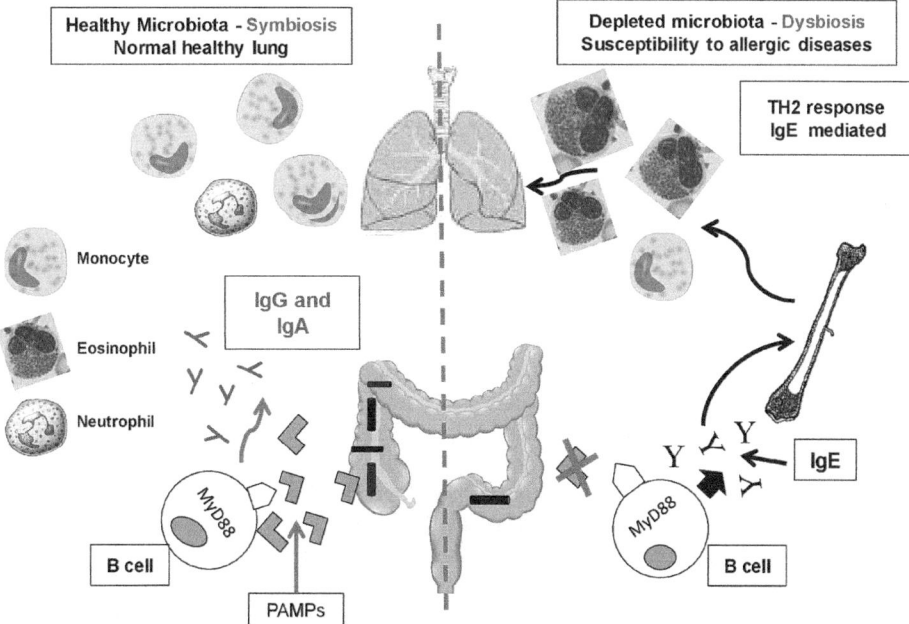

Figure 2.3. Microbiota and allergic inflammation.

also synergizes with IL-4 and stem cell factor to promote mast cell development. In concert with IL-13 and TGF-β it contributes to airway remodeling (Holgate 2012).

As seen in Fig. 2.2, in the presence of TGF-B and IL-6, THO cells differentiate into TH 17 cells. TH 17 cells secrete IL-17A, IL-17F and IL-22 which induce CXCL8 on epithelial and endothelial cells as well as fibroblasts. CXCL8 is a potent neutrophil chemokine and its expression is elevated in airway secretions in severe asthma. Thus, TH17 cells are implicated in neutrophilic airway inflammation and this forms the basis for the neutrophilic asthma phenotype.

The role of invariant Natural Killer T cells (iNKT) in human asthma is being explored based on the observations that iNKT can interact with TH2 cells and modulate the asthma phenotype (Holgate 2012).

Finally, the distinguished work of Hill et al in murine models shed light on the interrelationship of microbiota, hygiene hypothesis and emergence of asthma phenotype (Fig. 2.3). The microbiota inhabiting the normal, healthy colonic mucosa is predominantly gram negative and shed endotoxin as part of the spectrum of PAMPs. These PAMPS bind to TLR4 and in a MYD 88 dependent fashion activate the luminal B cells to preferentially produce IgA and IgG antibodies and thus maintain the integrity of the mucosal immunity. On the other hand, absence of MyD88 dependent-microbial stimulation, results in IgE production by B cells, expansion of basophils from the bone marrow and increased susceptibility to allergic disease (Hill et al. 2012). It remains to be studied if respiratory microbiota can similarly abrogate TH2 responses in the lung. TLR 9 activation by CpG oligodeoxynucleotides has been shown to inhibit IgE class switching by B cells and possibly mitigate airway hyper responsiveness in humans (Creticos et al. 2006, Pascal et al. 2018). CpG motifs are considered pathogen-associated molecular patterns (PAMPs) due to their abundance in microbial genomes but their infrequency in vertebrate genomes. The link between the hygiene hypothesis and susceptibility to allergic diseases, may be a reflection of multiple environmental hits to the microbiota, including antibiotics, infection and diet changes, paired with the possible genetic defects in the human host that prevent appropriate recovery of the microbiota after disruption.

The community of microorganisms that live on or inside another organism is termed as 'microbiome' Their interactions with each other and with the host may be beneficial (symbiotic) or detrimental (pathogenic). Alterations in the quantity (bacterial levels) or quality (diversity) is referred to as dysbiosis and as shown in Fig. 2.4 regulate immune tolerance or inflammation.

The gut microbiome represents a highly complex and dynamic ecosystem. While a diverse community of bacteria is the predominant species, it includes eukaryotic fungi and some viruses. Colonization begins in utero and expands in the first three years of life. The major phyla are *Actinobacteria, Bacteroidetes, Firmicutes* and *Proteobacteria*. Its composition is dynamic and dependent on host-associated factors such as age, diet and environmental conditions.

Children born by a Caesarian section have lower levels of *Escherichia Coli, Bifidobacterium and Bacteroides* species compared to those delivered vaginally. Further, children born by a Caesarian section have a microbiome enriched with *Staphylococcus* and *Streptococcus*, akin to the maternal skin microbiome. These differences appear to be associated with atopy and a higher risk of allergic diseases including asthma. Breast feeding promotes colonization with *Lactobacilli* and *Bifodbacteria*, and together with its content of oligosaccharides and fatty acids has been shown to promote T regs cells and confer protection against allergic diseases. Dietary derived Short Chain Fatty Acids (SCFAs) such as, acetate, butyrate and propionate, derived from fermentation of complex dietary carbohydrates exert anti-inflammatory effects by increasing epithelial barrier function, inducing T regs and IL-10 production (Pascal et al. 2018). Excessive and indiscriminate use of antibiotics promotes dysbiosis and contributes to the development of atopic dermatitis and asthma in some studies. The net result of microbial dysbiosis is a perturbation of the innate and adaptive immunity and together with alterations in microbial metabolites, results in loss of immune regulation, epithelial cell dysfunction, mucosal integrity and emergence of a immune system that is skewed to TH2 and TH17 mediated allergic diathesis and manifesting as allergic rhinitis, asthma, atopic dermatitis, food allergy and eosinophilic esophagitis (Fig. 2.4).

Given the concept that the upper respiratory airways and the lung are part of the 'united airway system' Fazlollahi and colleagues performed 16S ribosomal RNA sequencing on nasal swabs obtained from three cohorts—healthy controls, adults with exacerbated asthma and non-exacerbated asthma

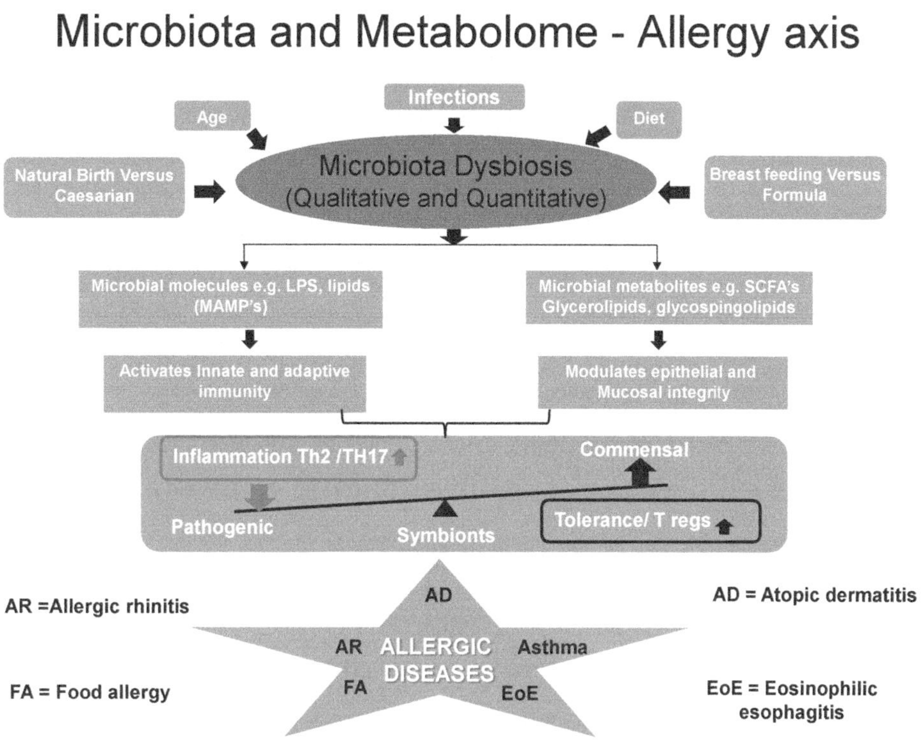

Microbiota and Metabolome - Allergy axis

Figure 2.4. Microbiota, metabolome and allergic inflammation.

(Fazlollahi et al. 2018). They found that relative to controls, the nasal microbiota of subjects with asthma was enriched with taxa from *Bacteroidetes* and *Proteobacteria*. Further four species were differently abundant based on asthma status after correction for multiple comparisons. These include *Prevotella buccalis, Dilister invisus, Gardnerella vaginalis* and *Alkanindges hongkongenesis*. This study is pivotal in that it sampled nasal or airway microbiota (rather than fecal or cutaneous communities) and demonstrated changes between normal controls and asthma. Such studies will pave the way in the understanding the role of microbiota in allergic diseases.

Given this homeostatic balance of microbiota, could modulation of microbial communities be a therapeutic approach for allergic diseases?

Probiotics are defined as "live microorganisms which, when administered in adequate amounts, confer a health benefit to the host". Prebiotics represent non-digestible food components that benefit the host by selectively stimulating the growth and activity of microorganisms. Foods rich in fibers and oligosaccharides have this property. Beneficial synergism resulting from a combination of prebiotics and probiotics is called synbiotics (Pascal et al. 2018). Early studies using probiotics, prebiotics and synbiotics shed light on the need to define the optimal time as well as composition of microbiota for these interventions, be it before, during or after the birth of the child or early childhood.

Insight into the future

The pathway to better preventive and therapeutic strategies for allergic diseases lies in the careful dissection of the atopic march, the immunological basis of the allergic inflammation in the context of genetic, epigenetic factors as well as environmental factors. Further elucidation of the mechanisms and pathways of allergic inflammation will be facilitated by the 'omics' era when, functional genomics, immunogenomics, immunoproteomics are integrated with nutritional genomics and pharmacogenomics in the context of translational research focused on individual and community health.

References

Bostock J. Case of periodic affection of the eyes and chest. Med Chir Trans 1819; 10: 161.
Chang YJ, Kim HY, Albacker LA, Baumgarth N, McKenzie ANJ, Smith DE, et al. Innate lymphoid cells mediate influenza-induced airway hyper-reactivity independently of adaptive immunity. Nat Immunol 2011; 12: 631–638.
Cohen SC, Samter M (Editors). Excerpts from classics in Allergy. Second edition. 1979; 4–5, Published by Symposia Foundation. Carlsbad, CA. (1979 a,b,c,d).
Cookson W. The immunogenetics of asthma and eczema: A new focus on the epithelium Nat Rev Immunol 2004; 4: 978–988.
Creticos PS, Schroeder JT, Hamilton RG, Balcer-Whaley SL, Khattignawong AP, Lindblad R, et al. Immunotherapy with a ragweed toll like receptor 9 agonist vaccine for allergic rhinitis. N Engl J Med 2006; 355: 1445–1455.
Fazlollahi M, Lee TD, Andrade J, Oguntuyo K, Chun Y, Grishina G, et al. The nasal microbiome in asthma. J Allergy Clin Immunol 2018; 142: 832–843.
Freeman J. Further observations on the treatment of hay fever by hypodermic inoculation of pollen vaccine. Lancet 1911; ii; 814–817.
Gell PGH, Coombs RRA (eds.). Clinical Aspects of Immunology. Philadelphia: F.A. Davis Company; 1963.
Hill DA, Siracusa MC, Abt MC, Kim BS, Kubuley D, Kubo M, et al. Commensal bacteria-derived signals regulate basophil hematopoiesis and allergic inflammation. Nature Medicine 2012; 18: 538–546.
Holgate ST, Davies DE, Lackie PM, Wilson SJ Puddicombe SM, Lordan JM. Epithelial-mesenchymal interactions in the pathogenesis of asthma. J. Allergy Clin. Immunol. 2000; 105: 193–204.
Holgate ST. A brief history of asthma and its mechanisms to modern concepts of disease pathogenesis. Allergy Asthma Immunol Res. 2010; 2: 165–171.
Holgate S. Innate and adaptive immune responses in asthma. Nature Medicine 2012; 18: 673–683.
Ishizaka K, Ishizaka T. Identification of gamma-E antibodies as a carrier of reaginic activity. J Immunol. 1967; 99: 1187.
Johansson SGO, Bennich H and Wide L. A new class of immunoglobulins in human serum. Immunology 1968; 14: 266–272.
Lambrecht BN and Hammad H. The airway epithelium in asthma. Nature Medicine 2012; 18: 684–692.
Leung DY, Nicklas RA, Li JT, Bernstein L, Blessing-Moore J, Boguniewicz M, et al. Disease management of atopic dermatitis: an updated practice parameter. Joint task force of Practice Parameters. Ann Allergy Asthma Immunol 2004; 93; S1.
McIntire JJ, Umetsu SE, Akbari O, Potter M, Kuchroo VK, Barsh GS, et al. Identification of Tapr (an airway hyperactivity regulatory locus) and the linked *TIM* gene family. Nature Immunol 2001; 2: 1109–1116.
Mossman TR, Cherwinski H, Bond MW, Giedlin MA, Coffman RL. Two types of helper T cell clone. J Immunol 1986; 136: 2348–2357.
Neil DR, Wong SH, Bellosi A, Flynn RJ, Daly M, Langford TKA, et al. Nuocytes represent a new innate effector leukocyte that mediates type-2 immunity. Nature 2010; 464: 1367–1370.
Noon L. Prophylactic inoculation against hay fever. Lancet 1911; i: 1572–1573.
Osler W. The Principles and Practice of Medicine. 1st ed. NY: D. Appleton and Company 1892. p. 497–501.
Pascal M, Perez-Gordo M, Caballero T, Escribese MM, Longo LL, Luengo O, et al. Microbiome and allergic diseases. Frontiers in Immunology 2018; 9: 1–9.
Pearce N. The use of beta agonists and the risk of death and near death from asthma. J Clin Epidemiol. 2009; 62: 582–587.
Portier P, Richet C. De l' action anaphylactique de certains venins. C R Soc Biol (Paris). 1902; 54: 170.
Prausnitz C. Clinical aspects of immunology. pp. 808–816. *In*: Gell PGH, Coombs RRA (eds.). Clinical Aspects of Immunology. Oxford: Blackwell Scientific Publications; 1962: 808–816.
Robinson DS, Hamid Q, Ying S, Tsicopoulos A, Barkans J, Bentley AM, et al. Predominant TH2-like bronchoalveolar T-lymphocyte population in atopic asthma. N Engl J Med 1992; 326: 298–304.
Saenz SA, Siracusa, MC, Perrigoue JG, Spencer SP, Urban JF Jr., Tocker JE, et al. IL-25 elicits a multipotent progenitor cell population that promotes TH2 cytokine responses. Nature 2010; 464: 1362–1366.
Semlali A, Jacques E, Koussih L, Gounni AS, Chakir J. Thymic stromal lymphopoietin-induced human asthma airway epithelial cell proliferation through an IL-13 dependent pathway. J. Allergy Clin. Immunol. 2010; 125: 844–850.
Soter NA, Austen KF. The diversity of mast cell-derived mediators: Implications for acute, subacute and chronic cutaneous inflammatory disorders. J Invest Dermatol 1976; 67: 313–319.
Spergel JM. From atopic dermatitis to asthma: the atopic march. Ann Allergy Asthma Immunol 2010; 105: 99.
Strachan DP. Hay fever, hygiene and household size. Brit. Med. J 1989; 299: 1259–1260.
Von Mutius E. The environmental predictors of allergic disease. J Allergy Clin. Immunol 2000; 105: 9–19.
Von Pirquet C. Allergie. Munch Med Wochenschr, 1906; 53: 1457 Translated from the German version by Prausnitz C.
Wenzel S. Asthma phenotypes: the evolution from clinical to molecular approaches 2012; 18: 716–725.
Ying S, O'Connor B, Ratoff J, Meng Q et al. Thymic stromal lymphopoietin expression is increased in asthmatic airways and correlates with expression of TH2 attracting chemokines and disease severity. J. Immunol 2005; 174: 8183–8190.

# 3

History Taking
Evaluation of Allergic Disorders

Gabriel K Wong* and Mamidipudi Thirumala Krishna

INTRODUCTION

Obtaining an accurate clinical history is fundamental to the holistic approach of modern day medicine. Together with clinical examination they spawn the original impression, differential diagnoses, initial investigations and management plan of the patient.

In allergology, clinical examination is usually unremarkable. Moreover, mass screening of potential allergens without knowledge of the nature of the reaction is meaningless; therefore clinicians need to place particular emphasis on the clinical history in allergology.

A detailed allergy history could provide a clear direction for specific IgE testing and avoid an unnecessary allergen challenge. It can also extract vital information that helps to effectively manage patients. If performed correctly, the clinician's effort will be rewarded by a positive outcome and patient satisfaction.

The approach is similar to the standard medical history and should follow the logical sequence of presenting a complaint, history of presenting a complaint, Past Medical History (PMH), Drug History (DH), Social History (SH), Family History (FH) and review of systems (RVS).

During the consultation, one should focus on addressing the key questions listed in Box 3.1.

Box 3.1. Questions to be addressed during the consultation
1. Is the presenting complaint consistent with an allergic or allergic-like disorder?
2. What are the underlying mechanisms for the reaction/s?
3. How severe are the reactions?
4. Is there a consistent identifiable trigger to the reaction/s?
5. Do co-factors play a role?
6. Consider other relevant information from PMH, DH, SH, FH, RVS.

Department of Allergy and Clinical Immunology. Birmingham Heartlands Hospital. Bordesley Green East. Birmingham. B9 5SS. UK, Email: thirumala.krishna@heartofengland.nhs.uk
* Corresponding author: g.wong@bham.ac.uk

General approach

Is this an allergy?

By definition, an allergic reaction is one of an immunological nature. However, the term 'allergy' may be loosely used by the general public particularly for cutaneous and gastrointestinal complaints. A patient may presume the cause of his/her symptoms and therefore it is important for the clinician to avoid this trap and remain open-minded. Paediatric patients will require additional attention since the history is usually obtained indirectly from the parents. (Many conditions including lymphoid malignancies and autoimmunity can mimic allergy.)

IgE versus non-IgE mediated reactions

Once a reaction of immunological nature is suspected, the focus should turn towards the mechanism of the reaction. Reactions can be divided into IgE mediated (Type 1) or non-IgE mediated (Type 2–4 and eosinophilic diseases). IgE mediated reactions are caused by mast cell degranulation and occur soon after (maximum up to 2 hours) allergen exposure. The hallmark symptoms of IgE mediated reaction include sneezing, pruritus, urticaria, angioedema, bronchospasm, hypotension and tachycardia and rarely full blown anaphylaxis (Table 3.1). Some patients may experience non-specific symptoms such as nausea, vomiting, GI disturbance and headaches. Rarely myocardial infarction and seizure may occur in conjunction with anaphylaxis as a consequence of severe hypotension. The severity of systemic reactions may be graded according to the Mueller classification 1990 (Table 3.2). On the other hand, non-IgE mediated reactions are usually delayed and seldom lead to anaphylaxis. They usually present with a maculopapular or purpuric or exanthematous rash, and rarely as Steven-Johnson's Syndrome (SJS) and Toxic Epidermal Necrolysis Syndrome (TENS). Eosinophilic diseases can occur with a multitude of symptoms and are difficult to diagnose (Bischoff 2010). Symptoms (such as weakness, facial flushing and tingling of the lips) that are not consistent with allergy should raise the consideration for other disorders.

Correctly diagnosing the nature of the reaction has significant implications on subsequence management. Serum and skin specific IgE testings are only suitable for the investigation of IgE mediated reactions and have no roles in other type of hypersensitivities (Portnoy 2011). Whilst the management of a non-IgE mediated reaction is mainly avoidance; allergen specific immunotherapy and anti-IgE monoclonal antibody may be an option for true IgE mediated reaction/s.

Table 3.1. Hallmark symptoms of type 1 hypersensitivity.

Hallmark symptoms of type 1 hypersensitivity
Itching
Erythema
Watering of the eyes
Sneezing
Nasal congestion
Urticaria
Throat itching and tightness
Hoarseness
Angioedema
Shortness of breath
Bronchospasm and wheezing
Impeding sense of doom
Vomiting
Diarrhoea
Dizziness secondary to hypotension
Palpitation
Collapse with loss of consciousness

Table 3.2. Classification of the severity of IgE medicated allergic reaction *(Muller 1990).

*Mueller grading	Clinical features
Grade I	Generalized urticaria, itching, malaise, anxiety
Grade II	Any of the above plus two or more of the following: angioedema, chest constriction, nausea, vomiting, diarrhoea, abdominal pain, dizziness
Grade III	Any of the above plus two or more of the following: dyspnoea, wheezing, stridor, dysarthria, hoarseness, weakness, confusion, feeling of impending disaster
Grade IV	Any of the above plus two or more of the following: fall in blood pressure, collapse, loss of consciousness, incontinence, cyanosis

Urticaria and angioedema

1) Urticaria

Urticaria is well demarcated, raised and erythematous with a pale centre and is often associated with intense itching. It may occur with or without the presence of angioedema. It is important to understand that urticaria is not diagnostic of a type 1 hypersensitivity and may also be seen in a number of non-allergic disorders. Individual lesions of simple urticaria usually last for < 24 hours with complete resolution. In contrast, urticarial vasculitis is painful, burning and on resolution usually leaves bruising, scarring and/or hyperpigmentation. According to the European Association of Allergology and Clinical Immunology (EAACI) urticaria can be categorized into acute (< 6 weeks) or chronic (> 6 weeks). Recurrent episodes lasting for more than 6 weeks are unlikely to be caused by allergy and should prompt the clinician to search for other physical, inflammatory or idiopathic causes of urticaria. Urticaria may occur on any cutaneous surface, determining whether it is localized or systemic could be helpful especially in the case of drug allergy, insect venom allergy and oral allergy syndrome. Cholinergic urticaria which is a type of physical urticaria mainly occurs under the armpits, groins and lower limbs. Rarely urticaria may be associated with periodic fever syndrome (Zuberbier et al. 2006).

Eczematous and maculopapular rashes are often T cell mediated and a photosensitive rash is suggestive of lupus and drug reaction. These cutaneous manifestations should not be confused with urticaria. One should bear in mind that patients could present with more than one type of rash.

(If possible, it is always useful to ask patients to provide photographic evidence of their symptoms. The details of urticaria will be discussed later in the chapter.)

2) Angioedema

Angioedema is deep tissue swelling affecting the mucocutaneous junction. It is acute and non-persistent but once established angioedema may take up to several days to resolve. It is important to determine the affected areas as facial and lip swellings, though vivid, do not have any life threatening consequences whereas oropharyngeal swelling could compromise the airway and warrant the use of adrenaline. Most cases of angioedema in adults are Angiotensin Converting Enzyme Inhibitor (ACE-I) induced or idiopathic but rarer causes such as hereditary angioedema (HAE) and acquired angioedema exist (Kanani et al. 2011). In the case of HAE, patients suffer from a non-pitting, non-pruritic (bradykinin mediated) peripheral (such as finger), intestinal, genital, urethral and/or oropharyngeal/laryngeal swelling which are uncommon with IgE mediated reactions. Typically patients with HAE do not experience urticaria (Bowen et al. 2010). Acquired angioedema is a rare condition secondary to the presence of auto antibodies against C1 esterase inhibitor for which an underlying lymph proliferative disorder or non-organ specific autoimmune disease can often be found (Breibart and Bielory 2010).

(Please refer later in the chapter for details of angioedema.)

Trigger of symptoms

Establishing a link between a potential trigger and the patient's reactions is an essential part in the allergy history. The clinician should question whether the culprit could consistently reproduce the symptoms within a similar time frame. For example, a patient with true peanut allergy will consistently develop an immediate systemic reaction when peanut is ingested. On the contrary, the lack of symptoms and temporal consistency could steer away from an allergy diagnosis. Equally, an IgE mediated reaction to food is highly unlikely if the patient has nocturnal symptoms or symptoms first thing in the morning.

(Caution: One should remember that it is only natural for patients to attempt a retrospective search for the possible causes of their symptoms. This information is often misleading and must be interpreted with caution especially when a number of culprits have been suggested.)

Box 3.2. Questions that could be useful in establishing or disproving a potential trigger
1. Were symptoms always associated with the same culprit? 2. Can symptoms occur without the culprit? 3. Were there any episodes when a reaction did not occur despite the definitive presence of the culprit? 4. Is the temporal association between exposure to culprit and reaction constant? (Always 15 minutes, 2 hours or 2 days after, etc.?)

The importance of co-factors

Although the mechanism is not clear, it is well known that co-factors such as Non-Steroidal Anti-Inflammatory Drugs (NSAIDs), exercise, alcohol, stress and menstruation can potentially trigger or exacerbate symptoms of allergy. Patients with salicylate intolerance may develop upper respiratory symptoms and/or bronchospasm (asthma, salicylate intolerance and nasal polyps—Samter's Triad) in response to NSAID/s and aspirin (Kowalski et al. 2011). These drugs may also lower the threshold of other allergic diseases without evidence of Samter's triad. Exercise-induced allergy or food dependent exercise-induced anaphylaxis should be considered when a patient's symptoms are clearly associated with the presence of co-factors (Wong et al. 2010). The connection between symptoms and physical factors such as pressure, change in temperature, solar exposure and even contact with water are well-described in specific disorders such as symptomatic dermographism, cholinergic urticaria, cold urticaria, solar urticaria and aquagenic urticaria respectively (Zuberbier et al. 2006). A detailed interrogation of these co-factors will allow the clinician to differentiate rarer diagnosis from chronic idiopathic diseases.

Disease progression and severity

Progression of clinical disease as evidenced by an increased frequency, duration, severity of symptoms or a need for increased medication requirement for symptom control or a delay in response to the same medications as compared to previous episodes are an important part of clinical history taking. On detailed history taking, majority of the patients will confirm that their allergies have progressed with time and the rate of progression will vary between individual patients. Halting the progression of disease should be an important part of the management plan. The current guidelines for allergic rhinitis (ARIA) (Pawankar et al. 2012) and asthma (GiNA) (Bousquet et al. 2007) do not include the rate of progression of allergic symptoms in the classification of disease severity. Individual rate of progression may vary, for example one may need 20 years to move from GINA II to GINA IV, while another could be as short as two years. It is important that these two types of patients are managed differently with the latter requiring a more aggressive approach.

Related past medical history

Atopic diseases such as eczema, asthma and rhinitis often occur in clusters within affected families with variable penetrance suggesting a genetic predisposition to these conditions. Moreover, the 'allergic march' hypothesis proposed a link between the development of eczema to food allergy to allergic rhinitis to asthma. Data from studying Australian siblings has provided strong evidence to support the causal effect of eczema in allergic rhinitis though the link between eczema and asthma is less evident (Hopper et al. 2012). Another recent study has observed that the highest risk for developing asthma is within the first few years after developing allergic rhinitis. In this study approximately 80% of children and 60% of adults develop asthma within 2 years after the onset of allergic rhinitis, whereas asthma is unlikely to develop in children or adults who have had allergic rhinitis for more than 10 years (Mahesh et al. 2009). These findings raise the debate of early immunological intervention for the prevention of asthma. It is therefore important during history taking to establish the duration of allergy symptoms to guide the decision on implementing secondary prevention of asthma; such as immunotherapy for allergic rhinitis.

The presence of eczema should alert the clinician to remain cautious when interpretating specific IgE results; as patients are often polysensitized but not necessarily allergic. As previously mentioned many immunological disorders can be associated with allergic disorders. Autoimmune thyroid disease is closely associated with chronic spontaneous urticaria and angioedema (Rumbyrt and Schoket 2004), while rheumatoid arthritis, systemic lupus erythematous and chronic hepatitis C infection may indicate an underlying vasculitic process (Davis and Brewer 2004). Lymphoproliferative disorders and non-organ specific autoimmune disease may also be responsible for recurrent episodes of angioedema *via* the consumption of complement C1q (Breibart and Bielroy 2010).

Treatment/Drug history

One should pay particular attention to the use of ACE-I and non steroidal anti-inflammatory drugs (NSAIDs). ACE-Is are well recognized causes of spontaneous angioedema by promoting the accumulation of bradykinnin. Its effect may last up to 6–8 weeks following the withdrawal of treatment (Vasekar and Craig 2011). Non-steroidal anti-inflammatory drugs may cause intolerance and lower the threshold of other allergic reactions. It is therefore important to question whether the use of NSAIDs preceded the reaction/s (Kowalski et al. 2011). The use of beta blockers may induce refractory anaphylaxis and therefore replacement with an alternative agent should be considered following a careful 'risk-benefit analysis'(Lang 2008). Other information such as drug, latex and food allergies and treatment history of allergic disorders could also be extracted during this section.

(Please also see Box 3.6 for example of drug allergy history taking.)

Social and occupational history

Details of an individual's housing/indoor environment may be helpful in diagnosing perennial allergic rhinitis. Damp humid environment fosters the growth of mould and house dust mite. Similarly information regarding pets and hobbies could be useful. Some allergic conditions are associated with certain occupations and therefore it is important to question the nature of the patient's job and whether symptoms improve while away from work (Fig. 3.1.) A history of smoking is also important in the evaluation for rhinitis and asthma. The clinician should assess the impact of the patient's symptoms on his or her quality of life as this will also influence the choice of treatments particularly with conditions which may require high risk therapy.

Family history

In addition to atopic diseases that were discussed in earlier, hereditary angioedema and periodic fever syndromes are genetic disorders that follow mendelian inheritance. A detailed family history is therefore essential if these conditions are suspected.

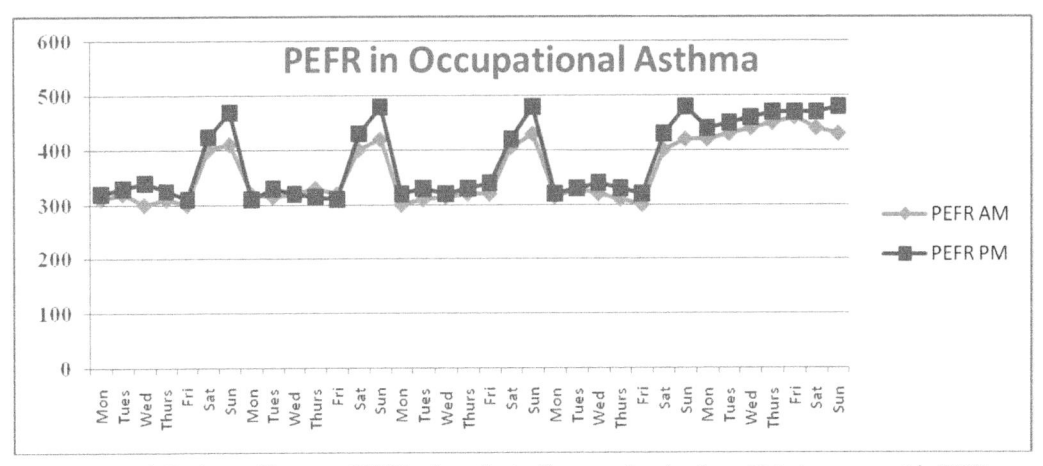

Figure 3.1. Peak Expiratory Flow rate (PEFR) of a patient with occupational asthma. Note improvement in PEFR over weekends and the last week in the chart when patient was away from work (a health care worker, had demonstrable specific IgE to latex), i.e., latex-induced occupational asthma which improved following institution of latex-free measures.

Review of systems

This section could reveal symptoms of associated disorders such as hypothyroidism and lymphoproliferative disorders. The severity of asthma along with other respiratory disorders should also be questioned but the details are beyond the scope of this chapter.

Case histories: how to direct a consultation

The following examples (Boxes 3.3–3.7) will outline the basic principle of allergy history taking with each scenario focusing on a specific aspect. The aim is to obtain crucial information for (1) making an accurate clinical diagnosis, (2) formulating an investigation plan, (3) assembling a holistic management plan and (4) carrying out a risk-benefit analysis for specific treatment.

In summary

An accurate detailed clinical history is vital for making a diagnosis in allergology. Skin and laboratory testing can only provide supportive evidence for clinical diagnosis. Clinicians should be aware of a wide range of differential diagnoses for symptoms in allergology (Table 3.3). One must keep an open mind about the patients' presenting symptoms and must never assume that all patients present at an allergy clinic will have an allergy. The approach should focus on working in partnership with the patient and if in doubt, inconsistent information should be challenged. Since the diagnosis of an allergic disorder is heavily dependent on the clinical history, the clinician should remain vigilant and be prepared to review the diagnosis should new information arise. It is not unusual that a diagnosis cannot be made on the first visit and only begins to shed light on subsequent visits. Finally, clinicians should also attempt to gather all information that is relevant for the formulation of an effective management plan.

Key points

- Keep an open mind, not everything is an allergy.
- Identifying the culprit correctly could aid target avoidance and minimize lifestyle disruption.
- Type 1 reaction is not the only type of allergy.

Box 3.3. Urticaria and angioedema.—**A 55 year old lady presents with a 3 year history of recurrent urticaria. She also had 4 episodes of facial swelling in the past 12 months**

Symptoms
- Identify the rash by detailed interrogation of its appearance, size, margin, colour, etc.
- Is the rash itchy?
- How long does each individual lesion last for (< or > 24 hours)?
- Is there any burning, scarring or hyperpigmentation following resolution?
- When did symptoms begin?
- How frequent are these lesions appearing (daily, weekly, monthly, every few months, etc.)?
- Where do they commonly affect (localized or systemic, scalp, armpits, legs and sun exposed areas)?
- Ask the patient to describe her angioedema in detail.
- Is there any upper airway involvement and/or anaphylaxis, and if so, how severe?

Possible trigger
- Is there a consistent trigger to her symptoms?
- What is the temporal relationship?
- If the patient is convinced that there is a common trigger use Box 3.2 to further clarify.
- Are there nocturnal symptoms or are symptoms noticeable first thing in the morning?
- Do co-factors such as physical activity, change in temperature, stress, alcohol, the use of NSAIDs and menstrual cycle play a role here?

Treatment response and severity
- Do symptoms respond to antihistamine?
- What treatment has the patient tried (regular or as required)?
- Is there recurrent use of corticosteroid?
- Has the patient been admitted to the hospital for her symptoms, if so, check if plasma tryptase was measured (if positive a true type 1 reaction should be considered).
- Was adrenaline ever needed? In some cases, scrutinization of emergency records would be valuable in distinguishing anaphylaxis from other mimics (e.g., vasovagal syncope).

Others
- Other past medical history (atopic disease, thyroid disease, autoimmunity and lymphoproliferative disorders).
- Is the patient on an ACE-I (will worsen angioedema)?
- Does the patient use NSAIDs?
- Known drug allergies—e.g., Penicillin?
- Are there any family history of allergies or allergic like disorders?
- Are there other symptoms to suggest a disorder that is closely related to urticaria and angioedema?

Box 4. Rhinoconjuctivitis—A 21 year old university student presents with a 5 year history of worsening nasal congestion and sneezing

Symptoms
- Ask the patient to describe his/her nose symptoms (itching, congestion, nasal discharge, and sneezing).
- Does the patient have sneezing?
- Ask the patient to describe his/her eye symptoms (itching, tearing).
- Does the patient suffer from loss of smell?
- Does the patient have unexplained post nasal drip (causing frequent clearing of the throat, cough)?

Allergen identification
- Is there seasonal variation to his/her symptoms or do symptoms occur all round the year (perennial or seasonal)?
- If there is seasonal variation, when are his/her symptoms worst (spring or summer) and map to calendar?
- Are his/her symptoms related to exposure to pets/animals?
- Is there diurnal variation of symptoms?
- Are symptoms worse or better at work?

Severity of symptoms
- What treatments has the patient tried so far and have they worked (antihistamine, mast cell stabilizer, antibiotics, nasal and/or oral/parenteral corticosteroid, leukotriene and surgery)?
- Also check compliance and correct nasal spray technique at this stage.
- Is wheezing part of the patient's symptoms (suggestive of allergic asthma)?
- Are symptoms impinging on the patient's work, study or sleep (quality of life in general)? In children, check regarding school performance and attendance.

Selecting the right candidate for immunotherapy
- If there is a history of asthma, its severity and level of control?
- Does the patient suffer from ischaemic heart disease, severe respiratory disease like COPD, autoimmune disease and malignancy?
- Does the patient use ACE-I or a beta-blocker?
- Is the patient pregnant (female patients only)?
- Is the patient likely to be poly or monosensitized?
- What is the patient's possible long term compliance to immunotherapy (standard programme is generally 3 years)?

Others
- As above

Box 5. Anaphylaxis—A 28 year old male presents with 2 episodes of collapse and generalized rash

Symptoms

- Meticulously gather details of the patient's reactions.
- A witness would be helpful as patient could be unconscious for the large part of it.
- If possible review the medical notes especially for vital signs.
- If the patient is admitted in hospital, check if there is a plasma tryptase measured.
- The key is to distinguish anaphylaxis from other causes of collapse.
- What treatment did the patient receive?
- Did the patient make a prompt recovery?
- Did a biphasic reaction occur?

Possible trigger

- Does physical activity, change in temperature, stress, alcohol, the use of NSAIDs and menstrual cycle play a role here (if so exercise induced or food dependent exercise induced anaphylaxis should be considered)?
- What could be the trigger (see previous)?
- Is the trigger avoidable (e.g., drug) or not (food and insect venom)?

Treatment option/s

- Does the patient suffer from ischaemic heart disease, severe respiratory disease like COPD, autoimmune disease and malignancy?
- Does the patient use ACE-I, NSAID or a beta-blocker (if so, suggest alternatives)?
- Is the patient compos mentis and able to manipulate an adrenaline auto-injection device?
- Is this the patient suitable for immunotherapy in cases of hymenoptera sting induced anaphylaxis?

Box 6. Drug allergy—A 40 year old male developed a full blown systemic reaction to antibiotics

Symptoms
- What were the symptoms?
- What was the temporal association between reactions and administration of the drug (minutes, hours or days)?
- Did the reaction happen with the first dose or during the course of treatment?
- How long was the total duration of the reaction?
- Are symptoms suggestive of an IgE mediated or a non-IgE mediated reaction?
- Was it SJS, TENS or systemic vasculitis (Further testing is not recommended as far as possible)?
- What treatment was given to reverse the reaction?
- If the patient was admitted to hospital was a plasma tryptase measured?
- Did the patient make a full recovery (severe non-IgE mediated reaction often leave residual signs)?

Identify the offending agent
- What exact drug/s were involved?
- What was the dose given?
- What was the route of administration (oral, IV, SC, IM)?
- Has the patient previously tolerated the drug/s?
- Has the patient previously reacted to the same drug/s, if so was it the same reaction?
- Has the patient subsequently tolerated the drug (exclusion)?
- If multiple drugs are involved, attempt to temporally relate the type of reaction back to the culprit. (For example if an IgE mediated reaction occurs, the offending drug is likely to be administrated within the last hour.) In case of peri-operative anaphylaxis careful scrutinization of anaesthetic charts is valuable.

(The patient may not be able to provide an answer to these questions, therefore it is important to review the medical notes and/or obtain the medical history from the patient's general practitioner.)

Avoidance or desensitization
- Rapid drug desensitization is an option for IgE medicated reactions (and aspirin intolerance) but a careful 'risk-benefit analysis' must be carried out.
- What was the clinical reason for the drug in the first place?
- Are there any alternatives?
- If there are no alternatives, how important is the treatment? (For example, penicillin is the treatment of choice for neurosyphilis, syphilis in pregnancy and bacterial endocarditis.)
- Ask about any potential contraindication for desensitization as above.

Please note that allergy to general anaesthesia is complex and is beyond the scope of this chapter.

Box 7. Oral Allergy Syndrome—A 19 year old girl present with recurrent oral swelling with multiple fruits and nuts.

Symptoms/Severity
- How severe are the oral swellings?
- Has the airway been threatened?
- Are there any signs to suggest systemic involvement (i.e., generalized urticaria, asthma and anaphylaxis—patients with non-specific Lipid Transfer Protein [nsLTP] allergy can be affected)? Do the reactions respond to antihistamine?
- Had there been any hospital admissions?
- Had adrenaline ever been administrated?

Identifying the cross reactive plant protein
- Where is the likely geographical location for sensitization (Mediterranean/northern Europe/western Europe/Asia/North America)?
- Does the patient suffer from seasonal allergic rhinitis, if so identify the pollen?
- What fruits, nuts and vegetables consistently trigger the patient's symptoms?
  (Apple, pear, peaches, hazelnut, cherries and celery)
  (Banana, latex, avocado)
  (Melons, figs, tomatoes, oranges)
- Can the patient eat cooked, tinned or processed form of the same fruits or vegetables?

Other related issues
- Other atopic diseases ('allergic march')?
- Is the patient's seasonal allergic rhinitis well controlled?
- Would the patient's symptoms warrant an adrenaline auto-injector device?
- Is the patient's diet adequate?
- Would she benefit from seeing a dietician?
- Does the patient have a fear of eating fruits and vegetable?

- Specific IgE testing and immunotherapy are suitable for IgE mediated only (except aspirin intolerance which is non-IgE mediated).
- Improvement of patients' symptomatology and preventing further life threatening events with minimal lifestyle disruption are the keys to the management of allergic disorders.

Table 3.3. Differential diagnoses of allergic symptoms.

Predominant feature	Differential diagnoses
Urticaria	• Type 1 allergy • Idiopathic urticaria • Physical urticaria (aquagenic, cold, solar, cholinergic, exercise induced) • Urticarial vasculitis • Periodic fever syndrome
Urticaria and angioedema	• Type 1 allergy • Chronic idiopathic (spontaneous) urticaria and angioedema
Angioedema	• Type 1 allergy • Oral allergy syndrome (type 1 allergy) • ACE-I induced • Idiopathic angioedema • Hereditary angioedema • Acquired angioedema
Rhinitis	• Seasonal allergic rhinitis (type 1 allergy) • Perennial allergic rhinitis (type 1 allergy) • Non-allergic rhinitis (chronic rhinosinusitis) • Nasal polyps
Asthma	• Allergic asthma to common aeroallergen (type 1 allergy) • Non-allergic asthma • Occupational asthma (type 1 allergy) • Aspirin/NSAID hypersensitivity • Sulphite hypersensitivity
Anaphylaxis	• Type 1 allergy—foods, drugs, insect sting, etc. • Drug induced • Exercise induced anaphylaxis • Food dependent exercise induced anaphylaxis (type 1 allergy) • Idiopathic anaphylaxis
Other rashes	• Delayed hypersensitivity • Steven Johnson Syndrome (SJS) • Toxic Epidermal Necrolysis (TENS) • Drug Reaction with Eosinophilia and Systemic Symptoms (DRESS)
Others	• Eosinophilic gastrointestinal or respiratory diseases

Reference

Bischoff SC. Food allergy and eosinophilic gastroenteritis and colitis. Curr Opin Allergy Clin Immunol 2010; 10(3): 238–45.

Bousquet J, Clark TJ, Hurd S, Khaltaev N, Lenfant C, O'byrne P, et al. GINA guidelines on asthma and beyond. Allergy 2007 Feb; 62(2): 102–12.

Bowen T, Cicardi M, Farkas H, Bork K, Longhurst HJ, Zuraw B, et al. 2010 international consensus algorithm for the diagnosis, therapy and management of hereditary angioedema. Allergy Asthma Clin Immunol 2010; 6(1): 24.

Breibart SI, Bielory L. Acquired angioedema: autoantibody associations and C1q utility as a diagnostic tool. Allergy Asthma Proc. 2010; 31(5): 428–34.

Davis MDP, Brewer JD. Urticaria vasculitis and hypocomplementemic urticaria vasculitis syndrome. Immunol Allergy Clin Am 2004; 24: 183–213.

Hopper JL, Bui QM, Erbas B, Matheson MC, Gurrin LC, Burgess JA, et al. Does eczema in infancy cause hay fever, asthma, or both in childhood? Insights from a novel regression model of sibling data. J Allergy Clin Immunol. 2012 Nov; 130(5): 1117–1122.e1.

Kanani A, Schellenberg R, Worrington R. Urticaria and angioedema. Allergy Asthma Clin Immunol 2011; 7 Suppl 1: S9.

Kowalski ML, Makowska JS, Blanca M, Bavbek S, Bochenek G, Bousquet J, et al. Hypersensitivity to non-steroidal anti-inflammatory drugs (NSAIDs)—classification, diagnosis and management: review of the EACCI/EDNA(#) and GA2LEN/HANNA*. Allergy 2011; 66(7): 818–29.

Lang DM. Do beta blockers really enhance the risk of anaphylaxis during immunotherapy? Curr Allergy Asthma Rep 2008; 8(1): 37–44.

Mahesh PA, Vedanthan PK, Holla AD, Jayaraj BS, Prabhakar AK. Time interval and the factors associated with the development of asthma in patients with allergic rhinitis. Lung 2009; 187(6): 393–400.

Muller U. Insect sting allergy: clinical picture, diagnosis and treatment. New York: Gustav Fischer Verlag; 1990.

Pawankar R, Bunnag C, Khaltaev N, Bousquet J. Allergic rhinitis and its impact on asthma in Asia Pacific and the ARIA update 2008. World Allergy Organ J 2012 Apr; 5(Suppl 3): S212–7.

Portnoy JM. Appropriate allergy testing and interpretation. Mo Med 2011; 108(5): 339–43.

Rumbyrt JS, Schocket AL. Chronic urticaria and thyroid disease. Immunol Allergy Clin Am 2004; 24: 215–223.

Vasekar M, Criag TJ. ACE inhibitor-induced angioedema. Curr Allergy Asthma Rep 2011 [Epub ahead of print].

Wong GKY, Huissoon AP, Goddard S, Collins DM and Krishna MT. Wheat dependent exercise induced anaphylaxis: is this an appropriate terminology? J Clin Pathol 2010; 63(9): 814–7.

Zuberbier T, Bindslev-Jensen C, Canonica W, Grattan CEH, Greaves MW, Henz BM, et al. EAACI/GA^{2}LEN/EDF guideline: definition, classification and diagnosis of urticaria. Allergy 2006; 61: 316–320.

4

Allergy Skin Testing

Pudupakkam K Vedanthan[1,*] *and Harold Nelson*[2]

INTRODUCTION

Allergy Skin test (AST) is the most common method to determine the sensitization to allergens. In this chapter, the basis underlying AST as well as the details of the procedure will be discussed in detail.

What is Allergy Skin Test (AST)?

AST is a bio assay to determine the presence of specific IgE antibodies on the surface of mast cells. A positive AST is elicited when a specific allergen is introduced into the skin and a wheal and flare reaction develop over a period of 15–20 minutes. 'Sensitization' is an immunologic term; it does not mean the person is 'allergic' which indicates the individual is not only sensitized, but also has symptoms on exposure to the allergen. Hence AST determines sensitization and confirms allergy based upon the clinical presentation.

> 'Sensitization' is an Immunologic term. 'Allergy' is a clinical term.
> Allergy Skin testing is an Immunologic test for sensitization.
> You can be sensitized but not allergic

The mechanism of Type 1 Hypersensitivity is depicted diagrammatically in Fig. 4.1. There are two phases in allergic reaction: 1. Sensitization, 2. Re-exposure.

Sensitization

In genetically prone individuals, initial exposure to the antigen (allergen) will initiate activation of T cells through its presentation by Antigen-Presenting Cells (APC). The differentiated T cell in turn causes class switching of the B cell through IL-4 and IL 13 to produce IgE. IgE that is released will circulate in the blood as free IgE as well as attach to the high affinity FCeRI receptor on the surface of mast cells and basophils. This phase, where the specific IgE is bound to the mast cells, is called sensitization.

---

[1] University of Colorado, Denver, Colorado USA.
[2] National Jewish Health, Denver, Colorado, USA, Email: nelsonh@njhealth.org
* Corresponding author: pkv1947@gmail.com

Allergy Skin Testing 33

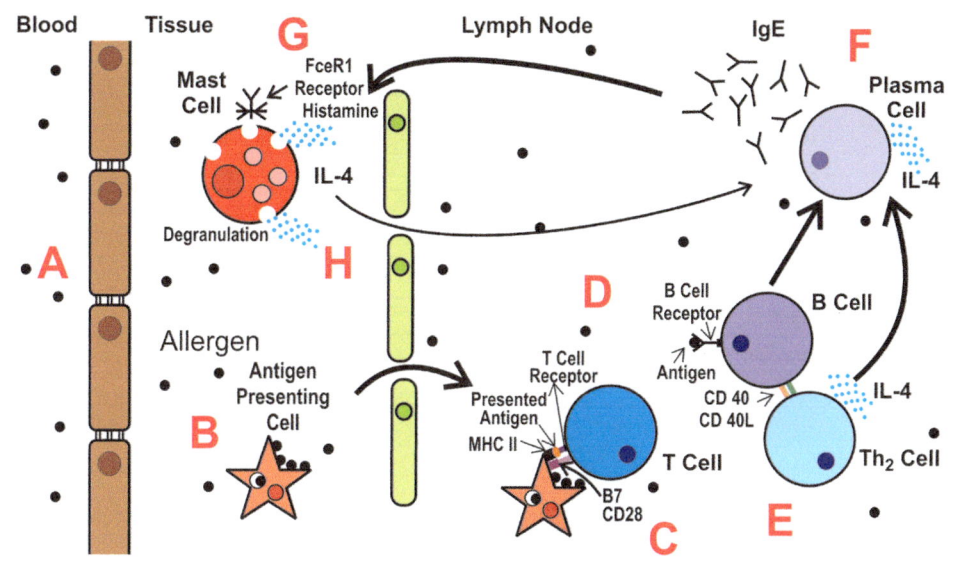

Figure 4.1. Allergic reaction mechanism.
(Source:https://commons.wikimedia.org/wiki/File:The_Allergy_Pathway.jpg)

A. The allergen enters the body. **B.** an Antigen-presenting cell takes up the allergen molecule and presents its epitopes, through the MHC II receptor, onto its surface. The activated antigen presenting cell then migrates to the nearest lymph node. **C.** where it activates T cells that recognize the allergen. They then give the decision for the T cell to differentiate to Th2 cell. **D.** at the same time, B cells recognize the allergen and through the activated Th2 cell **E.** the B cell would be activated. **F.** and differentiate into plasma cells, at which point they would actively synthesize antibodies of the IgE isotype. **G.** the IgE antibody, that now recognizes epitopes of the allergen molecule, circulates around the body through the lymphatic and cardiovascular systems and finally binds to its FcεRI receptor on mast and basophil cells. **H.** when the allergen re-enters the body at a later time, it binds to the IgE, which is on the cell surface, resulting in an aggregation of the receptor causing the cells to release pre-formed mediators. One of these mediators is histamine which causes the five symptoms of allergic inflammation: heat, pain, swelling, redness and itchiness. Another mediator is IL-4, which affects more B cells to differentiate into plasma cells and produce more IgE and thus the vicious cycle continues.

Re-exposure

During AST the mast cell is exposed to the antigen in the dermis. If the mast cells are sensitized, cross linking of the cell bound IgE by the antigen occurs with release of various mediators (histamine, tryptase, leukotrienes) which can cause vasodilatation, increased vascular permeability and smooth muscle spasm. The release of the mediators locally at the site in the skin causes the wheal and flare reaction of the AST.

Technique of skin testing

AST is a rapid, cost effective, clinically relevant, safe and simple method of detecting allergenic sensitization. There are different types of AST:

1. Epicutaneous skin test: Prick, puncture, scratch
2. Intradermal skin test

For reasons of safety, AST should ALWAYS start with epicutaneous testing. If the epicutaneous St is negative, and there is a strong clinical history suggestive of atopic sensitization, there may be some value to proceed further with Intradermal (ID) skin testing. The differences between epicutaneous and intradermal skin testing are detailed in the Table 4.1 (below).

Table 4.1. Epicutaneous skin test vs. intradermal skin test.

Item	Epicutaneous Skin Test	Intradermal Skin Test
Safety	Very Safe	Some Risk
Technique	Simple	Complicated
Speed	Good	Slower
False Positives	Low	High
Clinical Correlation	High	Low
Number Of St/Setting	Several	Few
Comfort	Good	Painful
Reproducibility	Poor	Good
Sensitivity	Good	Very High

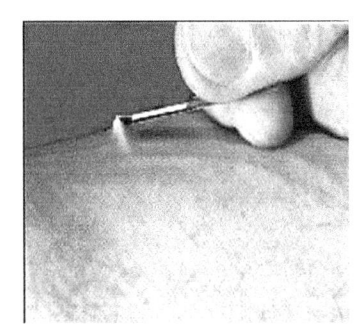

Figure 4.2. Allergy Prick skin test.

Epicutaneous ST

1. Scratch ST: A superficial abrasion is made with a needle or any other sharp instrument, and the extract is applied to the site. This approach is rarely used.
2. Puncture ST: The extract is placed on the skin first, and a superficial break in the epidermis is made by a perpendicular pressure through the drop, usually with a needle or a commercial plastic device.
3. Prick ST: A drop of the extract is placed on the skin and a sharp instrument is passed through the drop, penetrating the skin at approximately a 45 degree angle. The device is then lifted, creating a small break in the epidermis. It is estimated that 3 microliters of fluid is introduced into the skin (Squire 1950). The Prick ST has been the most popular and most commonly used. However, commercial devices are now available that allow performance of 6–8 puncture tests at one time. This has contributed to increased use of puncture testing, particularly in children.

Allergy Prick Skin test is a rapid, safe, simple, cost effective and clinically relevant method of detecting allergic sensitization.
ID STs are more sensitive, but more often detect sensitization that is not clinically relevant. They also are more apt to cause systemic reactions.

Intradermal Skin test (ID Skin test)

Intradermal Skin test (ID Skin test) is more sensitive than epicutaneous ST. It is performed ONLY when the Epicutaneous is NEGATIVE for a particular allergen. The test is performed using a 25–27 gauge needle. A small amount of allergen (0.02–0.05 ml) is injected into the skin to raise a small bleb 2–3 mm in diameter, the space between test sites should be minimum of 2 cms. The concentration of the allergen extract used for ID skin testing is generally 1: 1000 or 1: 500 weight per volume (Indrajana et al. 1971). There are several technical errors associated with ID ST including injecting too deeply, using too much extract and causing bleeding. These factors could potentially affect the results of the ID ST. ID ST is more risky than epicutaneous ST and adverse reactions including anaphylaxis have been reported. Hence extreme care should be undertaken in performing these ST and emergency tray cart with trained personnel and a physician's physical presence are mandatory.

Allergy testing 'in vitro'

An alternative to AST for detecting IgE sensitization is an *in vitro* test. *In vitro* tests are somewhat less sensitive, take longer to get the results and are more costly that prick STs, however, in certain circumstances (extensive eczema, interference by medications or recent anaphylaxis) when skin tests cannot be performed, the *in vitro* becomes the method of choice.

The *in vitro* method originally introduced was Radio Allergo Sorbent Test (RAST). This is a test for specific IgE for different allergens (inhalants, foods) using a patient's serum sample. A number of changes in the RAST assay have evolved over the past 45 years including, most notably, the use of enzyme conjugated antihuman IgE antibody in place of the radio labeled antibody. Thus the test is now properly called an enzyme-linked immunoassay (ELISA). One commercial method, the immunoCAP test is used extensively due to it's high accuracy and no use of radioactive material. The major differences between AST and ImmunoCAP are mentioned in Table 4.2 below.

Table 4.2. Comparison of immunoCap and allergy skin test (epicutaneous).

Item	ImmunoCap	Allergy Skin Test (Epicutaneous)
Sensitivity	Less	More
Specificity	High	High
Risk	None	Low
Delay in results	Yes	No
Antigen selection	Good	Excellent
Equipment	Extensive	Minimal
Cost to set up	Very high	Low
Patient perception	More scientific	Less scientific
Clinical Correlation	Excellent	Excellent
Interference by medications	None	Yes

How many ST need to be performed?

There is no standard number of ST recommended. The number of STs is based on the patient's age and history. Location, antigens suspected as well as socio-economic criteria. Testing for large numbers of allergens (> 100) is generally unacceptable and unnecessary. This is of crucial importance among general medical practitioners, as well as the general public, where there seems to be a perception that the number of STs directly correlates with the diagnostic acumen of the allergy specialist. This is not true and actually testing for a few relevant antigens is clinically and therapeutically more useful.

Selection of antigens for AST

There is no general rule regarding the selection of allergens for allergy skin testing. The local aerobiology data will be important in the selection of inhalants, especially tree pollens. Grass and weed pollens are spread in a common manner over wide areas and there is generally cross reactivity within botanical families. There is no need to include a large number of cross-reacting allergens, one or two locally important representatives of each group will suffice.

There are three different categories of allergens for AST: inhalants, ingestants (foods) and biting or stinging insects. The inhalants are further classified as (1) Indoor antigens: House dust mites, cockroaches, animal dander (cats, dogs), and molds and (2) Outdoor antigens: tree, grass, weed pollens and mold spores. Generally it is felt that indoor antigens like HD mites, cockroaches, and animal danders are common causes of allergic asthma. Hence, it is imperative all children and young adults, with significant respiratory symptoms suggestive of allergy need to be tested for these important indoor antigens. This information has both prognostic and therapeutic importance in the management of allergies.

Foods are classified as Class 1 (protein antigens) and Class 2 (plant derived).

Insect allergen extracts include venom for the flying hymenoptera, but for insects, such as ants, only whole body extracts are available.

Prick Skin testing procedure

Once the decision to perform ASTs has been taken, it is very important for the allergist or his/her assistant to fully explain the rationale, procedure, precautions, expectations and performance of the AST to the patient and the family. The following steps are generally recommended:

a. Documentation: Preparation of the allergy skin test recording sheet which needs to include the following information (Fig. 4.3): Patient's name, age, sex, address, contact information, clinic registration number, date, time ST are inserted, time St are read, signature/name of the person performing the AST, antigen name, concentration, manufacturer and batch number.

b. Self introduction to the patient by the allergy technician or person performing the test.

c. Explanation: Patient/family needs to be informed in detail regarding the exact procedure step by step.

d. Preparation of the site: the area of skin (either on the back, upper arm or forearm) by cleaning the site with 70% alcohol swab and then allowing it to dry. If the portion of skin is hairy, the patient is instructed to shave the area the day before.

e. Marking of the test sites: with a skin marking pen the sites are numbered in a consecutive order starting generally with Negative Saline control and ending with Positive Histamine control.

f. Minute drops of the allergen extract are placed on the sites marked. Taking extra precautions they match the exact order and numbering on the ST recording sheet.

g. Using a sharp instrument (for example a small pox needle) and with a firm grip on the needle, it is pushed through the drop of allergen extract swiftly making sure the skin is pressed lightly and the needle drawn upwards making a small nip (this is actually felt by the technician).

h. If the same device is to be used for all sites, the lancet is thoroughly wiped with a WET alcohol swab, before inserting through the next drop. If separate needles or lancets are being used, there is no need to wipe with the moist cotton swab.

i. The penetration of the allergen occurs with the pricking action; therefore the remaining liquid may be immediately wiped away with a cotton pledget without affecting the results of the test.

j. It is important to stress the importance of using very small amounts of allergen extracts for testing, since only 0.3 microliter will enter the dermis irrespective of the size of the drop of allergen extract. Hence, there is no need to use a full drop for AST and this will avoid unnecessary wastage of the antigen.

k. After 15–20 minutes, the test is read. First the negative saline control and positive histamine control test site should be examined. The acceptable reading of the saline test will be < 3 mm in diameter. The acceptable diameter for the histamine control will be 3 mm or above.

l. It is important to measure the maximum wheal diameters perpendicular to each other and record the readings. There is no need generally to measure the erythema area. Some allergists' offices use 1+, 2+, 3+ 4+ readings based upon the histamine reading or some arbitrary scale. This method is not recommended to avoid any potential ambiguity and inaccuracies.

AST proficiency testing

The results of AST are very dependent on the correct performance of the tests by the responsible technician. To confirm that the technician is using an acceptable technique it is suggested that they be periodically tested by having them blindly perform multiple positive and negative controls on a volunteer subject. They should be able to consistently achieve no reaction with saline and a reaction consistently > 3 mm with the positive histamine control.

Quality of extracts

Pollen extracts, even when not standardized are usually quite potent. Extracts of cat dander and house dust mites, even the FDA standardized extracts, are about one-fifth as potent as most pollen extracts. Dog dander, except for Acetone-Precipitated dog (Jubilant Hollister-Steir, Spokane, WA) is very weak, as are most cockroach and mold extracts. Cockroach and mold extracts also contain strong proteolytic activity which will digest the allergens in the extracts. For cockroach and fungi (mold) only 50% glycerin extracts should be used.

Many food extracts quickly lose their potency. Therefore, especially for fruits and vegetables, pricking the uncooked food and then pricking the patient's skin (prick and prick technique) will often given positive results when the test with the commercial preparation is negative.

Positive and negative controls

It is very important to perform and interpret the control ST reactions before going further with the reading of the allergens. The negative saline control is interpreted as acceptable if it is < 3 mm in diameter. The positive histamine control has to be 3 mm in diameter in size and 3 mm larger than the negative saline control for the test to be considered reliable. A positive ST is interpreted as ≥ 3 mm larger than the negative saline control. The negative control signifies the baseline reactivity of the skin. A histamine positive control less then 3 mm in diameter suggests interference such as suppression by antihistamines.

Representative skin tests are shown in Figs. 4.3, 4.4 and 4.5 at the end of this chapter for ready reference.

Table 4.3. Allergy skin test suppression by medication.

Anti histamines: H 1 blockers	3–10 days
Antihistamines: H2 blockers	No effect
Ketotifen	Upto 5 days
Imipramines (Tricyclic antidepressants)	Upto 21 days
Phenothiazines	Upto 10 days
Systemic Steroids	No effect
Topical steroids	Upto 7 days
LABA	No Effect

Factors influencing allergen skin tests

1. Medications: Significant suppression of the skin reactivity is seen following conventional doses of antihistamines (see Table 4.3). It is important to instruct all patients to avoid all antihistamine preparations for a minimum of 3 days prior to the AST appointment. It is very important to routinely double check with the patient or patient's family regarding this issue before starting with the test procedure.

2. Age: The skin reactivity generally declines with age, especially after 60 years of age (Tuft et al. 1955, Carey and Gay 1934). Reaction to histamine is generally smaller in infants and young children, resulting in smaller ASTs (Gallant and Maibach 1973).

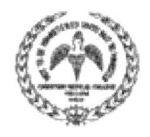

CHRISTIAN MEDICAL COLLEGE

VELLORE TOWN
ALLERGY PRICK SKIN TESTING
NAME: ID: REF.BY:
AGE: DATE: DR:
SEX: TIME DONE: (ANY OTHER INFO)
                         TIME READ: TECHNICIAN:

No.	Allergens	Wheal dia (in mm)	No	Allergens	Wheal dia (in mm)
1.	Dust mite mix (D&F)		1.	Milk	
2	Cockroach		2.	Potato	
3.	Prosopis		3.	Apple	
4.	Acacia		4.	Mutton	
5.	Partheium		5.	Ground nut	
6.	Cannabis sativa		6.	Soya	
7.	Amboosia		7.	Wheat	
8.	Amaranthus spinosus		8.	Bengal Gram	
9.	Sorghum Halipase		9.	Cashew nut	
10.	Artemesia Tulenta		10.	Chicken	
11.	Xanthium		11.	Citrus (Lemon)	
12.	Morus Alba		12.	Dal masoor	
13.	Cocos Nucifera		13.	Dal moong	
14.	Ricinis Communis		14.	Egg white	
15.	Alternaria Tenius		15.	Fish	
16.	Alternaria Alternata				
17.	Curvularia				
18.	Aspergillus fumigtus				
19.	Helminthosporium sativum				
20.	Fusarium				
21.	Pencillium				
22.	Rhizopus nigricans				
23.	Aspergillus niger				
24.	Aspergillus flavus				
25.	Dog Dander				
26.	Cat Dander				
27.	Cattle				
28.	Gram mill dust				
29.	Saline control				
30.	Histamine control				

INTERPRETATION:

Figure 4.3. Full adult skin test panel (inhalants and foods).

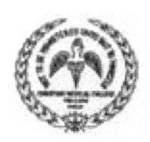

CHRISTIAN MEDICAL COLLEGE

VELLORE TOWN
ALLERGY PRICK SKIN TESTING
NAME: ID: REF.BY:
AGE: DATE: DR:
SEX: TIME DONE: (ANY OTHER INFO)
                              TIME READ: TECHNICIAN:

PAEDIATRIC ROUTINE PANEL

No.	Allergens	Wheal dia (in mm)
1.	Dust mite mix (D&F)	
2	Cockroach	
3.	Prosopis Julifora	
4.	Parthenium	
5.	Cynodon dactylon	
6.	Sorghum Halipase	
7.	Alternaria Tenius	
8.	Dog Dander	
9.	Cat Dander	
	FOODS	
1.	Chicken	
2.	Egg white	
3.	Fish	
4.	Milk	
5.	Ground nut	
6.	Soya	
7.	Wheat	
	Saline control	
	Histamine control	

INTERPRETATION:

Figure 4.4. Example for recording Pediatric skin test sheet results.

MODEL OF ALLERGY SKIN TESTING REPORT

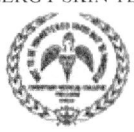

CHRISTIAN MEDICAL COLLEGE

VELLORE TOWN
ALLERGY PRICK SKIN TESTING

NAME: Child   ID: xxxxx   REF.BY:Dr ABC
AGE: 8 yrs   DATE: xx xx xxxx   DR:
SEX: Male   TIME DONE: xx xx   (ANY OTHER INFO)
   TIME READ: xx xx   TECHNICIAN:xyz

PAEDIATRIC ROUTINE PANEL
(should indicate whether the blanks represent negative reactions or tests that were no done_)

No.	Allergens	Wheal dia (in mm)
1.	Dust mite mix (D&F)	12×12 P E
2	Cockroach	10×10 PE
3.	Prosopis Julifora	6×8
4.	Parthenium	
5.	Cynodon Dactylon	
6.	Sorghum Halipase	
7.	Alternaria Tenius	3×4
8.	Dog Dander	
9.	Cat Dander	3×3
	FOODS	
1.	Chicken	
2.	Egg white	
3.	Fish	
4.	Milk	3×3
5.	Ground nut	
6.	Soya	
7.	Wheat	
	Saline control	1×1
	Histamine control	8×10

INTERPRETATION: Strongly Sensitized to House Dust Mite Mix, Cockroach and Prosopis with good positive and negative controls. (P: Pseudopod, E: Erythema)

Date: time   Signature of the technician

Figure 4.5. An example of the results of prick skin testing in a child.

3. Area of the body: The mid and upper back are more (33%) reactive than the lower back. The back as a whole is more (53%) reactive than the forearm (Voorhorst 1980). The ante-cubital area is the most reactive of the upper arm and the wrist is the least reactive (50% reduction). The radial side of the forearm is less (50%) reactive than the ulnar side.

4. Distance between the test sites: There has to be a minimum distance of 2 cm between test sites. This is to prevent a non specific enhancement through the axon reflex from a nearby strong reaction (Brown et al. 1979).

Correlation of allergy skin tests

1. *In vitro* measurement: There is good correlation between Prick St and *in vitro tests* (up to nearly 80%) (Sampson 2003).
2. There is positive correlationship in children between the size of the reaction of HD mite and the likelihood of having asthma.
3. There is a direct correlation of skin test reactivity and nasal and bronchial inhalation challenge to antigens like HD mite, Alternaria, and Bermuda grass.
4. There is a direct correlation of AST wheal size and immunocap grading as well as clinical sensitivity to food items like peanuts, milk, eggs and fish. This is of great clinical value in elimination as well as deciding on the performance of the food challenge (Sprecace et al. 1966).
5. Long term follow up studies by (Hagy and Settipane 1976) demonstrated a strong correlation of positive ST and subsequent development of allergic rhinitis/asthma (Nelson 1983).
6. There is a prompt decline in the ST reactivity with immunotherapy. In long-term studies, the decrease in ASTs correlates with clinical improvement and persistence of benefit following discontinuation of treatment (Nelson 1983). Specific IgE falls with long term immunotherapy but not with short term immunotherapy (Ownby and Naderson 1982).

Some practical points

1. It is preferable to express the AST measurements in mms rather than using a semi-quantitative grading system such as comparison with the histamine control (Ownby and Naderson 1982).
2. Vigorous wiping of the same testing needle with a wet sponge is definitely preferable to dry cotton. It also facilitates quicker testing compared to changing needles for each antigen to be tested (Ortolani et al. 1993).
3. Blotting of the test site immediately after pricking does not seem to influence the final size of the resulting reaction. This is very helpful especially in the pediatric age group Allergy Diagnostic Testing, Practice Parameters 2008).
4. ASTs can be positive in clinically asymptomatic subjects. A positive test only signifies sensitization, not clinical allergic disease.
5. In the case of food items like fruits and vegetables, use of fresh material by the prick and prick test should be used (Sampson 2003).
6. When reporting the results of the AST, the term ALLERGIC needs to be avoided; instead the term SENSITIZED needs to be used. Always report on the positive and negative controls.

Conclusions

Allergy Skin testing is extremely useful in diagnosing sensitization.
AST along with history will help in the appropriate management of the allergic patient.
AST is very helpful in determining the choice of allergen for allergen avoidance and immunotherapy.
AST is a highly reliable, safe, quick and a very useful tool in the hands of a trained allergy specialist.

References

Allergy Diagnostic Testing: An Updated Practice Parameter. Ann Allergy Asthma Immunol March 2008; 100(3): 3.
Brown WG, Halonen MJ, Kaltenborn WT, Barbee RA. The relationship of respiratory allergy, skin test reactivity, and serum IgEin a community population sample. J allergy Clin Immunol 1979; 63: 328.
Carey TN, Gay LN. Skin reactions in infants; comparison of the skin of the new born to passive atopic sensitization, comparison with reaction to histamine. J Allergy 1934; 5: 488.
Gallant SP, Maibach H. Reproducibility of allergy Epicutaneous test techniques. J Allergy & Clin Immuno 1973; 51: 245.

Hagy GW. Settipane GA. Risk factors for developing asthma and allergic rhinitis. A 7 year follow up study of college students. J Allergy & Clini Immunol 1976; 58: 330.

Indrajana T, Spieksma FT, Voorhorst R. Comparative study of Intracutaneous, scratch and prick tests in allergy. Ann of Allergy 1971; 29: 639.

Nelson H, Diagnostic procedures in allergy: allergy skin testing Annals of Allergy Oct 1983; 51(4): 411–418.

Ortolani C, Pastorello EA, Farioli L, Ispano M, Pravettoni V, Berti C et al. IgE mediated allergy from vegetable allergens. Ann Allergy 1993; 71: 470–6.

Ownby DR, Naderson JA: An improved Prick skin test procedure for young children. J Allergy & Clin Immuno 1982; 69: 533.

Sampson H. Food allergy. J Allergy Clin Immunol 2003;111: S 540-7.

Sprecace GA, Pamper SG, Sherman WB, Lemlich A, Ziffer H. The effect of antigen injections on skin reactivity to antigens. J Allergy 1966; 38: 9.

Squire JR. The relationship between horse dandruff and horse serum antigen in asthma. Clin Sci 1950; 9: 127.

Taylor G and Walker J. Charles Harrison Blackley (1820–1900) Clin Allerg 1973; 3: 103.

Tuft L, Heck VM, Gregory DC. Studies in sensitization as applied to skin test reactions, influence of age upon skin test reactivity. J Allergy 1955; 26: 359.

Voorhorst R. Perfection of skin testing technique. Allergy 1980; 35: 247.

5

In vitro Laboratory Tests for the Diagnosis of Allergy

Vijaya Knight,[1] *Preveen Ramamoorthy*[2] *and Ronald J Harbeck*[3,*]

INTRODUCTION

In the diagnosis of human allergic disease *in vitro* laboratory tests for total IgE and specific IgE antibodies are often used when a patient's clinical history identifies atopy and a relevant allergen exposure. This chapter will discuss the various *in vitro* tests that are available, their interpretations and pitfalls. Thorough reviews of this topic are available from a variety of sources (Hamilton 2006, Hamilton 2010).

Measurement of total IgE

The immunoglobulin, IgE, is associated with type I hypersensitivity and is an important component in allergic disorders (Gould et al. 2003). IgE is the least abundant isotype in the blood of normal, non-atopic individuals with typical levels of only 0.05% of the total immunoglobulin concentration. However, this low amount is capable of triggering powerful allergic reactions. Atopic individuals can have levels that far exceed those found in normal individuals.

IgE was discovered in 1966 by Ishizakas and Hornbrook (Ishizaka et al. 1966) (reviewed in (Johansson 2011)). IgE can specifically recognize allergens that are typically proteins, e.g., the dust mite DerP1, the cat Fel d 1 or components from grass, weed, tree pollens and certain foods. The symptoms of allergy are the result of the release of inflammatory mediators from basophils and mast cells that have IgE antibodies bound to their high-affinity receptor, FceR1. The crosslinking of specific IgE molecules by an allergen causes the release of chemicals such as histamine, leukotrienes and cytokines that result in many of the conditions seen in patients with allergy, asthma, eczema and allergic rhinitis.

Since the level of total serum IgE in individuals is lower than the other immunoglobulins, sensitive immunoassays have been applied to its measurement. Past methods which are no longer commonly used involve competitive-binding liquid-phase immunoprecipitation, competitive-binding solid-phase labeled-antigen immunoassays and noncompetitive solid-phase labeled-antigen immunoassays [reviewed

---

[1] Children's Hospital Colorado and University of Colorado, School of Medicine, Assoc. Professor, Department of Pediatrics, Section of Allergy and Clinical Immunology, Aurora, Colorado, USA, Email: vijaya.knight@childrenscolorado.org
[2] HealthTell Inc. and University of Colorado, School of Medicine, Adjunct Faculty Department of Medicine, Aurora, Colorado, USA, Email: preveenr@gmail.com
[3] Advanced Diagnostic Laboratories, Professor, Dept. of Medicine, Division of Pathology, National Jewish Health, Denver, Colorado, USA.
* Corresponding author: harbeckr@njhealth.org

in (Hamilton and Franklin Adkinson 2004)]. The one which is most commonly used in clinical and research laboratories is the noncompetitive solid-phase two-site immunoassay. As originally described, the assay employed a polyclonal anti-human IgE covalently bound to a solid support, e.g., a cellulose disk (Johansson and Yman 1988). After incubation with the patient's serum, followed by a buffer wash to remove unbound serum components, the amount of bound human IgE to the disk is determined by the addition of a radiolabeled anti-human IgE. The results are then compared to a calibrator or control. Thus the amount bound of the radiolabeled IgE is directly related to the amount of IgE present in the patient's serum. During the latter part of the 20th century, manufacturers of instruments and reagents developed non-radioactive immunoassays that replaced the older radiolabeled reagents. In the United States, the Food and Drug Administration (FDA) has approved several immunoassay methods for the measurement of total IgE using non-radioisotope labeled anti-IgE. Among these are the Thermo Fisher Phadia ImmunoCAP® (Uppsala, Sweden), the Siemens Immunolite® (Tarrytown, NY), Hycor Hytec® (Indianapolis, IN) and the Roche Diagnostics Cobas® (Indianapolis, IN).

Total serum IgE levels are age-related. The level increases during childhood and around 10 years of age total serum IgE levels reach values that are maintained throughout adult life, i.e., 22 + 85 kU IgE/l, where 1 kU equals 2.4 ng/mL (Barbee et al. 1981, Seagroatt and Anderson 1981). Individuals with levels of IgE greater than the upper 95% confidence limit often have atopic disorders such as allergic asthma, atopic dermatitis and bronchopulmonary aspergillosis. However, an elevated IgE does not prove that a patient's symptoms are due to allergy, and a normal IgE level does not exclude allergy.

In cases where the humanized monoclonal anti-IgE omalizumab (Xolair, Genentech, Inc., San Francisco and Novartis Pharmaceuticals Corp, East Hanover, NJ) is being initiated for treatment of atopic disease, the patients must first have a total IgE level measured to determine if they are candidates (Brownell and Casale 2004). If the level is determined to be between 30 and 700 kU/L then the total IgE level can be used to calculate the dose of Xolair. Xolair has also been reported to be beneficial in occupational asthma (Leynadier et al. 2004), non-allergic asthma with relatively lower concentrations of total IgE (Garcia et al. 2013), and exacerbations due to viral infection induced asthma (Teach et al. 2015).

Measurement of specific IgE

Shortly after the discovery of IgE, the radioallergosorbent test (RAST) was introduced for the detection of allergen specific IgE in patient's serum (Wide et al. 1967). As originally described this non-competitive, solid phase assay consisted of incubating a patient's serum with an allergen that is conjugated to a cellulose paper disk that has been activated with cyanogen bromide (Ceska and Lundkvist 1972). If allergen-specific IgE is present, it binds to the paper disk and unbound antibodies are washed away after the incubation period. IgE bound to the allergen is then detected by the addition of a radiolabeled (typically ^{125}I) antihuman IgE directed toward the Fc region. The amount of bound radiolabeled antihuman IgE is measured in a gamma counter and the radioactivity measured is proportional to the amount of allergen specific IgE present in the initial serum sample.

A number of changes in the RAST assay have evolved over the past 48 years including, most notably, the use of enzyme conjugated antihuman IgE antibody in place of the radiolabeled antibody. Thus while the term RAST is still used to describe an allergen specific IgE assay; it is technically incorrect since the assays used today no longer use a radioactive label. With the improvement in allergen extraction techniques and identification of relevant allergens, the number of allergens available has increased substantially since the assay was first employed. The use of cellulose as the binding matrix for allergens is still used by some companies (Hycor), however others have used a cellulose sponge matrix (ImmunoCAP, Thermo Fisher Phadia) or biotinylated allergens (Siemens Immulite) to increase the allergen-binding capacity. Automation of the process has also allowed for the clinical laboratory to run multiple allergens on multiple samples with rapid throughput. These changes have resulted in assays that have increased sensitivity, specificity and reproducibility compared to the earlier assays (Hamilton and Franklin Adkinson 2004).

In 2009, the Clinical Laboratory Standards Institute (CLSI) published guidelines for manufacturers of allergy testing platforms and reagents to establish uniform reporting of allergen-specific IgE results.

The establishment by manufacturers of a more uniform reporting of allergen specific IgE results was published in a 2009 by the Clinical Laboratory Standards Institute (Matsson et al. 2008). In this document it was suggested that manufacturers use a common unit, i.e., kUA/L (or kilounits of antibody per liter), using a calibration system linked to the World Health Organization IgE standard, 75/502. However, because of the use of extracts containing different allergen compositions, the inter-assay variation between manufacturers can be significant. Thus the results from one assay cannot necessarily be compared to the results from another system (Wood et al. 2007). Another pitfall in the measurement of allergen specific IgE include the potential for false positives in patients with high total IgE levels likely caused by the non-specific binding of the patient's IgE (Merkel et al. 2015). In addition, the measurement of the serum concentration of allergen specific IgE may not accurately reflect its biological relevance of the IgE associated with mast cells and basophils.

Testing for specific IgE initially employed crude allergen extracts that contained both allergenic and non-allergenic molecules. Some of these molecules may share structural features with other environmental allergens. For example, individuals who are positive for IgE to birch pollen may also show elevated IgE to peanuts and hazelnuts (Mittag et al. 2004). Using crude allergens to detect specific IgE, therefore, has the potential to lead to falsely elevated specific IgE. However, recent progress in molecular biological and biochemical techniques has now made possible the production of high purified or recombinant allergens as well as individual allergenic proteins for a particular allergen. For example, several well-defined peanut (Arachis hypogea, Ara h) proteins have been approved by the FDA and are now available for clinical testing. More than a few studies have shown Ara h2 to be superior to whole peanut extract in predicting clinical allergy (Nicolau et al. 2010, Dang et al. 2012, Lieberman et al. 2013). However, establishment of optimal cut-off values for sIgE to Ara h2 to predict or diagnose clinical allergy remains a challenge. Individual allergen components have also been identified for a variety of foods (peanuts, soy, cashew nuts, hazel nuts, walnuts, wheat, fruits including apples and peaches), grass and weed pollen and animal proteins. Using these allergen components in 'Component Resolved Diagnostics' or CRD tests studies are being conducted to determine if specific components of the allergen are superior correlates of true allergy, and whether reactivity to individual components has a role in predicting the progress or resolution of allergy (Nicolaou et al. 2010).

Defining patterns of allergic sensitization and disease with multiplex allergen assays has gained recent interest (Salcedo and Diaz-Perales 2010, Sastre 2010). Within the last decade an allergen microarray chip has been employed to measure IgE reactivity to native and component allergens (Skamstrup Hansen and Poulsen 2010). The current system offered by Thermo Fisher is a multi-array assay (ISAC, immune-solid phase allergen chip) that can be performed with 20 microliters of serum and provides semi-quantitative results for specific IgE to multiple native or recombinant allergen components.

Emerging diagnostics for allergy

Although CRD have significantly increased the scale of allergen testing from single-plex assays to measuring 112 allergen components and such technology represents a quantum leap in highly multiplexed allergy testing, they have high specificity but lower sensitivity than current first line tests (Flores Kim et al. 2018).

It is estimated that there are 3000 known allergens (Jakob et al. 2015) and there are no CRD panels that can measure all of those allergens in a multiplexed fashion. Developing new recombinant allergen reagents for CRD is not a very scalable process. Given this challenge, comprehensive allergy panels that can cover all known allergens (~ 3000) are not likely to be available as CRD panels. High density peptide arrays with tens of thousands of peptides have been applied to many disease states such as infectious diseases and cancer (Sykes et al. 2013, Rowe et al. 2017). Many low-density peptide arrays have been applied to epitope mapping of allergens (Flinterman et al. 2008, Dall'antonia et al. 2014, Matsuo et al. 2015). It is conceivable that high-density peptide arrays can be applied to discover novel allergen epitopes and massively parallel allergy testing of all known allergens.

Epigenetic modifications mediate the effect of various environmental exposures, both allergy-protecting and conferring susceptibility to allergic diseases. Hence, they are relevant diagnostic avenues to pursue for allergy testing (Potaczek et al. 2017). In one study 96 methylation blood DNA biomarker signature out-performed allergen-specific IgE and skin prick tests for predicting Oral Food Challenges (OFC) outcomes (Martino et al. 2015). Though these are still early days for blood-based DNA methylation tests for allergy testing, they have the potential to augment and enhance current allergy testing modalities.

Basophil activation tests (BAT) in the diagnosis of allergy

Basophils present in the peripheral blood generally represent less than 1% of the total leukocyte population. The granules of basophils contain histamine, proteoglycans, proteolytic enzymes, leukotrienes and several cytokines including IL-4. Basophils share many properties with tissue mast cells especially the histamine content and the presence on their surface of FceR1. Basophils can be activated by one of four different mechanisms: (1) cross-linking of the FceR1 via an allergen-IgE interaction, (2) cross-linking with specific anti-IgE or anti-FceR1 antibodies, (3) by lectins that cross-link by an antigen-independent manner or (4) independently of FceR1 cross-linking via different receptors. Historically basophil activation has been measured by the release of cysteinyl leukotriene or histamine (Haydik and Ma 1988). Recently investigators have used flow cytometry along with specific markers to examine basophil activation (MacGlashan 2010). These include CD63 which is present on the intracellular granules membrane and thus is not detected in unactivated basophils by surface staining with an anti-CD63 antibody. However, upon activation and exocytosis the granules fuse with the cell membrane resulting in CD63 expression on the cell surface in a relatively high density (Knol et al. 1991). CD203c is a lineage-specific marker which is constitutively expressed on the surface of basophil membranes and on activation is rapidly upregulated (Buhring et al. 1999). Antibodies to the FceR1 present in the serum of patients with chronic urticaria have been detected using CD203c as a marker of basophil activation (Yasnowsky et al. 2006). The usefulness of *in vitro* Basophil Activation Test (BAT) for the detection of allergen-induced expression of CD63 or the upregulation of CD203c has been demonstrated for various IgE-mediated allergies (Ebo et al. 2006, de Weck et al. 2008) and is being investigated for its utility as a diagnostic tool. As mentioned earlier, because homology among allergens can occur, IgE-mediated sensitization to one allergen may result in a positive IgE test to a related allergen in the absence of true clinical allergy. Since the BAT is a direct measure of the activity of specific- IgE sensitized basophils, it may correlate more accurately with *in vivo* responses such as the Skin Prick Test (SPT) results. While this correlation has not been conclusively proven, the BAT has been shown to have some utility in complementing specific IgE testing and SPT to allow improved discrimination between allergic and non-allergic individuals (Ocmant et al. 2009). Recently BAT has been shown to have a 95% positive predictive value and 98% negative predictive value which allowed for a two-thirds reduction in the number of oral food challenges to peanuts (Koplin et al. 2019).

Summary

In vitro allergy testing is a rapidly developing field for the diagnostic laboratory. Technological advances have converted conventional immunoassays into automated, high throughput processes and the definition of the molecular determinants of allergens has further refined and added specificity to testing for allergy. Measurement of cellular (both basophil and lymphocyte) responses is an emerging and exciting field. Current studies in this area are largely confined to research programs; however, the emerging data suggests that cell-based assays are likely to be important diagnostic tools for future laboratory—based testing for allergy. Molecular technologies such as peptide arrays have the potential to identify novel allergen epitopes. DNA methylation is an area of increased research focus that may yield epigenetic tests for allergy.

References

Barbee RA, Halonen M, Lebowitz M, Burrows B. Distribution of IgE in a community population sample: correlations with age, sex, and allergen skin test reactivity. J Allergy Clin Immunol 1981; 68(2): 106–111.
Brownell J, Casale TB. Anti-IgE therapy. Immunol Allergy Clin North Am 2004; 24(4): 551–568, v.

Buhring HJ, Simmons PJ, Pudney M, Muller R, Jarrossay D, van Agthoven A, et al. The monoclonal antibody 97A6 defines a novel surface antigen expressed on human basophils and their multipotent and unipotent progenitors. Blood 1999; 94(7): 2343–2356.

Ceska M, Lundkvist U. A new and simple radioimmunoassay method for the determination of IgE. Immunochemistry 1972; 9(10): 1021–1030.

Dall'antonia F, Pavkov-Keller T, Zangger K, Keller W. Structure of allergens and structure based epitope predictions. Methods 2014; 66(1): 3–21. doi:10.1016/j.ymeth.2013.07.024.

Dang TD, Tang M, Choo S, Licciardi PV, Koplin JJ, Martin PE et al. Increasing the accuracy of peanut allergy diagnosis by using Ara h 2. J Allergy Clin Immunol 2012; 129(4): 1056–1063.

de Weck AL, Sanz ML, Gamboa PM, Aberer W, Bienvenu J, Blanca M et al. Diagnostic tests based on human basophils: more potentials and perspectives than pitfalls. Int Arch Allergy Immunol 2008; 146(3): 177–189.

Ebo DG, Sainte-Laudy J, Bridts CH, Mertens CH, Hagendorens MM, Schuerwegh AJ, et al. Flow-assisted allergy diagnosis: current applications and future perspectives. Allergy 2006; 61(9): 1028–1039.

Flinterman AE, Knol EF, Lencer DA, Bardina L, den Hartog Jager CF, Lin J, et al. Peanut epitopes for IgE and IgG4 in peanut-sensitized children in relation to severity of peanut allergy. J Allergy Clin Immunol 2008; 121(3): 737–743 e710.

Flores Kim J, McCleary N, Nwaru BI, Stoddart A and Sheikh A. Diagnostic accuracy, risk assessment, and cost-effectiveness of component-resolved diagnostics for food allergy: A systematic review. Allergy 2018; 73(8): 1609–1621.

Garcia G, Magnan A, Chiron R, Contin-Bordes C, Berger P, Taille C, et al. A proof-of-concept, randomized, controlled trial of omalizumab in patients with severe, difficult-to-control, nonatopic asthma. Chest 2013; 144(2): 411–419.

Gould HJ, Sutton BJ, Beavil AJ, Beavil RL, McCloskey N, Coker HA, et al. The biology of IGE and the basis of allergic disease. Annu Rev Immunol 2003; 21: 579–628.

Hamilton RG, Franklin Adkinson N, Jr. In vitro assays for the diagnosis of IgE-mediated disorders. J Allergy Clin Immunol 2004; 114(2): 213–225; quiz 226.

Hamilton RG. Immunological methods in the diagnostic allergy clinical and research laboratory. In: Detrick B, Hamilton RG, Folds JD (eds.). Manual of Molecular and Clinical Laboratory Immunology. 7th ed. ASM Press, Washington, DC: 2006; 955–963.

Hamilton RG. Laboratory diagnosis and management of human allergic disease. In: Leung JYM, Sampson HA, Geha R, Szefler SJ (eds.). Pediatric allergy: principles and practices. 2nd ed. Elsevier, Edinburgh 2010; 240–249.

Haydik IB, Ma WS. Basophil histamine release. Assays and interpretation. Clin Rev Allergy 1988; 6(2): 141–162.

Ishizaka K, Ishizaka T, Hornbrook MM. Physico-chemical properties of human reaginic antibody. IV. Presence of a unique immunoglobulin as a carrier of reaginic activity. J Immunol 1966; 97(1): 75–85.

Jakob T, Forstenlechner P, Matricardi P, Kleine-Tebbe J. Molecular allergy diagnostics using multiplex assays: methodological and practical considerations for use in research and clinical routine: Part 21 of the Series Molecular Allergology. Allergo J Int 2015; 24: 320–332.

Johansson SG. The History of IgE: From discovery to 2010. Curr Allergy Asthma Rep 2011; 11(2): 173–177. doi:10.1007/s11882-010-0174-3.

Johansson SG, Yman L. In vitro assays for immunoglobulin E. Methodology, indications, and interpretation. Clin Rev Allergy 1988; 6(2): 93–139.

Knol EF, Mul FP, Jansen H, Calafat J and Roos D. Monitoring human basophil activation via CD63 monoclonal antibody 435. J Allergy Clin Immunol 1991; 88(3 Pt 1): 328–338.

Koplin JJ, Perrett KP, Sampson HA. Diagnosing peanut allergy with fewer oral food challenges. J Allergy Clin Immunol Pract 2019; 7(2): 375–380.

Leynadier F, Doudou O, Gaouar H, Le Gros V, Bourdeix I, Guyomarch-Cocco L, et al. Effect of omalizumab in health care workers with occupational latex allergy. J Allergy Clin Immunol 2004; 113(2): 360–361.

Lieberman JA, Glaumann S, Batelson S, Borres MP, Sampson HA, Nilsson C. The utility of peanut components in the diagnosis of IgE-mediated peanut allergy among distinct populations. J Allergy Clin Immunol Pract 2013; 1(1): 75–82.

MacGlashan D, Jr. Expression of CD203c and CD63 in human basophils: relationship to differential regulation of piecemeal and anaphylactic degranulation processes. Clin Exp Allergy 2010; 40(9): 1365–1377. doi: 10.1111/j.1365-2222.2010.03572.x.

Martino D, Dang T, Sexton-Oates A, Prescott S, Tang ML, Dharmage S, et al. Blood DNA methylation biomarkers predict clinical reactivity in food-sensitized infants. J Allergy Clin Immunol 2015; 135(5): 1319–1328 e1311–1312.

Matsson FH, Robert G. Hamilton, Per N. Matsson, Debra L. Hovanec-Burns, Mark Van Cleve, Sic Chan et al. Analytical performance characteristics and clinical utility of immunological assays for human IgE antibodies of defined allergen specificities. 2nd ed. Wayne, PA: Clinical Laboratory Standards Institute 2008. DOI:https://doi.org/10.1016/j.jaci.2014.12.961.

Matsuo H, Yokooji T, Taogoshi T. Common food allergens and their IgE-binding epitopes. Allergol Int 2015; 64(4): 332–343.

Merkel PA, O'Sullivan MD, Ridge C, Knight V. Critique on the quantitative nature of IgE antibody measurements. J Allergy Clin Immunol Pract 2015; 3(6): 973–975.

Mittag D, Akkerdaas J, Ballmer-Weber BK, Vogel L, Wensing M, Becker WM, et al. Ara h 8, a Bet v 1-homologous allergen from peanut, is a major allergen in patients with combined birch pollen and peanut allergy. J Allergy Clin Immunol 2004; 114(6): 1410–1417.

Nicolaou N, Poorafshar M, Murray C, Simpson A, Winell H, Kerry G, et al. Allergy or tolerance in children sensitized to peanut: prevalence and differentiation using component-resolved diagnostics. J Allergy Clin Immunol 2010; 125(1): 191–197 e191–113.

Ocmant A, Mulier S, Hanssens L, Goldman M, Casimir G, Mascart F, et al. Basophil activation tests for the diagnosis of food allergy in children. Clin Exp Allergy 2009; 39(8): 1234–1245.

Potaczek DP, Harb H, Michel S, Alhamwe BA, Renz H and Tost J. Epigenetics and allergy: from basic mechanisms to clinical applications. Epigenomics 2017; 9(4): 539–571.

Rowe M, Melnick J, Gerwien R, Legutki JB, Pfeilsticker J, Tarasow TM, et al. An ImmunoSignature test distinguishes Trypanosoma cruzi, hepatitis B, hepatitis C and West Nile virus seropositivity among asymptomatic blood donors. PLoS Negl Trop Dis 2017; 11(9): e0005882.

Salcedo G, Diaz-Perales A. Component-resolved diagnosis of allergy: more is better? Clin Exp Allergy 2010; 40(6): 836–838. doi:10.1111/j.1365-2222.2010.03506.x.

Sastre J. Molecular diagnosis in allergy. Clin Exp Allergy 2010; 40(10): 1442–1460. doi:10.1111/j.1365-2222.2010.03585.x.

Seagroatt V, Anderson SG. The second international reference preparation for human serum immunoglobulin E and the first British standard for human serum immunoglobulin E. J Biol Stand 1981; 9(4): 431–437.

Skamstrup Hansen K, Poulsen LK. Component resolved testing for allergic sensitization. Curr Allergy Asthma Rep 2010; 10(5): 340–348. doi:10.1007/s11882-010-0133-z.

Sykes KF, Legutki JB, Stafford P. Immunosignaturing: a critical review. Trends Biotechnol 2013; 31(1): 45–51.

Teach SJ, Gill MA, Togias A, Sorkness CA, Arbes SJ, Jr, Calatroni A, et al. Preseasonal treatment with either omalizumab or an inhaled corticosteroid boost to prevent fall asthma exacerbations. J Allergy Clin Immunol 2015; 136(6): 1476–1485.

Wide L, Bennich H, Johansson SG. Diagnosis of allergy by an *in-vitro* test for allergen antibodies. Lancet 1967; 2(7526): 1105–1107.

Wood RAS, N; Ahlstedt S, et al. A comparison of skin prick tests, intradermal skin tests and RASTs in the diagnosis of cat allergy. Ann Allergy Asthma Immunol 2007; 99: 34–41.

Yasnowsky KM, Dreskin SC, Efaw B, Schoen D, Vedanthan PK, Alam R, et al. Chronic urticaria sera increase basophil CD203c expression. J Allergy Clin Immunol 2006; 117(6): 1430–1434.

6

Aerobiology for the Clinician
Basic and Applied Aspects, Pollen Sources, Pollen Calendars

Shripad N Agashe

INTRODUCTION TO AEROBIOLOGY

The term Aerobiology was coined in the 1930s by F.C. Meier who was a plant pathologist in the Department of Agriculture, USA. Aerobiology is the study of airborne particles of plant and animal origin. These bio-particles get into the atmosphere after their release from the source. Prominent among the airborne particles are pollen grains and fungal spores. Pollen grains induce pollination and fertilization which lead to fruit setting and multiplication of plants. Fungal spores aid in the reproduction of fungi. Some of the airborne pollen and spores when inhaled by human beings produce allergic reactions.

The primary objective of aerobiological studies is to identify and monitor the occurrence of pollen and spores and their relative representation in the atmosphere. Airborne pollen and spores are trapped in pollen traps or air sampling devices and are microscopically scanned and identified in the laboratory.

Blackley (1873), a well known physician in the U.K., suffered from allergy to grass pollen and was the first to clinically prove the importance of airborne pollen in causing allergic symptoms.

Due to the enormous applications of aerobiology in public health and medicine, a new term has been added recently—'Medical Palynology'. This branch is concerned with the identification and study of airborne pollen and fungal spores, responsible for causing allergies. It also deals with various aspects of immunotherapy of allergy patients using pollen and fungal allergen extracts.

Palynology is an important component of aerobiology. Hence, it is pertinent to understand the basic importance of palynology.

Introduction to palynology

The term palynology is derived from the Greek verb 'palynein' meaning—to strew, to spread or to disseminate. Pollen grains are male reproductive structures of flowering plants which are meant to be disseminated.

Palynology involves the study of pollen and spores and includes their structural and applied aspects. Palynology obtained real impetus after the discovery of the microscope. This is logical because pollen grains are extremely tiny particles which cannot be seen clearly by the naked eye. They come in an infinite variety of shapes with complex surface ornamentation. They are ubiquitous in nature unlike other

University of Bangalore, Bangalore, India, Email: shri99@yahoo.com plant parts and are highly resistant to decay. They could be buried deep in rocks, ground surface, water, and the air indoors and outdoors including the upper atmosphere. Pollen and spores also find their way through the nasal and oral cavity to the respiratory and digestive tract of humans and animals causing various degrees of discomfort.

Basic aerobiology

Field botanical studies

In any particular locality the first step in the investigation of pollen responsible for pollinosis (inhalant allergy caused by pollen) is a thorough field botanical study for the various plants of that area.

All the plants of the area are identified. A list of the local plants classified into anemophilous, entomophilous and amphiphilous on the basis of their mode of pollination is made. Pollination is the transfer of the male reproductive structures (pollen) to the female structures of the same species. Pollination is accomplished by several methods. Most flowering plants are pollinated by insects (entomophilous). In such plants, the flowers may be colorful, fragrant and attractive to the pollinating agents. The pollen wall is covered by sculptures and often has a sticky coating. The pollen of importance in aerobiology are from plants in which the wind is the pollinating agent (anemophilous). In these plants, the flowers are usually small, inconspicuous, numerous and odorless. Pollen in these flowers are mostly small, smooth and non-sticky and so get airborne easily. In some plants the pollination may be by wind as well as by insects (amphiphilous).

Notes are prepared on the flowering periods of the plants, the distribution of the plants and their pollen production. Plants are also classified on the basis of their habitat as trees, shrubs or weeds. All these observations help to create a Flowering Calendar, also called a Pollination Calendar. Data about important plants responsible for pollinosis are obtained. All the above information is useful for the identification of airborne pollen.

A Pollen Calendar is constructed on the basis of field botanical studies as well as aeropalynological surveys (sampling of airborne pollen). The compilation of a Pollen Calendar is the ultimate objective of aerobiologists. It will be a very useful aid to clinicians for the diagnosis and treatment of allergy.

Pollen production

The amount of the pollen in the air depends on several factors, the most important being pollen production in the individual species. The amount of pollen production and methods of their dispersal are important factors in causing environmental pollution and allergy (Singh 1984). In general, pollen production is controlled not only by their size, but also by genetic and physiological factors.

Agashe and Soucenadin (1992) studied the pollen productivity of some allergenically significant plants in Bangalore. Pollen output or pollen production may be expressed as absolute number of pollen grains per anther or flower or inflorescence or for the entire plant. Most studies express the pollen production as the number of pollen grains per anther.

Pollen release and dispersal

The chance of pollen release and dissemination into the air is greater in trees because of their height and exposure. This release is compensated by greater production. However, entomophilous trees release less pollen into the air because of the fact that their pollen grains are heavy and sticky and their agents of pollination are insects. Anemophilous trees send out enormous quantities of pollen into the air. Their pollen grains being small and dry will remain longer in the air and will have a wider distribution. They will have greater chances of getting into the human respiratory system and so have a significant role in the cause of inhalant allergy. However, entomophilous plants may emit pollen in their immediate vicinity and may also cause allergy. *Carica papaya* (Papaya) with heavy pollen is entomophilous and allergic. Mridula et al. (2011) reported significant allergic reactions to the airborne pollen of the entomophilous avenue tree, *Dolichandroneplatycalyx* from Mysore and Bangalore, India.

Pollen release and dispersal are influenced by the prevailing weather, which in turn is influenced by the time of day. Subba Reddi and Reddi (1985) investigated pollen release and dispersal at different times of the day in certain plants.

Applied aerobiology

Compilation of a Pollen Calendar

A Pollen Calendar is distinct from a Pollination Calendar (Flowering Calendar). A pollination calendar indicates the nature of the flowering of plants like time of flowering and duration of flowering; whereas a pollen calendar gives information about the types of air borne pollen and their relative concentration in the atmosphere.

An aeropalynological survey (air sampling) involves the identification and estimation of airborne pollen and spores. Although the atmosphere contains an array of pollen and fungal spores, only a few of them are responsible for allergic manifestations. The knowledge of the occurrence and concentration of these allergenic pollen and spores, which can be inferred from the pollen calendar, can be of great help to e clinicians. A detailed pollen calendar of a region is a prerequisite for the immunological treatment of pollen allergies.

In India, several pollen calendars from major cities have been compiled (Deshpande and Chitaley 1976, Singh and Babu 1982, Mandal et al. 2008). They show the types of air borne pollen and their count in the air of these cities. The pollen calendar of Bangalore (Agashe and Abraham 1990) is shown in Fig. 6.1 and can be compared with a pollen calendar from Denver, Colorado, USA in Fig. 6.2. In Bangalore, airborne pollen of *Parthenium, Casuarina*, Grasses, *Eucalyptus, Ricinus* and Amaranth-Chenopod occurred throughout the year. The high pollen months were June and July attributable to the weeds. A comparison of the pollen calendars (Agashe and Abraham 1990) of Bangalore shows a shift in high pollen months from year to year. If there are good pre-monsoon showers in May then the pollen peak is seen during June, or else the peak is later in July. Most of the tree pollen occurs during February to May.

A sizeable number of residents in Bangalore suffer from allergies. From a retrospective statistical study done for three years on the number of cases of asthma admissions in Victoria Hospital, Bangalore, it was found that most of them showed symptoms during August to October, which correlated to the peak pollen season of *Parthenium, Casuarina, Ricinus* and Amaranth-Chenopod (Agashe and Philip 1990).

Pollen calendars compiled by aerobiologists provide knowledge about the occurrence and concentration of the allergenic airborne pollen, which is of great help to clinicians for proper diagnosis and treatment of allergy patients (Agashe and Caulton 2009). Hence collaboration of aerobiologists and allergologists is essential to tackle the problems of suffering patients. Using a pollen calendar, airborne pollen types which occur in significant numbers are selected and their antigenic extracts are used for

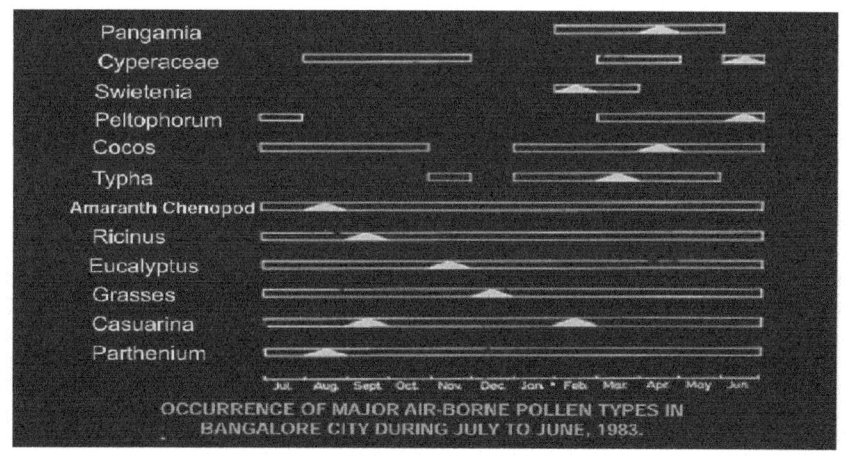

Figure 6.1. Pollen calendar of Bangalore, India.

52 *Textbook of Allergy for the Clinician*

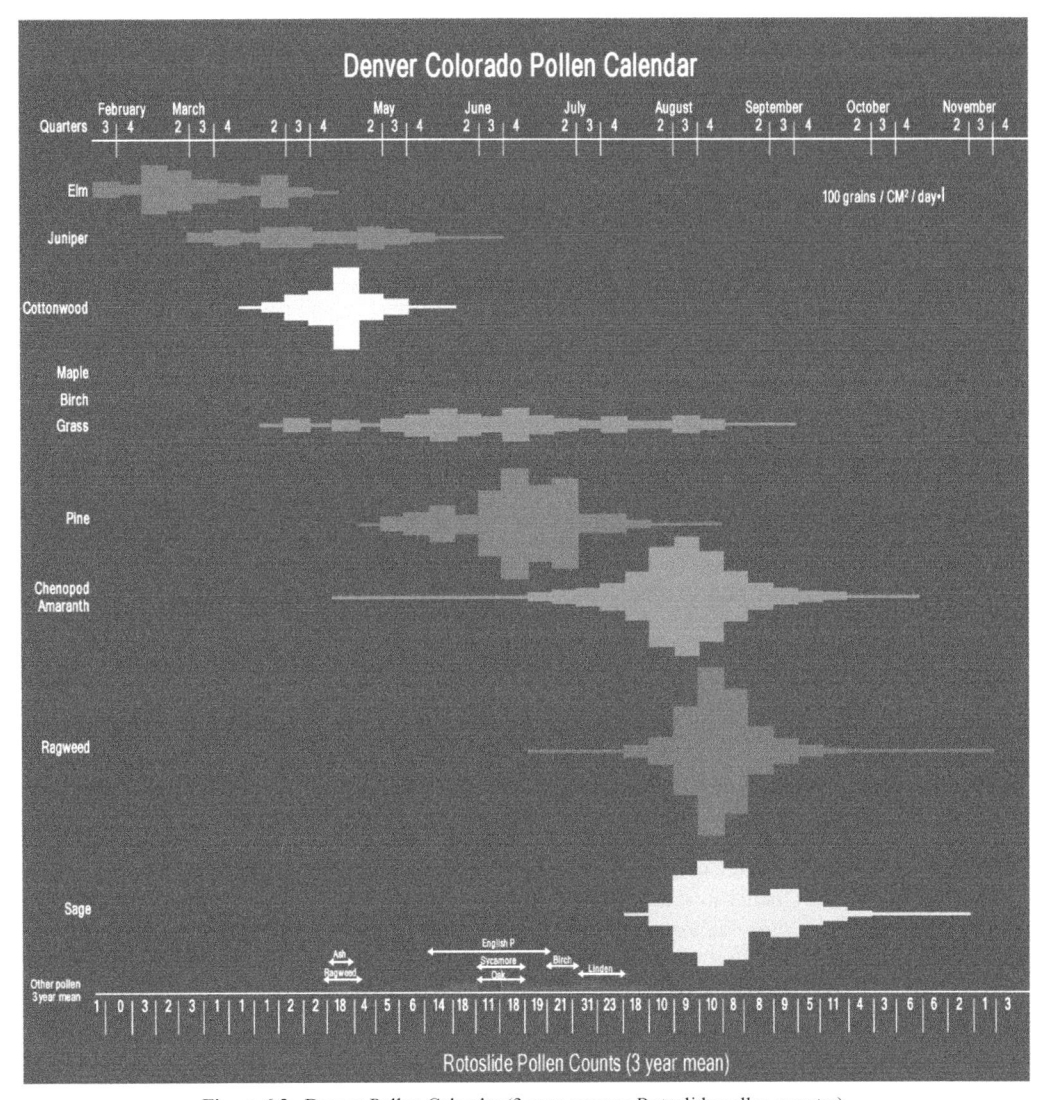

Figure 6.2. Denver Pollen Calendar (3 year average Rotoslide pollen counter).

testing on patients. Once the offending allergens are detected through various clinical tests, the patients are treated by immunotherapy ensuring that they get sufficient protection from the effects of airborne pollen and spores.

The knowledge of the pollen calendar of the local region is essential for two basic reasons. Firstly, only the relevant antigens need to be tested on the patients. There are many antigen kits available in the market and most of them will not be specific to the locality. Hence, selection of the right antigens is ensured by consulting the local pollen calendar. Secondly, many patients suffer from seasonal allergic manifestations due to the seasonal occurrence of pollen types. The seasonal pollen types are identified through the pollen calendar. The magnitude and the quality of the annual pollen load in the atmosphere vary significantly. Therefore, it is essential that the aerobiological survey of an area is conducted continuously over the years and the pollen calendars should be compiled and updated every year (Agashe 1994). In addition, awareness has to be created among clinicians, patients and the public about the results of the air being monitoring. In the western countries, particularly in the USA, daily counts of airborne pollen and spores are published through mass media such as radio, television and newspapers.

Common aeroallergens, their aerobiology, morphology and source

Acacia auriculiformis (Babhul, Wattle)

It is commonly called an Australian Acacia or golden shower plant. In India the plant was introduced from tropical Australia. The trees, without spines, grow 10–15 m high and produce drooping spikes of golden yellow flowers. The flowering period is from July to February. The mode of pollination is amphiphilous.

Albizialebbeck (Shishir, Lebbek) (Figure 6.3)

The plant is native to India, Sri Lanka, South East Asia and South China. It is usually grown as avenue trees for shade and has greenish white feathery flowers and long pods. The tree can grow as tall as 20 m. Mode of pollination: Anemophilous.

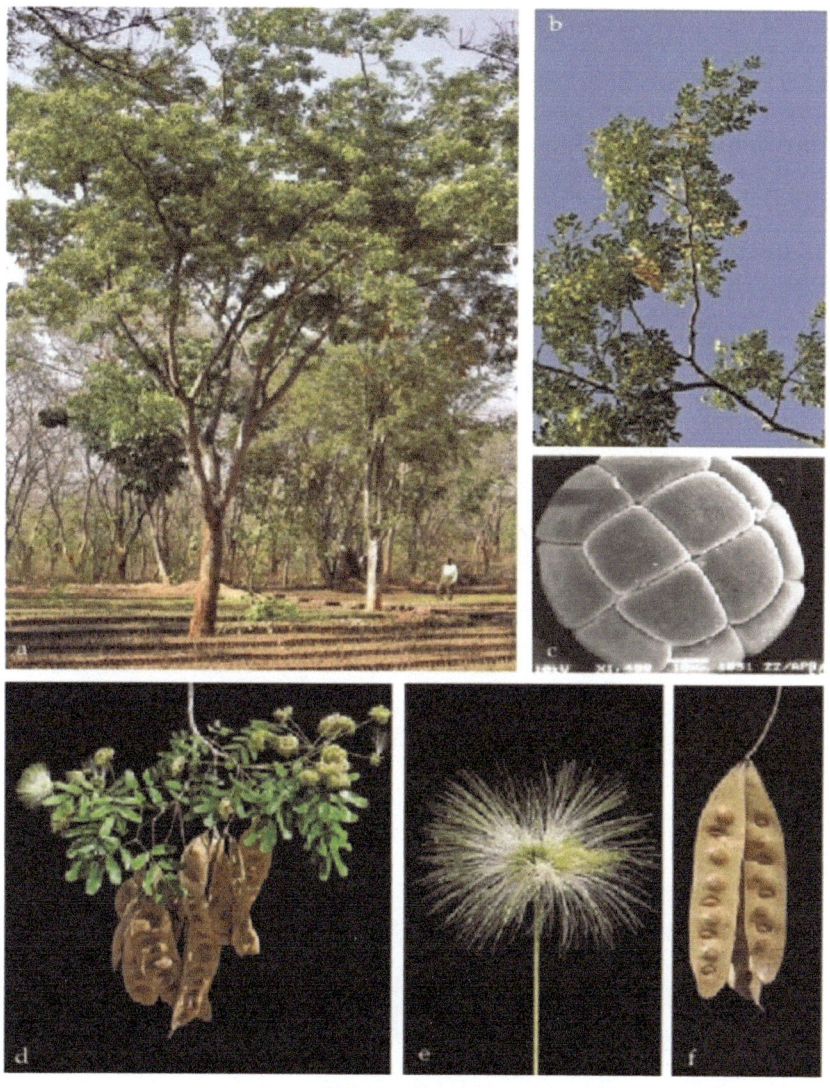

Figure 6.3. Albizia lebbeck.

Mimosa pudica (Sensitive plant or Touch me not)

These spreading procumbent herbs with prickly stems are native of South America but have been introduced and naturalized in India. The plant is referred to as 'Touch me not' on account of their leaves, which are sensitive to touch. Their leaflets fold in when touched. Flowers are pink, globose and 0.6 mm across. Pollination: Anemophilous

Cassia siamea

They are grown as avenue trees in many cities including Bangalore. They are moderately tall with numerous yellow colored blooms. Anthers are exposed for easy dispersal of pollen by wind.

Prosopisjuliflora (Kikar, Mesquite)

Though it is native to North and Central America, it invasively grows profusely in semiarid regions of both northern and southern regions of India and the Middle-East. The trees grow up to a height of 8 m. have small leaves and drooping inflorescence with very small creamy flowers. Pollination: Anemophilous

Amaranthusspinosus (Spiny Amaranth) (Figure 6.4)

This is a common notorious weed. The stems have thick spines and hence avoided by cattle. In many sites it appears to compete with *Parthenium* and can invade areas previously occupied by *Parthenium*. The plant flowers throughout the year. Pollen grains are spheroidal, 18–28 microns in diameter. They are pantoporate with more than 40 pores. Pollination: Anemophilous

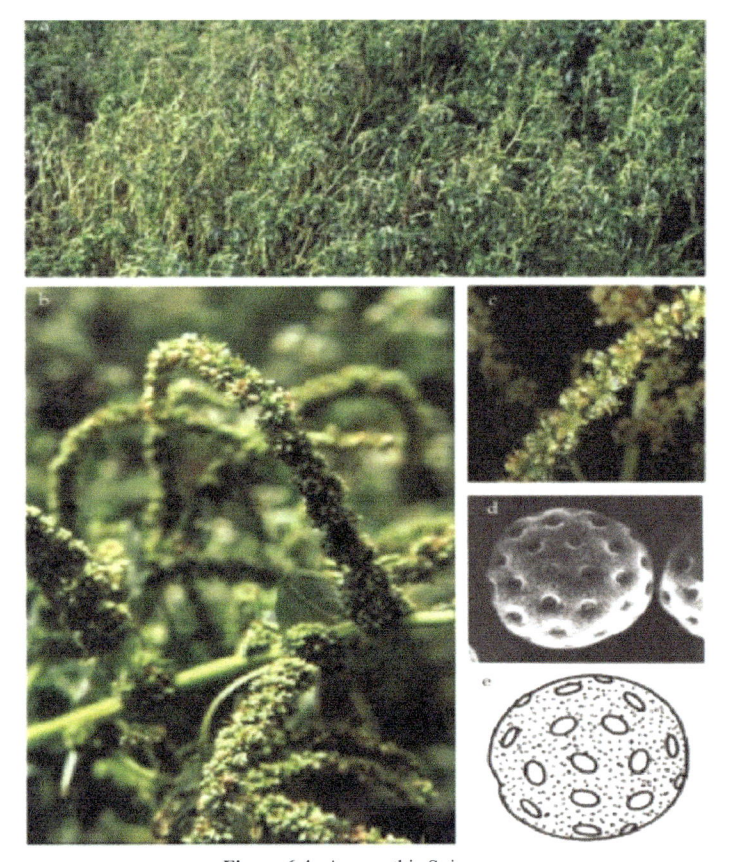

Figure 6.4. Amaranthis Spinosus.

Holopteleaintegrifolia (Chilbil, Indian Elm) (Figure 6.5)

The trees are distributed in tropical and sub tropical parts of Asia and Africa. The plants are widely distributed in India, particularly in the northern and the western parts of India. A handful of trees are observed in Bangalore. The plants are prolific pollen producers. In Bangalore, during its flowering nearly 70% of the pollen in the atmosphere comes from these plants. It flowers for a very short period of 2–3 weeks from mid March to early April. Pollination is very rapid and within a couple of weeks, winged fruits are produced.

It is an important pollen allergen of Lucknow, Jaipur, Aligarh, Bangalore and Delhi.

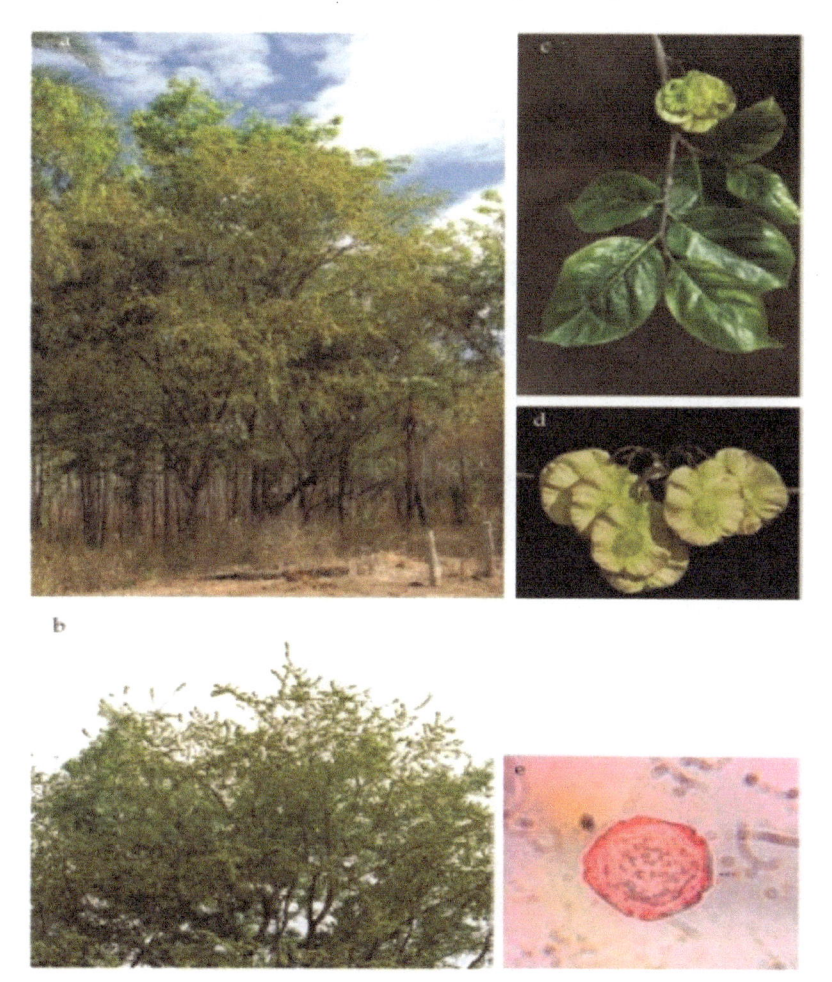

Figure 6.5. Heloptelea integrifolia (Ulmaceae).

Ricinuscommunis (Castor bean plant) (Figure 6.6)

Oil extracted from the seeds has applications in industries and medicine. The plants are large shrubs to small trees and have palmately compound leaves. They reach a height of 8–12 feet and grow abundantly in waste places. Figure 6.6 shows *Ricinuscommunis* plants growing profusely on either side of a railway track near Bangalore. Male flowers are loaded with numerous branched stamens and with anthers exposed to the air for easy pollen dispersal. Pollen grains are tricolporate, oblate-spheroidal, finely reticulate and 20 × 30 microns in diameter.

56 *Textbook of Allergy for the Clinician*

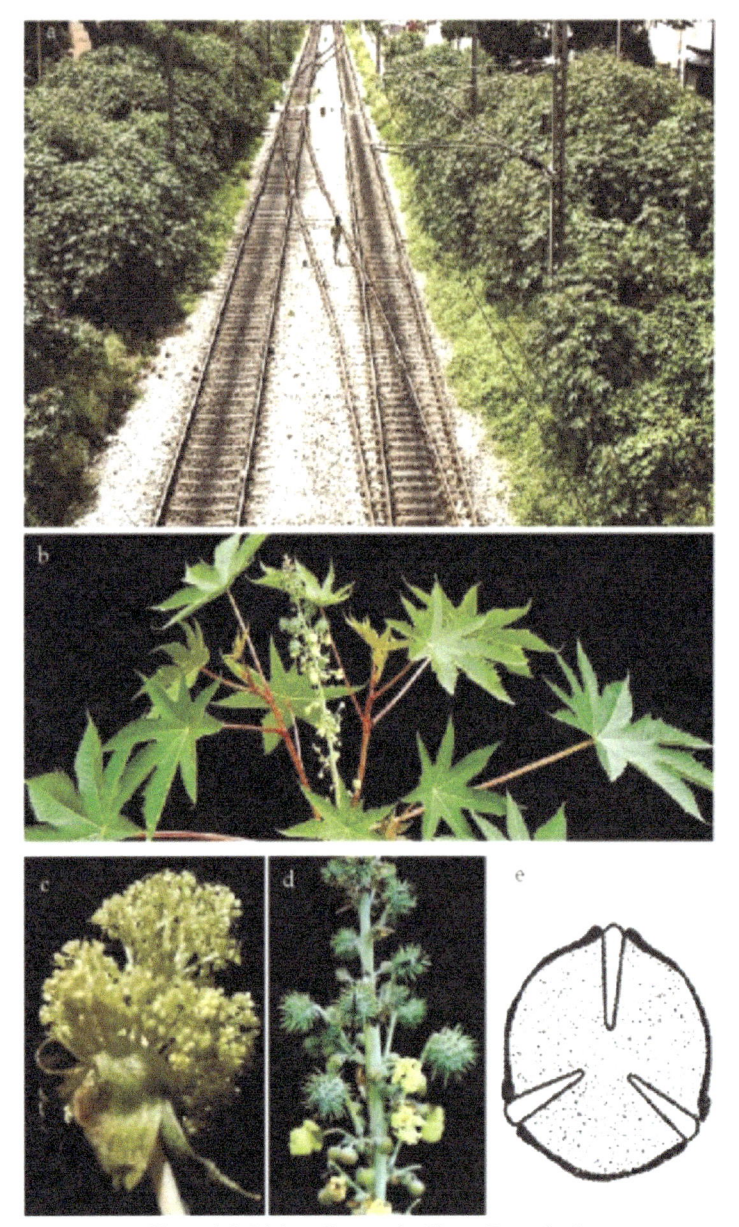

Figure 6.6. Ricinus Communis (Castor Bean plant).

Casuarinaequisetifolia (Australian Pine) (Figure 6.7)

They are tall tropical trees resembling pines. Leaves are absent as the branches are green and act as leaves. Branches are jointed. The trees grow profusely in coastal regions in South India. They serve as wind breaks. Agashe and Abraham (1990) reported large amounts of airborne pollen of this species in the atmosphere of Bangalore. Pollen extracts tested on the skin showed high positivity. Male flowers are on small drooping inflorescences. They are ideally situated for wind dispersal.

Pollen grains are suboblate, 22 × 30 um in diameter, 3 pororate, exine surface is granulate.

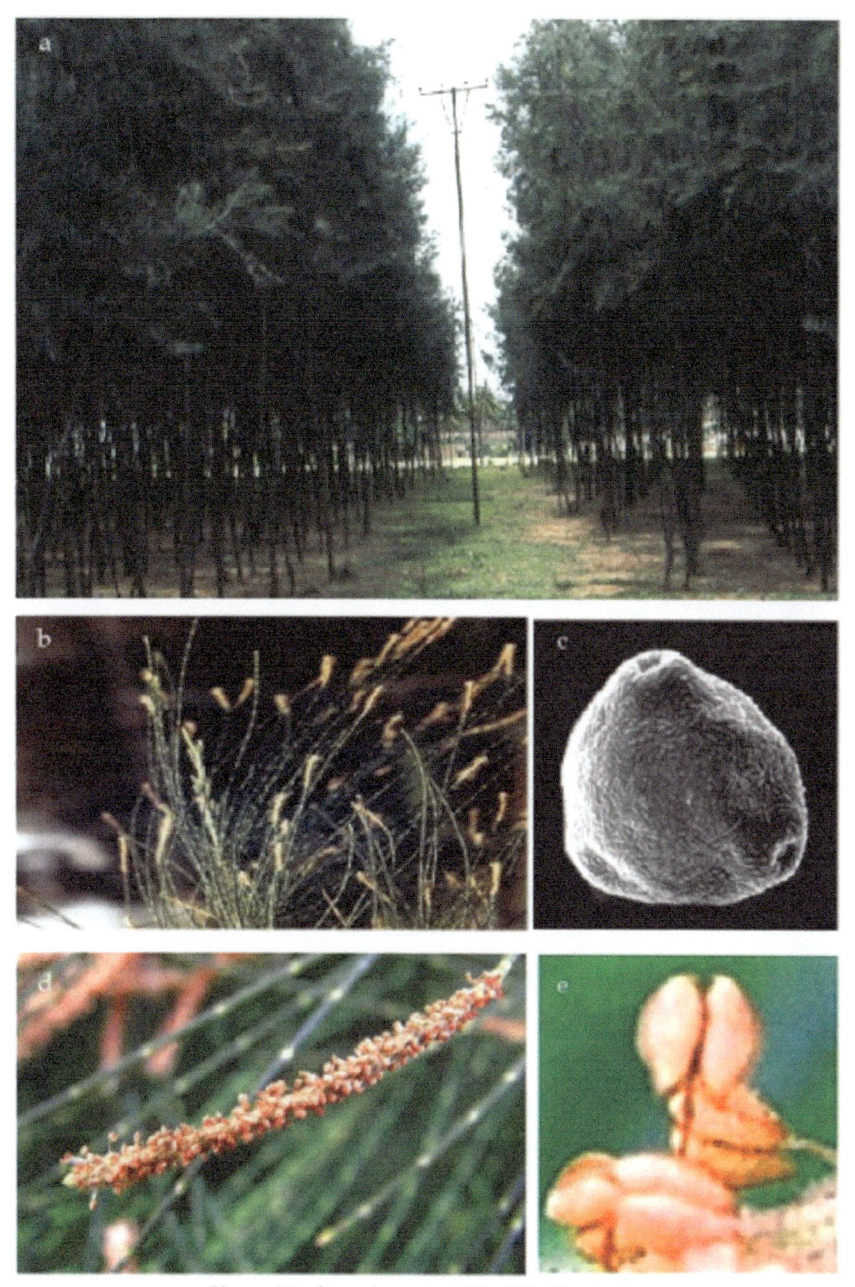

Figure 6.7. Casuarinaequisetifolia (Wind breaker).

Typhaangustata (Cattail) (Figure 6.8)

This weed is a prolific pollen producer. The plants with linear leaves grow profusely in marshy habitats. The flowering stalk ends in a long flowering spike. Pollen grains are spheroidal, 20–27 microns in diameter, monoporate and exine is reticulate.

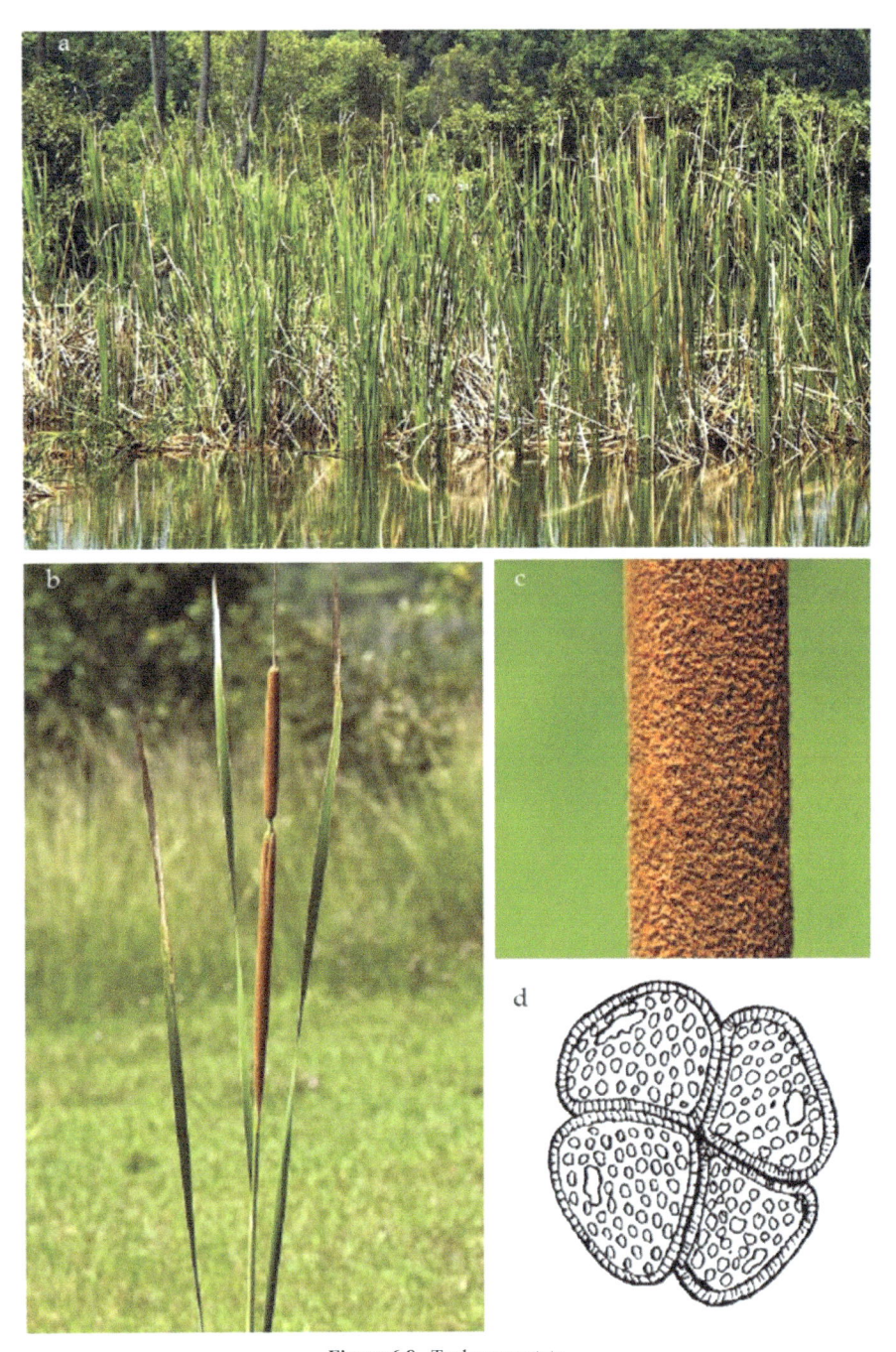

Figure 6.8. Typha augustata

Eucalyptusglobulus (Figure 6.9)

The species are tall trees with peeling bark. They are widely cultivated on account of their economic importance. The wood is used in the pulp and paper industry. Oil is extracted from leaves. Flowers are loaded with numerous long stamens carrying anthers at their tips. Pollen are wind dispersed. Pollen grains are oblate-spheroidal, smooth and trisyncolpate.

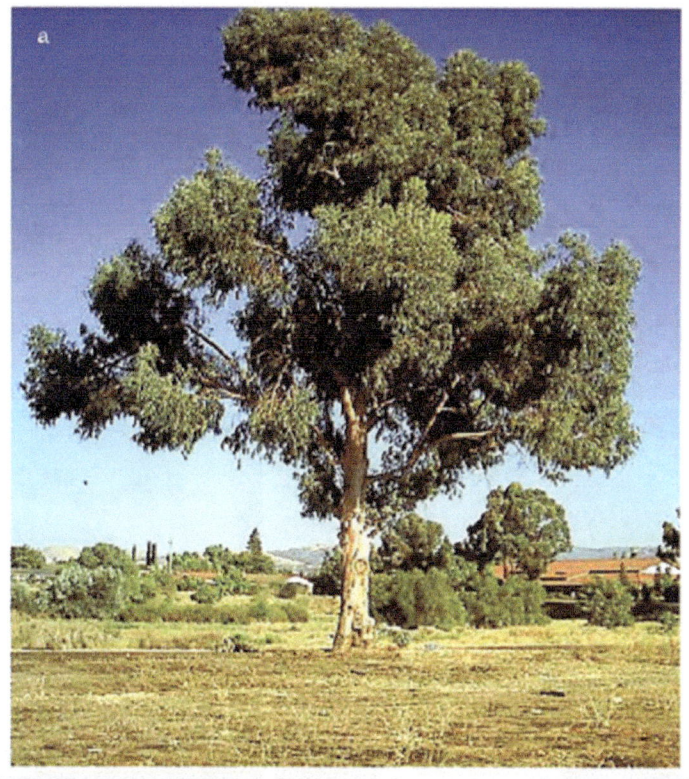

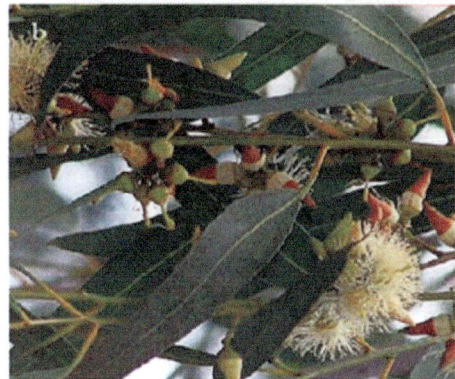

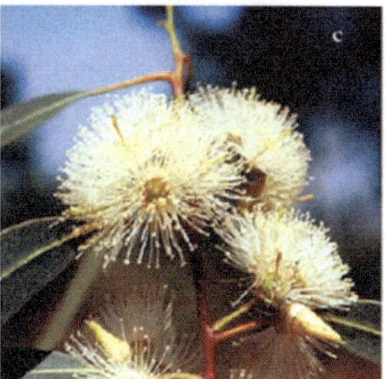

Figure 6.9. Eucalypyus Globulus

Partheniumhysterophorus (Congress grass, White top weed) (Figure 6.10)

Parthenium is a genus belonging to the family Asteraceae. It is related to the notorious weed—*Ambrosia* (ragweed). *Partheniumhysterophorus* is a ubiquitous annual weed native to the Gulf of Mexico region and West Indies but now disseminated in warm and semi arid subtropical regions of the United States and almost the entire Indian subcontinent. It believed that in 1956, *Partheniumhysterophorus* was introduced from the gulf regions of the U.S.A. to Pune in India (Agashe 1994).

Subsequently it spread like a wild fire to other regions of India resulting in serious agricultural problems and health hazards especially allergic dermatitis. The major offending chemical is the sesquiterpene lactone, parthenin is found throughout the plant body including the pollen. The plants produce a large quantity of pollen (an average 624 million/plant). The pollen becomes airborne to great heights in significant amounts either as individual grains or in clumps and cause nasobronchial allergy.

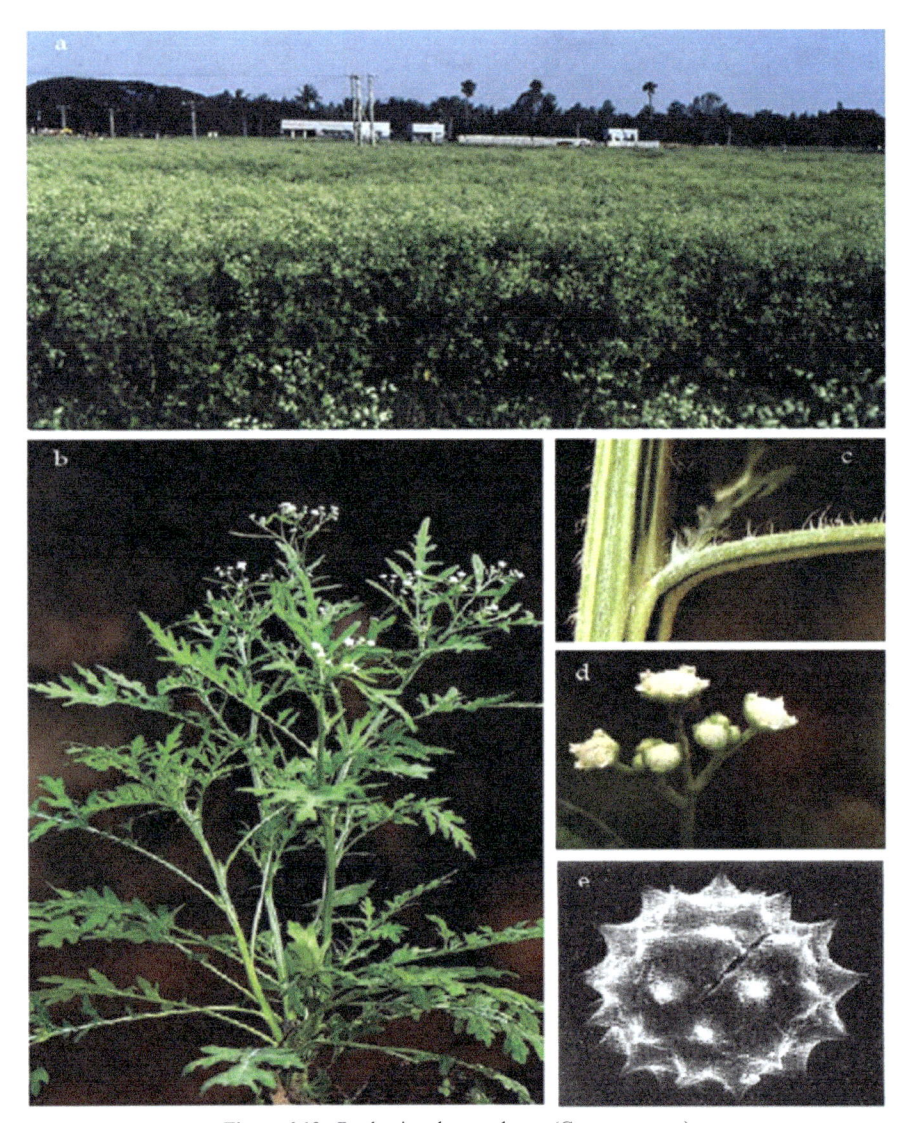

Figure 6.10. Parthenium hyterophorus (Congress grass).

In Bangalore, Subbarao et al. (1989) performed extensive studies on the allergenicity of *Parthenium hysterophorus*. Both skin tests and Radioallergosorbent test (RAST) were performed on patients with classic symptoms of allergic rhinitis during July and December. They demonstrated that 34% of patients with allergic rhinitis and 12% of patients with asthma were sensitive to extracts of *Parthenium* pollen.

Parthenium is amphiphilous and flowers profusely from July to September. The pollen are oblate spheroidal, tricolporate, echinate and about 15 microns in size. The rate of pollen production was found to be 9600-pollen/staminate flower or 345600 pollen per inflorescence.

Grass Pollen (Figure 6.12)

The Grass family Poaceae, earlier referred to as Gramineae is one of the largest families comprising more than 10,000 species. They have a worldwide distribution. The majority of grasses produce anemophilous or wind borne pollen and most of them are known to produce allergic symptoms.

Aerobiology for the Clinician: Basic and Applied Aspects, Pollen Sources, Pollen Calendars 61

Optical section of comman Ragweed pollen

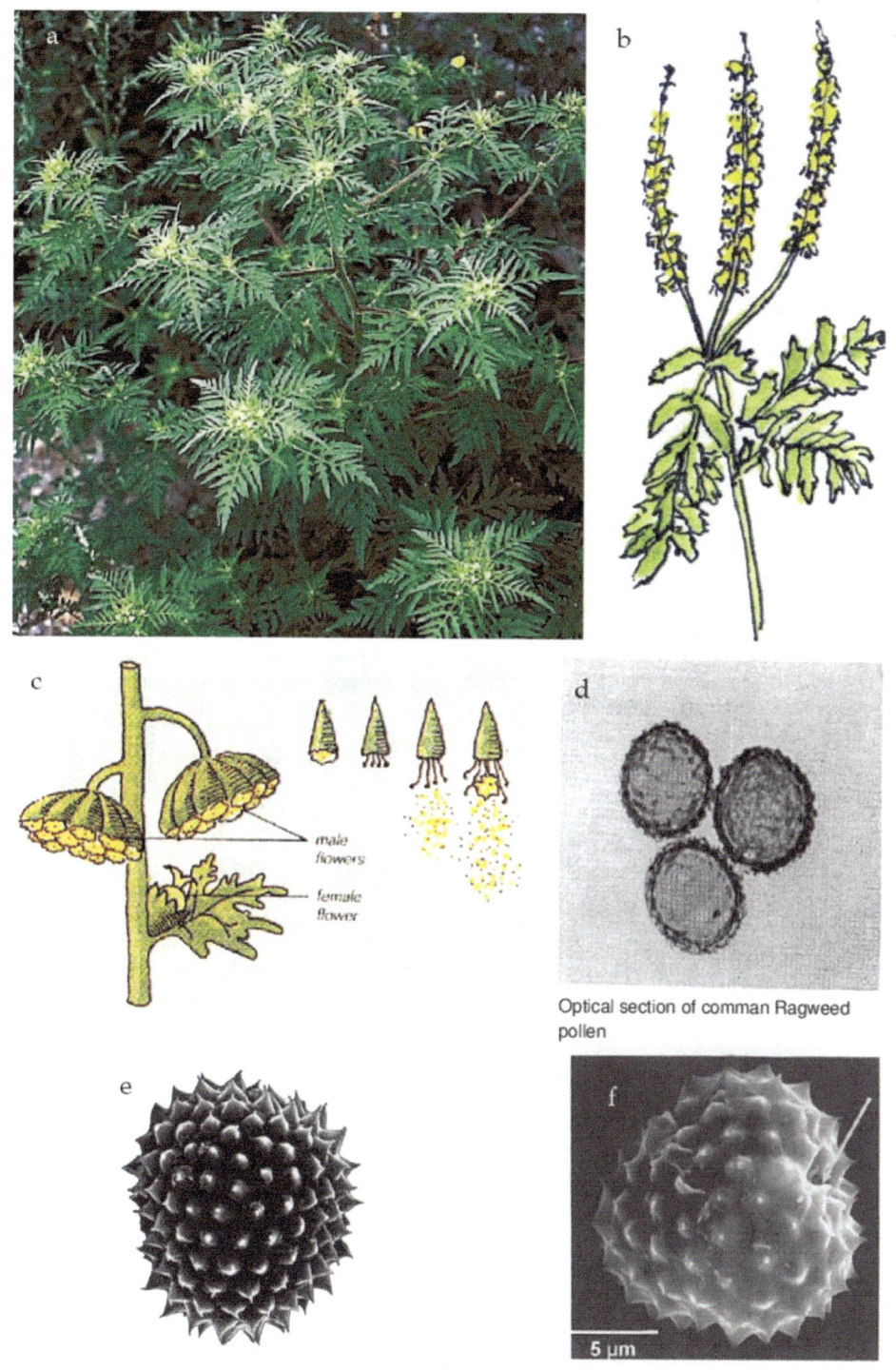

Figure 6.11. Ambrosia (Ragweed)

62 Textbook of Allergy for the Clinician

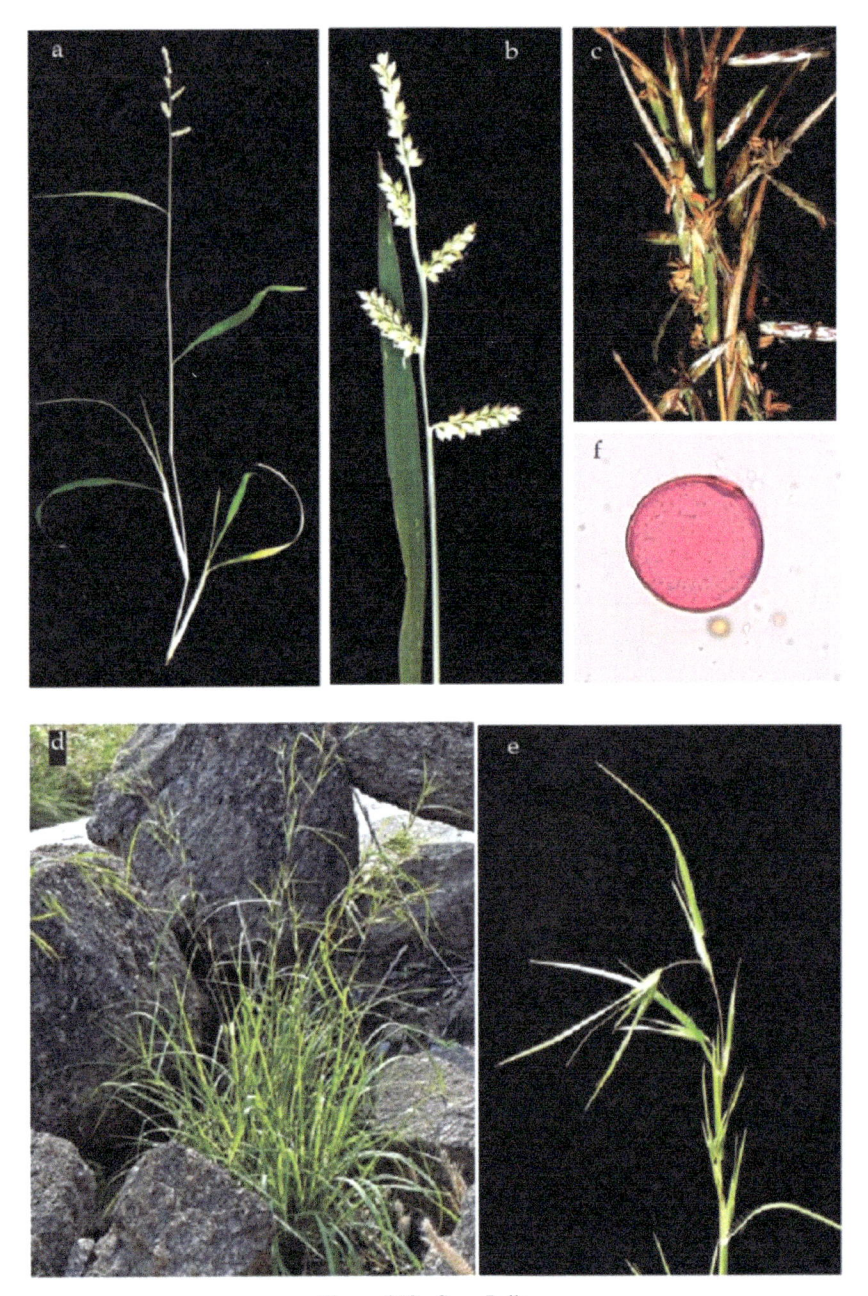

Figure 6.12. Grass Pollen

Pollen morphology is relatively similar in almost all species of grasses. Pollen are usually spheroidal 22–122 microns in diameter. The aperture is a single circular pore 2–8 microns in diameter (Fig. 6.12). The pore is surrounded by a thickened raised ring referred to as annulus.

Pollen of small size (around 35 microns) are seen in commonly occurring grasses such as *Agrostis* (bentgrass), *Cynodon* (Bermuda grass), *Poa* (Blue grass), *Dactylis* (orchard grass), *Holcus* (walnut grass). In contrast large sized pollen (above 50 microns) occurs in cultivated grasses (cereals).

The classical work of Charles H. Blackley (1873) on grass pollen entitled "Experimental researches on the causes and nature of Catarrhus Aestivus" is quoted by alaerobiologists as the first evidence of airborne pollen as the cause of hay fever.

Pollen sources from temperate regions

Ambrosia (Ragweed) (Figure 6.11)

Ragweed is a common allergenic weed in temperate regions of the world. Its abundant pollen production gives rise to high percentages of symptoms of seasonal rhinitis (hay fever). The plant is anemophilous. It is herbaceous and has both annual and perennial species. Ragweed has no economic value per se, but is a serious health hazard in temperate regions. It takes advantage of human habitat disturbance and grows profusely in cleared open spaces.

There are many species of *Ambrosia*. The most common and wide spread species is *Ambrosiaartemisiifolia* (*A. elatior*) which is the dwarf species. The plant body is characterized by opposite or alternate soft-green leaves, hairy stems, generally less than 1 meter in height bearing green to yellow inflorescences (Fig. 6.11). Each plant produces tens to hundreds of millions of pollen grains which get easily airborne.

In case of the common or dwarf ragweed and giant ragweed (*Ambrosiatrifida*) and probably the other species of *Ambrosia*, the peak pollen shedding time during dry weather is usually from 7 to 9 a.m. This two-hour period may shed 75% of the pollen in a day. Nearly all of the pollen will be shed before noon. At approximately 6 a.m. the mature flowers change shape; at 6:30 a.m. the anthers are exposed; if the humidity is low the flowers may open in 15 minutes; if high, it may take 2 or 3 hours; if it is raining they may not open at all. Dispersal may be divided into four phases:

(1) Ejection of pollen in clusters from flowers.
(2) Temporary attachment of pollen clumps to neighboring foliage.
(3) Reflotation by air currents.
(4) Final distribution in the atmosphere.

The pollen is typically echinate (spiny outer wall), spheroidal and measures around 20 microns (Fig. 6.11). It was known for long as the main cause of hay fever or pollinosis in North America. But was unknown in Europe. However, since 1960s *Ambrosia* has been reported growing in the Rhone valley, northern Italy, south of European Russia, Balkan states and in southern Austria.

Both giant and short ragweeds are found growing profusely throughout North America. Their pollen constitutes about 78% of the weed aeroallergens of St. Louis area.

Other common pollen sources in temperate regions of the world are: *Quercus* (Oak), *Alnus* (Alder), *Fraxinus* (Ash), *Ulmus* (Elm), *Betula* (Birch), *Fagus* (Beech), *Populus* (Aspen), *Chenopodium* (Goosefoot), *Amaranthus* (Pigweed), *Artemisia* (Mugwort/Sagebrush), Grass, etc.

Role of mold spores in aerobiology and allergy

Fungi are ubiquitous and so are the spores of various types produced by them. They occur indoors as well as outdoors. Outdoor fungal sources are soil, water or air. Aided by high temperature and humidity, fungi grow profusely on substrates like plant debris, organic mass, fallen leaves and dead flowers or fruits. As a part of their life cycle on these substrates they produce numerous spores which are small and light in weight. They get easily dispersed in the air. Some of these airborne spores may be breathed in or land onto the skin. Depending on the sensitivity of individuals they cause immediate allergic manifestation. In view of the above, a general knowledge of common allergenic fungal airborne spores is necessary and very useful for clinicians (Nilsson 1983).

Predominantly occurring airborne fungal spores belong to Ascomycetes, Deuteromycetes and Basidiomycetes. Unlike pollen most of the fungal spores are not restricted to any particular geographical region, though their concentration in air may differ from place to place. There is no sharp demarcation between types of airborne fungal spores indoors and outdoors.

Usually the source of indoor fungi are house grown plants, wooden furniture, old leather, old clothes, paper, left-over food, leaky bathrooms, damp walls, etc.

Classified list of allergically significant airborne fungal spores

Some of the commonly occurring and allergy causing fungal spores are:

Aspergillus niger, Aspergillus flavus and other species of *Aspergillus. Penicillium, Cladosporium, Curvularia, Mucor, Helminthosporium, Alternaria alternata,* Rust spores, Smut spores, *Nigrospora, Ganoderma* basidiospores, *Coprinus, Pithomyces, Chaetomium, Didymela, Pleospora, Botrytis, Dreschslera, Epicoccum, Tetraploa, Torula, Bispora, Periconia, Rhizopus.*

Conidia/spores of the following fungi having significance in allergy have been shown in Fig. 6.13a. *Alternaria* (two figures), *Cladosporium* (two figures), *Chaetomium, Cunninghemill, Trichoderma, Aspergillus flavus, Aspergillus niger, Mucor, Curvularia.*

Penicillium

It is a large genus of asexual fungi comprising of more than 250 species. They are more common in indoor air. In culture, *Penicillium* mycelia are white in color but pigmentation occurs at the time of spore production. The spore in mass looks blue, green, gray, yellow, brown or even black. *Penicillium* is frequently found in basements, attics or on e moldy oranges in the refrigerator.

In the air samples, it is almost impossible to distinguish the spores of *Asperguillus* and *Penicillium*. Both have either spherical or elliptical spores with attachment scars on either end of the spore. *Penicillium* causes a great deal of reactivity in an allergic host particularly during moist, high humidity times of the year.

Stachybotrys

Stachybotrys contamination in indoor environments is very common. The fungus is primarily soil fungus and hence spores can also occur outdoors. Indoors the fungus prefers water soaked buildings. It produces powerful mycotoxins. It occurs invariably on substrates containing cellulose but also requires a lot of water. It is frequently seen in areas where there have been leaks and the bathroom ceiling is soaked by a leak from the floor above.

Rhizopus nigricans

It is a commonly occurring fungus found in fruits stored in a refrigerator. Each spore can impact an allergy punch. It can occur on potted plants (indoors and outdoors) in a refrigerator on rotten fruit.

Botrytis

Spores are smooth, transparent, nonseptate egg shaped. They are found in large numbers during thunderstorms.

Aspergillus (Figure 6.13a)

It is often referred as a super bug. It is well known fact that *Aspergillus* causes infection or allergic symptoms which are referred as *Aspergillosis*. This fungus is less common in indoor environments. It frequently occurs in soil, dead leaves, stored grain, breads, food items such as peanuts, dry fruits, rotting vegetables, cheese, etc. In the indoor environments occasionally *Aspergillus* is found on the damp walls, cellulose rich material, floors, carpets, mattresses, dust, Heating Ventilation, Air-Conditioning(HVAC) system, etc.

Cladosporium (Figure 6.13b)

Cladosporium herbarum spores can cause allergy symptoms *Cladosporium cladosporides* colonies are dark olivaceous brown to blackish brown to compact, tough, velvety, reverse olivaceous black. Conidia 3–7 µm in diameter, ellipsoidal to lemon shaped, mostly smooth walled.

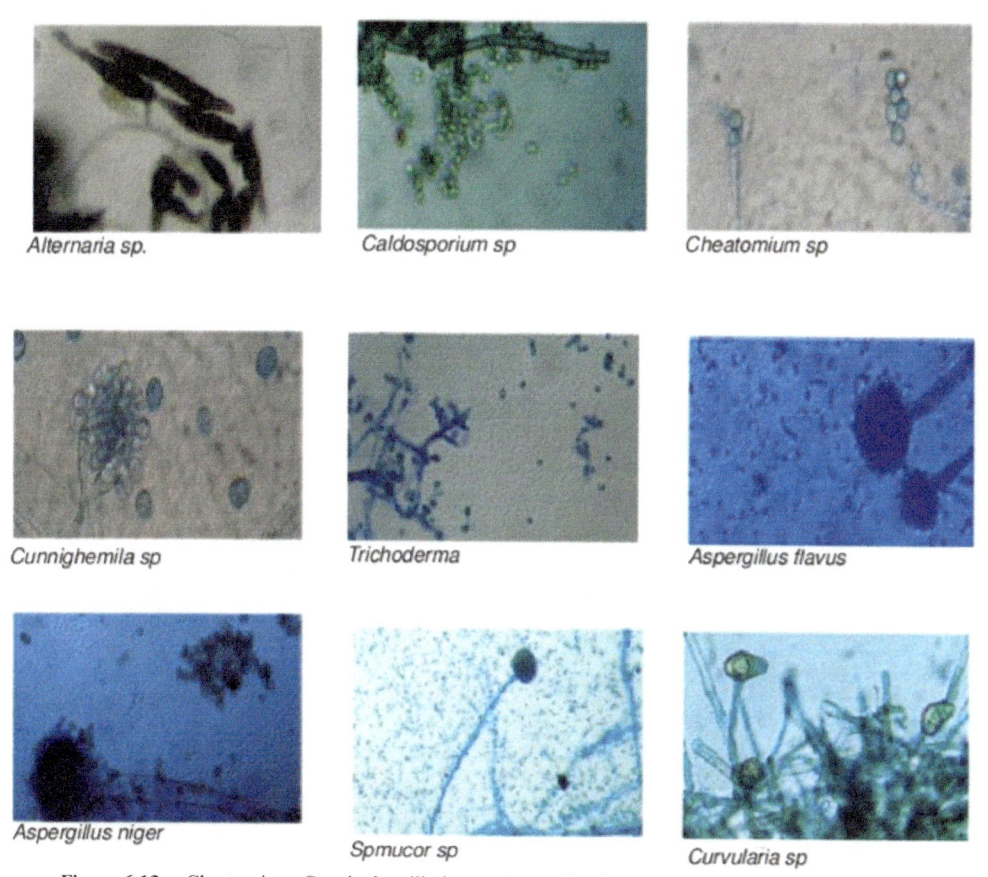

Aerobiology for the Clinician: Basic and Applied Aspects, Pollen Sources, Pollen Calendars 65

Alternaria sp. Caldosporium sp Cheatomium sp

Cunnighemila sp Trichoderma Aspergillus flavus

Aspergillus niger Spmucor sp Curvularia sp

Figure 6.13a. Chaetomium, Cunninghemill, derma, *Aspergillus flavus, Aspergillus niger*, Mucor, Curve.

Cladosporium Alternaria

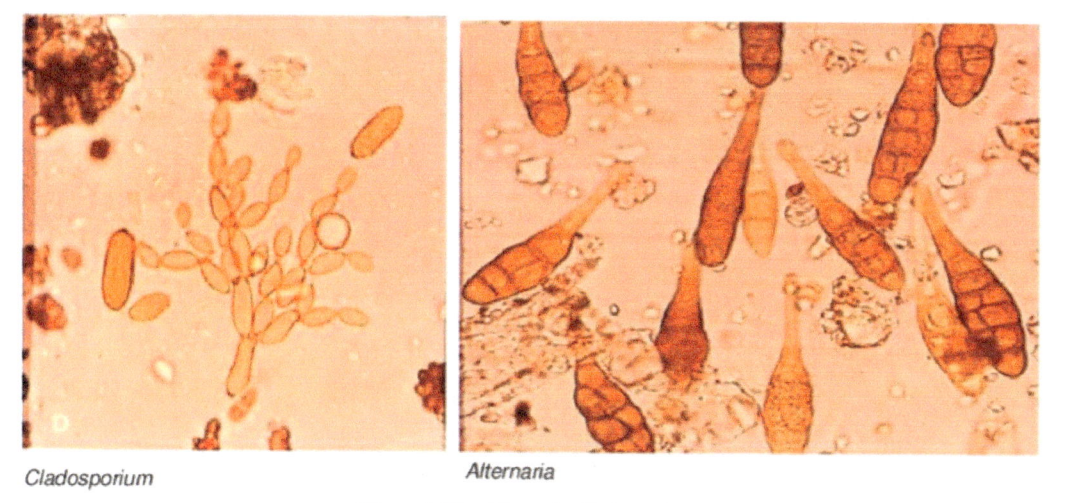

Figure 6.13b. Alternaria, Cladosporium.

Alternaria alternata (Figure 6.13b)

The colonies are spreading, olive green. Conidia are usually large, brown, tadpole-shaped formed in definite chains on conidiophores in acropetal succession.

Mucor

These spores cause allergy symptoms in patients sensitive to mold spores. Patients will experience sinus pressure, sinus headaches particularly during periods of high humidity when these are released to the air in abundance

Basidiospores (Figure 6.14a)

The basidiospores produced by bracket fungi are frequently found in the atmosphere when the humidity is highest somewhere between midnight and 6 a.m. On account of the smaller size of the Basidiosperes of *Coprinus, Ganoderma*, it is possible that they can penetrate deeper in the respiratory tract. This may explain why they cause more asthma than rhinitis.

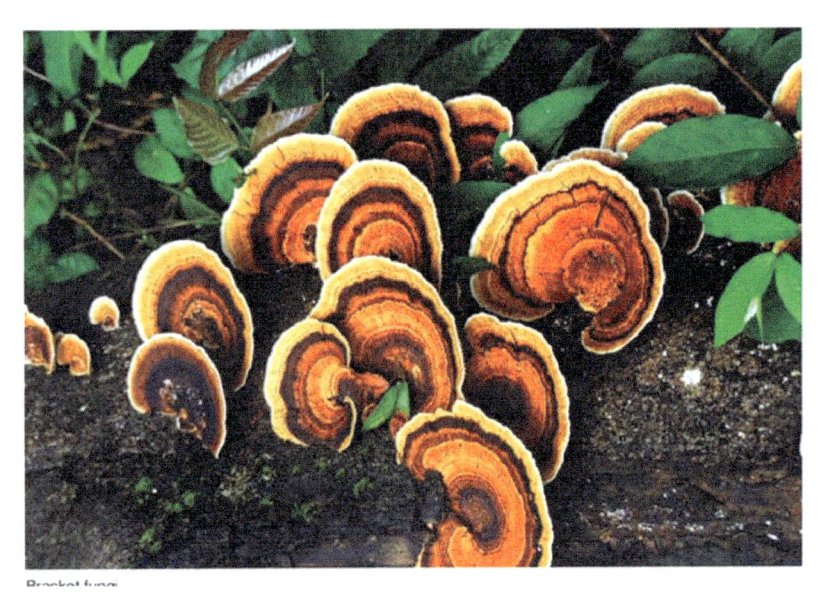

Figure 6.14a. Pleurotus Ostreatus.

Pleurotus ostreatus

It is called the oyster mushroom. The spores produced by this fungus are believed to be highly allergic.

Lichens (Figure 6.14b)

Lichens growing on rocks and tree branches are known to cause contact dermititis.

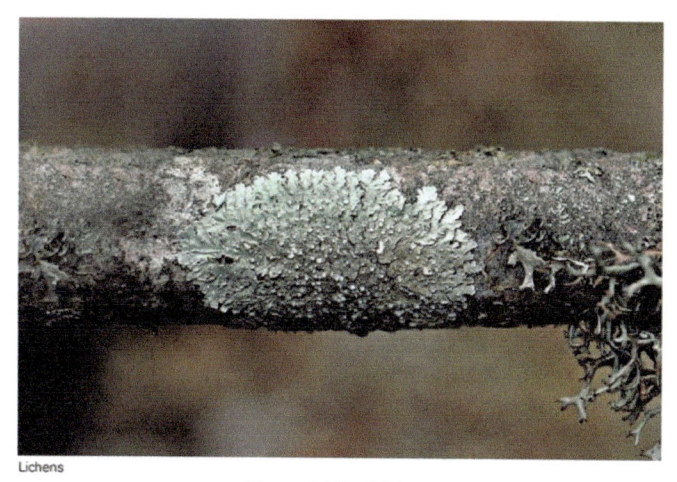

Aerobiology for the Clinician: Basic and Applied Aspects, Pollen Sources, Pollen Calendars 67

Figure 6.14b. Lichens

Pollen count report (Figure 6.15)

Pollen and mold counts are reported commonly in the local media as public information.

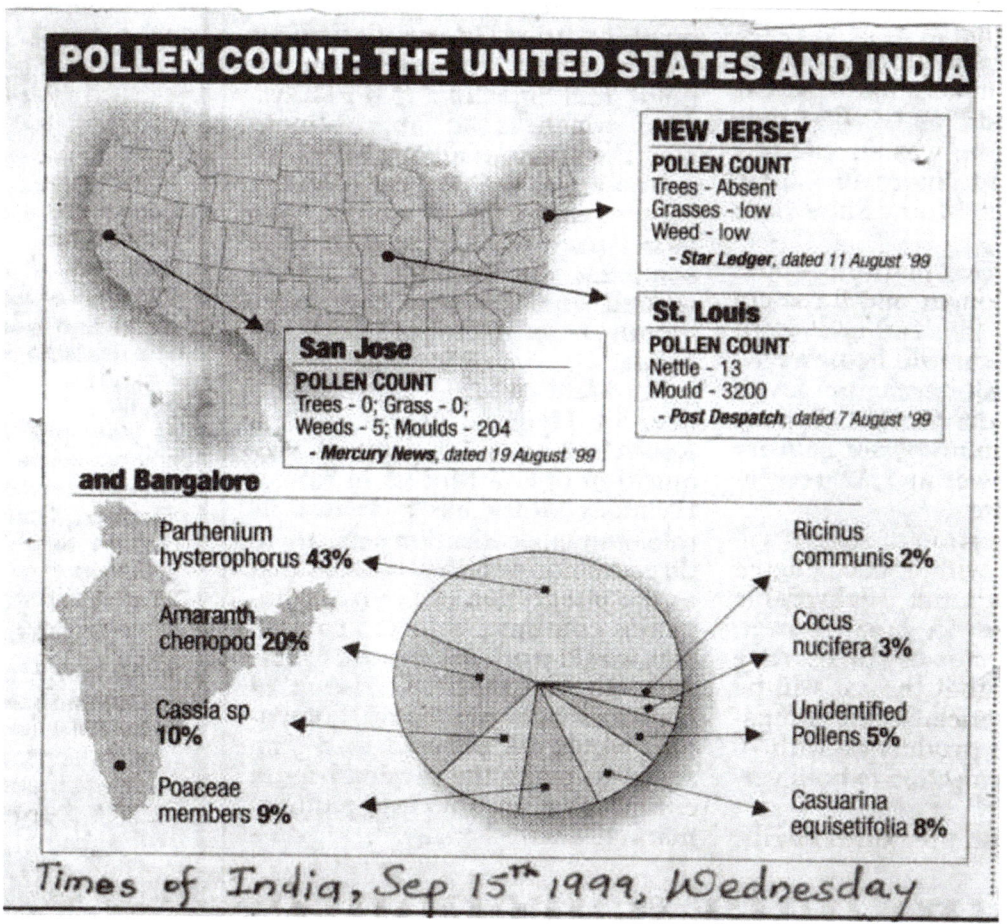

Figure 6.15. Pollen Count report: Local news media (USA and INDIA).

Conclusion

This chapter herewith gives an introduction to the various airborne particles of plant origin, which are of clinical significance to the practice of allergy.

References

Agashe SN, Abraham JN. Pollen calendar of Bangalore City: Part II. J Palynol 1990; 91: 297–304.

Agashe SN, Philip Elizabeth. Correlation of incidence of bronchial asthma and high pollen counts in Bangalore – A retrospective study. XIV Ann Convention of ICAI. Abst 1990.

Agashe SN, Soucenadin S. Pollen productivity in some allerginically significant plants in Bangalore. Ind J Aerobiol 1992; (Special Volume): 63–67.

Agashe SN. Importance of updating Pollen Calendars in the assessment of Allergy. Recent Trends in Aerobiology, Allergy and Immunology. Ed. Agashe, Shripad N. Oxford and IBH Pub. Co. New Delhi 1994, pp. 43–53.

Agashe SN, Caulton Eric. Pollen and Spores: Applications with special emphasis on Aerobiology and Allergy. Science Publishers, Enfield, NH, U.S.A. 2009, pp.397.

Blackley CH. Experimental Researches on the cause and Nature of Catarrhus Aestivus. Dawson (First printed by Baillieri, Tindall and Cox in 1873).

Deshpande SU, Chitaley SD. Pollen Calendar of Nagpur, India. Review of Paleobot and Palynol 1976; 21: 253–262.

Mandal Jyotshna, Chakraborty Pampa, Roy Indrani, Chatterjee Soma, Bhattacharya Swati Gupta. Prevalence of allergenic pollen grains in the aerosol of the city of Calcutta, India : A two year study. Aerobiologia 2008; 24: 151–164.

Mridula PA, Mahesh PA, Abraham JN, Amrutha DH, Agashe SN, Roy Sitesh, et al. *Dolichandrone platycalyx* : New entomophilous pollen-A report on pollen sensitization in allergic individuals. Am J Rhinol Allergy 2011; 25: 1–5.

Nilsson S (ed.). Atlas of Airborne Fungal spores in Europe, Springer – Verlag, Berlin 1983; P 139.

Singh AB, Babu CR. Survey of atmospheric pollen allergens in Delhi. Ann Allergy 1982; 48(2): 115–122.

Singh AB. Pollen production in common allergenic plants of Delhi and their atmospheric prevalence. Science and Cult 1984; 50: 65–67.

Subbarao M, Om Prakash, Subbarao PV. Reaginic allergy to *Parthenium* pollen: Evaluation by skin test and RAST. Clin Allergy 1989; 15: 449–454.

Subba Reddi C, Reddi NS. Relation of pollen release to pollen concentrations in air. Grana 1985; 24: 109–113.

7

Risk Factors for Allergies and Asthma

Harold Nelson

INTRODUCTION

The prevalence of allergies and asthma varies greatly in different countries. The International Study of Asthma and Allergies in Childhood (ISAAC) assessed the prevalence of symptoms of asthma, rhinitis and eczema in 463,801 children ages 13–14 years from 155 centers in 56 (ISAAC 1998). It was found that the prevalence of asthma in these children varied from 1.6% in Indonesia to 36.8% at one center in the United Kingdom. Similar differences were seen for the prevalence of symptoms of allergic rhinitis (1.4 to 39.7%) and eczema (0.3 to 20.5%). Furthermore, the prevalence rates of asthma have not been static. In the US, the prevalence of asthma increased from 3.1 in 1980, to 5.5 in 1996 and 8.4% in 2010, with the increase occurring in all age groups (CDC 2019). Over the same period, the prevalence of allergic sensitization in a representative sample of US residents, 6 to 59 years of age, measured by the presence of at least one positive reaction on prick skin testing to 6 allergens, increased from 21.8% in 1976–80 to 41.9% in 1998–2004 (Arbes et al. 2005). Similar increases in asthma were recorded in Europe at the same time (Haahtela et al. 1990, Ninan and Russel 1992). Although the genetic underpinning of allergies and asthma is well recognized (Castro-Rodriquez et al. 2016), radical changes in the DNA of the effected populations could not explain this sudden increase in allergies and asthma. However, epigenetic modifications in the DNA could and are being increasingly demonstrated as being associated with various environmental exposures (Joubert et al. 2016). Also, environmental factors can affect the gut microbiome of the mother, leading to a microbiome in the infant less capable of inducing a healthy development of its immune system (Buccigrossi et al. 2013). It is also now recognized that all asthma is not of the atopic, eosinophilic phenotype (Schleich et al. 2018). Many patients with asthma show predominantly neutrophilic or even paucicellular phenotypes. These realizations have led to a search for environmental exposures that may explain the country-to-country differences and the major increase within countries of allergies and asthma that have occurred in the last few decades. Table 7.1 lists the associations, both positive and negative, of environmental factors with the risk for developing asthma and, in some cases, also increased sensitization to environmental allergens. In this chapter, some of the more recent studies supporting these associations will be discussed. With two exceptions, fish oil and vitamin D where there are interventional studies, these associations are usually the result of multivariate analyses with adjustment for other possible confounders. The results are expressed as adjusted Odd Risk (aOR), Relative Risk (aRR) and Hazard Ratios (aHR).

National Jewish Health, Denver, Colorado.

Table 7.1: Factors Associated with the Risk for Asthma and Allergies

Prenatal Factors	Risk Factors

Protective:
1. Probiotics
2. Fish oil
3. Mediterranean diet
 	
Risk factors:
1. Obesity
2. Psychological factors
3. Hypothyroidism
4. Maternal diet;
   a. Fast foods
   b. Vitamin D
   c. Sugar sweetened beverages/free sugar
5. Maternal medications
   a. antibiotics
   b. acid suppressive drugs
   c. Acetaminophen
6. Exposures
   a. Environmental tobacco smoke
   b. Spray household cleaning products
   c. Air pollution (vehicle)
   d. Bisphenol A/phthalates
 	
Perinatal factors:
1. Caesarean section
2. Preterm/low birth weight
3. Neonatal hyperbilirubinemia
 	
Post-natal factors
Protective
 	
1. Hygiene factors
   a. Early animal and insect exposure
   b. Early farm animal and farm milk exposure
   c. H pylori infection
   d. Probiotics
   e. Contaminated water supply
   f. Older siblings
   g. Early daycare
   h. BCG vaccination
2. Diet
   a. Mediterranean diet
   b. Dietary fruits and vegetables
   c. Fish consumption
   d. Fish oil consumption
   e. Monosaturated fatty acids and oleic acid and olive oil.
   f. Breast feeding
	1. Diet
	   a. Vitamin D insufficiency
	   b. Fructose/sweetened beverages
	   c. Ultra-processed foods (meats)
	   d. Fast-foods
	   e. High animal protein and carbohydrate diet
	2. Obesity
	   a. Early weight gain in infancy.
	   b. Obesity in adults.
	3. Psychological factors
	   a. Maternal stress
	   b. Personal stress/depression
	4. Air pollution:
	   a. Air pollution (vehicles))
	   b. Particulates
	   c. Open fire cooking
	   d. Environmental tobacco smoke
	   e. Spray household cleaning agents
	   f. Mold/dampness in home
	   g. Unvented natural gas appliances.
	   h. Polyvinyl chloride exposure
	   i. Formaldehyde
	   j. Volatile organic compounds
	   k. Swimming pools
	5. Exposures (ingestion)
	   a. Pesticides
	   b. Bisphenol A/phthalates
	6. Inactivity (TV watching)
	7. Acetaminophen use:
	8. Early antibiotic use:
	9. Female hormone replacement
	10. Occupation
	11. Viral respiratory infections
	12. Heredity:

Prenatal factors

Protective

Mothers of 460 children provided information of their dietary intake during pregnancy (Chatzi et al. 2008). A high, as opposed to low, Mediterranean Diet Score during pregnancy was protective, after adjusting for potential confounders, for persistent wheeze (aOR 0.22), atopic wheeze (aOR 0.30) and atopy (aOR 0.55) at 6.5 years. Twelve hundred twenty-five pregnant women were given a mixture of probiotics or a placebo for 36 weeks of gestation, their infants then received the same product for the first six months (Kallio et al. 2019). In a follow-up of the children at 13 years, among the Caesarean-delivered subgroup those treated with probiotics fared better than the placebo group for allergy (41.5 versus 67.9%), for wheezing during the previous 12 months (8.5 versus 14.7%) and for eczema (18.9 versus 37.5%). A group of Danish women were placed on n-3 long-chain polyunsaturated fatty acids (n-3 PUFA) or olive oil starting at 24 weeks gestation (Bisgaard et al. 2016). The risk of a persistent wheeze or asthma at 3 years was significantly reduced in children of the fish-oil-treated mothers (16.9 versus 23.7% with olive oil). The effect was mostly in the women with the lowest third of blood levels for n-3 PUFA at baseline. Follow-up at 5–7 years confirmed the outcome.

Risk factors

In a systematic review of 14 studies including 108,321 women and off-spring, followed from 14 months to 16 years, obesity was associated with an increased risk for current asthma or wheeze (OR 1.21) with a dose response (Forno et al. 2014). Increased risk has also been reported with maternal untreated hypothyroidism (Lu et al. 2018). A review of 30 studies of maternal stress, including mood disorders, anxiety, exposure to violence, bereavement and socio-economic problems, found the presence of any of these in the mother during gestation increased the risk in the children of developing atopic dermatitis (OR 1.34), allergic rhinitis (OR 1.30), wheeze (Or 1.34) and asthma (OR 1.15) (Flanigan et al. 2018). Exposure to anxiety and depression had the greatest effect.

Several factors in the maternal diet during gestation have been shown to be associated with an increased risk for atopic outcomes in the offspring. Maternal intake of fast food was shown to be associated with increased risk for current asthma and rhinitis in the offspring at 3.5 years (von Ehrenstein et al. 2015). Information on maternal intake of sugar was collected during pregnancy and the presence of physician-diagnosed asthma in the child at 7.5 years in a large birth cohort (Bedard et al. 2017). There was a positive association between maternal intake of free sugar and allergic asthma (aOR 2.01, p for trend 0.004). In another birth cohort there was a significant association between current asthma in a child at age 7.7 years and higher pregnancy intake of sugar sweetened beverage (aOR 1.70) and total fructose (aOR 1.58) (Wright et al. 2018).

The evidence for an increased risk for asthma in children born of women with low vitamin D levels during pregnancy is not consistent (Hennessy et al. 2018, Mirzakhani et al. 2019). However, early results from double-blind, placebo-controlled trials of maternal supplementation with vitamin D suggest positive results. A group of women from New Zealand were given 1000 IU, 2000 IU or a placebo daily beginning at 27 weeks of gestation and the offspring were treated until age 6 months (Grant et al. 2016). There was a reduction in house dust mite sensitization and clinic visits for asthma up to age 18 months in offspring of mothers who had received vitamin D supplementation. In a merging of the results from two placebo-controlled studies of vitamin D supplementation in pregnancy, children of mothers receiving vitamin D supplementation had decreased risk for wheezing/asthma at 3 years (aOR 0.74) (Wolsk et al. 2017).

Intake of acid-suppressive drugs during pregnancy was found to be a risk for eczema (aOR 1.32), asthma (aOR 1.57) and allergic rhinitis (aOR 2.40) in the offspring at a mean age of 4.9 years (Mulder et al. 2014). A systematic review of antibiotic use during pregnancy, including 10 studies, found an OR for wheeze or asthma of 1.20, strongest with use in the 3rd trimester (Zhao et al. 2015). Two studies found that maternal use of acetaminophen during pregnancy was a risk for asthma in the offspring, but only in children with certain alleles for glutathione reductase, an important antioxidant (Shaheen et al. 2010, Perzanowski et al. 2010).

A meta-analysis of 79 studies showed prenatal maternal smoking was significantly associated with an increased incidence of asthma or wheeze in all age groups with ORs ranging from 1.28 in children 3–4 years old to 1.52 I children 5–18 years old (Castro-Rodriquez et al. 2016). Even tobacco smoking by a grandmother during their mothers' pregnancy was an increased risk for asthma not modified by maternal smoking (Lodge et al. 2017).

Exposure to household cleaning agents during pregnancy was a risk for non-allergic asthma in the children at age 8.5 years (Henderson et al. 2008). Particulate (PM_{10}) exposure during pregnancy and at 1 year of age showed significant associations with airway hyper responsiveness and risk of new diagnosis of asthma at age 7 years (aOR 2.06) (Yang et al. 2018).

Increased amounts of mono-n-butyl phthalate in the mother's urine at 34 weeks gestation was associated with a diagnosis of asthma (p = 0.009) and risk for allergic sensitization against inhalant allergens (p = 0.004) when the child was 6 years of age (Jahreis et al. 2017). A mouse model confirmed the results and demonstrated epigenetic changes (Jahreis et al. 2017).

Perinatal factors

Low birth weight and neonatal hyperbilirubinemia have both been associated with an increased risk for asthma (Castro-Rodriquez et al. 2016). Delivery by Caesarean section is a risk for asthma (Castro-Rodriquez et al. 2016). This could be due to the altered infant gut microbiome that results from the Caesarean section delivery or the stress associated with the procedure.

Postnatal factors

Protective

Related to the hygiene hypothesis

The protective effect of early close proximity to farm animals on allergic sensitization and asthma is well demonstrated by outcomes in Amish and Hutterite children, 2 groups closely similar genetically (Stein et al. 2016). Amish children have a close farm animal contact, while Hutterites do not. Sensitization and asthma occurred in 7.2 and 5.2% of the Amish children and 33.3 and 21.3% of the Hutterite children. Drinking unpasteurized farm milk is similarly protective (Loss et al. 2011). Also associated with a lower risk for asthma at age 7 years, was exposure of inner city children at an early age to higher concentrations of cockroach, mouse and cat allergens (O'Connor et al. 2018). Childhood infection with H. pylori was associated with significantly reduced odds of any allergic disease (Taye et al. 2017). Higher bacterial counts in drinking water in Russian Karelia compared to Finnish Karelia were significantly associated with the lower risk of atopy in Russian Karelia (Von Hertzen et al. 2007).

Both the presence of Older siblings in the home and entry of the child into day care during the first 6 months of life were associated with a reduced risk of physician-diagnosed asthma at age 6 to 13 years (Ball et al. 2000). A systematic review including 25 studies suggested a protective effect of BCG vaccination on childhood asthma (OR 0.86) (El-Zein et al. 2010).

Related to diet

A questionnaire-based evaluation of 1,784 school children found that following a Mediterranean diet was associated with a reduced risk of wheeze at 4 years (aOR 0.54) (Castro-Rodriquez et al. 2008). An assessment of 690 children, aged 7–18 years, living in Crete found adherence to a Mediterranean diet was protective for allergic rhinitis (OR 0.34) with a more modest protection against wheezing and atopy (Chatzi et al. 2007). In that same study, the intake of fruits and vegetables was protective for wheezing and rhinitis, while in Japan the prevalence of allergies, rhinitis and asthma was significantly reduced in children with increasing intake of fruit (Kusunoki et al. 2017).

A systematic review found a beneficial effect for fish intake on current asthma (OR 0.75) and current wheeze (OR 0.62) in children up to 4.5 years, and of 'fatty fish' on asthma development in children 8–14 years (or 0.35) (Papamichael et al. 2018). Introduction of fish oil to infants between 3 and 6 months reduced diagnosed food allergy (0.8%) compared to introduction between 7 and 9 months (1.4%) or not receiving fish oil (2.9%) (Clausen et al. 2018). In a study of 3,115 Dutch children, having received breast feeding for > 16 weeks, compared to no breast feeding, was associated with significantly less asthma from age 3 to 8 years (OR 0.57) (Scholtens et al. 2009).

Risks

Serum vitamin D levels were measured 6 times in the first 5 years in children in a high risk cohort (Hollams et al. 2017). Vitamin D deficiency in early childhood was associated with an increased risk for persistent asthma at age 10 years. Data from NHANES 2001–2010 was examined for 10,860 children ages 6–17 years and 14,115 adults (Han et al. 2017). Vitamin D insufficiency was associated with current asthma (OR 1.35) in children and current wheeze in children and adults (OR 1.17) as well as lower FEV1 and FVC.

Higher intake of fructose in 3–4 year olds was associated with greater odds of current asthma at 7.7 years (aOR 1.77) after adjustment for children's BMI (Wright et al. 2018). Among 2,406 11-year old Dutch children the consumption of > 21.5 glasses of fruit juice and sugar added drinks per week, compared to < 12.5 glasses/week was associated with an increased risk for physician-diagnosed asthma (aOR 1.91) (Berentzen et al. 2015). Data from NHANES reported excess free-fructose beverages were significantly associated with asthma in 2–9 year olds (OR 5.29) (DeChristopher et al. 2016).

In Brazilian adolescents the total consumptions of ultra-processed foods was positively associated with the presence of asthma and wheezing in a dose-response manner (Melo et al. 2018). In Korean middle and high school students a high intake of fast food was related to recent asthma (OR 2.05) (Kang et al. 2018). In Korean adults there was an association of physician-diagnosed asthma and high consumption of processed meat (OR 13.85) and instant noodles (Or 9.49) (Kang et al. 2018). In adolescents and adults from nine European countries a high animal protein/carbohydrate diet was associated with a higher risk for current asthma (RR 2.03), atopic status (RR 1.68) and decreased lung function (RR 4.57) (Bakolis et al. 2018).

Systematic reviews have repeatedly demonstrated that obesity in children and adults is associated with an increased risk for asthma both cross sectionally and prospectively (Castro-Rodriguez et al. 2016). Studies also suggest that the asthma associated with obesity occurs in children with low, but not elevated fractional exhaled nitric oxide (Han et al. 2014).

Maternal depression during the child's first 6–7 years was a risk for a child having asthma (OR 2.36) (Giallo et al. 2015). In both Puerto Rican and Swedish mothers with asthma and depression, compared to those with asthma alone were twice as likely to have offspring with asthma (Medsker et al. 2017). Children 0–17 years of age were assessed for the presence of six types of Adverse Childhood Experience (ACE) (divorce, death, jail time, mentally ill, suicidal, depression, alcohol or drugs or physical assault) (Wing et al. 2015). The number or ACE exposures was associated with increased risk for asthma (one ACE a OR 1.28, 5 or 6 ACE aOR 1.61).

Studies in children, adolescents and adults have shown that living in close proximity to a road with heavy vehicle use is a risk for having or developing asthma (Baumann et al. 2011, Bowatte et al. 2018). In over 7 million children receiving Medicaid, increased exposure to particulate matter, particularly 2.5 microns ($PM_{2.5}$), was associated with increased asthma prevalence (Keet et al. 2018). Open-fire cooking, another exposure to particulate matter, was found to be a risk of asthma in both children 6–7 years and adolescents 13–14 years (Silverwood et al. 2019).

Passive exposure to tobacco smoke is a risk for asthma in adolescents (aOR 1.33) and in adults (aHR 1.21) (Castro-Rodriguez et al. 2016).

In a prospective study of 3,503 adults, using spray household cleaning agents at least once per week was an increased risk for new onset asthma over 9 years follow-up (RR 2.11) (Zock et al. 2007).

In a systematic review, household dampness and mold was found to be associated with increased odds of childhood wheeze (aOR 1.53) (Castro-Rodriguez et al. 2016). In another systemic review of 61 studies reporting signs of mold in the home, there were increased odds of asthma (OR 1.49) and wheeze (Or 1.68) (Castro-Rodriguez et al. 2016).

Cooking with natural gas produces nitrogen dioxide. A survey of 15,000 young adults in the UK found that women who regularly used gas for cooking were at increased risk for current wheeze (aOR 2.07) and asthma attacks (aOR 2.60) (Jarvis et al. 1996).

Children ages 6 months to 3 years with asthma in an emergency department were shown to have been exposed in their home to higher levels of volatile organic compounds than matched controls (Rumchev et al. 2004). Adults who had had indoor surfaces painted within the past 12 months more often reported asthma symptoms (OR 1.5) (Wieslander et al. 1997). Longitudinal studies showed an association between the presence of polyvinyl chloride surface materials in the home and an increased risk of asthma (OR 1.45) (Castro-Rodriguez et al. 2016). Among adolescents the prevalence of current asthma and allergic sensitization significantly increased with the lifetime number of hours spend in outdoor swimming pools (Bernard et al. 2008).

Data from NHANES 2005/2006 showed that > 90% of participants 6 years of age and older had detectable levels of 2 dichlorophenols in their urine. Comparing the highest to the lowest tertile for 2, 5 dichlorophenol there was a higher prevalence of physician-diagnosed asthma in allergic individuals (Or 4.7) (Jerschow et al. 2014).

In a birth cohort, children's urine was tested for bisphenol A (BPA) at ages 3, 5, and 7 years. Higher concentrations were associated with asthma at each time with ORs of 1.4 or 1.5 (Sordillo et al. 2015). In Korean children BPA urine concentrations at age 7–8 years were associated with wheezing (OR 2.48) and asthma (HR 2.13) at 11–12 years of age (Kim et al. 2014).

Children free of wheezing at 3.5 years of age had parent-reported hours/day of television viewing record. The odds ratio for physician-diagnosed asthma at 7.5 years persisting at age 11.5 years was 0.7 for < 1 hour view, 1.0 for 1–2 hours viewing and 1.89 for > 2 hours viewing (Sherrif et al. 2009).

Use of acetaminophen is early childhood is associated with an increased risk for later development of asthma. When the presence of early infections is factored-in, the increased risk is usually eliminated (Sordillo et al. 2015). There is still disagreement, however, whether there remains an increased risk (Silverwood et al. 2019). In a prospective study of 121,700 adult women, increased frequency of acetaminophen use was positively associated with newly diagnosed asthma (p for trend = 0.006) (Barr et al. 2004). The multivariate rate ratio for asthma for participants who received acetaminophen for more than 14 days per month was 1.63 (95% confidence interval, 1.11–2.39) compared with non users.

Because of its association with respiratory infections, a risk factor itself for asthma, the independent risk associated with early life use of antibiotics is also controversial (Silverwood et al. 2019).

In the same prospective study of women that found a risk for asthma with use of acetaminophen, use of estrogen-containing products was associated with an increased risk of asthma (aOR 2.29) (Gomez Real et al. 2006). In a postal questionnaire in Denmark, hormone replacement therapy was associated with increased risk of asthma (OR 1.57) and hay fever (Or 1.48) (Kogevinas et al. 2007).

It is well recognized that certain occupations are associated with increased risk of developing asthma (Kogenivas et al. 2007, Jaakkola et al. 2003).

Children with asthma at age 7 years were reported to have had more respiratory tract infections and antibiotic use in the first 24 months of life (Toivonen et al. 2019). In a birth cohort wheezing illness due to rhinovirus in the first 3 years was associated with an increased risk for having asthma at age 13 years (OR 3.3) (Rabner et al. 2017). It is not clear whether acute respiratory tract infections (URIs) in early childhood predispose the child to the development of asthma or whether the susceptibility to URIs and asthma share common pathophysiologic mechanisms.

Finally, all these environmental exposures that are associated with decreased or increased risk of developing asthma act on the hereditary disposition of the individual. The contribution of hereditary predisposition to the development of allergies and asthma is well established (Castro-Rodriguez et al. 2016, Mirzakhani et al. 2019).

Conclusions

- There has been a marked increase in the prevalence of allergies and asthma in many developing and developed countries over the past few decades.
- In epidemiologic studies many environmental factors are positively associated with the prevalence of allergies and asthma.
- Some maternal exposures during pregnancy are associated with allergies and asthma in the offspring. The mechanism may be by epigenetic alterations in the DNA or through changes in the gut microbiome.
- Important environmental factors associated with an increased risk for allergies and asthma include:
    1. Dietary changes, particularly less fruits and vegetables, more processed foods and more fructose and free sugar.
    2. Obesity.

3. Air pollution, including vehicle emissions, tobacco smoke and outgassing from building materials.
4. Chemicals including pesticides and those derived from plastic containers.
5. Psychological factors including stress and depression.

References

Arbes SJ Jr, Gergen PJ, Elliott L, Zeldin DC. Prevalence of positive skin test responses to 10 common allergens in the US population. J Allergy Clin Immunol 2005; 116: 377–83.

Bakolis I, Hooper R, Bachert C, Lange B, Haahtela T, Keil T, et al. Dietary patterns and respiratory health in adults from nine European countries – evidence from the GA²LEN study. Clin Exp Allergy 2018; 48: 1474–1482.

Ball TM, Castro-Rodriuez JA, Griffith KA, Holberg CJ, Martinez FD, Wright AL. Siblings, Day-care attendance, and the risk of asthma and wheezing during childhood. N Engl J Med 2000; 343: 538–43.

Barr RG, Wentowski CC, Curhan GC, Somers SC, Stampfer MJ, Schwartz J, et al. Prospective study of acetaminophen use and newly diagnosed asthma among women. Am J Respir Crit Care Med 2004; 169: 836–41.

Baumann LM, Robinson CL, Combe J, Gomez A, Romero K, Gilman RH, et al. Effects of distance from a heavily transited avenue on asthma and atopy in a periurban shantytown in Lima Peru. J Allergy Clin Immunol 2011; 127: 875–82.

Berentzen NE, van Stokkom VL, Gehring U, Koppelman GH, Schaap LA, Smit HA, et al. Associations of sugar-containing beverages with asthma prevalence in 11-year-old children: the PIAMA birth cohort. Eur J Clin Nutr 2015; 69: 303–8.

Bedard A, Northstone K, Henderson AJ, Shahee, SO. Maternal intake of sugar during pregnancy and childhood respiratory and atopic outcomes. Eur Respir J. 2017; 50: 1700073.

Bernard A, Nickmilder M, Voisin C. Outdoor swimming pools and the risks of asthma an allergies during adolescence. Eur Respir J 2008; 32: 979–88.

Bisgaard H, Vissing NH, Carson CG, Bischoff AL, Faisgaard NV, Kreiner Moller E, et al. Fish oil-derived fatty acids in pregnancy and wheeze and asthma in offspring. N Engl J Med 2016; 375: 2530–9.

Bowatte G, Erbas B, Lodge CJ, Knibbs LD, Gurrin LC, Marks GB, et al. Traffic related air pollution and development and persistence of asthma and low lung function. Environ Int 2018; 113: 170–176.

Buccigrossi V, Nicastro E, Guarino A. Functions of intestinal microflora in children. CurrOpinGastroenterol 2013; 29: 31–8.

Castro-Rodriquez JA, Garcia-Marcos L, Alfonseda-Rojas JK, Valverde-Molina J, Sanchez-Solis M. Mediterranean diet as a protective factor for wheezing in preschool children. J Pediatr 2008; 152: 823–8.

Castro-Rodriquez JA, Forno E, Rodriquez-Martinez CE, Celedon JC. Risk and protective factors for childhood asthma: What is the evidence? J Allergy Clin Immunol Pract 2016; 4: 1111–22.

CDC. gov—National Asthma Surveillance Data. (Accessed 18 May 2019).

Chatzi L, Apostolaki G, Bibakin I, Skypala I, Bibaki-Liakou V, Tzanakis N, et al. Protective effect of fruits, vegetables and the Mediterranean diet on asthma an allergies among children in Crete. Thorax 2007; 62: 677–81.

Chatzi L, Torrent M, Romieu I, Garcia-Esteban R, Ferrer C, Vioque J, et al. Mediterranean diet in pregnancy is protective for wheeze and atopy in childhood. Thorax 2008; 63: 507–13.

Clausen M, Jonasson K, Keil T, Beyer K, Sigurdardottir SR. Fish oil in infancy protects against food allergy in Iceland-Results from a birth cohort study. Allergy 2018; 73: 1305–1312.

DeChristopher LR, Uribarri J, Tucker KL. Intakes of apple juice, fruit drinks and soda are associated with prevalent asthma in US children aged 2–9 years. Pub Health Nutr 2016; 19: 123–30.

Donohue KM, Miller RL, Perzanowski MS, et al. Prenatal and postnatal bisphenol A exposure and asthma development among inner-city children. J Allergy Clin Immunol 2013; 131: 736–42.

El-Zein M, Parent M-E, Benedetti A, Rousseau M-C. Does BCG vaccination protect against the development of childhood asthma? A systematic review and meta-analysis of epidemiological studies. Int J Epidemiol 2010; 39: 469–86.

Flanigan C, Sheikh A, DunnGaivin A, Brew BK, Almqvist C, Nwaru BI. Prenatal maternal psychosocial stress and offspring's asthma and allergic disease: A systematic review and meta-analysis. Clin Exp Allergy 2018; 48: 403–414.

Forno E, Young OM, Kumar R, Simhan H, Celedon JC. Maternal obesity in pregnancy, gestational weight gain, and risk of childhood asthma.Pediatrics 2014; 134: e535–46.

Giallo R, Bahreinian S, Brown S, Cooklin A, Kingston D, Kozyrskyj A. Maternal depressive symptoms across early childhood and asthma in school children: findings from a longitudinal Australian population based study. PLoS ONE 2015; 10: e0121459.

Gomez Real F, Svanes C, Bjornsson EH, Franklin KA, Gislason D, Gislason T, et al. Hormone replacement therapy, body mass index and asthma in perimenopausalwomen: a cross sectional survey. Thorax 2006; 61: 34–40.

Grant CC, Crane J, Mitchell EA, Sinclair J, Stewart A, Milne T, et al. Vitamin D supplementation during pregnancy and infancy reduces aeroallergen sensitization; a randomized controlled trial. Allergy 2016; 71: 1325–1334.

Haahtela T, Lindholm H, Bjorksten F, Koskenvuo K, Laitinen LA. Prevalence of asthma in Finnish young men. Br Med J 1990; 301: 266–8.

Han YY, Forno E, Celedon JC. Adiposity, fractional exhaled nitric oxide, and asthma in US children. Am J Respir Crit Care Med 2014; 190: 32–9.

Han YY, Forno E, Celedon JC. Vitamin D insufficiency and asthma in a US nationwide study. J Allergy Clin Immunol Pract 2017; 5: 790–6.

Henderson J, Sherriff A, Farrow A, Ayres JG. Household chemicals, persistent wheezing and lung function: effect modification by atopy? Eur Respir J 2008; 31: 547–54.

Hennessy A, Hourihane JO, Malvisi L, Irvine AD, Kenny LC, Murray DM, et al. Antenatal vitamin D exposure and childhood eczema, food allergy, asthma and allergic rhinitis at 2 and 5 years of age in the atopic disease-specific Cork BASELINE Birth cohort Study. Allergy 2018; 73: 2182–2192.

Hollams EM, Teo SM, Kusel M, Holt BJ, Holt KE, Inouye M, et al. Vitamin D over the first decade and susceptibility to childhood allergy and asthma. J Allergy Clin Immunol 2017; 139: 472–481.

International Study of Asthma and Allergies in Childhood (ISAAC) Steering Committee. Worldwide variation in prevalence of symptoms of asthma, allergic rhinoconjunctivitis, and atopic eczema: ISAAC. Lancet 1998; 351: 1225–1232.

Jaakkola JJK, Piipari R, Jaakkola MS. Occupation and asthma: a population-based incident case-control study. Am J Epidemiology 2003; 158: 981–7.

Jahreis S, Trump S, Bauer M, Thurmann L, Feltens R, Wang Q, et al. Maternal phthalate exposure promotes allergic airway inflammation over 2 generations through epigenetic modifications. J Allergy Clin Immunol 2017; 141: 741–753.

Jarvis D, Chinn S, Luczynska C, burney P. Association of respiratory symptoms and lung function in young adults with use of domestic gas appliance. Lancet 1996; 347: 426–31.

Jerschow E, Parikh P, McGinn AP, de Vos G, Jariwala S, Hudes G, et al. Relationship between urine dichlorophenol levels and asthma morbidity. An Allergy Asthma Immunol 2014; 112: 511–18.

Joubert BR, Felix JF, Yousefi P, Bakulski KM, Just AC, Breton C, et al. DNA methylation in newborns and maternal smoking in pregnancy: genome-wide consortium meta-analysis. Am J Human Genetics 2016; 98: 680–696.

Kallio S, Kukkonen AK, Savilahti E, Kuitunen M. Perinatal probiotic intervention prevented allergic disease in a Caesarean-delivered subgroup at 13-year follow-up. Clin Exp Allergy 2019; 49: 506–514.

Kang S-Y, Song W-J, Kim M-H, Kim S-H, Cho S-H, Chang Y-S, et al. Dietary assessment and the development of asthma in Korean adolescents and adults. Allergy 2018; 73: 2254–2256.

Keet CA, Keller JP, Peng RD. Long-term coarse particulate matter exposure is associated with asthma among children in Medicaid. Am J Respir Crit Care Med 2018; 197: 737–746.

Kim KN, Kim JH, Kwon HJ, Hong SJ, Kim BJ, Lee SY, et al. Bisphenol A exposure and asthma development in school-age children: a longitudinal study. PLoS One 2014; 9: e111383.

Kogevinas M, Zock JP, Jarvis D, Kromhout H, Lillienberg L, Plana E, et al. Exposure to substances in the workplace and new-onset asthma: an international prospective population-based study (ECRHS-II). Lancet 2007; 370: 336–41.

Kusunoki T, Takeuchi J, Morimoto T, Sakuma M, Yasumi T, Nishikomori R, et al. Fruit intake reduces the onset of respiratory allergic symptoms in schoolchildren. Ped Allergy Immunol 2017; 28: 793–800.

Lodge CJ, Braback L, Lowe AJ, Dharmage SC, Olsson D, Forsberg B. Grandmaternal smoking increases asthma risk in grandchildren: a nationwide Swedish cohort. Clin Exp Allergy 2017

Loss G, Apprich S, Waser M, Kneifel W, Genuneit J, Buchele G, et al. The protective effect of farm milk consumption on childhood asthma and atopy: the GABRIELA study. JACI 2011; 128: 766–73.

Lu X, Andersen SL, Olsen J, Agerbo E, Schlunssen V, Dharmage SC, et al. Maternal hypothyroidism in the perinatal period and childhood asthma in offspring. Allergy 2018; 73: 932–939.

Medsker BH, Brew BK, Forno E, Olsson H, Lundholm C, Han YY, et al. Maternal depressive symptoms, maternal asthma, and asthma in school-aged children. Ann Allergy Asthma Immunol 2017; 118: 55–60.

Melo B, Razende L, Machado P, Gouveia N, Levy R. Associations of ultra-processed food and drink products with asthma and wheezing among Brazilian adolescents. Ped Allergy Immunol 2018; 29: 504–511.

Mirzakhani H, Carey VJ, Zeiger R, Bacharier LB, O'Connor GT, Schatz MX, et al. Impact of parental asthma, prenatal maternal asthma control and vitamin D status on risk of asthma and recurrent wheeze in 3-year old children. Clin Exp Allergy 2019; 49: 419–429.

Mulder B, Schuiling-Veninga CC, Bos HJ, De Vries TW, Jick SS, Hak E. Prenatal exposure to acid-suppressive drugs and the risk of allergic disease in the offspring: a cohort study. Clin Exp Allergy 2014; 44: 261–9.

Ninan TK, russel G. Respiratory symptoms and atopy in Aberdeen schoolchildren: evidence from two surveys 25 years apart. Br. Med J 1992; 304: 873–5.

O'Connor GT, Lynch SV, Bloomberg GR, Kattan M, Wood RA, Gergen PJ, et al. Early-life home environment and risk of asthma among inner-city children. J Allergy Clin Immunol 2018; 141: 1468–75.

Papamichael MM, Shrestha SK, Itsiopoulos C, Erbas B. The role of fish intake on asthma in children: A meta-analysis of observational studies. Ped Allergy Immunol 2018; 29: 350–360.

Perzanowski MS, Miller RL, Tang D, Ali D, Garfinkel RS, Chew GL, et al. Prenatal acetaminophen exposure and risk of wheeze at age 5 years in an urban low-income cohort. Thorax 2010; 65: 118–123.

Rabner FJ, Jackson DJ, Evans MD, Gangnon RE, Tisler CJ, Pappas TE, et al. Early life rhinovirus wheezing, allergic sensitization and asthma risk at adolescence. J Allergy Clin Immunol 2017; 139: 501–7.

Rumchev K, Spickett J, Bulsara M, Phillips M, Stick S. Association of domestic exposure to volatile organic compounds with asthma in young children. Thorax 2004; 59: 746–51.

Schleich FN, Zanelia D, Stefanuto PH, Bessonov K, Smokinskaj A, Dallinga JW, et al. Exhaled volatile organic compounds are able to discriminate between neutrophilic and eosinophilic asthma. Am J Respir Crit Care Med 2019; doi 10.1164/rccm.201811-22110C. Epub ahead of publication.

Scholtens S, Wijga AH, Brunekreef B, Kerkhof M, Hoekstra MO, Gerritsen J, et al. Breast-feeding, parental allergy and asthma in children followed for 8 years. The PIAMA birth cohort study. Thorax 2009; 64: 604–9.

Shaheen SO, Newson RB, Ring SM, Rose-Zerilli MJ, Holloway JW, Henderson AJ. Prenatal and infant acetaminophen exposure, antioxidant gene polymorphisms, and childhood asthma. J Allergy Clin Immunol 2010; 126: 1141–8.

Sherrif A, Maitra A, Ness AR, Mattocks C, Riddoch C, Reilly JJ, et al. Association of duration of television viewing in early childhood with the subsequent development of asthma. Thorax 2009; 64: 321–5.

Silverwood RJ, Rutter CE, Mitchell EA, Asher MI, Garcia-Marcos L, Strachan DP, et al. Are environmental risk factors for current wheeze in the International Study of Asthma and Allergies in childhood (ISAAC) phase three due to reverse causation? Clin Exp Allergy 2019; 49: 430–441.

Sordillo JE, Scirica CV, Rifas-Shiman SL, Gillman MW, Bunyavanich S, Camargo CA, Jr, et al. Prenatal and infant exposure to acetaminophen and ibuprofen and the risk for wheeze and asthma in children. J Allergy Clin Immunol 2015; 135: 370–8.

Stein MM, Hrusch CL, Gozdz J, Igartua C, Pivniouk V, Murray SE, et al. Innate immunity and asthma risk in Amish and Hutterite farm children. N Engl J Med 2016; 375: 411–421.

Taye B, Enquselassie F, Tsegaye A, Amberbir A, Medhin G, Fogarty A, et al. Association between infection with Helicobacter pylori and atopy in young Ethiopian children: a longitudinal study. Clin Exp Allergy 2017; 47: 1299–1308.

Toivonen L, Forsstrom V, Waris M, Peltola V. Acute respiratory infection in early childhood and risk of asthma at age 7 years. J Allergy Clin Immunol 2019; 143: 407–10.

vonEhrenstein OS, Aralis H, Flores ME, Ritz B. Fast food consumption in pregnancy and subsequent asthma symptoms in young children. Ped Allergy Immunol 2015; 26: 571–7.

Von Hertzen L, Laatikainen T, Pitkanen T, Viasoff T, Makela MJ, Vartiainen E, et al. Microbial content of drinking water in Finnish and Russian Karelia – implications for atopy prevalence. Allergy 2007; 62: 288–92.

Wieslander G, Norback D, Bjornsson E, Janson C, Boman G. Asthma and the indoor environment: the significance of emission of formaldehyde and volatile organic compounds from newly painted indoor surfaces. Int Arch Occup Environ Health 1997; 69: 115–24.

Wing R, Gielsvik A, Nacera M, McQuaid EL. Association between adverse childhood experiences in the home and pediatric asthma. Ann Allergy Asthma Immunol 2015; 114: 379–384.

Wolsk HM, Chawes BL, Litonjua AA, Hollis BW, Waage J, Stokholm J, et al. Prenatal vitamin D supplementation reduces risk of asthma/recurrent wheeze in early childhood: A combined analysis of two randomized controlled trials. PloSONE e 2017; 12: e0186657.

Wright LS, Rifas-Shirman SL, Oken E, Litonjua AA, Gold DR. Prenatal and early-life fructose, fructose-containing beverages and mid-childhood asthma. Ann Am ThoracSoc 2018; 15: 217–224.

Yang SI, Lee SY, Kim HB, Kim HC, Leem JH, Yang HJ, et al. Prenatal particulate matter affects new asthma via airway hyperresponsiveness in school children Allergy 2018; 74: 675–684.

Zhao D, Su H, Cheng J, Wang X, Xie M, Li K, et al. Prenatal antibiotic use and risk of childhood wheeze/asthma: A meta-analysis. Ped Allergy Immunol 2015; 26: 756–64.

Jan-Paul Zock J-P, Plana E, Jarvis D, Antó JM, Kromhout H, Kennedy SM, et al. The use of household cleaning sprays and adult asthma: an international, longitudinal study. Am J Respir Crit Care Med 2007; 176: 735–41.

8

Rhinitis
Allergic and Nonallergic

Vinay Mehta,[1,*] *Srinivasan Ramanuja*[2] *and Pramod S Kelkar*[3]

INTRODUCTION

Rhinitis is among the most common chronic conditions in both children and adults for which medical care is sought. It is a heterogenous disorder resulting in inflammation of the nasal mucosa and characterized by symptoms of sneezing, rhinorrhea, nasal congestion and nasal itching. Cough, irritability and fatigue are other common complaints. An estimated 400 million people worldwide suffer from allergic rhinitis and another 200 million suffer from nonallergic rhinitis, which to a large extent remains underdiagnosed and undertreated. Although rhinitis is not life-threatening, it can significantly impact one's quality of life, and is responsible for loss of work and school productivity. Chronic rhinitis may also contribute to fatigue, sleep disorders and learning difficulties. All of these aspects make chronic rhinitis an important global health issue.

Classification

Allergic rhinitis

Allergic Rhinitis (AR) is caused by immunologic sensitization to one or more environmental allergens, which leads to production of allergen-specific IgE antibodies that bind high-affinity IgE receptors on the surface of mast cells and basophils. Upon re-exposure, the allergen cross-links allergen-specific IgE antibodies, resulting in mast cell and basophil degranulation and release of preformed histamine and newly synthesized mediators, namely prostaglandins, leukotrienes and kinins. This early phase response is characterized by itching, sneezing and congestion due to increased vascular permeability, vasodilatation and mucus production. Further release of inflammatory mediators results in a late-phase reaction that occurs 4–6 hours after allergen exposure. Cytokines and chemokines generated during this phase recruit T lymphocytes, basophils and eosinophils, which in turn, release further inflammatory mediators which worsen nasal symptoms and prime the nose so that future allergen exposure leads to more severe symptoms. Mediators involved in allergic rhinitis are listed in Table 8.1.

---

[1] Allergy, Asthma & Immunology Associates, P.C., Lincoln, NE, USA.
[2] Mankato Clinic, Allergy/Asthma/Immunology, Mankato, MN, USA, Email: vasanr@mankato-clinic.com
[3] Allergy and Asthma Care. Maple Grove, MN, USA, Email: pramodkelkar@gmail.com
* Corresponding author: drvinaymehta@gmail.com

Table 8.1. Mediators involved in allergic rhinitis.

	Symptoms	Mediators
Early Phase	Sneezing, itching, rhinorrhea	Histamine, cysteinyl leukotrienes, prostaglandins, platelet-activating factor
Late phase	Nasal congestion and mucus hypersecretion	Inflammatory cells: basophils, eosinophils, neutrophils, mononuclear cells; IL-4, IL-5, IL-13

Although AR can begin at any age, most individuals develop symptoms during childhood. Sensitization, followed by clinical allergy, develops first to allergens that are continually present in the environment (e.g., dust mites or animal dander), then to pollens and other seasonal allergens. In a study of approximately 600 children, at least two seasons of pollen exposure were required before most children developed allergic symptoms (Kulig et al. 2000). After the age of two years, the prevalence of AR steadily increases, demonstrating a bimodal peak in early school and early adult years. AR is usually persistent throughout adulthood, then improves starting in the 6th decade.

AR rarely presents for the first time in older adults, unless there is a significant change in allergen exposure (i.e., new pet or new climate). Thus, in an older adult with new symptoms of rhinitis symptoms, alternative causes of rhinitis should be considered first.

The Allergic Rhinitis and its Impact on Asthma (ARIA) guidelines classify AR both by a temporal pattern (intermittent vs. persistent) and by severity (mild vs. moderate-severe) (Brożek et al. 2017). This classification system was proposed by an international workshop of 34 specialists in respiratory allergy in collaboration with the World Health Organization. Intermittent rhinitis is defined by symptoms less than four days per week or for less than four weeks, whereas persistent rhinitis is defined by symptoms more than four days per week and for more than four weeks. The severity of rhinitis is considered as being moderate-severe if one or more of the following items are present: (1) sleep disturbance; (2) impairment of school or work performance; (3) impairment of daily activities, leisure, and/or sport activities; and (4) troublesome symptoms. If none of these items are present, allergic rhinitis is defined as being mild.

Other commonly used terms are 'seasonal' when symptoms occur at a particular time of the year and 'perennial' when symptoms are present year-round. Seasonal allergens, which include pollens from trees, grasses and weeds, as well as outdoor molds, can contribute to intermittent rhinitis, whereas perennial allergens, which include dust mites, animal dander, cockroaches and indoor molds, can contribute to persistent rhinitis. However, in tropical climates, pollens can be present throughout the year and thus cause persistent rhinitis. Table 8.2 lists common biologic aeroallergen sources. For further details regarding aeroallergens, the reader is referred to Chapter 6: Aerobiology for the Clinician.

Table 8.2. Common biologic aeroallergen sources.

Source	Particle Type
Plant	
Bacteria, algae	Metabolites in droplets; cells, fragments
Fungi	Spores, mycelial fragments
Ferns, club mosses	Spores
Grass, weeds, shrubs, trees	Pollens
Animal	
Protozoa	Metabolites in droplets
Arthropods	Fecal particles, body parts, saliva
Birds	Fecal material, feathers
Mammals	Dander, saliva, urine

Nonallergic rhinitis

Nonallergic Rhinitis (NAR) is a heterogeneous group of disorders involving symptoms such as sneezing, rhinorrhea, nasal congestion and post-nasal drainage without an obvious allergic trigger (Lieberman and Pattanaik 2014). Although the pathogenesis for NAR remains unknown, it has been postulated to involve abnormalities in the autonomic nervous system, including the adrenergic, cholinergic and/or non adrenergic-non cholinergic innervation of the nose.

Nonallergic rhinitis can be classified into nine subtypes: (1) drug-induced rhinitis (including rhinitis medicamentosa); (2) gustatory rhinitis; (3) hormonal-induced rhinitis; (4) infectious rhinitis; (5) non-allergic rhinitis with eosinophilia; (6) occupational rhinitis; (7) senile rhinitis; (8) atrophic rhinitis; (9) vasomotor rhinitis.

The most prevalent form of NAR is vasomotor rhinitis (VMR), which is characterized by intermittent symptoms of congestion and/or rhinorrhea, and an exaggerated reaction to nonspecific irritants such as tobacco smoke, perfumes, air pollution, diesel particles, cleaning products, cold, dry air, temperature changes and barometric pressure changes. These triggers do not involve IgE cross-linking or histamine release. VMR is clinically distinguished from AR by a later age of onset (> 20 years of age), less prominent nasal and ocular itching and sneezing, more prominent nasal congestion and postnasal drainage. Unlike AR, VMR is usually not worsened by exposure to allergens such as pollen, house dust mite or animal dander. However, because VMR may be caused by changes in temperature and humidity, patients may experience seasonal symptoms during spring and fall.

Rhinitis medicamentosa is another common form of NAR. It is caused by overuse of topical nasal decongestants such as oxymetazoline or phenylephrine. When used briefly (less than 3–5 days consecutively), these medications provide significant relief of nasal congestion. However, with chronic use, rebound nasal congestion can occur as the medication wears off. In addition to nasal decongestants, a variety of systemic medications can induce nasal symptoms, namely oral contraceptives, antihypertensives (alpha-blockers, beta-blockers, angiotensin-converting enzyme inhibitors), nonsteroidal anti-inflammatory drugs and antipsychotic medications. Rhinitis symptoms caused by these medications generally subside within a few weeks of discontinuation.

Mixed rhinitis

Mixed rhinitis is the combination of allergic and nonallergic rhinitis. It is the most common form of rhinitis in adults.

Comorbidities

Both allergic and nonallergic rhinitis can be associated with a number of other disorders, including conjunctivitis, asthma, nasal polyps, acute and chronic sinusitis, acute and chronic otitis media, atopic dermatitis and frequent upper respiratory tract infections. Additionally, individuals who are strongly sensitized to pollens may develop oral allergy syndrome. Nasal obstruction due to severe rhinitis can also result in sleep-disordered breathing and anosmia. In addition, there may be an increased prevalence of migraine headache in patients with allergic rhinitis (Ku et al. 2016).

Anatomy and physiology

The internal ostium is the entrance to the nasal cavity. The turbinates (inferior, middle and superior) are located laterally and lined with pseudostratified columnar respiratory epithelium. They are important in air filtration and air conditioning. The nasal septum, which forms the medial wall of the nasal cavity, divides the nose into two nostrils, and is composed of membranous, cartilaginous and bony components.

The nasal epithelium rests on the basement membrane, below which is the lamina propria which is highly vascularized. The arterioles have a porous basement membrane, increasing permeability and allowing greater access for pharmacologic agents. The capillaries are fenestrated, allowing for rapid transfer of fluid across the capillary wall. Vascular sinusoids in the turbinates contribute to heating and humidification of inspired air. Periosteum and bone are located beneath the lamina propria.

The trigeminal nerve provides sensory fibers to the nasal mucous membrane; when these fibers are activated, it produces sensations of irritation or pain, which can result in sneezing. Sympathetic fibers, which follow the blood vessels release noradrenaline and neuropeptide Y, causing vasoconstriction. The nasal cycle involves increasing patency in alternate nostrils (every 2–4 hours), reflecting fluctuations in a sympathetic tone throughout the day.

Vasodilation and glandular secretion are under the control of parasympathetic fibers, which release acetylcholine and vasoactive intestinal peptide. Vasodilation with transudation can cause thickening of the nasal mucosa.

Nasal mucus acts as a barrier against external pathogens and has antioxidant, antiprotease and antimicrobial properties. Major constituents of nasal mucus are the mucins, which play an important role in antimicrobial and anti-inflammatory defenses and in mucociliary clearance. Ciliated epithelium traps foreign bodies in a thin layer of surface mucus that migrates towards the posterior nasopharynx.

During airflow through the nose, the turbinates, septum and ostiomeatal complex contribute to natural turbulence of the air column. This turbulence contributes to impaction of potentially harmful inhaled particles in the upper airway, protecting against inhalation into the lower airways.

United airway hypothesis

Asthma and allergic rhinitis often coexist and may in fact represent a spectrum of the same disease. Indeed, AR is a strong risk factor for the development of allergic asthma (Braunstahl 2009). In the same way, patients with NAR are at increased risk of developing nonallergic asthma. Over 80% of asthmatics have rhinitis, and 10–40% of patients with rhinitis have asthma, suggesting the concept of 'one airway, one disease'. Furthermore, 30% of patients with AR without asthma have increased airway hyper responsiveness to methacholine.

The upper and lower airways are not only contiguous but also have anatomic and physiologic similarities. Postulated mechanisms through which they may interact include the nasal bronchial reflex, disturbance of nasal mucosa conditioning, nitric oxide effects, drainage of irritants and inflammatory material and systemic propagation of inflammation. The latter is currently thought to be the primary mechanism. This is supported by studies demonstrating increased production and release of eosinophils from the bone marrow into the systemic circulation after a nasal allergen challenge (Denburg et al. 2000).

Diagnosis

A careful, detailed history is important; questions should assess the specific symptoms (e.g., nasal itching, sneezing, rhinorrhea, nasal congestion), timing of symptoms (seasonal versus perennial), relieving factors and triggers for symptoms, family history of atopy and living/working environments (e.g., pets at home). Additional details regarding history taking are discussed in Chapter 3: History taking: Evaluation of Allergic Diseases.

Physical examination may reveal several characteristic facial features; these include 'allergic facies', (highly arched palate, open mouth due to mouth breathing, and dental malocclusion), 'allergic shiners' (infraorbital dark circles related to subcutaneous venodilatation), 'allergic gape' (open-mouth breathing from nasal blockage), and 'allergic salute' (a transverse nasal crease caused by repeated rubbing and pushing the tip of the nose up with the hand).

Examination of the nose may reveal pale or bluish edematous turbinates and clear rhinorrhea; examination of the eyes may reveal palpebral and bulbar conjunctival injection, and examination of the oropharynx may reveal post-nasal drip and hyperplastic lymphoid tissue ('cobblestoning').

In patients older than five years of age, flexible fiberoptic rhinoscopy is helpful but not essential for diagnosis. It is helpful in detecting abnormalities such as nasal septal deviation, nasal ulcers, nasal polyps, tumors and foreign bodies. Additional details regarding rhinolaryngoscopy are found in Chapter 11: Rhinolaryngoscopy for the Allergist.

Table 8.3. Physical examination findings suggestive of rhinitis.

General	• Appearing tired
Eyes	• Conjunctivitis • Dark circles under the eyes
Ears	• Chronic congestion indicated by air fluid levels
Nose	• Polyps or septum irregularities • Bloody or purulent discharge (sinusitis related)
Mouth	• Enlarged tonsils • Pharyngeal postnasal discharge • (these are usually associated with nonallergic rhinitis)
Neck	• Lymphadenopathy (infectious)
Chest	• Asthma or other allergic/atopic disease
Skin	• Eczema or other allergic/atopic disease

Physical examination should also include assessment of the ears (since otitis media and middle ear effusions occur with increased frequency in children with allergic rhinitis), chest (since asthma frequently is present in patients with allergic rhinitis), and skin (since eczema is common in patients with allergic rhinitis). Common physical examination findings indicative of rhinitis are listed in Table 8.3.

Although testing for allergen-specific IgE is not absolutely necessary, the identification of culprit allergens has been associated with improved patient outcomes (Szeinbach et al. 2005). Identifying the allergens that are important to patient facilitates allergen avoidance and identifies candidates for allergen immunotherapy. It also helps differentiate between allergic and nonallergic causes of rhinitis.

Skin prick testing is a quick and cost-effective way to identify the presence of allergen-specific IgE (Wallace et al. 2008). The skin testing panel should include a positive and a negative control (typically histamine and saline, respectively) and the major airborne allergens for the area in question. The results should be correlated with clinical history. Intradermal testing has lower specificity but higher sensitivity than percutaneous testing, and can be useful when there is increased clinical suspicion about a particular allergen which shows a negative percutaneous skin test result. Additional details regarding skin testing are discussed in Chapter 4: Allergy Skin Testing.

In vitro allergen-specific IgE immunoassays provide similar information as that obtained with skin testing, although they are more expensive and less sensitive. They are usually obtained when skin testing cannot be performed because a patient has extensive skin disease, cannot discontinue antihistamines or other interfering medications or has extensive dermatographia. On the other hand, measurement of total IgE is not as useful in determining the presence or absence of allergic disease. Additional details regarding allergen-specific IgE immunoassays are found in Chapter 5: *In vitro* Laboratory Tests for Diagnosis of Allergy.

Nasal cytology is performed by some clinicians to help differentiate rhinitis due to allergy from that due to infection. Nasal secretions may be obtained with a cotton swab or by asking the patient to blow the nose on waxed paper. Wright stain of nasal secretions usually reveals a predominance of eosinophils in cases of allergic rhinitis. By comparison, the presence of neutrophils suggests an infectious process.

Plain sinus x-rays are rarely useful, since a minor degree of mucosal swelling in the maxillary sinuses can be seen in patients with allergic rhinitis, and by itself, is not indicative of sinusitis; however, the presence of fluid in one or more sinuses, or their complete opacification should raise suspicion of sinusitis. Computed Tomography (CT) scans can remain abnormal for several weeks following a common cold; however, CT scans can be helpful if endoscopic surgery is anticipated or if malignancy is suspected.

Differential diagnosis

Because allergic sensitization takes at least two consecutive seasons to develop, one should consider other diagnoses in children under age 2 years of age. These include adenoidal hypertrophy, acute or chronic sinusitis, congenital abnormalities (i.e., choanal atresia), foreign bodies and nasal polyps. In older children and adults, in addition to acute and chronic infections, one must consider the various subtypes of nonallergic rhinitis, especially vasomotor rhinitis and drug-induced rhinitis.

Atrophic rhinitis is a syndrome of progressive atrophy of the nasal mucosa seen in older adults. Such individuals report chronic nasal congestion and smell a persistent bad odor. This condition is associated with mucosal colonization with Klebsiella ozaenae. A variant occurs in patients who have had multiple sinus surgeries resulting in loss of normal mucociliary function.

Unilateral rhinitis suggests the possibility of nasal obstruction by a foreign body, tumor or polyp. The presence of nasal polyps suggests nonallergic rhinitis with eosinophilia syndrome (NARES), chronic sinusitis with nasal polyps, allergic fungal sinusitis, aspirin hypersensitivity, cystic fibrosis or primary ciliary dyskinesia. Additional details are provided in Chapter 9: Chronic Rhinosinusitis, Nasal Polyps and AERD.

Treatment

Allergen avoidance

Allergen avoidance is appropriate for all patients with documented positive skin tests or allergen-specific IgE immunoassays, regardless of disease severity. Therefore, the clinician should spend adequate time educating patients on specific interventions to help reduce allergen exposure. However, the clinician should be mindful that major environmental modifications, such as removing carpeting, modifying heating systems, professional pest management or replacing old upholstered furniture, are expensive and may not be affordable. Recognition of this and an initial emphasis on low-cost interventions should enhance patient cooperation.

For house dust mite sensitivity, it is recommending to cover pillows and mattresses in dust-mite proof encasings; wash sheets, pillowcases and blankets in hot water every week; remove dust-collecting items (e.g., stuffed animals) from the bedroom; wear a filter mask when dusting or cleaning; and to keep the relative humidity indoors below 50% (Portnoy et al. 2013a).

For cockroach sensitivity, we recommend integrated pest management (professional cleaning, bait traps, insecticides and HEPA filter) to eliminate and prevent cockroach infestations (Portnoy et al. 2013b). Reservoirs of cockroach contaminants should be cleaned or removed. Factors that facilitate infestation such as standing water or access to refuse should be eliminated.

For rodent sensitivity, we recommend integrated pest management. Habitat modification should be performed to remove means of rodent ingress, food, water and shelter (Phipatanakul et al. 2012).

Every indoor environment has some mold present and moisture control is the key to mold growth control. Therefore, for indoor mold sensitivity, we recommend keeping the relative humidity indoors below 50%, covering cold surfaces such as water pipes with insulation and increasing the air temperature. Visible mold can be remediated using several simple measures. The least expensive and most effective means of removing surface mold involves scrubbing contaminated nonporous hard surfaces with detergent and water and then drying the area completely. Disinfectants or biocides, such as a diluted chlorine bleach solution are not usually necessary. Any contaminated areas in which mold has embedded itself, such as a porous wall, floor, carpet or upholstered area, need to be removed or replaced. A certified industrial hygienist is preferred if professional remediation is required.

The most effective measure in controlling allergens derived from animals is to persuade the family not to keep animals in the house. Scales shed from the animal's skin and particularly in cat saliva are the major source of animal allergens. Keeping a pet outdoors is effective, but restricting the animal to certain rooms is ineffective because animal allergens, particularly those from cats, are easily carried on clothing (Portnoy et al. 2012). Both cat and dog allergens can remain airborne for extended periods of time due to the carriage on particles that, because of their small size, settle very slowly. Removing carpeting, keeping upholstered furniture to a minimum, replacing drapes with blinds, vacuuming weekly using a vacuum with a HEPA filter and installing HEPA air filters can be beneficial. In addition, washing dogs twice a week may help, but washing cats does not reduce allergen levels significantly.

For pollen and outdoor mold sensitivity, we recommended checking pollen counts and staying indoors when the counts are high. We also recommend keeping home and car windows closed, using air conditioners to filter the air, and showering before bed to remove allergens from hair and skin to help reduce contamination of the bedding.

Pharmacotherapy

The most effective single therapy for patients with rhinitis is an intranasal corticosteroid spray (Bousquet et al. 2019). Other therapies include oral antihistamines, antihistamine nasal sprays, oral decongestants, mast cell stabilizers, leukotriene modifiers and nasal anticholinergics. These medication categories will be briefly reviewed (Table 8.4). Further details are found in Chapter 14: Pharmacotherapy of Rhinitis and Asthma. Nasal decongestants and systemic corticosteroids should be avoided due to potential deleterious side effects.

Intranasal corticosteroids are the most effective single maintenance therapy for allergic and nonallergic rhinitis. They are effective in controlling the four major symptoms of rhinitis, namely sneezing, itching, rhinorrhea and nasal congestion. They have an onset of action of a few hours, but their maximal effect may require several days or weeks. When used correctly (directed away from the septum) and at the recommended doses, they cause few side effects. The first-generation agents are beclomethasone, flunisolide, triamcinolone and budesonide while the second-generation agents (lower systemic bioavailability) are fluticasone propionate, mometasone furoate, fluticasone furoate, and ciclesonide (Table 8.5.). In most countries, these agents are available without a prescription.

The most common side effects, burning or stinging, are due to local irritation and is more commonly associated with alcohol or propylene glycol-containing solutions. Nasal biopsies after five years of continuous therapy found no signs of tissue atrophy or change. Nasal septal perforations are very rare. Growth in children should be monitored, especially when intranasal corticosteroids are taken with other corticosteroids preparations such as inhaled corticosteroids for asthma or topical corticosteroids for atopic dermatitis.

Oral antihistamines can reduce itching, sneezing and rhinorrhea, but with less impact on nasal congestion compared with intranasal corticosteroids. They are divided into first- and second-generation agents. Second-generation antihistamines are preferred and even mandated in some segments of the transportation industry over first-generation antihistamines due to fewer unwanted anticholinergic and central nervous system effects. Onset of action is within one hour for most agents and peak serum levels are attained in two to three hours. The commonly used agents and their respective dosage are listed in Table 8.6. Clinical experience and limited clinical studies suggest that they not as effective in the treatment of nonallergic rhinitis.

Intranasal antihistamines (Table 8.7), in contrast to oral antihistamines, possess anti-inflammatory effects and may help improve nasal congestion. Furthermore, unlike intranasal corticosteroids, intranasal antihistamines (azelastine and olopatadine) have a rapid onset of action (less than 15 minutes) and can be administered 'on demand'. Thus, these agents can be used for the symptoms of both allergic and nonallergic rhinitis. The combination of an intranasal antihistamine with an intranasal corticosteroid appears to confer greater efficacy than either agent used alone (Berger and Meltzer 2015). A combination spray containing azelastine and fluticasone propionate is commercially available under the brand name Dymista.

Oral decongestants such as pseudoephedrine and phenylephrine can reduce nasal congestion caused by both allergic and nonallergic rhinitis. However, they do not possess anti-inflammatory properties and are generally not effective in the treatment of other symptoms. Furthermore, decongestants can have a variety of adverse effects, including hypertension, insomnia, irritability and headache. They are relatively contraindicated in patients with hypertension, and should be used with caution in patients with closed angle glaucoma, cardiovascular or cerebrovascular disease, hyperthyroidism or bladder neck obstruction.

Cromolyn sodium is a mast cell stabilizer (Table 8.8), which prevents mast cells from releasing histamine. It has no serious side effects and is available over-the-counter as a nasal spray. However, most studies show it to be less effective than intranasal corticosteroids, intranasal antihistamines and even second-generation oral antihistamines. In addition, compliance is hampered by its short duration of

Table 8.4. Efficacy profile of pharmacologic agents.

Agent	Eye Symptoms	Itching	Sneezing	Rhinorrhea	Congestion
Intranasal corticosteroids	+	++	++	++	++
Oral antihistamines	++	++	++	++	-
Intranasal antihistamines	-	++	++	++	+
Oral decongestants	-	-	-	-	+
Intranasal mast cell stabilizers	-	+	+	+	+
Leukotriene modifiers	+/-	+/-	+/-	+/-	+/-
Intranasal anticholinergics	-	-	-	++	-
Intranasal decongestants	-	-	-	-	++

- = provides no benefit
+/- = provides little or minimal benefit
+ = provides modest benefit
++ = provides substantial benefit

Table 8.5. Intranasal corticosteroids.

Generic Drug Name	Adult Dosage	Children Dosage
Beclomethasone dipropionate (42 mcg/spray)	1–2 sprays in each nostril twice daily	6–12 years: Intially 1 spray in each nostril twice daily, may increase to 2 sprays in each nostril twice daily; once symptoms are adequately controlled, decrease to 1 spray in each nostril twice daily. 12 years and older: same as adult dosing.
Budesonide (32 mcg/spray)	2 sprays in each nostril twice daily; once control is achieved, may decrease to 1 spray in each nostril once daily	6 years and older: same as adults.
Flunisolide (25 mcg/spray)	2 sprays in each nostril twice daily; may increase to 2 sprays in each nostril 3–4 times daily (maximum of 8 sprays in each nostril per day).	6–14 years: 1 spray in each nostril 3 times daily or 2 sprays in each nostril twice daily (maximum of 4 sprays in each nostril per day) 14 years and older: same as adults.
Fluticasone propionate (50 mcg/spray)	2 sprays in each nostril once daily or 1 spray in each nostril twice daily	4 years and older: 1 spray in each nostril once daily (can increase to 2 sprays in each nostril once daily, but once adequate control is achieved, decrease back to 1 spray in each nostril once daily). 12 years and older: same as adults.
Fluticasone furoate (27.5 mcg/spray)	2 sprays in each nostril once daily; once symptoms are adequately controlled, may reduce to 1 spray in each nostril once daily.	2–11 years: 1 spray in each nostril once daily (can increase to 2 sprays in each nostril once daily, but once adequate control is achieved, decrease back to 1 spray in each nostril once daily). 12 years and older: same as adults.
Mometasone furoate monohydrate (50 mcg/spray)	2 sprays in each nostril once daily; once symptoms are adequately controlled, may reduce to 1 spray in each nostril once daily.	2–11 years: 1 spray in each nostril once daily. 12 years and older: same as adults.
Triamcinolone acetonide (55 mcg/spray)	2 sprays in each nostril once daily; once symptoms are adequately controlled, may reduce to 1 spray in each nostril once daily.	2–5 years: 1 spray in each nostril once daily. 6–11 years: 1 spray in each nostril once daily (can increase to 2 sprays in each nostril once daily, but once adequate control is achieved, decrease back to 1 spray in each nostril once daily). 12 years and older: same as adults.
Ciclesonide (50 mcg/spray)	2 sprays in each nostril once daily	6 years and older: same as adults.

Table 8.6. Oral second-generation antihistamines.

Generic Drug Name	Adult Dosage	Children Dosage
Fexofenadine	60 mg twice daily or 180 mg once daily	6 months to less than 2 years: 15 mg twice daily 2–11 years: 30 mg twice daily 12 years and older: same as adults
Loratadine	10 mg once daily	2–5 years: 5 mg once daily 6 years and older: same as adults
Desloratadine	5 mg once daily	6–11 months: 1 mg once daily 12 months to 5 years: 1.25 mg once daily 6–11 years: 2.5 mg once daily 12 years and older: same as adults
Cetirizine	5–10 mg once daily	12 months to less than 2 years: 2.5 mg once daily; may increase to 2.5 mg every 12 hours if needed 2–5 years: start with 2.5 mg once daily; may increase to 5 mg once daily or 2.5 mg every 12 hours if needed 6–11 years: same as adults
Levocetirizine	2.5–5 mg once daily (in the evening)	6 months to less than 6 years: 1.25 mg once daily (in the evening) 6–11 years: 2.5 mg once daily (in the evening) 12 years and older: same as adult dosing

Table 8.7. Intranasal antihistamines.

Generic Drug Name	Adult Dosage	Children Dosage
Azelastine	0.1%: 1–2 sprays (137 mcg/spray) in each nostril twice daily 0.15%: 1–2 sprays (205.5 mcg/spray) once daily.	0.1%: 1 spray in each nostril once daily for 5–11 years; for 12 years and older, dosage is same as adults 0.15%: for 12 years and older, dosage is same as adults
Olopatadine 0.6%	2 sprays in each nostril (665 mcg/100 microliter spray) twice daily.	6–11 years: 1 spray in each nostril twice daily 12 years and older: same as adults

Table 8.8. Intranasal mast cell stabilizer.

Generic Drug Name	Adult Dosage	Children Dosage
Cromolyn Sodium	One spray (5.2 mg/spray) in each nostril 3–4 times/ day (every 4–6 hours); may increase up to 6 times/day (maximum dose: 1 spray in each nostril 6 times/day, symptomatic relief may require 2–4 weeks)	2 years and older: same as adults

action, which necessitates topical administration up to six times daily. Studies of intranasal chromones in the treatment of nonallergic rhinitis are lacking.

Of the three available leukotriene modifiers, only montelukast is approved for the treatment of allergic rhinitis. However, its efficacy is inferior to that of intranasal corticosteroids and antihistamines (Bousquet et al. 2019). A previous meta-analysis suggested that montelukast reduced total nasal symptom score by a mere 3.4% when compared with a placebo (Grainger and Drake-Lee 2006). In addition, there are no data to support the addition of montelukast to nasal corticosteroid or intranasal antihistamine sprays. Also, studies of montelukast in the treatment of nonallergic rhinitis are lacking. Although the overall safety profile of leukotriene agents is good, neuropsychiatric changes have been reported in association with montelukast, including dream abnormalities, insomnia, anxiety, depression, thinking of suicide and in rare cases, suicide. It is therefore important to advise patients to stop the medication if they perceive adverse mood effects.

Ipratropium bromide nasal spray is an anticholinergic that is specifically useful for decreasing rhinorrhea in both allergic and nonallergic rhinitis. It is less effective for the treatment of other symptoms.

Intranasal decongestants include phenylephrine, oxymetazoline, xylometazoline and naphazoline. Although available over-the-counter, they are not meant to be used as monotherapy or for long-term use, as downregulation of alpha-adrenergic receptor develops after 3 to 7 days, and can result in rebound nasal congestion. In contrast, the combination of a topical nasal decongestant and topical corticosteroid may effectively treat symptoms without causing rhinitis medicamentosa.

Short courses (3–7 days) of oral corticosteroids may be appropriate for severe or intractable nasal symptoms that prevent the patient from sleeping or working. However, they should not be given repeatedly or for prolonged periods of time. Moreover, the administration of parenteral corticosteroids is discouraged because of unpredictable absorption and the inability to adjust the dose, if side effects occur.

Allergen immunotherapy

Allergen immunotherapy (AIT) alters the immune system's reaction to causative allergens and induces long-lasting tolerance to these allergens. In patients with allergic rhinitis, AIT has been shown to not only reduce the risk of developing asthma, but also to help prevent *de novo* allergic sensitizations. AIT is therefore indicated for patients with allergic rhinitis who have (a) severe symptoms; (b) a poor response to medications; (c) comorbid atopic conditions; (d) a desire to prevent worsening of their disease; or (e) a desire to prevent the onset of asthma. AIT can be given sublingually (SLIT) or subcutaneously (SCIT). Selection of the patient's immunotherapy extract should be based on a correlation between the presence of allergen-specific IgE antibodies (demonstrated by skin testing or *in vitro* testing) and the patient's clinical history (Cox et al. 2011). The typical duration of therapy is 3–5 years. Long-lasting benefits are generally observed for many years after the discontinuation of treatment. A more detailed discussion on allergen immunotherapy is found in Chapter 15: Allergen Immunotherapy.

Summary

Although rhinitis is not life-threatening, it can significantly impact one's quality of life and is responsible for loss of work and school productivity. Chronic rhinitis may also contribute to fatigue, sleep disorders and learning difficulties. The task for the clinician involves differentiating between allergic and nonallergic rhinitis through history-taking, physical examination and skin testing, formulating patient-specific allergen avoidance strategies, prescribing appropriate pharmacotherapy, and when suitable, initiating allergen immunotherapy. Skin testing and allergen-specific IgE testing results should always be interpreted in the context of the clinical history to determine relevance.

References

Berger WE, Meltzer EO. Intranasal spray medications for maintenance therapy of allergic rhinitis. Am J Rhinol Allergy 2015; 29: 273–282.

Bousquet J, Schünemann HJ, Togias A, Bachert C, Erhola M, Hellings PW, et al. Next-generation Allergic Rhinitis and Its Impact on Asthma (ARIA) guidelines for allergic rhinitis based on Grading of Recommendations Assessment, Development and Evaluation (GRADE) and real-world evidence. J Allergy Clin Immunol 2019, article in press.

Braunstahl GJ. United Airways Concept: What does it teach us about systemic inflammation in airways disease? Proc Am Thorac Soc 2009; 8: 652–654.

Brożek JL, Bousquet J, Agache I, Agarwal A, Bachert C, Bosnic-Anticevich S, et al. Allergic Rhinitis and its Impact on Asthma (ARIA) guidelines—2016 revision. J Allergy Clin Immunol 2017; 140: 950–958.

Cox L, Nelson H, Lockey R, Calabria C, Chacko T, Finegold I, et al. Allergen immunotherapy: A practice parameter third update. J Allergy Clin Immunol 2011; 127: S1–S55.

Denburg JA, Sehmi R, Saito H, Pil-Seob J, Inman MD, O'Byrne PM. Systemic aspects of allergic disease: bone marrow responses. J Allergy Clin Immunol 2000; 106: S242–246.

Grainger J, Drake-Lee A. Montelukast in allergic rhinitis: a systematic review and meta-analysis. Clin Otolaryngol 2006; 5: 360–367.

Ku M, Silverman B, Prifti N, Ying W, Persaud Y, Schneider A. Prevalence of migraine headaches in patients with allergic rhinitis. Ann Allergy Asthma Immunol 2016; 97: 226–30.

Kulig M, Klettke U, Wahn V, Forster J, Bauer CP, Wahn U, et al. Development of seasonal allergic rhinitis during the first 7 years of life. J Allergy Clin Immunol 2000; 106: 832–839.

Lieberman P, Pattanaik D. Nonallergic rhinitis. Curr Allergy Asthma Rep 2014; 14: 439.

Phipatanakul W, Matsui E, Portnoy J, Williams PB, Barnes C, Kennedy K, et al. Environmental assessment and exposure reduction of rodents: a practice parameter. Ann Allergy Asthma Immunol 2012; 109: 375–387.

Portnoy J, Kennedy K, Sublett J, Phipatanakul W, Matsui E, Barnes C, et al. Environmental assessment and exposure control: a practice parameter–furry animals. Ann Allergy Asthma Immunol 2012; 108: 223.e1–15.

Portnoy J, Miller JD, Williams PB, Chew GL, Miller JD, Zaitoun F, et al. Environmental assessment and exposure control of dust mites: a practice parameter. Ann Allergy Asthma Immunol 2013a; 111: 465–507.

Portnoy J, Chew GL, Phipatanakul W, Williams PB, Grimes C, Kennedy K, et al. Environmental assessment and exposure reduction of cockroaches: A practice parameter. J Allergy Clin Immunol 2013b; 132: 802–808.

Szeinbach SL, Williams PB, Kucukarslan S, Elhefni H. Influence of patient care provider on patient health outcomes in allergic rhinitis. Ann Allergy Asthma Immunol 2005; 95: 167–74.

Wallace, D.V., M.S. Dykewicz, D.I. Bernstein, J. Blessing-Moore, L. Cox, D.A. Khan, et al. The diagnosis and management of rhinitis: an updated practice parameter. J Allergy Clin Immunol 2008; 122: S1–84.

9

Chronic Rhinosinusitis, Nasal Polyps and Aspirin Exacerbated Respiratory Disease

Farshad N Chowdhury[1] and *Todd T Kingdom*[2,*]

INTRODUCTION

Chronic Rhinosinusitis (CRS)

- CRS is a highly prevalent disease, affecting over 15% of the US population and accounting for a significant patient and health-care economic burden with over US $8.6 billion in direct costs (Bhattacharyya 2011, Hamilos 2011).
- Quality Of Life (QOL) impairments in CRS patients are comparable in severity to disease states such as congestive heart failure, chronic obstructive pulmonary disease and chronic low back pain leading to significant lost productivity (Gliklich and Metson 1995, Bhattacharyya 2009, Sahlstrand-Johnson et al. 2011, Soler et al. 2011, Stankiewicz et al. 2011, Rudmik et al. 2014).
- The diagnosis of CRS is made by history, physical examination, nasal endoscopy or CT scan as shown in Table 9.1 (Rosenfeld et al. 2007).
- CRS is a complex, multifactorial disease where the structural host, environmental and infectious factors combine to produce a disorder of sustained inflammation falling within neutrophilic (T helper 1, Th1), eosinophilic (T helper 2, Th2) or mixed inflammatory endotypes (Akdis et al. 2013). The etiologic factors for CRS are listed in Table 9.2.
- Surgery can provide measurable benefits in appropriately selected patients and surgical goals vary by CRS subtype (i.e., with or without nasal polyps). Surgery is rarely a 'cure' and continued medical management in the postoperative setting is generally required (Rudmik et al. 2016, Patel et al. 2017).

---

[1] Department of Otolaryngology-Head and Neck Surgery, University of Colorado School of Medicine, Aurora, Colorado. USA, Email: farshad.chowdhury@cuanschutz.edu
[2] Department of Otolaryngology-Head and Neck Surgery, University of Colorado School of Medicine & National Jewish Health Denver. Colorado USA.
* Corresponding author: todd.kingdom@cuanschutz.edu

Table 9.1. Diagnostic criteria for CRS, which requires both symptoms and objective evidence of disease (Orlandi et al. 2016).

Twelve or More Weeks of:		
Two or More Symptoms	AND	**One or More Findings**
Nasal congestion		Sinus inflammation on CT Scan or exam
Nasal obstruction		Nasal Endoscopy with Purulence
Facial pain/pressure/fullness		
Purulent discharge		
Hyposmia/Anosmia		

Table 9.2. Etiologic factors in CRS. (Adapted from Kennedy DW and Ramakrishnan VR. Functional Endoscopic Sinus Surgery: Concepts, Surgical Indications, and Techniques. Chapter in: *Rhinology: Diseases of the Nose, Sinuses and Skull Base*; Editors Kennedy and Hwang. Thieme 2012.)

Environmental Factors	Local Host Factors	Systemic Host Factors
Smoking	Anatomic abnormality	Atopy
Pollution	Persistent local inflammation	Mucosal hyperreactivity
Allergens	Biofilms	Immune deficiency
Viruses	Osteitis	Ciliary dysfunction
Bacteria	Obstructing lesion	Cystic Fibrosis
Fungi	Granulomatous disease	Stress

Nasal polyps

- Nasal polyps are found in a subset of patients with CRS (CRSwNP) (Fig. 9.1). The majority of CRSwNP patients demonstrate a Th2 pattern of inflammation, though atopic patients are not definitively at increased risk for development of nasal polyps as the association between atopy and nasal polyposis is unclear. However, CRS patients with asthma are more likely to have nasal polyps than those without asthma.
- Multiple inflammatory mechanisms are implicated in the development of nasal polyps. Th2-mediated inflammation and eosinophilic disease is most usually present, however Th1-mediated pathways and neutrophilic disease predominate in some patients. Overall, the inflammatory processes are likely to exist on a spectrum and emerging evidence also supports the notion of regional variations in inflammatory endotypes (Wang et al. 2016, Gurrola and Borish 2017). As a result, subgroups of CRSwNP patients may respond to different medications.
- Steroids—systemic and/or topical—are the mainstay of medical therapy for nasal polyps.
- CRSwNP patients often continue to have symptoms despite aggressive medical therapies and may benefit from surgical intervention. Surgery itself is not curative, but is often a useful adjunct to medical therapy.

Aspirin Exacerbated Respiratory Disease (AERD)

- Aspirin Exacerbated Respiratory Disease (AERD), also known as aspirin-sensitive asthma or Samter's triad, is characterized by the clinical tetrad of aspirin sensitivity, asthma, nasal polyps and eosinophilia. Aspirin/NSAID ingestion triggers acute upper and lower airway reactions.
- The resulting pro-inflammatory state results in upper and lower airway remodeling. Chronic rhinosinusitis with nasal polyps (CRSwNP) is an upper airway manifestation of AERD.

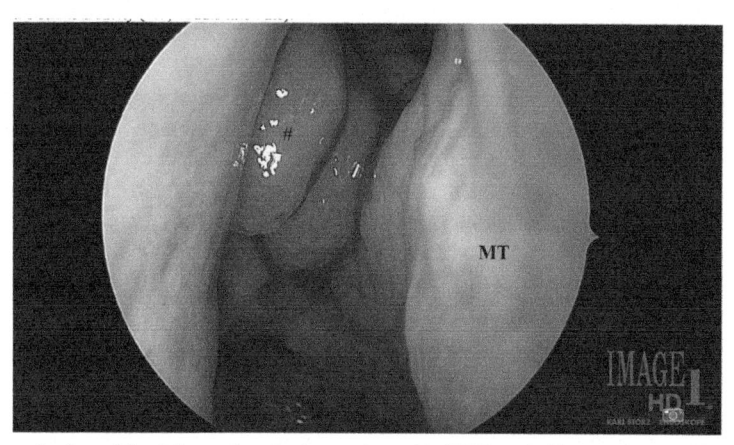

Figure 9.1. Endoscopic view of the right nasal cavity in a patient with AERD and a history of previous sinus surgery. Polyp recureence (#) is clearly visible in the ethmoid cavity (IT inferior turbinate, MT Middle turbinate).

- The disorder is most often diagnosed clinically and is confirmed with an observed aspirin challenge (White and Stevenson 2018).
- Disease in these patients is often refractory to medical therapies, causing progressive asthma symptoms and rapid polyp recurrence after surgical intervention in some.
- The incidence of aspirin sensitivity in the general population ranges from 0.6–2.5%, and can affect up to 10% of all patients with asthma and 24% of patients with severe asthma (Moloney 1977, Pfaar and Klimek 2006). AERD affects 9.7% of patients with CRSwNP (Rajan et al. 2015). In aspirin-sensitive asthmatics, nasal polyps are found in 36–96% of patients (Larsen 1996).
- AERD is more frequent in men than women, and generally presents with an adult onset at an average age of 30 years. A classic history begins with the appearance of rhinorrhea and congestion, possibly associated with an upper respiratory infection and subsequent development of nasal polyps. Nasal and sinus symptoms frequently present first, with later onset of asthma and aspirin sensitivity. Intolerance to other Non Steroidal Anti-inflammatory Drugs (NSAIDs) may be present, and ingestion of aspirin or NSAIDS results in an asthma exacerbation that is usually accompanied by nasal congestion and rhinorrhea (Asad et al. 1984).
- Alterations in the eicosanoid pathway are hypothesized to mediate this dysfunctional reaction. Normally cyclooxygenase (COX)-1 and COX-2 maintain homeostasis through prostaglandin E_2 (PGE_2). A baseline state of inflammation exists in AERD patients in which COX-2-dependent PGE_2 production is compromised and COX-1-mediated PGE_2 production is required for homeostasis. When COX-1 is inhibited by aspirin and other NSAIDs, loss of PGE_2 leads to increased cysteinyl leukotriene (e.g., LTC_4)-mediated airway obstruction as well as recruitment of TH2-type effector cells by cysteinyl leukotrienes, interleukin-22 and prostaglandin D_2 (Laidlaw and Boyce 2016).

Medical management

- Medical therapies are central to the management of CRS with and without nasal polyps.
- Corticosteroids are the mainstay of medical therapy for airway inflammation, particularly in the setting of eosinophilia. Regular use of intranasal steroids has been shown to decrease mucosal eosinophilia, reduce polyp size and improve sinonasal symptoms (Mastalerz et al. 1997, Ogata et al. 1999, Nores et al. 2003).
- The use of anti-leukotriene therapy in the management of CRSwNP is an off-label treatment option used by some clinicians as an adjunct to glucocorticoid therapy. Recent meta-analyses and consensus statements support the use of leukotriene modifying drugs as an optional agent in treating CRSwNP in AERD patients based on improvement in symptoms and limited objective measures of disease

(Orlandi et al. 2016, Beswick et al. 2017). However, additional studies to clarify the cost-benefit as well as the degree and stability of therapeutic benefit is needed.

- Biologic agents consist of monoclonal antibodies targeting selected components of the inflammatory pathway. Dupilumab (anti-interleukin-4/anti-interleukin-13) is the only biologic agent thus far with US Food and Drug Administration (FDA) approval as a treatment for CRSwNP. Other agents have demonstrated reductions in symptom scores and measures of polyp size in small, short-term trials. Omalizumab (anti-IgE), Mepolizumab (anti-interleukin-5) and Reslizumab (anti-interleukin-5) have shown promise in this regard and several phase III trials are underway. In addition to the need for Phase III level evidence for the use of these agents, high cost, need for subcutaneous injection and the risk for anaphylaxis have limited the widespread adoption of these biologic agents (Beswick et al. 2017, Hopkins 2019).

- Aspirin desensitization is recommended for CRSwNP with AERD following surgery. Though the reported desensitization regimen is variable in published literature, high quality evidence supports the use of aspirin desensitization to reduce polyp recurrence and number of surgical revisions, reduce the need for other medications and improve quality of life scores (Orlandi et al. 2016, White and Stevenson 2018, Chu et al. 2019).

- In CRSwNP patients as a whole, continued symptoms despite appropriate use of medical therapies merits the consideration of surgical intervention. Surgery may consist of simple polypectomy or progressively more thorough techniques such as Endoscopic Sinus Surgery (ESS) or rarely nasalization (Table 9.3).

Table 9.3. Endoscopic Sinus Surgery (ESS) techniques.

Polypectomy	Removal of obstructing nasal polyps, does not address underlying sinus tissues.
Endoscopic sinus surgery (ESS)	Mucosal preservation, removal of diseased sinus tissue and bone, possible enlargement of natural ostia.
Nasalization (Radical Sphenoethmoidectomy)	Middle turbinectomy, total ethmoidectomy with mucosal removal.
Minimally invasive surgical technique (MIST)	Enlarging transition spaces without manipulation of ostia. Does not treat nasal polyps.
Balloon Sinus Surgery	Balloon catheter used to dilate transition spaces and ostia without tissue removal. Does not treat nasal polyps.

Surgical management of CRS and nasal polyps

- Endoscopic sinus surgery (ESS) remains the treatment of choice for medically refractory CRS with and without nasal polyposis. Since its introduction in the 1980s, ESS has undergone substantial technical refinement with recent outcome studies firmly supporting its efficacy. When considering a wide range of patient subgroups, overall success rates have been reported to range from 85 to 97% (Levine 1990, Kennedy 1992, Senior et al. 1998, Metson and Gliklich 2000, Poetkar and Smith 2007b).

- It has been suggested in the past that the presence of nasal polyps is predictive of worse surgical outcome and poor response to therapy. Recent reports in the literature, however, have re-examined this issue.

- Published prospective data has demonstrated the benefits of ESS in patients with and without nasal polyps (Ragab et al. 2004, Smith et al. 2005). Poetker et al. reported on the subjective and objective outcomes of 43 polyp and 76 non-polyp patients undergoing ESS (Poetker et al. 2007a). In this study all the patients, regardless of polyp status, had significant improvement in both subjective and objective parameters. Notably, patients with polyps showed a greater degree of improvement than patients without polyps despite worse pre-operative and post-operative CT and endoscopy scores.

Polypectomy

- Polypectomy refers to the removal of obstructing nasal polyps from the nasal cavity. This may be performed in the clinic setting under local anesthesia or in the operating room under general anesthesia. The goal of polypectomy is to restore patency to the nasal airway without incurring risks of more aggressive surgery such as extended time under general anesthesia, significant bleeding, injury to the orbit or penetration of the skull base.
- A retrospective review of 101 patients with AERD who underwent polypectomy showed improvements in the nasal airway one-year after the procedure in 60% of patients (Brown et al. 1979). In the same study, asthma status one-year after polypectomy was subjectively improved in 30%, worse in 14%, and unchanged in the remainder.
- Another early study demonstrated benefit of polypectomy on asthma in AERD patients (English 1986). In this retrospective review of 205 suspected AERD patients, surgeries such as polypectomy with or without ethmoidectomy, Caldwell-Luc and Caldwell-Luc antral fat obliteration were performed. Decreased prednisone use was noted in all but the most severe asthma patients.
- Because the underlying ethmoid sinuses are not addressed, quick regrowth of nasal polyps is known to occur after simple polypectomy (Hosemann 2000, Masterson et al. 2010).

Endoscopic Sinus Surgery (ESS)

- The ESS technique stresses mucosal preservation and complete dissection of the involved sinuses, including removal of bony partitions and inflammatory foci, as well as identification and possible enlargement of sinus ostia (Kennedy et al. 1985). This technique is the most widely used for CRS and CRSwNP, and most current studies are performed using this technique.
- Most complete ESS cases are performed under general anesthesia and risks of complications such as severe hemorrhage, injury to the orbit and penetration of the skull base are exceedingly rare (Ramakrishnan et al. 2012).
- The more complete surgical dissection is thought to address the underlying disease of ethmoid cells, improve sinus ventilation, improve mucociliary clearance and significantly improve postoperative topical drug distribution within the sinuses (Senior et al. 1998, Wormald et al. 2004, Harvey et al. 2008).
- A number of studies have documented benefits of ESS on the lower airway in patients with chronic rhinosinusitis and asthma (Nishioka et al. 1994, Dunlop et al. 1999, Uri et al. 2002). Several retrospective analyses of polyp patients undergoing ESS have compared aspirin-sensitive to aspirin-tolerant patients and found ESS to have improved sinus and asthma symptoms, improved nasal endoscopy scores, improved FEV1 and decreased use of inhaled corticosteroids in both groups (Smith et al. 2005, Awad et al. 2008a, Awad et al. 2008b).
- AERD patients were compared to CRSwNP patients with Aspirin-Tolerant Asthma (ATA) in three retrospective ESS studies. In two large cohorts, AERD patients were found to have more improvement in nasal endoscopy scores, larger improvement in asthma severity scores and less need for inhaled corticosteroids than their ATA counterpart (Smith et al. 2005, Awad et al. 2008a).
- However, these results may not last as long as they do in ATA polyp patients. When measured by CT scan, only 63% of AERD patients had persistent improvement when compared to 96% of ATA patients (Awad et al. 2008a).
- Long-term asthma outcomes were assessed by a survey of 65 patients with AERD who underwent ESS, with a mean 10-year follow-up (Loehrl et al. 2006). Out of 34 respondents, 29 (94%) of patients with asthma preoperatively noticed a subjective asthma improvement at 1-year postoperatively. Improvements were also noted in use of oral and inhaled steroids, frequency of asthma attacks, frequency of physician visits for asthma-related concerns and hospitalizations for asthma exacerbations.

- ESS in patients with CRS is known to have long-lasting benefits if performed in a thorough and meticulous manner in appropriately selected patients (Senior et al. 1998).

Nasalization or radical ethmoidectomy

- Nasalization surgery includes radial sphenoethmoidectomy, including resection of the middle turbinate and removal of associated mucosa.
- With this technique, Jankowski and colleagues retrospectively compared polyp recurrence in 39 patients who underwent the nasalization procedure to 37 patients who underwent FESS (Jankowski et al. 1997). They found an overall functional benefit greater than in the more conservative ESS group, as documented by improved symptom, asthma, endoscopy and CT scores, as well as decreased use of systemic steroids. A follow-up study showed over a 50% reduction in polyp recurrence rate with those undergoing more aggressive surgery at 5-years postoperatively, implying that radical surgery is more likely to have improved symptoms over a longer course (Jankowski et al. 2006).
- The retrospective nature of these studies with a heterogeneous polyp population (some asthma, unclear AERD) and non-standardized postoperative medical regimens have led to reservations in adopting such an aggressive surgical technique.
- Although this procedure has not been widely accepted in general surgical practice, it nonetheless does support the notion that more aggressive surgery may have longer lasting results.

Specific outcomes measurements

Symptoms

- Measuring outcomes with chronic rhinosinusitis has been challenging for many years, and only recently have a number of validated, rhinology-specific, patient-based Quality Of Life (QOL) measurements become commonly used. As a result, many older studies have irregular and/or poorly-supported methodologies for measurements of disease severity and outcomes after intervention (Smith 2004). Many of these studies employed irregular and subjective outcomes, such as time to recurrence of disease or time to revision surgery.
- CRS patients suffer from a number of symptoms—namely nasal congestion, fatigue, headache, decreased sense of smell and nasal drainage. In a prospective study of medical management for CRS, modest gains were demonstrated in all domains except headaches (Hessler et al. 2007). In a recent systematic review and meta-analysis, sinus surgery demonstrates universal improvement in quality of life outcomes measured by the validated Sino-Nasal Outcome Test (SNOT-22), though the degree of improvement varies with the patient and disease factors (Soler et al. 2018).
- A landmark multi-institutional prospective study comparing the results of continued medical therapy versus surgery in CRS patients who failed initial medical management found significantly better symptoms control, less medication usage and fewer missed work/school days in the group who underwent surgery (Smith et al. 2013). A recent systematic review with meta-analysis also demonstrates improvement in both objective endoscopic scores and subjective quality of life measures in patients with medically refractory CRS who undergo surgery when compared to continued medical therapy alone (Patel et al. 2017).
- Special attention should be given to the sense of smell and nasal polyps, although this is an area of relatively little data. In a prospective study of CRS patients undergoing FESS, the Smell Identification Test (SIT) was performed preoperatively, and at 6- and 12-months postoperatively (Litvack et al. 2009). The authors found that patients with severe olfactory dysfunction had significant improvements with surgery, whereas those with more mild dysfunction did not. Patients with nasal polyps, asthma and/or aspirin sensitivity were more likely to be anosmic preoperatively. Interestingly, anosmic patients with nasal polyps had significant improvement in smell after surgery, whereas anosmic nonpolyp patients did not.

- In early studies, it was thought that patients with AERD are more likely to have preoperative anosmia, which appeared less likely to resolve after surgery (Thomassin and Korchia 1991). In a more recent study utilizing the Sniffin' Sticks smell test on polyp patients who underwent FESS, the presence of AERD was found to significantly limit olfactory restoration when compared to ATA patients (Katotomichelakis et al. 2009).

Objective outcomes

- Recent investigations have stressed the importance of using an objective measurement of disease, in addition to subjective QOL outcome measurements, as the two may not always correlate. Objective measurements of disease include CT scan staging systems and nasal endoscopy scoring systems.
- When comparing CRSwNP and CRSsNP populations, polyp patients have worse disease preoperatively on both CT and nasal endoscopy scoring, not surprisingly (Poetker et al. 2007a). After ESS, polyp patients gained more significant improvements in the endoscopic score, but still remained worse than those without polyps.
- When specifically comparing AERD polyp patients to aspirin-tolerant polyp patients, AERD patients tend to have significantly worse preoperative CT and nasal endoscopy scores (Robinson et al. 2007). But after ESS, there was no difference between the two groups in their degree of improvement on nasal endoscopy at a mean follow-up of 18 months, suggesting that significant benefits can be obtained in AERD patients with surgery.

Effects on asthma

- As mentioned earlier, primary studies on polypectomy had moderate subjective benefits on asthma and postoperative oral steroid use.
- Subsequent rigorous studies using a more thorough surgical technique (ESS) have demonstrated sustained improvement in asthma symptoms, spirometry measurements, corticosteroid use and associated health-care expenditure (Ragab et al. 2006, Ehnhage et al. 2012, Schlosser et al. 2017, Cao et al. 2019).

Summary

Endoscopic Sinus Surgery (ESS) is safe and efficacious for patients with CRS, nasal polyps and AERD, although the degree and duration of benefit may differ between patient populations. Nonetheless, significant improvements are seen in subjective and objective measurements of both the upper and lower airway.

The majority of studies available for review consist of retrospective studies with small patient cohorts. Surgical technique has improved over time, making studies published before 2000—describing follow-up of patients operated on in the early 1990s—less comparable to surgeries performed in modern practice. Additionally, the postoperative medical management of these patients varies between studies. Clearly, continued medical treatment after sinus surgery appears to reduce the need for repeat operations, particularly in the setting of AERD.

There is sufficient evidence to conclude that medical therapies and surgery in those patients refractory to medical therapy, prove beneficial to AERD patients. Furthermore, there a growing body of evidence and experience that biological agents may play an important role in the management of this disease, however further studies are required before fully understanding the optimal use of the family of medications. In these patients, the approach to surgery may require careful consideration as an advanced stage or recalcitrant disease may be associated with variations in the usual sinonasal anatomy leading to a more challenging approach (Fig. 9.2). More extensive surgery leads to improved distribution of topical medications, and may have as-of-yet undefined effects on the pathophysiology of the disease (Jankowski et al. 1997, Snidvongs et al. 2012). Additional prospective, randomized, controlled studies

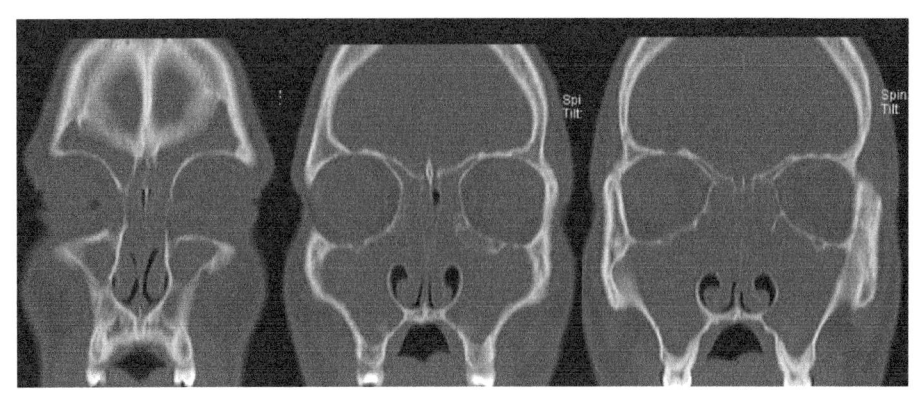

Figure 9.2. Coronal (left) and axial (right) CT scans of ethmoid mucocele. This patient was a 37 year old female with AERD and one previous surgery, who presented with recurrence of nasal obstruction and proptosis.

are necessary for examination of the additive benefits of emerging medical therapies (e.g., biological agents) in combination with the known benefits of surgery and postoperative maintenance therapy.

Conclusion

Our knowledge of CRS with and without nasal polyposis and in particular AERD, has advanced tremendously. Refinement in surgical technique and a deeper understanding of the pathophysiology have moved us beyond the time when polypectomy was believed to exacerbate or even induce asthma attacks (Francis 1928). The surgical management of nasal polyposis, including patients with AERD, has progressed from reluctance to perform surgery to the reliable expectation for measurable benefits with surgical management. Published data suggests that surgical intervention may lead to improved outcomes for both sino-nasal and asthma symptoms. Patients with AERD and nasal polyposis represent a complex cohort of patients that require multi-modality therapy for optimal control of upper and lower airway disease.

References

Akdis CA, Bachert C, Cingi C, Dykewicz MS, Hellings PW, Naclerio RM, et al. Endotypes and phenotypes of chronic rhinosinusitis: a PRACTALL document of the European Academy of Allergy and Clinical Immunology and the American Academy of Allergy, Asthma & Immunology. J Allergy Clin Immunol 2013; 131(6): 1479–1490.

Asad SI, Kemeny DM, Youlten LJ, Frankland AW, Lessof MH. Effect of aspirin in "aspirin sensitive" patients. Br Med J (Clin Res Ed) 1984; 288(6419): 745–748.

Awad OG, Fasano MB, Lee JH, Graham SM. Asthma outcomes after endoscopic sinus surgery in aspirin-tolerant versus apsirin-induced asthmatic patients. Am J Rhinol 2008a; 22(2): 197–203.

Awad OG, Lee JH, Fasano MB, Graham SM. Sinonasal outcomes after endoscopic sinus surgery in asthmatic patients with nasal polyps: a difference between aspirin-tolerant and aspirin-induced asthma? Laryngoscope 2008b; 118(7): 1282–1286.

Beswick DM, Gray ST, Smith TL. Pharmacological management of chronic rhinosinusitis: current and evolving treatments. Drugs 2017; 77(16): 1713–1721.

Bhattacharyya N. Contemporary assessment of the disease burden of sinusitis. American Journal of Rhinology & Allergy 2009; 23(4): 392–395.

Bhattacharyya N. Incremental health care utilization and expenditures for chronic rhinosinusitis in the United States. Annals of Otology, Rhinology & Laryngology 2011; 120(7): 423–427.

Brown BL, Harner SG, Van Dellen RG. Nasal polypectomy in patients with asthma and sensitivity to aspirin. Arch Otolaryngol 1979; 105(7): 413–416.

Cao Y, Hong H, Sun Y, Lai Y, Xu R, Shi J, et al. The effects of endoscopic sinus surgery on pulmonary function in chronic rhinosinusitis patients with asthma: a systematic review and meta-analysis. European Archives of Oto-Rhino-Laryngology 2019; 276(5): 1405–1411.

Chu DK, Lee DJ, Lee KM, Schunemann HJ, Szczeklik W, Lee JM et al. Benefits and harms of aspirin desensitization for aspirin-exacerbated respiratory disease: a systematic review and meta-analysis. Int Forum Allergy Rhinol 2019.

Dunlop G, Scadding GK, Lund VJ. The effect of endoscopic sinus surgery on asthma: management of patients with chronic rhinosinusitis, nasal polyposis, and asthma. Am J Rhinol 1999; 13(4): 261–265.

Ehnhage A, Olsson P, Kölbeck K-G, Skedinger M, Stjärne P. One year after endoscopic sinus surgery in polyposis:asthma, olfaction, and quality-of-life outcomes. Otolaryngology–Head and Neck Surgery 2012; 146(5): 834–841.

English GM. Nasal polypectomy and sinus surgery in patients with asthma and aspirin idiosyncrasy. Laryngoscope 1986; 96(4): 374–380.

Francis C. The prognosis of operations of nasal polypi in cases of asthma. Practitioner 1928; 123: 272–278.

Gliklich RE, Metson R. The health impact of chronic sinusitis in patients seeking otolaryngologic care. Otolaryngol Head Neck Surg 1995; 113(1): 104–109.

Gurrola J, Borish L. Chronic rhinosinusitis: Endotypes, biomarkers, and treatment response. Journal of Allergy and Clinical Immunology 2017; 140(6): 1499–1508.

Hamilos DL. Chronic rhinosinusitis: epidemiology and medical management. J Allergy Clin Immunol 2011; 128(4): 693–707; quiz 708–699.

Harvey RJ, Goddard JC, Wise SK, Schlosser RJ. Effects of endoscopic sinus surgery and delivery device on cadaver sinus irrigation. Otolaryngol Head Neck Surg 2008; 139(1): 137–142.

Hessler JL, Piccirillo JF, Fang D, Vlahiotis A, Banerji A, Levitt RG, et al. Clinical outcomes of chronic rhinosinusitis in response to medical therapy: results of a prospective study. Am J Rhinol 2007; 21(1): 10–18.

Hopkins C. Chronic rhinosinusitis with nasal polyps. N Engl J Med 2019; 381(1): 55–63.

Hosemann W. Surgical treatment of nasal polyposis in patients with aspirin intolerance. Thorax 2000; 55 Suppl 2: S87–90.

Jankowski R, Pigret D, Decroocq F. Comparison of functional results after ethmoidectomy and nasalization for diffuse and severe nasal polyposis. Acta Otolaryngol 1997; 117(4): 601–608.

Jankowski R, Pigret D, Decroocq F, Blum A, Gillet P. Comparison of radical (nasalisation) and functional ethmoidectomy in patients with severe sinonasal polyposis. A retrospective study. Rev Laryngol Otol Rhinol (Bord) 2006; 127(3): 131–140.

Katotomichelakis M, Riga M, Davris S, Tripsianis G, Simopoulou M, Nikolettos N, et al. Allergic rhinitis and aspirin-exacerbated respiratory disease as predictors of the olfactory outcome after endoscopic sinus surgery. Am J Rhinol Allergy 2009; 23(3): 348–353.

Kennedy DW, Zinreich SJ, Rosenbaum AE, Johns ME. Functional endoscopic sinus surgery. Theory and diagnostic evaluation. Arch Otolaryngol 1985; 111(9): 576–582.

Kennedy DW. Prognostic factors, outcomes and staging in ethmoid sinus surgery. Laryngoscope 1992; 102(12 Pt 2 Suppl 57): 1–18.

Laidlaw TM, Boyce JA. Aspirin-exacerbated respiratory disease—new prime suspects. N Engl J Med 2016; 374(5): 484–488.

Larsen K. The clinical relationship of nasal polyps to asthma. Allergy Asthma Proc 1996; 17(5): 243–249.

Levine HL. Functional endoscopic sinus surgery: evaluation, surgery, and follow-up of 250 patients. Laryngoscope 1990; 100(1): 79–84.

Litvack JR, Mace J, Smith TL. Does olfactory function improve after endoscopic sinus surgery? Otolaryngol Head Neck Surg 2009; 140(3): 312–319.

Loehrl TA, Ferre RM, Toohill RJ, Smith TL. Long-term asthma outcomes after endoscopic sinus surgery in aspirin triad patients. Am J Otolaryngol 2006; 27(3): 154–160.

Mastalerz L, Milewski M, Duplaga M, Nizankowska E, Szczeklik A. Intranasal fluticasone propionate for chronic eosinophilic rhinitis in patients with aspirin-induced asthma. Allergy 1997; 52(9): 895–900.

Masterson L, Tanweer F, Bueser T, Leong P. Extensive endoscopic sinus surgery: does this reduce the revision rate for nasal polyposis? Eur Arch Otorhinolaryngol 2010; 267(10): 1557–1561.

Metson RB, Gliklich RE. Clinical outcomes in patients with chronic sinusitis. Laryngoscope 2000; 110(3 Pt 3): 24–28.

Moloney JR. Nasal polyps, nasal polypectomy, asthma, and aspirin sensitivity. Their association in 445 cases of nasal polyps. J Laryngol Otol 1977; 91(10): 837–846.

Nishioka GJ, Cook PR, Davis WE, McKinsey JP. Functional endoscopic sinus surgery in patients with chronic sinusitis and asthma. Otolaryngol Head Neck Surg 1994; 110(6): 494–500.

Nores JM, Avan P, Bonfils P. Medical management of nasal polyposis: a study in a series of 152 consecutive patients. Rhinology 2003; 41(2): 97–102.

Ogata Y, Okinaka Y, Takahashi M. Detection of activated eosinophils in nasal polyps of an aspirin-induced asthma patient. Rhinology 1999; 37(1): 16–20.

Orlandi RR, Kingdom TT, Hwang PH, Smith TL, Alt JA, Baroody FM, et al. International Consensus Statement on Allergy and Rhinology: Rhinosinusitis. Int Forum Allergy Rhinol 2016; 6 Suppl 1: S22–209.

Patel ZM, Thamboo A, Rudmik L, Nayak JV, Smith TL, Hwang PH. Surgical therapy vs continued medical therapy for medically refractory chronic rhinosinusitis: a systematic review and meta-analysis. Int Forum Allergy Rhinol 2017; 7(2): 119–127.

Pfaar O, Klimek L. Eicosanoids, aspirin-intolerance and the upper airways—current standards and recent improvements of the desensitization therapy. J Physiol Pharmacol 2006; 57 Suppl 12: 5–13.

Poetker DM, Mendolia-Loffredo S, Smith TL. Outcomes of endoscopic sinus surgery for chronic rhinosinusitis associated with sinonasal polyposis. Am J Rhinol 2007a; 21(1): 84–88.

Poetker DM, Smith TL. Adult chronic rhinosinusitis: surgical outcomes and the role of endoscopic sinus surgery. Curr Opin Otolaryngol Head Neck Surg 2007b; 15(1): 6–9.

Ragab S, Scadding GK, Lund VJ, Saleh H. Treatment of chronic rhinosinusitis and its effects on asthma. European Respiratory Journal 2006; 28(1): 68–74.

Ragab SM, Lund VJ, Scadding G. Evaluation of the medical and surgical treatment of chronic rhinosinusitis: a prospective, randomised, controlled trial. Laryngoscope 2004; 114(5): 923–930.

Rajan JP, Wineinger NE, Stevenson DD, White AA. Prevalence of aspirin-exacerbated respiratory disease among asthmatic patients: A meta-analysis of the literature. J Allergy Clin Immunol 2015; 135(3): 676–681 e671.

Ramakrishnan VR, Kingdom TT, Nayak JV, Hwang PH, Orlandi RR. Nationwide incidence of major complications in endoscopic sinus surgery. Int Forum Allergy Rhinol 2012; 2(1): 34–39.

Robinson JL, Griest S, James KE, Smith TL. Impact of aspirin intolerance on outcomes of sinus surgery. Laryngoscope 2007; 117(5): 825–830.

Rosenfeld RM, Andes D, Bhattacharyya N, Cheung D, Eisenberg S, Ganiats TG, et al. Clinical practice guideline: adult sinusitis. Otolaryngol Head Neck Surg 2007; 137(3 Suppl): S1–31.

Rudmik L, Smith TL, Schlosser RJ, Hwang PH, Mace JC, Soler ZM. Productivity costs in patients with refractory chronic rhinosinusitis. Laryngoscope 2014; 124(9): 2007–2012.

Rudmik L, Soler ZM, Hopkins C, Schlosser RJ, Peters A, White AA, et al. Defining appropriateness criteria for endoscopic sinus surgery during management of uncomplicated adult chronic rhinosinusitis: a RAND/UCLA appropriateness study. Int Forum Allergy Rhinol 2016; 6(6): 557–567.

Sahlstrand-Johnson P, Ohlsson B, Von Buchwald C, Jannert M and Ahlner-Elmqvist M. A multi-centre study on quality of life and absenteeism in patients with CRS referred for endoscopic surgery. Rhinology 2011; 49(4): 420–428.

Schlosser RJ, Smith TL, Mace J, Soler ZM. Asthma quality of life and control after sinus surgery in patients with chronic rhinosinusitis. Allergy 2017; 72(3): 483–491.

Senior BA, Kennedy DW, Tanabodee J, Kroger H, Hassab M, Lanza D. Long-term results of functional endoscopic sinus surgery. Laryngoscope 1998; 108(2): 151–157.

Smith TL. Outcomes research in rhinology: chronic rhinosinusitis. ORL J Otorhinolaryngol Relat Spec 2004; 66(4): 202–206.

Smith TL, Mendolia-Loffredo S, Loehrl TA, Sparapani R, Laud PW, Nattinger AB. Predictive factors and outcomes in endoscopic sinus surgery for chronic rhinosinusitis. Laryngoscope 2005; 115(12): 2199–2205.

Smith TL, Kern R, Palmer JN, Schlosser R, Chandra RK, Chiu AG et al. 2013. Medical therapy vs surgery for chronic rhinosinusitis: a prospective, multi-institutional study with 1-year follow-up. Int Forum Allergy Rhinol 3(1): 4–9.

Snidvongs K, Pratt E, Chin D, Sacks R, Earls P, Harvey RJ. Corticosteroid nasal irrigations after endoscopic sinus surgery in the management of chronic rhinosinusitis. Int Forum Allergy Rhinol 2012; 2(5): 415–421.

Soler ZM, Wittenberg E, Schlosser RJ, Mace JC, Smith TL. Health state utility values in patients undergoing endoscopic sinus surgery. Laryngoscope 2011; 121(12): 2672–2678.

Soler ZM, Jones R, Le P, Rudmik L, Mattos JL, Nguyen SA, et al. Sino-Nasal outcome test-22 outcomes after sinus surgery: A systematic review and meta-analysis. 2018; 128(3): 581–592.

Stankiewicz J, Tami T, Truitt T, Atkins J, Winegar B, Cink P, et al. Impact of chronic rhinosinusitis on work productivity through one-year follow-up after balloon dilation of the ethmoid infundibulum. Int Forum Allergy Rhinol 2011; 1(1): 38–45.

Thomassin JM, Korchia D. [Nasosinusal polyposis. Indications. Results. Apropos of 222 ethmoidectomies]. Ann Otolaryngol Chir Cervicofac 1991; 108(8): 455–464.

Uri N, Cohen-Kerem R, Barzilai G, Greenberg E, Doweck I, Weiler-Ravell D. Functional endoscopic sinus surgery in the treatment of massive polyposis in asthmatic patients. J Laryngol Otol 2002; 116(3): 185–189.

Wang X, Zhang N, Bo M, Holtappels G, Zheng M, Lou H, et al. Diversity of TH cytokine profiles in patients with chronic rhinosinusitis: A multicenter study in Europe, Asia, and Oceania. Journal of Allergy and Clinical Immunology 2016; 138(5): 1344–1353.

White AA, Stevenson DD. Aspirin-exacerbated respiratory disease. N Engl J Med 2018; 379(23): 2281–2282.

Wormald PJ, Cain T, Oates L, Hawke L, Wong I. A comparative study of three methods of nasal irrigation. Laryngoscope 2004; 114(12): 2224–2227.

10

Allergic Diseases of the Eye

Andrew Braganza* and Alo Sen

INTRODUCTION

This chapter deals with the common forms of ocular surface allergies, affecting the conjunctiva and cornea. The conjunctiva is usually the primary tissue affected, with the cornea suffering secondary effects that can be sight threatening. Discomfort of the ocular surface is a much under-emphasized cause of decreased productivity in the workplace, and can even be life threatening for those involved in controlling heavy machinery. Understanding the condition and rational care can go a long way towards providing relief from symptoms.

Allergic conjunctivitis is extremely common; it is estimated that 15–20% of the adult population will have at least one episode of symptomatic allergic conjunctivitis per year. Some forms are highly seasonal, related to pollen release by plants or dust and mites. The ocular surface, being in direct contact with the external environment, can react directly and specifically to some antigens. There are also perennial forms of ocular surface allergy (Butrus and Portela 2005).

Diagnosis

The diagnosis of allergic conjunctivitis is clinical (Table 10.1). Itching is the characteristic and most prominent symptom, and is directly related to mast cell degranulation and histamine release. Redness, tearing, swelling of the eyes are other symptoms. Infectious forms of conjunctivitis and dry eye are the main differential diagnoses. These can be distinguished from allergies by the presence of discharge associated with infections and by the signs of deficient ocular surface wetting in the dry eye (Butrus and Portela 2005). It must be emphasized that the diagnosis is best left to an ophthalmologist. Thus, all patients with ocular symptoms should be referred to a specialist. As the condition is chronic and subject to periodic or seasonal exacerbations, the role of the primary care physician is to monitor and adjust treatment and refer to the specialist in the event of complications.

Allergic rhinitis is often associated with tearing, photophobia and some redness of the eyes. Itching is usually absent. This is generally considered a secondary effect of the nasal mucosal reaction and has been shown to have associated histamine release and activation of conjunctival eosinophils and mast cells, though with possibly different chemical mediators of inflammation (Pelikan 2012, 2013). Treatment of the rhinitis is generally successful in resolving the ocular symptoms, which may have proved refractory to the standard topical ocular medications. Allergic rhinitis is also common with some primary ocular

---

Department of Ophthalmology, Christian Medical College, Vellore, India, Email: alosen8281@hotmail.com
* Corresponding author: andrew@cmcvellore.ac.in

Table 10.1. Types of allergic conjunctivitis.

	Types of Conjunctivitis			
	Allergic conjunctivitis	Vernal Kerato-conjunctivitis	Atopic Kerato-conjunctivitis	Giant Papillary conjunctivitis
Chemosis	+	±	±	±
Large papillae	-	++	++	++
Discharge	Clear mucoid	Stringy mucoid	Stringy mucoid	Clear white
Eyelid Involvement	-	+	+	-
Lymph Node Swelling	-	-	-	-
Predominant Cell Type	Mast cell Eosinophil	Lymphocyte Eosinophil	Lymphocyte Eosinophil	Lymphocyte Eosinophil

+=Present; ± = may or may not be present; - = not present

allergies such as Vernal Keratoconjunctivitis (VKC), but each condition may manifest independently (Butrus and Portela 2005).

Giant papillary conjunctivitis is a special form of allergy that does not generally present with itching. There is a definite association with atopy, though the condition results from chronic mechanical insult usually by the use contact lens. Sandy and dusty environments are also presumed to be causative factors.

Classification of allergic conjunctivitis

- Seasonal Allergic Conjunctivitis (Fig. 10.1)
    - Most common form of allergic conjunctivitis
    - Usually concurrent with allergic rhinitis
    - Usually symptoms present bilaterally
    - Symptoms may include:
        - Tearing and itching
        - Burning or stinging
        - Bilateral ocular and periocular pruritus
        - Milky or pinkish conjunctiva
- Perennial Allergic Conjunctivitis (Fig. 10.2)
    - Less prevalent and with milder symptoms than those associated with seasonal allergic conjunctivitis
    - Sensitivity response to allergens present year round
- Atopic Keratoconjunctivitis (Figs. 10.3 and 10.4)
    - Symptoms may include:
        - Bilateral itching
        - Photophobia
        - Stringy, ropy or watery discharge
        - Redness, burning, tearing
        - Corneal vascularization, ulceration or scarring
        - Lower and upper tarsal conjunctiva exhibit papillary hypertrophy
    - Associated with atopic dermatitis of the face and eyelids
    - Onset usually late teens to early twenties
    - Patient history of allergy is very common (especially allergic rhinitis/ asthma)
- Vernal Keratoconjunctivitis (Figs. 10.5–10.9)
    - Most patients have a history of atopic disease, and/or allergy (especially allergic rhinitis/ asthma)
    - If left untreated, scarring can lead to vision loss
    - Usually occurs in childhood, most commonly seen in boys

Allergic Diseases of the Eye 101

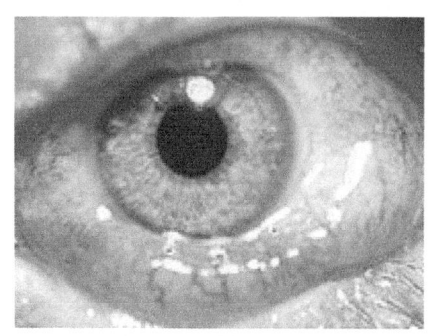

Figure 10.1. Seasonal allergic Conjuctivitis.

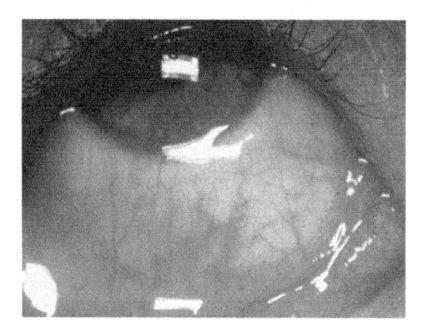

Figure 10.2. Seasonal and perennial allergic conjunctivitis.

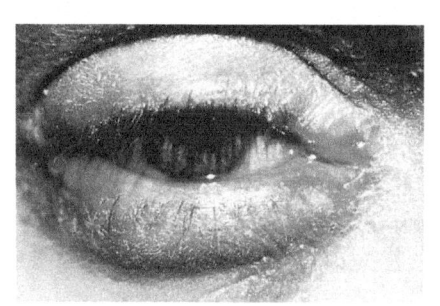

Figure 10.3. Atopic Keratoconjuctivitis.

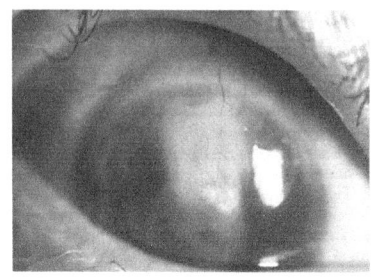

Figure 10.4. Anterior stromal scarring seen in atopic keratoconjuctivitis.

102 *Textbook of Allergy for the Clinician*

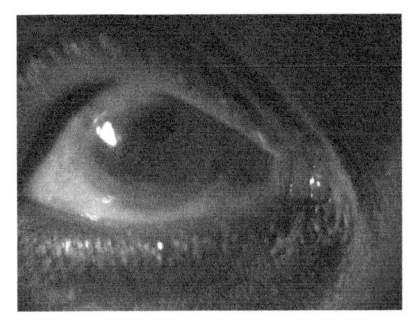

Figure 10.5. Vernal keratoconjuctivitis.

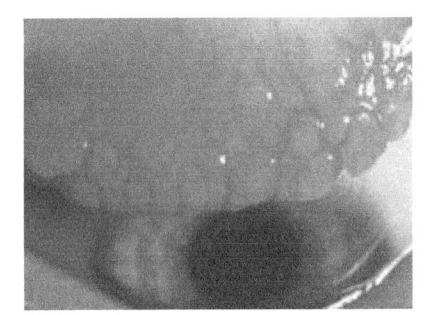

Figure 10.6. Vernal conjunctivitis.

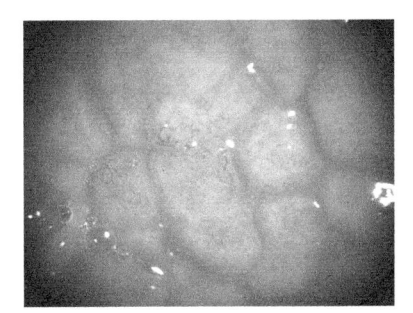

Figure 10.7. Cobblestone papillae.

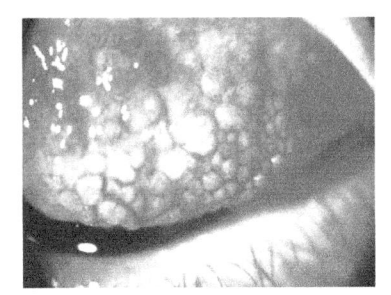

Figure 10.8. Papillary hypertrophy.

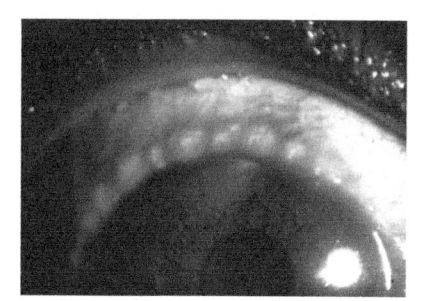

Figure 10.9. Horner-Tranta's dots (indicated by arrow).

- ○ Usually seasonal
- ○ Symptoms may include:
  - Intense itching
  - Chronic bilateral inflammation of conjunctiva
  - Photophobia
  - Stringy, ropy discharge
  - Foreign body sensation
  - Blurred vision
  - Blepharospasm
  - Horner-Trantas dots
  - Giant papillae on palpebral conjunctiva
- Giant Papillary Conjunctivitis
  - ○ This reaction may be an allergy involving proteins that adhere to surfaces of contact lenses, sutures, ocular prostheses
  - ○ Symptoms and signs include:
    - Foreign body sensation
    - Ocular itching
    - Small strand of mucus and/or stringy discharge
    - Slight blurring of vision
    - Mild pruritus
    - Mild hyperemia
    - Macro- and giant papillae on upper tarsal conjunctiva
    - Abnormal thickening of conjunctiva
    - Opacification of conjunctiva
- Contact Allergy
  - ○ The frequency of ocular contact allergy incidence is increasing due to increasing use of products like contact lens solutions and topical medications
  - ○ May involve both conjunctiva and eyelid skin
  - ○ May be caused by inadvertent spreading of cosmetics used on hands, hair, face or fingernails.
  - ○ Symptoms may include
    - Itching
    - Burning
    - Photophobia
    - Fine epithelial punctate keratitis
    - Conjunctival vasodilation and chemosis
    - Corneal opacity (rare)

Pathogenesis

- Common airborne antigens (grass and weed pollens, etc.) may provoke symptoms of allergic conjunctivitis. These symptoms may include ocular itching, redness, burning and tearing. This is most common in seasonal allergic conjunctivitis.
- Perennial Allergic Conjunctivitis may also be caused by seasonal allergens, but not exclusively. Common household allergens such as dust mites, pet dander and cockroaches may also play a role.
- Vernal keratoconjunctivitis is commonly associated with personal or familial history of atopy. More than 90% of these patients exhibit one or more atopic conditions.
- Atopic keratoconjunctivitis has a strong association with atopic dermatitis, which is a hereditary disorder.
- Giant Papillary Conjunctivitis (GPC) is an inflammatory condition characterized by the presence of large ('giant') papillae in the palpebral conjunctiva. Prolonged mechanical irritation from foreign bodies is thought to be a contributing factor. Contact lenses are the most common irritants associated with GPC (Butrus and Portela 2005).
    - A diagnostic flow chart for conjunctivitis is provided in Fig. 10.10
    - The characteristics of vernal and atopic keratoconjunctivitis are listed in Table 10.2.

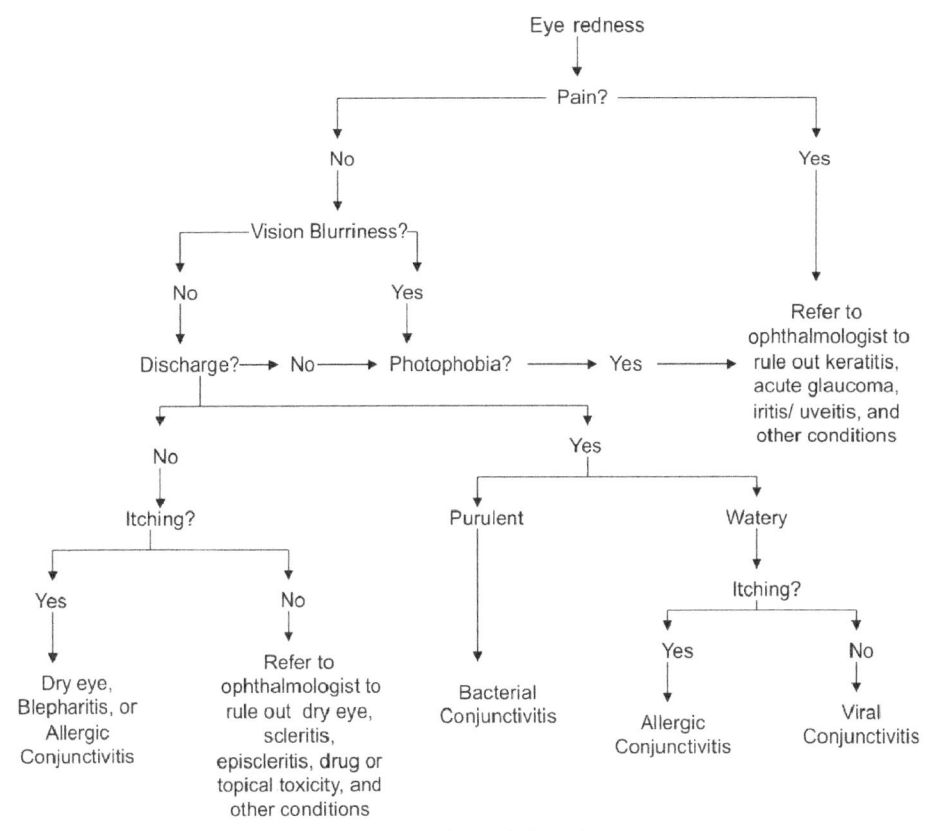

Figure 10.10. Diagnostic flow chart.

Table 10.2. Comparison between Vernal Keratoconjunctivitis (VKC) and Atopic Keratoconjunctivitis (AKC).

Characteristics	AKC	VKC
Gender Predilection	-	Males affected preferentially
Onset Age	20 to 50 years	3 to 20 years
Corneal neovascularization	Present (usually deep)	Not Present
Discharge	Watery and Clear	Thick mucoid
Variance by season	Perennial	Typically seen in spring months
Conjunctival Scarring	Yes (high incidence)	-
Eosinophils present in conjunctival scraping	Unlikely	More likely
Horner-Trantas Dots***	Rare	Dots and shield ulcers commonly seen

***Horner-Trantas Dots are small, white and calcareous like cellular infiltrates occurring on the edge of the conjunctiva. These are clusters of necrotic eosinophils, neutrophils and epithelial cells.

Management

With primary ocular allergies it is not usually possible to identify the allergen, though pollens, suspended particulate matter, secondary cigarette smoke and others have been implicated (Butrus and Portela 2005). No clinical test is available to identify the cause, nor is specific desensitization available for the eye (AIT is effective for nasal allergy associated conjunctivitis); hence treatment is directed at controlling the signs and symptoms. Where possible, avoidance of contact with the allergen should be encouraged, but this is not often practical or feasible.

Topically administered drugs for the treatment of allergic conjunctivitis are listed in Table 10.3. This list is by no means comprehensive, but covers the classes of drugs used.

For patients presenting with acute symptoms, it is usual to prescribe a moderately potent topical steroid with low ocular penetration, such as fluorometholone or loteprednol, three or four times a day for around two weeks. Along with this a mast cell stabilizer or a dual action drug is started as a preventive medication, intended for long term instillation (Mantelli et al. 2007). Prophylactic treatment is usually continued through the expected period of allergen exposure. As drugs such as olopatadine and alcaftadine are available as once-a-day preparations for this purpose, compliance is usually good.

Most patients respond to the above treatment. However, there are a few who need more potent steroids and a small proportion of patients become steroid dependent, with recurrence of symptoms if a steroid dose is missed. Obviously, these patients are at a risk of losing their vision to ocular steroid side-effects such as glaucoma or cataract and must be followed up by an ophthalmologist.

Mast cell inhibitors, once the mainstay of prophylactic treatment, are now being replaced by the dual action drugs. As the latter are of once or twice daily dosage, they are easier to use and more effective than pure mast cell inhibitors and are likely to entirely supplant this class of drug.

NSAIDs are not useful in treating acute presentations. Their main use is in the treatment of chronic PAC, usually in combination with a dual action prophylactic drug (Butrus and Portela 2005). Topical Cyclosporine has been tried with limited success and is not routinely recommended (Daniell et al. 2006). Tacrolimus, however, has been successful as a primary treatment and in treating steroid dependent cases and is now available as a topical preparation that is increasingly being prescribed (Fukushima et al. 2014).

- Specialist Referral
- Refer to an ophthalmologist when:
    - This is the first episode of the ocular condition
    - Long term use of topical corticosteroids is needed
    - Allergic origin is in question and symptoms are severe
    - Any corneal lesion is noted or vision is affected
    - Vernal conjunctivitis is increasingly difficult to control
    - Giant papillary conjunctivitis is difficult to control

Table 10.3. Classification of topical medications used with some examples.

○ Mast Cell stabilizers 　■ Cromolyn sodium 　■ Lodoxamide
○ Antihistamines 　■ Emedastine 　■ Azelastine 　■ Epinastine
○ Vaso-constrictors 　■ Phenylephrine 　■ Antazoline
○ Dual Action agents (Antihistamine + mast cell stabilizers) 　■ Levocabastine 　■ Olopatadine 　■ Ketotifen 　■ Alcaftadine
○ Non-steroidal Anti-inflammatory Drugs 　■ Ketorolac 　■ Nepafenac
○ Corticosteroids 　■ Fluorometholone 　■ Rimexolone 　■ Loteprednol 　■ Dexamethasone 　■ Prednisolone
○ Immuno-modulating agents 　■ Cyclosporin A 　■ Tacrolimus

Case study 1

A 7-year old boy presented with severe itching and swelling of the eyes of two days duration. He had recently been to his grandfather's farm in the country, in anticipation of a longer stay for the approaching summer vacation.

He was noted to have conjunctival congestion and chemosis with Horner-Trantas dots clearly seen. Large papillae were seen in the palpebral conjunctiva. He was started on topical loteprednol four times a day along with 0.2% Olopatadine once daily in the mornings. He was advised to see an ophthalmologist as soon as possible for confirmation of the diagnosis and planning of further management.

He was not able to get an appointment for the ophthalmologist, but returned a week later with complete resolution of the symptoms and disappearance of the conjunctival redness and swelling. Topical steroids were stopped and he was asked to continue the Olopatadine till he could see the ophthalmologist. He returned in three days with a recurrence of the symptoms and signs. Loteprednol was restarted, and this time continued for two weeks, before reduction in dosage and gradual tapering. A visit to the ophthalmologist confirmed the diagnosis of vernal conjunctivitis. The boy remained symptom free through the summer on Olopatadine, apart from one episode of itching which responded to addition of loteprednol for two weeks. Olopatadine was discontinued when he rejoined school in the fall term, with no recurrence. His parents have been told that it will probably be advisable to restart the drop in March-April of the following year.

Case study 2

A 25-year old male reported with itchy, watery and red eyes for the past two years in spring, summer and fall. He also had nasal congestion and sneezing. The symptoms were virtually absent in winter. He had tried over-the-counter eye drops and lubricants without benefit. The physical examination was suggestive of allergic rhinitis and conjunctivitis. What would you do next?

This patient underwent allergy evaluation and was counseled about the typical allergens that are present seasonally (trees in spring, grasses in summer and weeds such as ragweed in the fall in the USA). He was tried on dual action (antihistamine-mast-cell stabilizer) eye drops and had only partial benefit. He was given steroid nose spray and that helped partially as well. The antihistamine caused dry eyes and he discontinued them. At this point, he was prescribed a low-dose topical steroid eye drop—loteprednol which helped significantly but still not a hundred percent. The patient returned to the allergist's office for further evaluation. Based on his allergy skin tests and severe seasonal allergies, he was counseled about allergen immunotherapy and he elected to begin the treatment. Within about one year of starting immunotherapy, he was dramatically better and hardly needed allergy medications to control the symptoms.

Photographs of allergic ocular disorders have been provided courtesy of P.K. Vedanthan, MD.

Conclusion

A summary of the common allergic types of allergic conjunctivitis with different diagnosis and treatment has been discussed. The classification of the common opthalmic preparations comes in very handy.

References

Butrus S, Portela R. Ocular Allergy: Diagnosis and Treatment. Ophthalmol Clin N Am 2005; 18: 485–492.
Daniell M, Constantinou M, Vu HT, Taylor HR. Randomised controlled trail of topical Ciclosporin A in steroid dependent allergic conjunctivitis. Br. J Ophthalmol 2006; 90: 461–464.
Fukushima A, Ohashi Y, Ebihara N, Uchio E, Okamoto S, Kumagai N, et al. Therapeutic effects of 0.1% Tacrolimus eye drops for refractory allergic ocular diseases with prolifrative lesion or corneal involvement. Br J Ophthalmol 2014; 98: 1023–1027.
Mantelli F, Santos MS, Petitti T, Sgruletta R, Cortes M, Lambiasi A, et al. Systematic review and meta-analysis of randomized clinical trials on topical treatments for vernal keratoconjunctivitis. Br J Ophthalmol 2007; 91: 1656–1661.
Pelikan Z. Cytological change in tears during the secondary conjunctival response induced by nasal allergy. Br J Ophthalmol 2012; 96: 941–948.
Pelikan Z. Inflammatory mediator profiles in tears accompanying keratoconjunctival responses induced by nasal allergy. Br J Ophthalmol 2013; 97: 820–828.

11

Rhinolaryngoscopy for the Allergist

Jerald W Koepke[1] *and William K Dolen*[2,*]

INTRODUCTION

Routine upper airway examination usually consists of inspection of the anterior nares with an otoscope or nasal speculum and examination of the pharynx with a tongue depressor. The otoscope permits only limited examination of the proximal structures. The traditional speculum and head mirror allow examination of large portions of the nasal cavity as well as part of the nasopharynx. Use of a tongue depressor permits evaluation of parts of the posterior pharyngeal wall, and an indirect mirror examination allows a more complete inspection of the nasopharynx, hypopharynx and the glottic structures. These conventional examination skills do not permit examination of the recessed structures of the upper airway, such as the sinus ostia, sphenoethmoidal recess and Eustachian tube ostium, and they are difficult to master.

The flexible fiberoptic rhinoscope (Fig. 11.1) makes upper airway examination a simple and convenient procedure, permitting comprehensive evaluation of the upper airway. The endoscopist can quickly and thoroughly examine most areas of the upper airway without discomfort to the patient. Examinations may be recorded for permanent record keeping, and recordings may be replayed and explained to patients. The performance of fiberoptic rhinolaryngoscopy requires a basic understanding of relevant anatomy, physiology and pathology, and relatively frequent use of the endoscope.

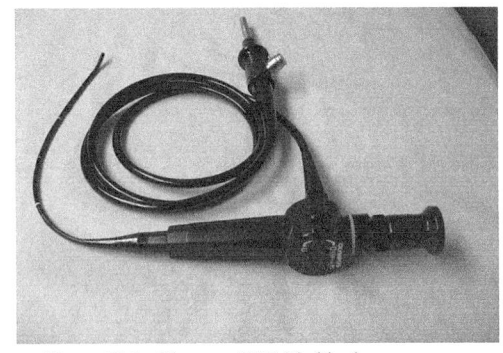

Figure 11.1. Olympus ENF-P3 rhinolaryngoscope.

---

[1] Colorado Allergy and Asthma Centers, Denver, Colorado, Email: jw.koepke@coloradoallergy.com
[2] Allergy-Immunology and Pediatric Rheumatology Division, Departments of Pediatrics and Medicine, Medical College of Georgia at AugustaUniversity, Augusta, Georgia 30912.
* Corresponding author: bdolen@augusta.edu

An overview of normal upper airway anatomy

The upper airway may be divided into regions (Fig. 11.2). In adults, the nasal cavity is a channel approximately 9 to 10 centimeters in length from the meatus to the posterior choana. The posterior choana separates the nasal cavity from the nasopharynx. The oropharynx, in which the palatine tonsils are located, extends from the inferior margin of the soft palate to the upper edge of the epiglottis. The hypopharynx is located posterior to the aperture of the larynx. The triangular inlet of the larynx (*aditus laryngis*) is formed by the superior margin of the epiglottis, the aryepiglottic folds and the arytenoid cartilages. The larynx becomes continuous with the trachea.

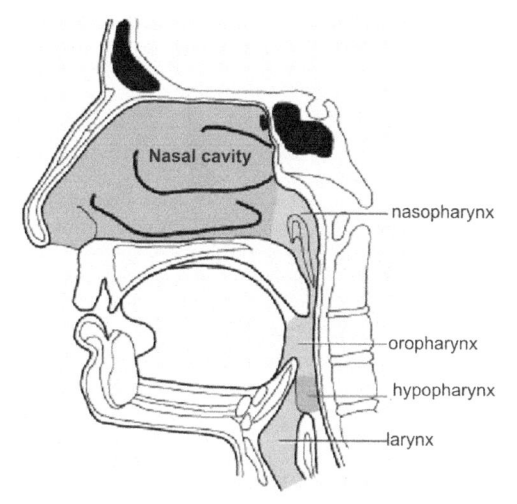

Figure 11.2. The anatomic divisions of the upper airway. All five divisions may be inspected with a fiberoptic endoscope.

Anterior nasal structures

The septum divides the nasal cavity into right and left chambers. The nasal vestibule is the most anterior and inferior portion of the nasal cavity (Fig. 11.3). It is bounded medially and laterally by the alar cartilages and extends to the inferior border of the lateral nasal cartilage. Above the vestibule and in front of the middle meatus is the nasal atrium, and above this is the *agger nasi*, a prominence which generally contains anterior ethmoid air cells. The nasal floor is formed anteriorly by the maxillary bone and posteriorly by the palatine bone. It is slightly concave and passes horizontally from the vestibule to the choana. The nasal vault narrows superiorly to form the roof of the nose.

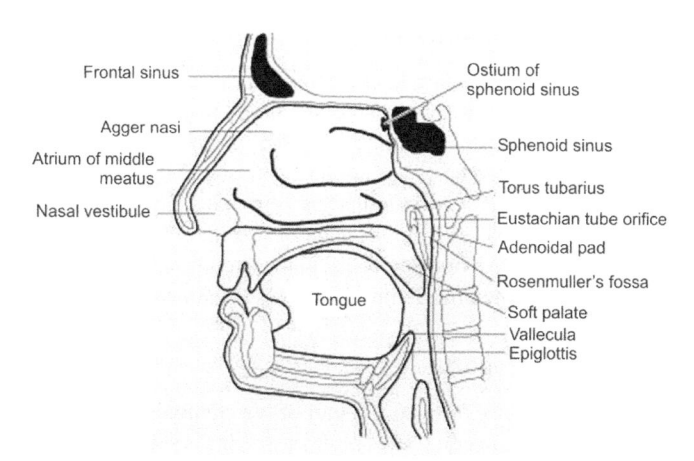

Figure 11.3. A sagittal section of the head demonstrating lateral structures of the nasal cavity and pharynx.

Nasal septum

The nasal septum, rarely straight in normal adults, consists of both cartilaginous and bony components (Fig. 11.4), with mucous membrane overlying perichondrium or periosteum of the underlying cartilage or bone. The mobile, anterior portion of the septum is composed of a quadrangular septal cartilage resting in a groove on the maxillary bone and articulating posteriorly with the thin, delicate bone of the perpendicular plate of the ethmoid and inferiorly with the thicker, more rigid bone of the vomer. The vomer forms the medial border of the choanae and rests on the crest of the maxillary bone anteriorly and the crest of the palatine bone posteriorly. The perpendicular plate of the ethmoid extends superiorly, attaching to the cribriform plate (*lamina cribosa*). A superior projection of the hard palate, the maxillary ridge (crista nasalis maxillae; nasal crest of maxilla) often forms a 'T' anteriorly at the base of the septum. The lateral wings of the 'T' may project into the nasal cavity.

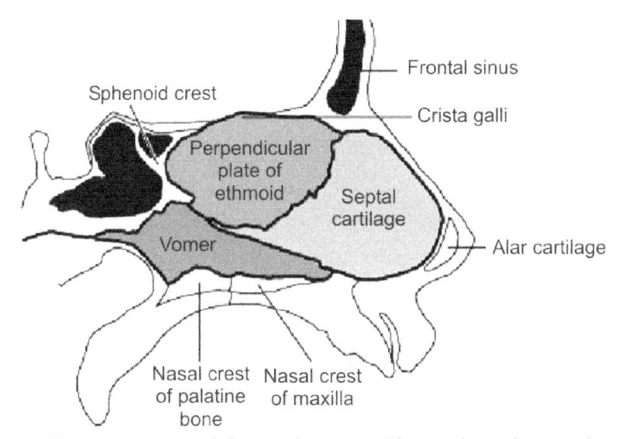

Figure 11.4. Cartilaginous and bony structures of the nasal septum. The quadrangular septal cartilage and the vomer articulate with bones of the nasal floor. The thin perpendicular plate of the ethmoid extends upward to the cribriform plate.

Turbinates

Three or four turbinates provide filtration, heating and cooling and humidification of inspired air and offer resistance to air flow. The turbinates are comprised of a scroll-shaped bony supporting structure, called a concha and overlying mucosa. Clefting or segmentalization of the turbinates may occur both horizontally and sagittally, and clefting of a middle turbinate may be difficult to distinguish from a nasal polyp on anterior examination. The space created by a turbinate and the lateral wall of the nose is called a meatus.

Inferior turbinate and inferior meatus

The inferior concha is a separate bone sitting in an opening in the maxilla and resting in the lateral wall of the nasal passage. It is attached to the palate and maxilla by membranous soft tissue. The turbinate follows the lower lateral wall of the nose in a course parallel to that of the nasal floor. In patients with nasal septal deviation, the inferior turbinates are not the same size. The only structure opening into the inferior meatus is the nasolacrimal duct which drains tears through a large opening in the anterior roof of the meatus (Fig. 11.5), located about 1 cm from the anterior margin of the turbinate. The orifice is almost never seen by fiberoptic rhinoscopy. An opening found in the lateral wall at this location is most likely an antral window surgically placed in the inferior meatus to provide drainage for the maxillary sinus.

Middle turbinate and middle meatus

The middle turbinate, like the superior turbinate, is part of the ethmoid bone and is suspended from the roof of the nose rather than from the lateral wall. The anterior edge is superior and posterior to that of the inferior turbinate.

Rhinolaryngoscopy for the Allergist 111

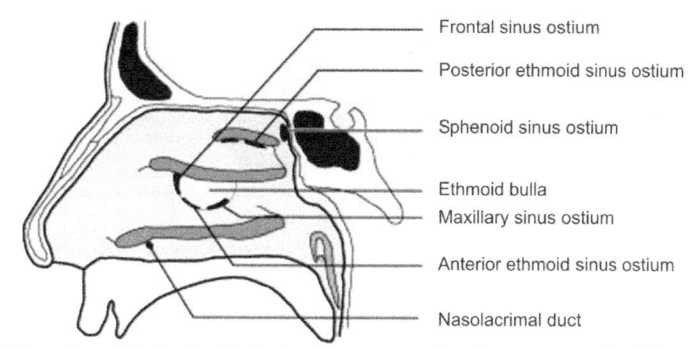

Figure 11.5. A sagittal section of the head with the turbinates removed to demonstrate ostia of the paranasal sinuses and nasolacrymal duct.

The semilunar hiatus (*hiatus semilunaris*), is a crescent-shaped cleft located in the middle meatus (Fig. 11.5). The ostium of the nasofrontal duct and the anterior ethmoid sinus ostia typically are located in the anterior and midportions of the hiatus. The nasofrontal duct may have a separate opening anterior to the semilunar hiatus. The maxillary sinuses open into the posteroinferior portion of the semilunar hiatus. The ostium of the maxillary sinus varies in size in normal individuals from pinpoint to several millimeters in diameter and large accessory ostia may be present. The ethmoid bulla (*bulla ethmoidalis*) is a bulge containing anterior and middle ethmoid air cells, located posterior and superior to the semilunar hiatus.

Superior and supreme turbinates

The superior turbinate is a short, oblique structure located superior and posterior to the middle turbinate. The posterior ethmoid sinuses drain into the superior meatus (Fig. 11.5). A supreme turbinate medial to the superior turbinate is occasionally noted.

Sphenoethmoidal recess

The sphenoethmoidal recess is a deep groove located superior, posterior and medial to the superior turbinate. It contains the ostium of the sphenoid sinus (Fig. 11.5).

Nasopharynx

The torus tubarius is located on the lateral wall of the nasopharynx, defining and protecting the Eustachian tube orifice (Fig. 11.5). Rosenmueller's fossa is a vertical cleft, a potential space, between the posterior lip of the torus tubarius and the adenoidal pad. Many of the insidious malignancies of the pharynx have their origin in this space. The adenoid or pharyngeal tonsil, is a primary lymph node of first line defense for inflammation involving the upper airway.

Oropharynx

The lingual tonsils are located on either side of the dorsum of the tongue anterior to the epiglottis (Fig. 11.6). The median glossoepiglottic fold and the two lateral glossoepiglottic folds attach the epiglottis to the base of the tongue.

Hypopharynx

The valleculae are cup shaped spaces, separated by the median glossoepiglottic fold, posterior to the base of the tongue and anterior to the epiglottis. To the right and to the left of the larynx are the piriform sinuses, gutter-like structures that direct food to the esophagus.

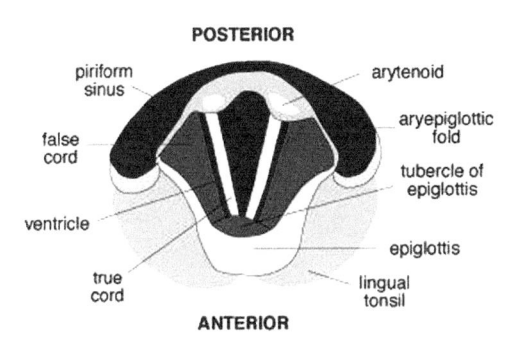

Figure 11.6. The larynx as viewed from above and oriented as it would be seen with a fiberoptic endoscope.

Larynx

The framework of the larynx is formed by the thyroid, cricoid and epiglottic cartilages and by pairs of arytenoid, corniculate and cuneiform cartilages. The aryepiglottic folds and the arytenoids are located immediately behind the epiglottis (Fig. 11.6). The aperture of the glottis (*rima glottidis*) is formed by the true vocal folds (*plicae vocales*) and the posterior commissure between the arytenoids. The anterior ligament of the true vocal folds is located at the anterior angle of the vocal folds. Between the true vocal folds and the false vocal folds (vestibular folds; *plicae ventriculares*) is the laryngeal ventricle. The nodular swellings located medially in the aryepiglottic folds are the corniculate cartilages which sit on top of the arytenoid cartilages. Lateral to the corniculate cartilages are the cuneiform cartilages.

The true vocal folds are anteriorly attached to the thyroid cartilage. The posterior attachment is to the vocal processes of the arytenoid cartilages. The true vocal folds often reflect light in such a manner that they appear whiter than the surrounding mucosa. The strong vocal ligaments are covered by a connective tissue and a thin layer of epithelium. Reinke's space is the potential space between the vocal ligaments and the subepithelial connective tissue layer. The mobile arytenoid cartilages move in and out with respiration and phonation.

Selected examples of upper airway pathology

Without a thorough upper airway examination, a patient complaining of nasal congestion or other upper airway symptoms might be placed on decongestant therapy, antibiotics or allergen immunotherapy when symptoms are largely due to anatomic obstruction of the nasal passage or other conditions primarily managed by surgery. A complete discussion of upper airway pathology is beyond the scope of this chapter, which will present examples of upper airway pathology that might be encountered in an outpatient allergy practice (Table 11.1).

Mucosa

The upper airway mucosa are normally moist and reddish-pink in color, shrinking easily when topical decongestants are applied. The differential diagnosis of mucosal dryness includes various systemic diseases (such as sicca syndrome), living in a low humidity environment, atrophic rhinitis and rhinitis sicca. Allergic rhinitis classically produces a bluish discoloration of the nasal mucosa in association with clear rhinorrhea. So-called cobblestoning of the mucosa is a sign of chronic inflammation.

Nasal Cavity

Turbinates

Hypertrophy of the nasal turbinates may occur secondary to chronic inflammation of the nasal mucosa, or in cases of septal deviation as a compensatory mechanism in the nasal passage opposite to the obstructed

Table 11.1. Findings and pathology evident on fiberoptic endoscopy of the upper airway.

Region	Findings
Mucosa	Mucus (clear vs. purulent)
	Color, vascular changes
	Inflammation, cobblestoning
	Moist or dry
	Mucosal atrophy
Nasal Cavity	
Turbinates	Bony or mucosal hypertrophy
	Compression from septal deviation
	Surgical resection
	Clefting (horizontal and sagittal)
	Polypoidal extension, degeneration
	Concha bullosa
Septum	Deviation, dislocation, perforation, spurs
	Maxillary ridge (may contribute to obstruction)
Polyps	Origin in paranasal sinuses
	Turbinate degeneration
	Mucocele
Paranasal sinuses	Direct inspection of maxillary sinus
	Postoperative evaluation of sinus surgery
Nasopharynx and Superior Oropharynx Choana	Atresia or stenosis (unilateral or bilateral)
Torus, Eustachian tube orifice	Cystic degeneration
	Incorporation of lymphoid tissue
	Edematous obstruction
	Poor function with ear clearing
	Postsurgical scarring and retraction resulting in patulous orifice
Adenoids	Adenoiditis, Rathke's pouch cyst
	Hypertrophy, anterior herniation through choana
Pharyngeal wall	Osteophytes, carotid aneurysm
	Constrictor muscle spasm
Malignancies	Carcinomas originating in Rosenmueller's fossa
Oropharynx, Hypopharynx, Larynx	
Posterior tongue	Cystic circumvallate papillae, mucocele
	Papillomata, Candida infection
Lingual tonsils	Hypertrophy
Epiglottis	Edema, positional deformity
	Inflammation of petiole
Glottis	Erythema, edema, laryngocele
Arytenoids	Contact ulcers, edema
Vocal folds	Contact ulcers, webs, paralysis
	Vocal cord dysfunction syndrome

side. Turbinate hypertrophy may also occur without an obvious underlying cause. Complete or partial turbinectomy may have been performed in an attempt to relieve obstructive symptoms or as part of more complicated nasal or sinus surgery.

Horizontal or sagittal clefting of a turbinate is a normal anatomic variant that may be mistaken for polypoidal degeneration. It may also be difficult to distinguish polypoidal degeneration of a turbinate from polyps that emanate from the anterior group of ethmoid air cells and enter the nose via the middle meatus. In either case, manipulation of the suspected polyps under direct visualization may be useful.

A concha bullosa results when misplaced ethmoid air cells localize in the concha of a middle turbinate. A concha bullosa may produce significant obstruction of the nasal airway.

Septum

The nasal septum is not normally a perfectly straight midline structure. In normal people, one side of the nasal cavity is larger than the other, but differences are not perceived. More prominent septal deviation will result in obstructive symptoms, and complex deviation will produce bilateral nasal blockage. Occasionally, severe deviation of the septum will not even permit passage of the rhinoscope. Septal deviation may compress the nasal turbinates, causing facial pain.

A septal spur (Fig. 11.7) is a displacement of the perpendicular plate of the ethmoid bone and the quadrangular septal cartilage into the nasal cavity. If this spur impinges on adjacent mucosal tissues, facial pain will result. Occasionally, the maxilla will form a shelf or ridge, on which the cartilaginous portion of the septum rests. This maxillary ridge is a common finding, but may be sufficiently large to cause symptomatic obstruction.

Patients with septal perforation may complain of nasal congestion, intermittent bleeding and a whistling sound with nasal breathing. Septal perforation may be caused by a variety of pathological conditions. Infection of a posttraumatic septal hematoma will cause perforation. Septal perforation may also be associated with cocaine abuse or prolonged use of topical nasal decongestants.

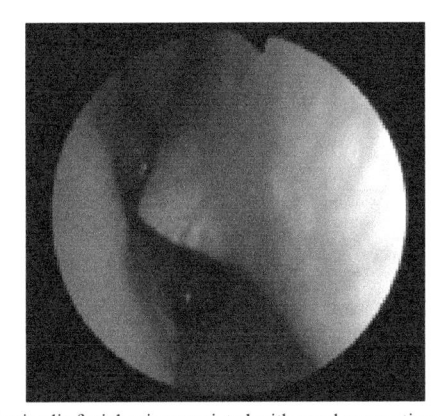

Figure 11.7. This patient reported episodic facial pain associated with nasal congestion. Examination of the superior portion of the mid nasal passage showed a septal spur impinging on the medial surface of the middle turbinate. A past direct blow to the nose had caused the posterior portion of the quadrangular cartilage of the septum to displace from its articulation with the bony structures of the septum. The symptom of facial pain of intranasal originis sometimes called Sluder syndrome.

Nasal polyps

Polyps (Fig. 11.8) characteristically are smooth, avascular structures, appearing slightly yellow or translucent. They can originate from degeneration of the mucosa of any structure in the nasal cavity or from any of the sinuses. Most originate in the ethmoid air cells. Polyps from the anterior and middle ethmoid air cells enter the nasal cavity from the meatus of the middle turbinate. They are usually easy to visualize on routine anterior examination of the nose, may extend anteriorly and can produce total nasal obstruction. It is not possible to detect posterior ethmoid polyps on routine examination unless they have reached huge proportions. Polyps located in the middle meatus originate from the anterior ethmoid or maxillary sinuses. Polyps extending from the sphenoethmoidal recess originate from the sphenoid or posterior ethmoid sinuses.

Polyps can often be moved with a cotton-tipped applicator so that their origin may more clearly be defined. Squamous metaplasia results as a consequence of dry air that induces keratinization of the mucosa covering the polyp.

Rhinolaryngoscopy for the Allergist 115

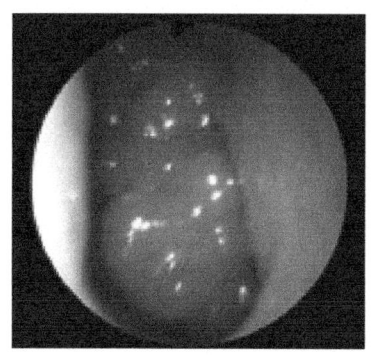

Figure 11.8. This adult patient complained of nocturnal awakenings associated with nasal .blockage. Examination showed a choanal nasal polyp of posterior ethmoid origin. Removal of this obstruction necessitated dissection of the polyp into three segments.

Neoplasms

Malignancy in the nose is an uncommon finding, but complaints as common as pain, burning or rhinorrhea can be the initial symptoms of malignant degeneration. Any lesion suspicious for malignancy should be evaluated by an otolaryngologist.

Nasal surgery

Procedures usually encountered in an allergy practice include repair of deviation or perforation of the septum, placement of antral windows and turbinectomy. It is often helpful to examine the results of surgical intervention.

Paranasal sinus surgery

Surgical creation of an antral window in the middle meatus (less commonly the inferior meatus) and exteriorization (or marsupialization) of the ethmoid and sphenoid sinuses can establish drainage in selected patients with chronic sinusitis, when other measures have failed. With the fiberoptic endoscope, one may assess patency of the antral window and inspect the surrounding mucosa for signs of inflammation or polypoidal growth. It may be possible to insert the endoscope into the maxillary sinus to examine the mucosa. Ethmoidectomy and sphenoidectomy are performed to establish drainage from and provide aeration to these areas in order to treat chronic inflammation and infection. At times, extensive surgery is indicated.

Nasopharynx, superior oropharynx

Choana

The posterior choana marks the beginning of the nasopharynx. Although complete bilateral choanal atresia almost always presents at birth, unilateral atresia or choanal stenosis might not be diagnosed until adulthood.

Torus tubarius

The torus is a partial ring of tissue protecting the ostium of the Eustachian tube. A variety of conditions involving the torus could produce symptoms and signs of Eustachian tube dysfunction, which interferes with equalization of pressure between the middle ear and the environment. A cyst of the torus blocking the Eustachian tube orifice would be evident on fiberoptic endoscopy, as would lymphoid infiltration from chronic inflammation and edema of the torus. Since adenoidectomy is often done by blind curettage,

116 *Textbook of Allergy for the Clinician*

damage to the Eustachian tube and torus with resulting formation of scar tissue and adhesions could lead to Eustachian tube dysfunction.

Rosenmueller's fossa

This vertical cleft, a potential space between the posterior lip of the torus tubarius and the adenoidal pad, is of considerable importance because many of the insidious malignancies of the pharynx have their origin here. It is impossible to examine this space without direct visualization.

Adenoid

The adenoid is a primary lymph node of first-line defense for inflammation involving the upper airway. The torus tubarius and Eustachian tube orifice are in close proximity to the adenoidal pad. Eustachian tube function may be compromised by adenoidal hyperplasia.

Adenoidal hyperplasia (Fig. 11.9) is a frequent cause of nasal obstruction in children, sometimes encountered in adults. In extreme cases, anterior herniation of adenoidal tissue through the choanae may result in total obstruction. In addition to producing discomfort, obstruction may result in hyponasal speech, other variations in voice quality, orthodontic difficulties due to abnormal development of facial bones (adenoidal facies) and sleep disturbances. A nasopharyngeal angiofibroma may mimic the obstruction of adenoidal hypertrophy and may be associated with recurrent epistaxis.

Severe adenoidal hyperplasia or other obstructing lesions of the nasopharynx can cause anterior rhinorrhea, a cardinal feature of rhinitis. Chronic adenoiditis may result in posterior rhinorrhea and halitosis and adenoidal tissue may block the orifice of the Eustachian tube causing chronic otitis media, otalgia and variation in hearing. When obstruction recurs following adenoidectomy, re-examination is indicated.

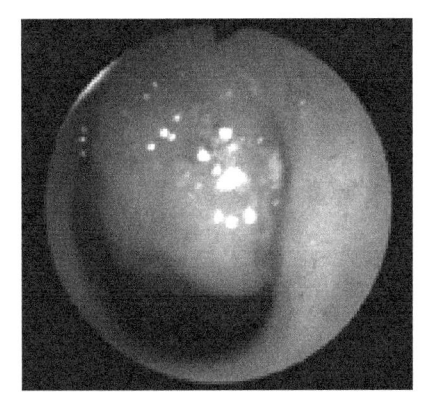

Figure 11.9. Partial obstruction of the right nasal cavity by adenoidal hyperplasia can result in snoring with apnea and mouth breathing with maxillofacial and dental growth abnormalities. The small aperture inferiorly may disappear when the patient is sleeping and the palate moves superiorly.

Pharyngeal wall

Anterior bony protrusions (osteophytes) from the vertebral bodies behind the posterior pharyngeal wall can cause obstruction; mucus that collects on these projections can lead to chronic pharyngeal symptoms. The pulsations of a carotid aneurysm might be noted on examination of the oropharynx. Cobblestoning of the mucosa (Fig. 11.10) results from hypertrophy of lymphoid tissue and is a sign of upstream inflammatory reaction. One of the most striking abnormalities of the pharyngeal walls is spasm of the pharyngeal constrictor muscles associated with anxiety or chemical irritation of the upper airway. The patient complaining of a tight throat may indeed have a tight throat; this might be difficult to understand on direct pharyngeal examination and the symptoms and signs might otherwise be confused with those of asthma.

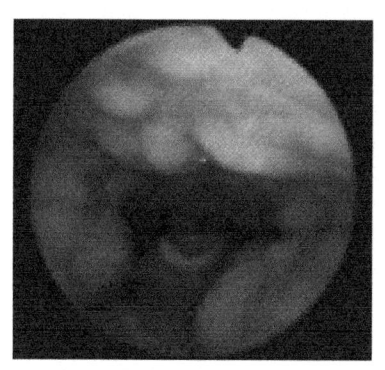

Figure 11.10. In this patient with long standing chronic rhinosinusitis, cobblestoning of the posterior pharyngeal wall is prominent. The tip of the examining scope is in the nasopharynx, directed inferiorly. At 12 o'clock is the posterior pharyngeal wall. The tip of the epiglottis is seen in the distance in the center of the slide. The palatine tonsils protrude from the lateral walls at 4 o'clock and 9 o'clock.

Malignancies

Since most of the pathology originating in the nasopharynx is painless, insidious development of malignancies is possible, with the first sign of pathology being metastasis to the regional lymph nodes. Trigeminal neuralgia may result from malignancy involving the trigeminal nerve (V). Palsy of cranial nerves III, IV, and VI are also ominous signs of malignancy that may originate in the nasopharynx.

Oropharynx, hypopharynx, larynx

Hoarseness or other changes in the quality of the voice suggest hypopharyngeal or laryngeal pathology. These symptoms are often the result of vocal fold polyps, nodules, contact ulcerations and granulomas. A sensation of tightness in the throat or dysphagia may be the direct result of hypertrophy of lymphatic tissue, edema or muscle spasm. Gastroesophageal reflux can result in chronic inflammation of the airway, chronic cough and dysphagia. Patients presenting with a history of severe asthma with an atypical clinical course may have dysfunction of the vocal folds. Examination of the upper airway during an acute episode will be diagnostic.

Posterior tongue, lingual tonsils

The circumvallate papillae form prominent pink nodules on the posterior tongue. The filiform papillae may appear white as a result of drinking coffee, cigarette smoking and other exposures. A white discoloration of the filiform papillae can be mistaken for Candida infection. Hypertrophy of the lingual tonsils may cause dysphagia, a globus sensation or a feeling that something is stuck in the throat.

Epiglottis

A variety of circumstances can lead to irritation, with hypervascularity and edema of the epiglottis. Gastroesophageal reflux, chronic sinusitis and irritants such as chemicals and tobacco smoke may produce irritation of the epiglottis. Edema of the glottic structures may be present in patients with acute urticaria and angioedema of the buccal mucosa, tongue and pharynx. When facilities for intubation or tracheotomy are available, the fiberoptic endoscope may be used to diagnose acute epiglottitis.

Glottis

Any change in the quality of the voice, including hoarseness, is a direct indication for examination of the hypopharynx and larynx. In *dysphonia plicae ventriculares*, abnormal quality of the voice results from use of the false vocal folds for speech. Laryngoceles may produce a muffled voice; infection of laryngoceles may produce acute airway obstruction.

118 *Textbook of Allergy for the Clinician*

True vocal folds

Paralysis of the left vocal fold may be due to malignancy in the mediastinum, thyroid or the glottic structures. The most common cause of nodules is voice abuse. A nodule is an accumulation of fibrous tissue in the submucosa, producing a small sessile lesion that may be hemorrhagic or pale gray in color. The surface mucosa covering the nodule is usually intact and indistinguishable from the surrounding mucosa. Often the mucosa over the nodule may appear hypertrophied. Vocal fold nodules and polyps are characteristically found at the junction of the anterior and middle third of the membranous vocal fold. When a nodule is present, a vocal polyp may be located on the opposite vocal fold at the position of contact with the nodule when the vocal folds are adducted.

Reinke's edema or diffuse polyposis of the vocal folds, results from filling of Reinke's space with fluid, usually as the result of voice abuse or smoking. It is characterized by harsh, low-pitched dysphonia, often in a middle-aged individual.

Contact ulcers and granulomas result from trauma that causes denudation of the mucosa overlying the cartilaginous structures. Usually, contact ulcers are on the inner surface of the vocal process of the arytenoids. Ulcers are most often seen as the result of loud talking, over singing or shouting for prolonged periods and result from the vocal process being forcefully pushed together. Mucosal integrity is compromised and infection of the underlying tissue may follow. Granulomas are more often the result of intubation.

Paralysis of one or both vocal folds should prompt further investigation. Paralysis of the left vocal fold may be associated with dysfunction of the left recurrent laryngeal nerve and mediastinal malignancy.

In vocal cord dysfunction syndrome (Fig. 11.11), endoscopy will be normal during asymptomatic periods, but during an episode of wheezing there will be nearly total adduction of the vocal folds during inspiration and expiration, producing a small posterior diamond-shaped chink. The arytenoids remain in a normal lateral position, and the false vocal folds tend to bunch together to a variable degree obscuring the laryngeal ventricles. When the patients and normal subjects are asked to reproduce the sound voluntarily, they are not able to produce the small posterior chink, bunching of the false vocal folds or maintain the arytenoids in abduction. More subtle clinical presentations without complete adduction have been reported.

Many patients with well characterized asthma note tightness in the throat as well as in the chest during episodes and expiratory constriction of the glottis has been observed during histamine or nebulized water bronchial challenge in asymptomatic asthmatic patients. Visualization of the larynx will distinguish this apparently normal phenomenon from the vocal cord dysfunction syndrome.

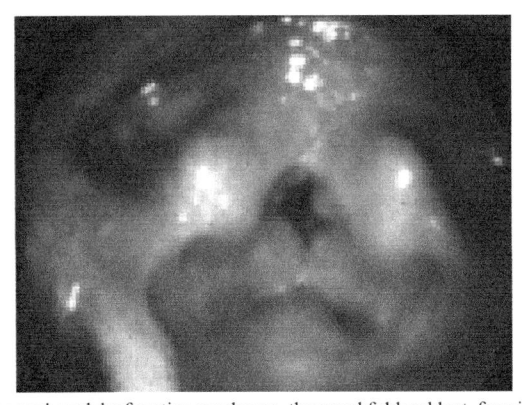

Figure 11.11. In patients with vocal cord dysfunction syndrome, the vocal folds adduct, forming a posterior diamond-shaped opening. This finding is not present in asthma.

Examination technique

Indications

Virtually any symptom or historical complaint referable to the upper airway could be an indication for fiberoptic examination (Table 11.2). The information obtained will almost always directly influence interpretation of patient complaints, establishment of a diagnosis and selection of treatment strategies.

Table 11.2. Selected Indications for Examination.

General
    any symptom or historical complaint referable to the upper airway

Nose and Nasopharynx
    nasal obstruction (particularly if unilateral)
    headaches
    facial pain
    epistaxis
    rhinorrhea
    sinusitis
    earache, recurrent or chronic otitis media
    difficulty equalizing middle ear pressure with the environment
    regional adenopathy
    assess result of surgical intervention

Hypopharynx and Larynx
    dysphagia or globus
    hoarseness, other changes in voice quality
    chronic cough
    atypical asthma (laryngeal dysfunction)

Preparation for examination

Other than explanation of the procedure to the patient, the only special preparation required is decongestion and anesthesia; the patient is not on a fast.

The patient is seated in an examining chair, preferably one with an adjustable headrest. A small child may sit in a parent's lap. Before administration of decongestant and anesthesia, it is appropriate to perform a preliminary nasal examination to determine patency of the nose and to identify pathology that might be visible on routine examination. The patient is then asked to clear secretions from the nose by gentle blowing of the nose; on occasion, saline irrigation may be necessary to clear the nasal passage of mucus and debris.

Topical decongestants such as phenylephrine or oxymetazoline, delivered by a standard nasal atomizer, may be used to shrink the nasal mucosa. Nasal anesthesia is provided with 4% xylocaine solution, also delivered by a nasal atomizer. Pharyngeal and laryngeal anesthesia is not necessary. In general, one or two sprays of each drug should be directed straight back, and the same amount superiorly and posteriorly at about a 45-degree angle. If desired, the rhinoscope may be lubricated with 2% viscous xylocaine or a water-based lubricant.

Examination sequence

Examination should proceed in a consistent, logical sequence (Table 11.3) that may be varied as needed in individual patients. It is usually convenient to examine structures of the anterior nasal cavity first, followed by examination of the pharynx and larynx. The sphenoethmoidal recess and middle meatus are more difficult to examine and may be less well anesthetized than other structures. Thus, they are generally examined last.

Table 11.3. Examination sequence.

Preliminaries
    Explain procedure to patient
    Nasal examination
    Clear secretions from nose; lavage may be necessary
    Decongestion, anesthetic; lubricate endoscope if desired

Nose, nasopharynx
    Nasal vestibule, septum, nasal floor, inferior turbinate, mucosa
    Superior portions of anterior nose
    Nasal roof
    Middle turbinate
    Nasal floor to choana
    Sphenoethmoidal recess (now, or after laryngeal examination)
    Nasopharynx: adenoidal pad; torus-both sides; Rosenmueller's fossa

Pharynx, larynx
    Lateral and posterior pharyngeal walls, soft palate
    Posterior tongue, lingual tonsils
    Epiglottis, vallecula, aryepiglottic folds
    Arytenoids, associated cartilages, piriform sinuses
    False vocal folds, true vocal folds, ventricles
    Transglottic look at trachea

Remaining nasal structures
    Sphenoethmoidal recess (if not previously examined)
    Middle meatus (if not previously examined)
    Contralateral nasal cavity

The patient is reminded that he may talk to the examiner during the examination. With good anesthesia, the procedure is not painful although the patient may report pressure from the endoscope. The patient should be asked to communicate any discomfort to the examiner so that the endoscope may be withdrawn from that area.

In the beginning, the endoscope is placed into the nasal vestibule. The examiner's left hand is placed against the patient's forehead approximately at the base of the nose and the thumb and index finger are used to hold the endoscope at the patient's nostril. If the examining chair has a headrest, the examiner will have some control of the patient's head. Since many patients will tense the frontalis muscle when more sensitive areas of the airway are examined, it is possible to perceive patient discomfort. Also, changes in skin temperature may be an early sign of a vasovagal reaction.

The right hand is used to advance the endoscope into the nasal cavity. The fingers should grasp and support the endoscope, leaving the thumb free to manipulate the tip of the endoscope with the lever. The endoscope is maintained in a straight anterior-posterior position, allowing it to adjust to the contours of the nasal passage as it is advanced, perhaps with slight manipulation of the endoscope tip. The endoscope tip may be flexed with the lever controlled by the thumb of the right hand or moved by altering the position of the endoscope in the nasal passage using the index finger and thumb of the left hand. It is important to remember that, in general, the endoscope will travel towards whatever structure is in the center of the eyepiece or video screen as it is advanced, and that slight flexing or moving the endoscope tip can result in a marked change in the direction of travel. All movements should be performed gently, and the endoscope should not be advanced when distant structures are not visible. Rather than advancing blindly, the examiner should withdraw the endoscope slightly, until anatomic landmarks can be seen and recognized.

With the endoscope approximately 1 cm into the nose, the nasal vestibule with its hairs (vibrissae) will be encountered and often a medial protrusion on the floor of the nose (the lateral feet of the medial crura) will be noted. The inferior turbinate, floor of the nose and septum will be in view (Fig. 11.12). If the endoscope tip is flexed slightly upward, the middle turbinate will be seen in the distance; with

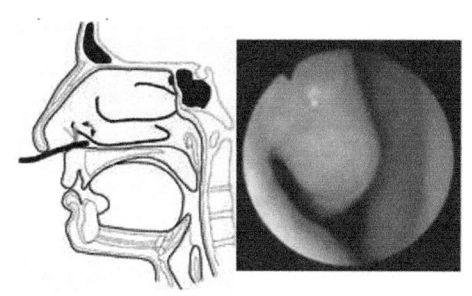

Figure 11.12. With the endoscope approximately 1 cm into the nose, the inferior turbinate, floor of the nose, and septum will be in view. If the endoscope tip is flexed slightly upward, the middle turbinate will be seen in the distance; with upward flexing upward to 60-90 degrees, the superior portion of the anterior nose can be evaluated.

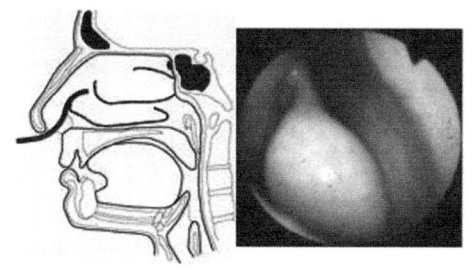

Figure 11.13. In this view of the anterior portion of the middle turbinate, the tip of the endoscope is directed over the inferior turbinate. While the endoscope is usually advanced to the choana along the floor of the nose, this position may be alternatively used if the lower route is obstructed.

upward flexion to 60–90 degrees, the superior portion of the anterior nose can be evaluated. If the inferior turbinate is large or swollen, it may be necessary to advance the tip of the endoscope over the anterior margin of the inferior turbinate in order to view the middle turbinate. A large maxillary ridge or displaced septal cartilage may similarly impede advancement of the endoscope. With the endoscope placed in the middle portion of the nasal cavity, the roof of the nose may be viewed by directing the endoscope upwards; this is the region of the cribriform plate. It is not usually possible to advance the endoscope towards the superior turbinate from this position.

To view the anterior portion of the middle turbinate, the tip of the endoscope is directed over the inferior turbinate (Fig. 11.13). The endoscope is usually advanced to the choana along the floor of the nose, but this position may be used if the lower route is obstructed.

Having been returned to the floor of the nose, the endoscope is directed posteriorly along the nasal floor until it is approximately 4–5 cm into the nasal fossa (Fig. 11.14). At this point, the posterior choana of the nose is usually in view. Septal deviation may interfere with observation of the posterior structures. At this point, the tip of the endoscope is directed upward (Fig. 11.13), and the inferior margin of the middle turbinate comes into view. It is usually possible to direct the endoscope superiorly and laterally into the middle meatus either at this point in the examination, or later after examination of the larynx and sphenoethmoidal recess. At this point, identification of the uncinate process and ethmoid bulla, which define the semilunar hiatus, is often possible. The ostium or accessory ostia, of the maxillary sinus may be identified. The ostia of the nasofrontal duct and the anterior and middle ethmoid air cells are more difficult to locate and ordinarily will not be seen on routine fiberoptic examination of the nose.

The endoscope tip is returned to the nasal floor and advanced to the posterior margin of the inferior turbinate with the choana clearly in view. It is advanced slightly so that structures of the nasopharynx may be viewed through the choana. The adenoidal pad appears on the posterior wall of the nasopharynx and the torus tubarius, which surrounds the Eustachian tube orifice, is well visualized. The endoscope is advanced into the nasopharynx. Once the vomer (the posterior margin of the septum) is lost from view, the tip of the endoscope may be flexed and rotated 90 degrees toward the ipsilateral torus to examine the Eustachian tube orifice and Rosenmueller's fossa. The patient may be asked to sing 'eeee' or say 'k-k-k-k'

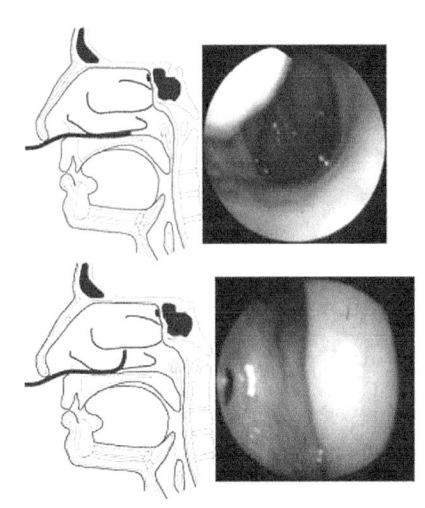

Figure 11.14. With the endoscope along directed posteriorly along the nasal floor approximately 4–5 cm into the nasal foosa, one should see the nasal choana (posterior naris) in the distance. When the tip of the endoscope is directed upward, the inferor margin of the middle turbinate comes into view. It may also be able to direct the endoscope superiorly and laterally into the middle meatus.

to make the orifice more visible. If the endoscope is advanced slightly into the nasopharynx and the tip is flexed 180 degrees behind the septum, the contralateral Eustachian tube orifice and Rosenmueller's fossa may be examined. After these structures have been examined, the endoscope is rotated back to midline and the tip is flexed inferiorly. The patient is asked to breathe through the nose in order to keep the soft palate from obstructing the view. The lateral and posterior walls of the pharynx, the soft palate and uvula are inspected for mucosal irregularities, pulsations, and protrusions into the pharynx. The endoscope is advanced into the oropharynx (Fig. 11.15). Structures of the posterior tongue, the epiglottis, valleculae, and glossoepiglottic and lateral epiglottic folds are examined.

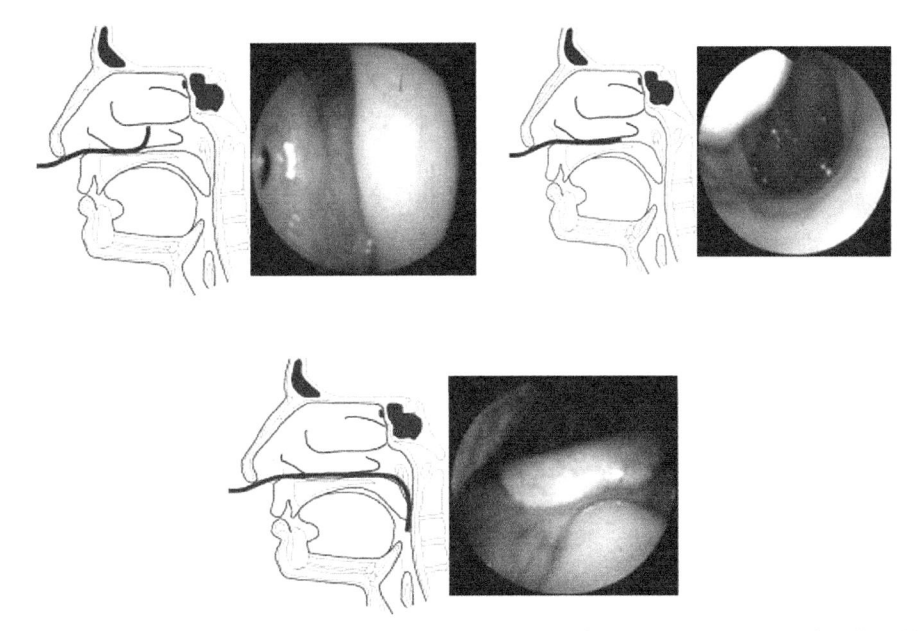

Figure 11.15. As the endoscope is advanced into the oropharnyx, structures of the posterior tongue, the epiglottis, valleculae and the glosso-epiglottic and lateral epiglottic folds are examined. The endoscope is kept close to the posterior wall of the pharynx as it is directed into the hypopharnyx.

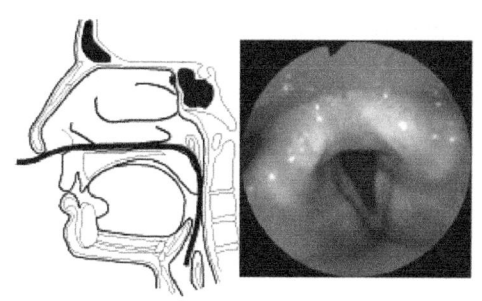

Figure 11.16. The endoscope is directed along the posterior pharyngeal wall in the midline, over the epiglottis. In this position, the arytenoids, the superior projections of the corniculate and cuneiform cartilages, the aryepiglottic folds, the true and false vocal cords and the ventricles are well visualized. Slight rotation of the endoscope in this position will very clearly reveal the piriform sinuses.

The endoscope tip is kept close to the posterior wall of the pharynx as it is directed into the hypopharynx. The patient is encouraged to breathe gently and asked not to swallow, but reassured that swallowing will merely result in the sensation of attempting to swallow the endoscope, not in discomfort. In the process of swallowing, the epiglottis can strike the endoscope; should this happen, the endoscope may be withdrawn slightly until the sensation of swallowing the endoscope has been lost. At this point, the examination may continue. The endoscope is directed along the posterior pharyngeal wall in the midline, over the epiglottis (Fig. 11.16). In this position, the arytenoids, the superior projections of the corniculate and cuneiform cartilages, the aryepiglottic folds, the true and false vocal folds and the ventricles are well visualized. Slight rotations of the endoscope in this position will very clearly reveal the piriform sinuses. From this position, the examiner often can clearly look into the trachea.

To examine the vocal folds in adduction, the patient is asked to sing 'eeee'. Often polypoidal changes and edematous distortion of the vocal folds can be identified with this maneuver. Displacement of the bony structures of the glottis, asymmetrical functioning (including paralysis) of the vocal folds and pathology such as polypoidal changes, granulomas, contact ulcerations will be apparent at this stage of the examination. Sometimes the endoscope must be withdrawn to just above the epiglottis before the patient is asked to phonate.

The endoscope is withdrawn under direct visualization to a position just anterior to the choana. As the endoscope is directed superiorly, the anterior margin of the sphenoid bone comes into view (Fig. 11.17). As the endoscope is advanced superiorly and anteriorly by flexing the tip 90–120 degrees, the posterior and then anterior margins of the superior turbinate may be examined (Fig. 11.17). The sphenoethmoidal recess is medial to the superior turbinate, and the ostium of the sphenoid sinus will often be visualized. The ostia of the posterior ethmoid air cells are less likely to be seen. Since this area may not be well

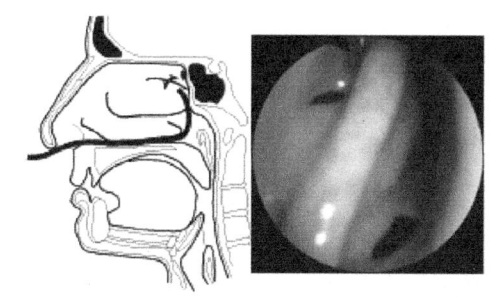

Figure 11.17. The endoscope is withdrawn to a position just anterior to the choana. As the endoscope is directed superiorly, the anterior margin of the sphenoid bone comes into view. As the endoscope is advanced superiorly and anteriorly by flexing the tip 90–120 degrees, the posterior and then anterior margins of the superior turbinate may be examined. The sphenoethmoidal recess is medial to the superior turbinate and the ostium of the sphenoid sinus will often be visualized. Lateral to the superior turbinate, posterior ethmoid ostia can be seen.

anesthetized in some patients, this portion of the examination may be done after examination of the laryngeal structures.

If structures of the middle meatus were not previously examined, they are studied at this time. It is usually easier to examine the middle meatus from posterior to anterior. Following withdrawal of the endoscope under direct visualization, examination of the other side of the nose is carried out. When possible, a video recording of the examination may be replayed and explained to the patient. Recordings can also be used to review findings with an otolaryngologist. Later the equipment is cleaned and disinfected in preparation for the next examination.

Conclusion

The surgical anatomy of the upper airway can be easily examined using a fiberoptic rhinolaryngoscope. The fiberoptiscope allows one to do a compete examination of the upper airway with minimal discomfort to the patient and be performed in a cost-effective manner. This is a relatively simple procedure to learn. Rhinoscopic examination of the structures in the nasal passage and larynx increases your ability to diagnose and treat conditions affecting the upper airway which will enhance the quality of life of your patients

Acknowledgements

Text, illustrations, and photographs in this chapter are from Selner J.C., Dolen W.K., Spofford B., Koepke J.W. Rhinolaryngoscopy. 2nd ed. Denver, CO: Allergy Respiratory Institute of Colorado; 1989. An updated online version of the text, images, and instructional videos may be found at http://www.augusta.edu/mcg/pediatrics/allergy/rhino/index.html. Used with permission.

In memoriam, John Canty Selner, MD (1936–2006).

12
Pediatric Asthma

Michael Teik Chung Lim,[1,2,*] *Mahesh babu Ramamurthy*[1,2] *and Daniel Yam-Thiam Goh*[1,2]

INTRODUCTION

Asthma is the most common chronic childhood disease in developed countries. The definitions of asthma are usually descriptive and tend to encompass both adult and childhood asthma. While airway obstruction is usually the end result, pathophysiological processes and natural history can vary between patients. The term 'airway hyper reactivity' refers to the tendency of the airways to narrow following exposure to the appropriate stimuli (such as allergens or pollutants).

It is important that asthma is recognized and promptly managed as the condition carries a high burden of morbidity in children, with a significant impact on quality of life and cost. For example, children with asthma report significantly more school absenteeism than healthy children (van Gent et al. 2007).

Special consideration is made for preschool children (defined as children less than six years of age) who present with wheezing. Wheezing as a result of respiratory viral illnesses is common in the preschool group, but not all children in this age group go on to develop asthma. Around two-thirds of children who have an episode of wheezing in the first 3 years of life will no longer wheeze by six years of age. The European Respiratory Society has classified these children according to two main groups depending on their triggers for wheeze (Brand et al. 2008). Children who wheeze in response to viral infections and at least one other stimulus (e.g., exercise) are referred to as having multiple-trigger wheeze, while those who wheeze only with viral infections and are well in between have episodicviral wheeze. Those with multiple-trigger wheeze tend to have wheezing later into their school years and develop atopic asthma, while the latter group will more likely stop wheezing by the age of 6 years. Even so, some preschool children display symptom patterns that change over time, and therefore overlaps exist between the two groups of children (Brand et al. 2014).

> **Introduction**
> - Asthma is a heterogenous disease with symptoms of airway obstruction as a result of underlying airway inflammation.
> - Wheezing is common in preschool children, but not all go on to develop school-age asthma.

---

[1] Khoo Teck Puat – National University Children's Medical Institute, National University Hospital, Singapore.
[2] Department of Paediatrics, Yong Loo Lin School of Medicine, National University of Singapore.
  Emails: mahesh_babu_ramamurthy@nuhs.edu.sg; paegohyt@nus.edu.sg
* Corresponding author: michael_tc_lim@nuhs.edu.sg

Prevalence

The prevalence of asthma varies widely around the world, ranging from 2.8 to 37.6% in children aged 6–7 years of age (To et al. 2012). Based on the International Study of Asthma and Allergies in Childhood (ISAAC) which looked at the prevalence of asthma in 56 countries, the latest phase of the study showed a peak in asthma symptom prevalence in high-burden countries 5–10 years on from the first phase of the study, while most low-prevalence countries had increases in prevalence since the first phase of the study (Pearce et al. 2007). In Singapore, the prevalence of current wheezing in 6–7 year-old children fell from 16.6 to 10.2%, but increased in 12–15 year-old children from 9.9 to 11.9% between 1994 to 2001 (Wang et al. 2004).

The burden of disease is high even in the very young as wheezing is a common presentation in the preschool age group. In one prospective birth cohort from Tucson, USA, 33.6% of children below 3 years of age had at least one episode of wheezing (Martinez et al. 1995). In another study from the UK, parents—reported preschool wheezing was 29% (Kuehni et al. 2001). Fortunately, mortality rates for childhood asthma are low, with a decrease over the past decade in the United States (Akinbami et al. 2016).

The prevalence of asthma is higher in boys in the first decade of life, but new-onset asthma is more common in girls during the teenage years (de Marco et al. 2000, Gissler et al. 1999).

Mild asthma with infrequent wheezing in childhood does not tend to progress to severe disease in adulthood (Tai et al. 2014). Remission of asthma for more than 3 years was mostly seen in those with intermittent childhood asthma (64%) compared to those with severe childhood asthma (15%). The Childhood Asthma Management Program, which studied children with mild to moderate persistent asthma, identified several factors that were associated with disease remission. These included the lack of allergen sensitivity, milder asthma and older age of onset (Covar et al. 2010).

Adults with asthma as children may have more airway hyper reactivity when challenged compared to those who only had infection-related wheezing, despite clinical remission. Evidence of airway inflammation may also be present even when the patient is asymptomatic. They also tended to have lower FEV1 values and more persistence of symptoms (van den Toorn et al. 2001).

Prevalence

- Asthma can begin at any age.
- Asthma is children is common, with prevalence peaking in high-burden countries, but rising in low-prevalence countries.

Pathogenesis

Asthma is caused by chronic inflammation and airway hyper responsiveness, although it is yet unclear whether one causes the other or vice versa. These processes lead to airflow limitation due to narrowing of the large and smaller airways (to variable degrees), resulting in hyperinflation and increased work of breathing. Hypoxic vasoconstriction leads to suboptimal ventilation-perfusion ratio and hypoxia occurs early in the process. A fall in carbon dioxide levels result from hyperinflation initially (and an ensuing respiratory alkalosis), but if the attack becomes more severe, CO_2 retention eventually occurs.

Asthma can begin at any age and most often has its origins in early childhood. There is variability in the extent of inflammatory cell involvement, timing of symptoms and specific triggers. These processes can lead to chronic airway remodelling. Postmortem specimens of asthmatic patients show thickening of the basement membrane (due to deposition of materials such as collagen), mucosal oedema, thick mucus plugging, hyperplasia of smooth muscles and hyperinflation. Features of airway remodelling can be seen in endobronchial samples even in children less than 2 years of age with a wheeze, particularly when wheezing is severe and persistent (Saglani et al. 2007). Following exposure of antigen-presenting cells to allergens, naïve T helper (TH0) cells differentiate into T helper 2 (TH2) cells which migrate back to the pulmonary tissue, leading to immunoglobulin E (IgE) synthesis and allergen sensitization (Holgate and Polosa 2008). In subsequent allergen exposure, IgE recognizes the allergen, and IgE-sensitized mast cells degranulate and release mediators such as histamine and cytokines as a result of a type 1 immediate reaction, resulting in smooth muscle contraction, mucus production and increased vascular permeability. There is a late, more chronic allergic response mediated by chemokines released following chronic activation of mast cells where there is an influx of eosinophils and Th2 cells, resulting in further release of pro-inflammatory mediators by eosinophils (such as IL-4, IL-5 and IL-13). There may also be impairment in airway defence mediators which normally control inflammation within the airway walls, resulting in chronic asthma.

In school-age children, asthma is predominantly an eosinophilic condition, as evidenced by endobronchial biopsy and broncho-alveolar lavage findings. Structural airway changes that are seen include thickening of the reticular basement membrane, increase in size and quantity of smooth muscles in the airway, and increased proliferation of blood vessels lead to airway hyper responsiveness (Holgate and Polosa 2006). The inflammatory profile varies from person to person, and the picture may not always be purely eosinophilic, particularly when acute respiratory infections which can cause a neutrophil predominant or mixed picture lead to wheezing.

In preschool children, a history of wheezing does not always lead to asthma in school-age. Multiple factors are at play in this age group. The airway microbiome, the underlying genetic susceptibility, exposure to allergens and pollutants and infections lead to the development of asthma symptoms. There is still a poor understanding of the mechanisms underlying wheezing in preschool children, and this is reflected by how they are managed clinically. Treatment is based mainly on the symptom pattern, yet clinical symptoms can change over time and is therefore of limited use when deciding on the appropriate treatment. About a quarter of children with preschool wheeze have eosinophilic airway disease, recognized by positive aeroallergen sensitivity and peripheral eosinophilia. These children tend to respond well to inhaled corticosteroids (ICS). However, three quarters of them may have neutrophilic predominance in their airways. These children do not respond very well to ICS. There is no consensus regarding management of these children at present (Fitzpatrick et al. 2016).

> **Pathogenesis**
> - Asthma is caused by chronic inflammation and airway hyper responsiveness, leading to airflow limitation and increased effort of breathing.
> - Exposure of antigen-presenting cells to allergens sets off a cascade of events that lead to allergen sensitization and subsequent allergen exposure results in asthma exacerbation.

Etiology

Genetic influence on asthma development and phenotype shows great heterogeneity, with the development of asthma stemming from a complex interplay between genetics and environment (Guilbert et al. 2004).

Some children wheeze when they contract a viral respiratory tract infection or are exposed to aeroallergens. There are several risk factors for increased risk of childhood wheezing, including first-degree relatives with atopy, low birth weight, prematurity, household smoking, aeroallergen sensitivity and a personal history of eczema. The immunopathological pathways that lead to allergic rhinitis are similar to those that result in asthma, and treatment of allergic rhinitis with intranasal corticosteroids and antihistamines has been shown to lead to improvement in asthma symptoms and lung function (Corren et al. 2004, Lohia et al. 2013). Protective factors include a history of breastfeeding and living in a rural location. There is good evidence that the environmental impact of living on a farm reduces the risk of developing asthma by affecting the innate immune system of the airway epithelium. The evidence of reduced risk from living in large family households conflicts with the development of more wheezing in attendance at day-care, where both environments are associated with increased exposure to infection, but conflict in the association with the development of asthma (Caudri et al. 2009, Karmaus and Botezan 2002). Animal studies have shown that early exposure to aeroallergen can lead to the presence of eosinophilia and airway hyper responsiveness and early exposure to respiratory virus infections in mice models can lead to increasing TH2 cytokine production (Krishnamoorthy et al. 2012, Saglani et al. 2009).

Exposure to tobacco smoking is one of the strongest environmental risk factors for the development of asthma in childhood (Martinez et al. 1995). Maternal smoking while pregnant increases the risk of wheezing in early life (Moshammer et al. 2006). Increased air pollution can also result in increased risk of asthma development in susceptible children (Gauderman et al. 2005, Millstein et al. 2004).

Breastfeeding could provide health benefits to the mother and child, but its impact on asthma is less clear, with inconsistent results from previous studies and methodological limitations (Miliku and Azad 2018). Potential mechanisms of protection from asthma include an influence in infant oral and gut microbiota, modulation of the infant's immune system development and support for lung growth.

In the preschool age group, the Asthma Predictive Index (API) is a validated tool to identify factors that predicted the likelihood of preschool children developing asthma in later life (Castro-Rodriguez et al. 2000). This was based on the Tucson Children's Respiratory Study, which was a longitudinal study of respiratory disease in children. Major criteria for the development of asthma were asthma in a parent and a personal history of eczema. Minor criteria were a personal history of allergic rhinitis, wheezing unrelated to viral respiratory infections and peripheral eosinophilia greater than or equal to 4%. A modified API has since been designed to include more objective criteria—adding allergic sensitization to at least one aeroallergen as a major criterion and allergic sensitization to milk, eggs or peanuts as a minor criterion (while removing allergic rhinitis as a minor criterion from the original API) (Guilbert et al. 2004). Those with a viral-associated wheeze with no atopic risk factors will usually stop having wheezing episodes by 6 years of age.

> **Etiology**
> - The development of asthma stems from an interplay between genetics and environment.

Diagnosis of asthma

Clinical—history and examination

Asthma is a heterogenous condition with a wide spectrum of manifestations. It is a symptom complex rather than a single disease entity. There are many terminologies applied to asthma and its related conditions. Increasingly, there is a need to differentiate various asthma phenotypes and even asthma endotypes, with the latter being an attempt at further refining the condition by including pathophysiologic mechanisms along with the identification of relevant cellular or molecular biomarkers in the pursuit to better understand and develop new therapeutic modalities.

Asthma is largely a clinical diagnosis. Central to all definitions of asthma is the presence of symptoms such as a wheeze, tightness of the chest, breathlessness or cough and variable airflow obstruction. Fundamental to these are the presence of airways hyper responsiveness and airways inflammation.

Wheezing is a central feature of asthma. This is, however, a common finding in children, with approximately a third of children wheezing during their first three years of life. While the majority of these children would have stopped wheezing by the age of six years, 40% will continue to wheeze, having already developed asthma or developing asthma at a later stage in life. It is also important to recognize that 'not all that wheezes is asthma'. For the younger children, the diagnosis is usually suspected based on a typical history of recurrent wheezing, cough, tightness of the chest and breathlessness. These symptoms are certainly not pathognomonic for asthma (Weinberger and Abu-Hasan 2007).

Childhood asthma often coexists with allergy and with other atopic diseases. The possible association between allergic sensitization and asthma in children led to the allergic march paradigm. Approximately 60–75% of school-aged children with asthma have an allergy (Guilbert et al. 2004).

The clinical examination in asthma is often negative, apart from evidence of atopy or concomitant allergies. Evidence of chest hyperinflation from air-trapping and the presence of wheezing may be found only in symptomatic periods.

There are no specific diagnostic tools or surrogate markers for asthma especially in a young child. In the diagnostic investigation of patients of all ages, clinical observations (i.e., suggestive symptoms) should be complemented by objective measurements where possible. These tests add support to the diagnosis of asthma and/or rule out important differential diagnoses by identifying variable airway obstruction or airway inflammation.

There is no single reliable test ('gold standard') and there are no standardized diagnostic criteria for asthma. Several predictive models have been proposed to aid in the diagnosis of asthma in the young, yet few (the API, the modified API and the Prevention and Incidence of Asthma and Mite Allergy or PIAMA risk score) have been externally validated (Castro-Rodriguez et al. 2000).

The clinical response to a treatment trial with an inhaled short-acting beta$_2$ agonist reliever or inhaled corticosteroid is not diagnostic either but may lend some support for the diagnosis.

Lung function tests/challenge tests

Peak expiratory flow readings can be used to identify airflow obstruction as well as increased variability in airflow dynamics over time. By itself, it is not a reliable way to confirm or rule out asthma in children. It can however be useful to obtain an objective assessment of asthma control over time.

Spirometry is the most commonly performed lung function test that can be used to support the diagnosis if airway obstruction is found reversible based on an FEV_1 (Forced Expiratory Volume in 1 second) increase of > 12% (and > 200 ml in adults) after administering 200–400 µg of inhaled salbutamol.

If there is clinical suspicion, but the spirometry is normal, bronchial challenge testing (e.g., with methacholine or indirect tests such as running exertion or inhalation of hyperosmolar solutions) may be helpful, especially to determine bronchial hyper responsiveness in older children and adults. Furthermore, an FEV_1 increase of +12% (and > 200 ml in adults) after 4 weeks of anti-inflammatory therapy may be suggestive of a diagnosis.

Other tests—FeNO, X-rays, allergy testing, sputum tests

Measuring Fractional exhaled Nitric Oxide (FeNO) is not yet an established practice in general asthma management and is not recommended in the current guidelines for a general therapy decision. There are however several indications in which an FeNO measurement may be helpful; as another supportive component in the asthma diagnosis when features may not be entirely typical, to check on therapeutic adherence to inhaled corticosteroid (ICS) or for the early detection of worsening asthma (Lu et al 2015).

A chest X-ray is not routinely done in the diagnosis of asthma. Apart from non-specific air-trapping and lung hyperinflation, the chest radiograph does not add any diagnostic evidence although it can potentially exclude some differential diagnoses. X-rays of the paranasal sinuses also add little value to the diagnosis of asthma. Its sensitivity in picking up sinusitis is itself in question.

The presence of allergen sensitization in the presence of clinical features may lend support to the diagnosis of atopic asthma. It can also identify the potential triggers and aid in allergen avoidance measures as well as provide prognostic information. Skin prick tests or blood tests for allergen-specific IgE can be performed. The former is most often recommended, being simple, quick and low cost and safe. Appropriate techniques in skin prick testing and proper selection of allergens are however important, and so are the interpretation of the results—to avoid reaching wrong conclusions.

Sputum eosinophil counts have been found to correlate with airway inflammation and are a marker of disease severity. It can also be used for predicting control status of asthma (Bandyopadhyay et al. 2013).

Differential diagnoses

Recurrent wheezing is frequently reported in preschool children. Usually these symptoms are triggered by frequently occurring viral upper airway infections. These upper airway infections may occur between six and eight times per year. Martinez et al. (1995) demonstrated that only 40% of these initial wheezers continue to wheeze at an older age and have or develop asthma. Unfortunately, the ability to predict which children will have *transient* and which will have *persistent* problems is poor. As such, epidemiologic data such as these have limited clinical applicability. In this regard, prospective studies in which subjects were also phenotyped using a number of different clinical measures (e.g., lung function, bronchoalveolar lavage, etc.) showed considerable overlap between the groups. Therefore, at present, there are no diagnostic tools that can reliably predict the development of asthma among wheezing infants.

In 2008, a task force from the ERS defined two phenotypes, 'episodic viral wheeze' and 'multiple-trigger wheeze' (Brand et al. 2008). The former is defined as a phenotype where wheezing only occurs during viral colds, while the latter better resembles asthma, with wheezing also occurring without colds and during physical strain, laughing and so forth. Unfortunately, there is no prospective validation of the two phenotypes, episodic viral wheeze and multiple-trigger wheeze. The 'allergic wheezing' phenotype, defined by the expert panel, and the 'multiple-trigger wheezing', as defined by the ERS task force, are more or less similar.

Asthma may be mimicked by other diseases such as dysfunctional breathing (hyperventilation or Vocal Cord Dysfunction, VCD), malformations of the airway anatomy such as a tracheomalacia or vascular anomalies such as a vascular ring. Other diseases that should be excluded are cardiac anomalies, immune deficiencies, primary ciliary dyskinesia, cystic fibrosis, bronchiectasis, bronchiolitis obliterans, inhaled foreign body, allergic rhinitis and gastroesophageal reflux.

Findings that increase or decrease the probability of asthma in children are listed in Table 12.1. ("British Thoracic Society (BTS), Scottish Intercollegiate Guidelines Network (SIGN). Guideline on the management of asthma : A national clinical guideline," 2012; "National Asthma Council Australia. Australian Asthma Handbook, Version 2.0. National Asthma Council Australia, Melbourne," 2019).

Conditions that can be confused with asthma in children are listed in Table 12.2 ("National Asthma Council Australia. Australian Asthma Handbook, Version 2.0. National Asthma Council Australia, Melbourne," 2019; Weinberger and Abu-Hasan 2007).

Common differential diagnoses of asthma in various age groups are listed in Table 12.3 (GINA 2019).

Table 12.1. Findings that increase or decrease the probability of asthma in children.

Asthma more likely	Asthma less likely
More than one of: • Wheeze • difficulty breathing • feeling of tightness in the chest • cough	Any of: • symptoms only occur when child has a cold, but not between colds • isolated cough in the absence of wheeze or difficulty breathing • history of moist cough • dizziness, light-headedness or peripheral tingling • repeatedly normal physical examination of chest when symptomatic • normal spirometry when symptomatic (children old enough to perform spirometry) • no response to a trail of asthma treatment • clinical features that suggest an alternative diagnosis
AND	
Any of: • Symptoms recur frequently • symptoms worse at night and in the early morning • symptoms triggered by exercise, exposure to pets, cold air, damp air, emotions, laughing • symptoms occur when child doesn't have a cold • history of allergies (e.g., allergic rhinitis, atopic dermatitis) • family history of allergies • family history of asthma • widespread wheeze heard on auscultation • symptoms respond to treatment trail of reliever, with or without a preventer • lung function measured by spirometry increases in response to rapid-acting bronchodilator • lung function measured by spirometry increases in response to a treatment trail with inhaled corticosteroid (where indicated)	
Sources British Thoracic Society (BTS). Scottish intercollegiate Guidelines Network (SIGN). *British Guildeline on the management of Asthma. A national clinical guideline*. BTS'SIGN, Edinburgh, 2012. Available from: https://www.brit-thoracic.org.uk/guidelines-and-quality-standards/asthma-guidline Respiratory Expert Group, Therapeutic Guideline Limited. *Therapeutic Guidelines: Respiratory, Version 4*. Therapeutic Guidelines Limited, Melbourne, 2009.	

Table 12.2. Conditions that can be confused with asthma in children.

Conditions characterised by cough
Pertussis (whooping cough) Post-viral cough Cystic fibrosis Airways abnormalities (e.g., tracheobronchomalacia) Protracted bacterial bronchitis in young children Habit-cough syndrome
Conditions charactrised by wheezing
Upper airway dysfunction Inhaled foreign body causing partial airway obstruction Tracheobronchomalacia
Condition characterised by difficulty breathing
Hyperventilation Anxiety Breathlessness on exertion due to poor cardiopulmonary fitness Upper airway dysfunction
Sources Weinberger M, Abu-Hassan M. Pseudo-asthma: when cough, wheezing, and dyspnea are not asthma. *Pediatrics* 2007; 120: 855–64. Available from: http://pediatrics.aappublications.org/content/120/4/855.full

Table 12.3. Common differential diagnoses of asthma in various age groups.

	≤ 5 years	6–11 years	12–39 years
Recurrent viral infections	X		
Gastroesophageal reflux	X		
Congenital malformations (tracheomalacia, vascular ring, etc.)	X		
Tuberculosis	X		
Protracted bacterial bronchitis	X		
Immunodeficiency	X		
PCD	X	X	
BPD	X	X	
Foreign body aspiration	X	X	X
Congenital heart defects	X	X	X
Cystic fibrosis	X	X	X
Chronic cough (upper respiratory tract)		X	X
Bronchiectasis		X	X
VCD			X
Hyperventilation			X
Alpha 1-antitrypsin deficiency			X
COPD			
Left ventricular heart failure			
Drug-related cough			
Parenchymatous lung disease			
Pulmonary embolism			
According to GINA update 2015, modified by the author team			

Adapted from GINA 2019.
(PCD primary ciliary dyskinesia, *BPD* bronchopulmonary dysplasis, *VCD* vocal cord dysfunction, *COPD* chronic obstructive pulmonary disease)

> **Diagnosis**
> - Asthma is largely a clinical diagnosis.
> - Symptoms of asthma may be mimicked by other diseases and differential diagnoses of childhood asthma should be considered when evaluating the patient.

Treatment

There are many international guidelines available for good asthma management. The basic principles are similar across all of them. While it is important to follow any one guideline, it is equally important to understand the basic principles of asthma management, so that implementation of guidelines becomes easy.

Tripod of asthma management

Optimal management control comprises of parent/patient education, environment control and pharmacotherapy. It can be visualized as a tripod, with each leg having to be addressed to gain good control of chronic disease.

Parent/Patient education: This is arguably the first and most important aspect. It is imperative to mention the term 'asthma' to the patient and to the family at the time of diagnosis. This will set the stage for further discussions and will improve parents' adherence for long-term management. Explaining the diagnosis and its pathogenesis in simple words helps to demystify the diagnosis. Addressing the usual trigger factors and the parental or child's concerns will help chronic asthma management. Explaining the need for long-term medication and the importance of adherence to treatment is of utmost importance. Addressing some of the common myths around asthma is useful even if parents do not bring it up. Education can sometimes take a long time and in a busy practice, it may be useful to see these patients either as a group or individually at specified times when there is adequate time for both the doctor and parent. In certain circumstances, it might even be acceptable if the education component is spread over two consultations or during a follow-up visit.

Environmental control: This includes avoidance of external triggers and addressing the co-morbidities that affect asthma control.

Allergic asthma symptoms occur in response to allergic triggers such as house dust mite and pollen. Non-allergic triggers including cigarette smoke (first, second and third hand exposure), air pollution, strong odours, stress and physical activity can play a prominent role. Though avoidance of triggers makes perfect sense, the evidence behind it is mixed. Problems arise particularly when looking at the impact of dust mite as it is impossible to eliminate the trigger completely. However, it is possible to reduce dust mite load in the environment. It is unlikely that any single intervention will yield significant benefits. One study, using an integrated approach (parent education, use of allergen impermeable covers, HEPA air filters and pest control measures at home) showed a decrease in symptoms, medication usage and improvement in lung function test in children with dust mite allergy and asthma(Morgan et al. 2004).

Similarly, cessation of active smoking improves lung function and reduces airway inflammation. Even a reduction in passive smoke exposure has been shown to improve asthma control and has shown to reduce asthma-related admissions in children (Rayens et al. 2008). While exercise has been shown to cause symptoms of asthma, it reflects control of the underlying asthma. This is one trigger that patients are told not to avoid. Regular medication will get exercise trigger under control and children should be encouraged to take part in physical activity.

Pharmacotherapy: The long-term goals of asthma management are to achieve good control of symptoms, maintain normal activity levels and to minimize the risk of asthma-related death, exacerbations, persistent airflow limitation and treatment side-effects (GINA 2019). Medication may be needed to achieve these goals.

On diagnosis of asthma in a medication-naïve child, it is important to diagnose whether it is intermittent or persistent asthma.

Intermittent asthma is defined when: ("National Heart, Lung, and Blood Institute National Asthma Education and Prevention Program Expert Panel Report 3: Guidelines for the Diagnosis and Management of Asthma Full Report," 2007).

- Symptoms (difficulty breathing, wheezing, tightness of the chest and coughing) occur fewer than 2 days a week and do not interfere with normal activities.
- Night time symptoms occur fewer than 2 days a month.

Children with intermittent asthma do not need regular long-term medication and can be treated as and when required with a bronchodilator such as salbutamol (a short-acting β_2-agonist).

Children categorized with persistent asthma symptoms will need long-term daily controller anti-inflammatory medication. Inhaled corticosteroids (ICS) is the recommended first-line controller. The other controller medications used in paediatrics are leukotriene pathway modifiers and combinations of ICS with long-acting b_2-agonist (LABA). Daily ICS is the preferred first-line medication in most children with persistent asthma irrespective of severity of chronic asthma. Most children will respond to a low-dose of ICS, which is equivalent to 100–200 mg of fluticasone, budesonide or beclomethasone (these being commonly used ICS in children). ICS has been shown to improve symptom control, reduce exacerbations, improve lung function, reduce hospitalisations and reduce asthma mortality (Hui 2019, Suissa et al. 2000). A list of currently available inhaled corticosteroids is shown in Table 12.4 (GINA 2019).

Any of the equivalent doses of low-dose ICS can be selected depending on local availability and cost considerations.

Intermittent ICS has been tried in asthmatic children but have not been shown to be equivalent to daily ICS (Castro-Rodriguez et al. 2016).

The use of ICS in low to medium doses is considered safe. A few studies have shown a small reduction in height with the use of ICS in asthma (Kelly et al. 2012). This effect is mostly seen in the first year of use and is generally not cumulative. Additionally, it should be emphasized that uncontrolled asthma can lead to a greater suppression of height compared to ICS use to control asthma. Some of the other side-effects that have been associated with ICS use are oral candidiasis and dysphonia, but these are minimized with the usage of spacers. Other systemic side effects of steroids are not clinically significant with low to medium doses of ICS.

Inhaler therapy, whether with ICS, salbutamol or other medications, must be given with proper inhaler devices and techniques. The various inhaler devices suitable for use in various age groups are listed in Table 12.5.

Leukotriene pathway modifiers like montelukast, have been shown to improve both daytime and night time asthma symptoms as well as reduce the need for β_2 stimulants and oral steroids in children with persistent asthma (Knorr et al. 2001). However, these are not as efficacious as ICS as primary controllers (Szefler et al. 2007). They are recommended as second-choice treatment to ICS or as add-on therapy.

Table 12.4. Currently available inhaled corticosteroids.

Drug	Daily low dose (mcg)	Daily medium dose (mcg)	Daily high dose (mcg)
Beclometasone dipropionate	100–200	> 200–400	> 400
Budesonide	100–200	> 200–400	> 400
Fluticasone propionate	100–200	> 200–500	> 500
Ciclesonide	80	> 80–160	> 160
Mometasone furoate	110	> 220–< 440	> 400
Triamcinolone acetonide	400–800	> 800–1200	> 1200

Table 12.5. Inhaler devices suitable for use in various age groups.

Age	Delivery devices
0–3 years	MDI (Metered dose inhaler) + spacer + mask
3–6 years	MDI + spacer
6–18 years	MDI + spacer DPI (Dry powder devices)

Long-Acting β_2-Agonists (LABA) such as salmeterol and formeterol are always used in conjunction with ICS. Most children respond to monotherapy with ICS alone, but when treatment needs to be escalated in children above 6 years, combinations of LABA and ICS are used.

Once controller medications are started, it is good practice to continue these for a prolonged period (3–6 months) at the same dose. Children need to be regularly monitored while on treatment. At each of the subsequent visits, the following need to be monitored (using the SPICE mnemonic):

Symptoms during the interval period

Parental concerns (if any)

Inhaler technique

Compliance (or adherence)

Environmental control

At each clinic visit, asthma control is assessed using the questions in Table 12.6 (GINA 2019).

For children with well-controlled asthma, controller medications are continued for up to 6 months before doses are gradually tapered, e.g., ICS doses are reduced by 50% every 3 months until the lowest dose is reached. If the child's asthma is well-controlled on the lowest dose of controller medication for 3 months, then the medication can be stopped. Exceptions to this rule are children who have relapsed in the past following dose reduction and high-risk children who have had previous ICU admissions; these patients will require a longer duration of ICS in the lowest possible dose.

For children with partly controlled and uncontrolled asthma, it is important to look out for the reasons why control is sub optimal. Sequentially, these steps may be taken to identify the reasons:

1. Check diagnosis
2. Check dose of controllers (to ensure they are adequate)
3. Check adherence (to ensure they are taking the medications)
4. Check inhaler technique (to ensure medications are reaching the intended target destination)
5. Check for co-morbid conditions such as allergic rhinitis and gastro-esophageal reflux disease (uncontrolled co-morbid conditions can interfere with control of asthma)
6. Check for psychosocial factors (conditions such as vocal cord dysfunction can mimic asthma)

Checking and correcting these six steps usually help to achieve better asthma control in most children. However, a minority of children will still have persistent symptoms. These are the difficult-to-

Table 12.6. Questions used to assess asthma control.

Asthma symptom control			Level of asthma symptom control		
In the past 4 weeks, has the patient had			Well controlled	Partly controlled	Uncontrolled
Day time symptoms more than twice a week?	Yes	No	None of these	1–2 of these	3–4 of these
Any night waking due to asthma?	Yes	No			
Reliever needed for symptoms more than twice/week?	Yes	No			
Any activity limitation due to asthma?	Yes	No			

treat asthmatics who will need escalation of medications. In children less than 5 years of age, either the dose of ICS is doubled or montelukast is added. In children over 6 years of age, LABA is added to ICS.

In a small percentage of difficult asthmatics, newer medications like Omalizumab (humanized monoclonal anti-IgE antibody), Mepolizumab (humanized monoclonal anti IL-5 antibody) and Benzralizumab (monoclonal anti IL-5 receptor antibody) may be considered.

Managing acute exacerbations

Management at home: It is important to give all patients diagnosed with asthma a written action plan. This is a document with advice on actions to be taken by the parent and child when they have symptom exacerbations at home. The written action plan also serves to reiterate the daily medication plan. Early recognition and prompt treatment of asthma can often curtail progression of the disease. The initial symptoms may start with a persistent cough and wheeze. It can however progress to more severe exacerbations manifested by breathlessness, increased use of accessory muscles leading to supra-sternal and subcostal indrawing, signs of hypoxia (irritability or drowsiness, tachypnoea, tachycardia, cyanosis) and a silent chest with impaired gas exchange.

Parents are encouraged to start using a salbutamol inhaler when their child becomes symptomatic. Two to four puffs of salbutamol 100 mcg inhaler is given every 4 hours as required. If symptoms persist or worsen, despite salbutamol, parents are requested to seek medical attention as soon as possible.

Management in clinic/emergency department: When a child presents to the emergency department or the doctor's clinic with an asthma exacerbation, the severity of the child's condition is established. The vital parameters including oxygen saturation are measured and monitored. If oxygen saturation is less than 92% in room air, supplemental oxygen is started. Upto 6 puffs of salbutamol 100 mcg inhaler are given every 20 minutes. However, if the child is hypoxic and requires oxygen, then salbutamol can be nebulized. In children less than 6 years of age, the dose is 2.5 mg salbutamol (0.5 ml of 0.5% salbutamol) mixed in with 2.5 ml of 0.9% sodium chloride solution. In older children, 5 mg salbutamol (1 ml of 0.5% salbutamol) mixed in with 2 ml of 0.9% sodium chloride solution is used. This can be repeated up to 3 times every 20 minutes. If the symptoms and wheeze persist, then a second round of salbutamol in combination with ipratropium bromide (250 to 500 mcg) is nebulized every 20 minutes up to 3 times. A dose of oral prednisolone (1–2 mg/kg body weight) is given as well. If the child improves, the child is monitored in the clinic and sent home with a 3-day course of oral prednisolone and salbutamol 100 mcg inhaler with an MDI with spacer (2–4 puffs to be taken every 4 hours as required). A follow-up appointment should be made to see the child in the clinic in 3 days' time.

If the child has not improved in the emergency department or clinic after 2 rounds of salbutamol nebulization and oral steroids, a bolus dose of magnesium sulphate, $MgSO_4$, at 25–75 mg/kg with a maximum dose of 2 grams is given as a slow intravenous bolus over 20 minutes. If the child still fails to improve, the child should be transferred to a Paediatric Intensive Care Unit (PICU).

Management in intensive care: In the PICU, the child is monitored closely. Continuous cardio-respiratory monitoring is mandatory. An arterial blood gas sample is taken to look for the degree of hypoxia and an accurate measurement of carbon dioxide (CO_2) levels. CO_2 levels are expected to be lower than normal as the child would have been hyperventilating. A normal or high CO_2 should alert the clinician to impending type 2 respiratory failure. Continuous nebulization with salbutamol is preferred using special large nebulizing chambers (5–15 mg/hour). If this is not possible, then a normal nebulizer can be used, and back to back nebulization with salbutamol is given. Further doses of $MgSO_4$ can be given every 6–8 hours from the first dose given in the emergency department. Nebulized ipratropium can be added to salbutamol and given every 6 hours. Oxygen supplementation and systemic steroids should be continued. If the child is sick and is not able to take medication orally, intravenous hydrocortisone is given (5–10 mg mg/kg). Serum electrolyte measurement is important as frequent use of salbutamol can cause hypokalaemia and severe asthma can also lead to Syndrome of Inappropriate Antidiuretic Hormone Secretion, or SIADH. A chest x-ray (should be done to look for air leak syndromes and infection. The hydration status of the child must be monitored and maintained. If bronchospasm is still severe and persistent, then an intravenous β_2-agonist (salbutamol or terbutaline) is started as a continuous infusion. Some centres prefer to use intravenous methylxanthines (aminophylline), though it is important to note the narrow therapeutic index for this medication.

Rarely, the exacerbation is resistant to therapy and the child progresses to frank respiratory failure requiring ventilatory support. Currently, the use of Non-Invasive Ventilation (NIV) is increasing in the management of severe asthma in PICU (Rampersad et al. 2018). While it decreases the work of breathing, but remains controversial whether this can avoid intubation in the majority of patients. The indications for intubation include cardiac arrest, respiratory arrest, altered sensorium, progressive exhaustion, a PaO_2 of less than 60 mmHg on 100% oxygen via a non-rebreather mask and a $PaCO_2$ of greater than 55 mmHg or $PaCO_2$ rising by more than 5 mmHg/hour (Brenner et al. 2009). Volume-cycled pressure-limited ventilation, with short inspiratory and long expiratory times and minimal PEEP (Peak End Expiratory Pressure) are recommended initial settings. Careful monitoring for air leaks is imperative. Once the child starts improving, the support systems including medications are sequentially tapered and stopped following the 'last in, first out' adage, with the most recently added support being the first to be stopped.

Any admission to ICU is considered a red flag, and these children need closer monitoring over time. They will usually require long-term controller therapy with a very slow taper down of doses.

Treatment

- Optimal management control involves parent/patient education, environment control and pharmacotherapy.
- At each clinic visit, monitor for symptoms during the interval period, parental concerns, inhaler technique, compliance to treatment and the environment that the child lives in.
- Co-morbid conditions and psychosocial factors need to be addressed as part of childhood asthma management.

Clinical pearls

- Asthma can begin at any age.
- About a third of children wheeze during their first three years of life, but not all go on to develop school-age asthma.
- Episodic viral preschool wheezing does not respond as well to conventional asthma treatments.
- The modified Asthma Predictive Index can help identify factors that predict the likelihood of preschool children developing asthma in later life.
- Asthma largely remains a clinical diagnosis. While there are several investigation options to help with the diagnosis, they are largely supportive to clinical findings.
- Features suggestive of other causes of cough and wheeze should be sought when conducting the history and examination to avoid misdiagnosing asthma.
- Before escalating treatment, ensure that the diagnosis of asthma is correct, that adherence to treatment and technique of drug delivery are optimal, and that co-morbid conditions and psychosocial factors are addressed.

Summary

Childhood asthma remains a heterogenous disease with variable presentation. The diagnosis of asthma in children is largely clinical, with symptoms of airway obstruction a result of underlying airway inflammation. A history of wheezing in the preschool age does not always lead to asthma in school-age. Clinical assessment should include consideration for other potential differential diagnoses of asthma, particularly if the child does not respond to escalating asthma treatment, regardless of age. The treatment of asthma is holistic and involves patient and caregiver education, environmental trigger avoidance and appropriate use of asthma medication.

References

Akinbami LJ, Simon AE, Rossen LM. Changing trends in asthma prevalence among children. Pediatrics 2016; 137(1). doi: 10.1542/peds.2015-2354.

Bandyopadhyay A, Roy PP, Saha K, Chakraborty S, Jash D, Saha D. Usefulness of induced sputum eosinophil count to assess severity and treatment outcome in asthma patients. Lung India 2013; 30(2): 117–123. doi: 10.4103/0970-2113.110419.

Brand PL, Baraldi E, Bisgaard H, Boner AL, Castro-Rodriguez JA, Custovic A, et al. Definition, assessment and treatment of wheezing disorders in preschool children: an evidence-based approach. Eur Respir J 2008; 32(4): 1096–1110. doi: 10.1183/09031936.00002108.

Brand PL, Caudri D, Eber E, Gaillard EA, Garcia-Marcos L, Hedlin G, et al. Classification and pharmacological treatment of preschool wheezing: changes since 2008. Eur Respir J 2014; 43(4): 1172–1177. doi: 10.1183/09031936.00199913.

Brenner B, Corbridge T, Kazzi A. Intubation and mechanical ventilation of the asthmatic patient in respiratory failure. Proc Am Thorac Soc 2009; 6(4): 371–379. doi: 10.1513/pats.P09ST4.

British Thoracic Society (BTS), Scottish Intercollegiate Guidelines Network (SIGN). Guideline on the management of asthma : A national clinical guideline. 2012.

Castro-Rodriguez JA, Holberg CJ, Wright AL, Martinez FD. A clinical index to define risk of asthma in young children with recurrent wheezing. Am J Respir Crit Care Med 2000; 162(4 Pt 1): 1403–1406. doi: 10.1164/ajrccm.162.4.9912111.

Castro-Rodriguez JA, Custovic A, Ducharme FM. Treatment of asthma in young children: evidence-based recommendations. Asthma Res Pract 2016; 2: 5. doi: 10.1186/s40733-016-0020-z.

Caudri D, Wijga A, Scholtens S, Kerkhof M, Gerritsen J, Ruskamp JM, et al. Early daycare is associated with an increase in airway symptoms in early childhood but is no protection against asthma or atopy at 8 years. Am J Respir Crit Care Med 2009; 180(6): 491–498. doi: 10.1164/rccm.200903-0327OC.

Corren J, Manning BE, Thompson SF, Hennessy S, Strom BL. Rhinitis therapy and the prevention of hospital care for asthma: a case-control study. J Allergy Clin Immunol 2004; 113(3): 415–419. doi: 10.1016/j.jaci.2003.11.034.

Covar RA, Strunk R, Zeiger RS, Wilson LA, Liu AH, Weiss S, et al. Predictors of remitting, periodic, and persistent childhood asthma. J Allergy Clin Immunol 2010; 125(2): 359–366 e353. doi: 10.1016/j.jaci.2009.10.037.

de Marco R, Locatelli F, Sunyer J, Burney P. Differences in incidence of reported asthma related to age in men and women. A retrospective analysis of the data of the European Respiratory Health Survey. Am J Respir Crit Care Med 2000; 162(1): 68–74. doi: 10.1164/ajrccm.162.1.9907008.

Fitzpatrick AM, Jackson DJ, Mauger DT, et al. Individualized therapy for persistent asthma in young children. J Allergy Clin Immunol. 2016; 138(6): 1608–1618.e12. doi:10.1016/j.jaci.2016.09.028.

Gauderman WJ, Avol E, Lurmann F, Kuenzli N, Gilliland F, Peters J, et al. Childhood asthma and exposure to traffic and nitrogen dioxide. Epidemiology 2005; 16(6): 737–743. doi: 10.1097/01.ede.0000181308.51440.75.

GINA. Global Strategy for Asthma Management and Prevention 2020.

Gissler M, Jarvelin MR, Louhiala P, Hemminki E. Boys have more health problems in childhood than girls: follow-up of the 1987 Finnish birth cohort. Acta Paediatr 1999; 88(3): 310–314. doi: 10.1080/08035259950170088.

Guilbert TW, Morgan WJ, Krawiec M, Lemanske RF, Jr, Sorkness C, Szefler SJ, et al. The Prevention of Early Asthma in Kids study: design, rationale and methods for the Childhood Asthma Research and Education network. Control Clin Trials 2004; 25(3): 286–310. doi: 10.1016/j.cct.2004.03.002.

Guilbert TW, Morgan WJ, Zeiger RS, Bacharier LB, Boehmer SJ, Krawiec M, et al. Atopic characteristics of children with recurrent wheezing at high risk for the development of childhood asthma. J Allergy Clin Immunol 2004; 114(6): 1282–1287. doi: 10.1016/j.jaci.2004.09.020.

Holgate ST, Polosa R. The mechanisms, diagnosis, and management of severe asthma in adults. Lancet 2006; 368(9537): 780–793. doi: 10.1016/S0140-6736(06)69288-X.

Holgate ST, Polosa R. Treatment strategies for allergy and asthma. Nat Rev Immunol 2008; 8(3): 218–230. doi: 10.1038/nri2262.

Hui RWH. Inhaled corticosteroid-phobia and childhood asthma: Current understanding and management implications. Paediatr Respir Rev 2019; doi: 10.1016/j.prrv.2019.03.009.

Karmaus W, Botezan C. Does a higher number of siblings protect against the development of allergy and asthma? A review. J Epidemiol Community Health 2002; 56(3): 209–217. doi: 10.1136/jech.56.3.209.

Kelly HW, Sternberg AL, Lescher R, Fuhlbrigge AL, Williams P, Zeiger RS, et al. Effect of inhaled glucocorticoids in childhood on adult height. N Engl J Med 2012; 367(10): 904–912. doi: 10.1056/NEJMoa1203229.

Knorr B, Franchi LM, Bisgaard H, Vermeulen JH, LeSouef P, Santanello N, et al. Montelukast, a leukotriene receptor antagonist, for the treatment of persistent asthma in children aged 2 to 5 years. Pediatrics 2001; 108(3): E48. doi: 10.1542/peds.108.3.e48.

Krishnamoorthy N, Khare A, Oriss TB, Raundhal M, Morse C, Yarlagadda M, et al. Early infection with respiratory syncytial virus impairs regulatory T cell function and increases susceptibility to allergic asthma. Nat Med 2012; 18(10): 1525–1530. doi: 10.1038/nm.2896.

Kuehni CE, Davis A, Brooke AM, Silverman M. Are all wheezing disorders in very young (preschool) children increasing in prevalence? Lancet 2001; 357(9271): 1821–1825. doi: 10.1016/S0140-6736(00)04958-8.

Le Bourgeois M, Goncalves M, Le Clainche L, Benoist MR, Fournet JC, Scheinmann P, et al. Bronchoalveolar cells in children < 3 years old with severe recurrent wheezing. Chest 2002; 122(3): 791–797. doi: 10.1378/chest.122.3.791.

Lohia S, Schlosser RJ, Soler ZM. Impact of intranasal corticosteroids on asthma outcomes in allergic rhinitis: a meta-analysis. Allergy 2013; 68(5): 569–579. doi: 10.1111/all.12124.

Lu M, Wu B, Che D, Qiao R, Gu H. FeNO and asthma treatment in children: a systematic review and meta-analysis. Medicine (Baltimore) 2015; 94(4): e347. doi: 10.1097/MD.0000000000000347.

Martinez FD, Wright AL, Taussig LM, Holberg CJ, Halonen M, Morgan WJ. Asthma and wheezing in the first six years of life. The Group Health Medical Associates. N Engl J Med 1995; 332(3): 133–138. doi: 10.1056/NEJM199501193320301.

Miliku K, Azad MB. Breastfeeding and the Developmental Origins of Asthma: Current Evidence, Possible Mechanisms, and Future Research Priorities. Nutrients 2018; 10(8). doi: 10.3390/nu10080995.

Millstein J, Gilliland F, Berhane K, Gauderman WJ, McConnell R, Avol E, et al. Effects of ambient air pollutants on asthma medication use and wheezing among fourth-grade school children from 12 Southern California communities enrolled in The Children's Health Study. Arch Environ Health 2004; 59(10): 505–514. doi: 10.1080/00039890409605166.

Morgan WJ, Crain EF, Gruchalla RS, O'Connor GT, Kattan M, Evans R, et al. Results of a home-based environmental intervention among urban children with asthma. N Engl J Med 2004; 351(11): 1068–1080. doi: 10.1056/NEJMoa032097.

Moshammer H, Hoek G, Luttmann-Gibson H, Neuberger MA, Antova T, Gehring U, et al. Parental smoking and lung function in children: an international study. Am J Respir Crit Care Med 2006; 173(11): 1255–1263. doi: 10.1164/rccm.200510-1552OC.

National Asthma Council Australia. Australian Asthma Handbook, Version 2.0. National Asthma Council Australia, Melbourne 2019. from http://www.asthmahandbook.org.au.

National Heart, Lung, Blood Institute National Asthma Education and Prevention Program Expert Panel Report 3: Guidelines for the Diagnosis and Management of Asthma Full Report 2007.

Pearce N, Ait-Khaled N, Beasley R, Mallol J, Keil U, Mitchell E, et al. Worldwide trends in the prevalence of asthma symptoms: phase III of the International Study of Asthma and Allergies in Childhood (ISAAC). Thorax 2007; 62(9): 758–766. doi: 10.1136/thx.2006.070169.

Rampersad N, Wilkins B, Egan JR. Outcomes of paediatric critical care asthma patients. J Paediatr Child Health 2018; 54(6): 633–637. doi: 10.1111/jpc.13855.

Rayens MK, Burkhart PV, Zhang M, Lee S, Moser DK, Mannino D, et al. Reduction in asthma-related emergency department visits after implementation of a smoke-free law. J Allergy Clin Immunol 2008; 122(3): 537–541 e533. doi: 10.1016/j.jaci.2008.06.029.

Saglani S, Payne DN, Zhu J, Wang Z, Nicholson AG, Bush A, et al. Early detection of airway wall remodeling and eosinophilic inflammation in preschool wheezers. Am J Respir Crit Care Med 2007; 176(9): 858–864. doi: 10.1164/rccm.200702-212OC.

Saglani S, Mathie SA, Gregory LG, Bell MJ, Bush A, Lloyd CM. Pathophysiological features of asthma develop in parallel in house dust mite-exposed neonatal mice. Am J Respir Cell Mol Biol 2009; 41(3): 281–289. doi: 10.1165/rcmb.2008-0396OC.

Suissa S, Ernst P, Benayoun S, Baltzan M, Cai B. Low-dose inhaled corticosteroids and the prevention of death from asthma. N Engl J Med 2000; 343(5): 332–336. doi: 10.1056/NEJM200008033430504.

Szefler SJ, Baker JW, Uryniak T, Goldman M, Silkoff PE. Comparative study of budesonide inhalation suspension and montelukast in young children with mild persistent asthma. J Allergy Clin Immunol 2007; 120(5): 1043–1050. doi: 10.1016/j.jaci.2007.08.063.

Tai A, Tran H, Roberts M, Clarke N, Gibson AM, Vidmar S, et al. Outcomes of childhood asthma to the age of 50 years. J Allergy Clin Immunol 2014; 133(6): 1572–1578 e1573. doi: 10.1016/j.jaci.2013.12.1033.

To T, Stanojevic S, Moores G, Gershon AS, Bateman ED, Cruz AA, et al. Global asthma prevalence in adults: findings from the cross-sectional world health survey. BMC Public Health 2012; 12: 204. doi: 10.1186/1471-2458-12-204.

van den Toorn LM, Overbeek SE, de Jongste JC, Leman K, Hoogsteden HC, Prins JB. Airway inflammation is present during clinical remission of atopic asthma. Am J Respir Crit Care Med 2001; 164(11): 2107–2113. doi: 10.1164/ajrccm.164.11.2006165.

van Gent R, van Essen LE, Rovers MM, Kimpen JL, van der Ent CK, de Meer G. Quality of life in children with undiagnosed and diagnosed asthma. Eur J Pediatr 2007; 166(8): 843–848. doi: 10.1007/s00431-006-0358-y.

Wang XS, Tan TN, Shek LP, Chng SY, Hia CP, Ong NB, et al. The prevalence of asthma and allergies in Singapore; data from two ISAAC surveys seven years apart. Arch Dis Child 2004; 89(5): 423–426. doi: 10.1136/adc.2003.031112.

Weinberger M, Abu-Hasan M. Pseudo-asthma: when cough, wheezing, and dyspnea are not asthma. Pediatrics 120(4): 855–864. doi: 10.1542/peds.2007-0078.

13

Adult Asthma

Flavia CL Hoyte,[1,*] *Eugene M Choo*[2] *and Rohit K Katial*[1]

INTRODUCTION

Asthma is a complex heterogeneous disease characterized by chronic airway inflammation, airway hyper responsiveness and variable airflow obstruction that reverses either spontaneously or with treatment. The hallmark respiratory symptoms that result include shortness of breath, wheezing, coughing and chest tightness; symptoms are often worst in the night or early morning (NIH 2002). Asthma is a common condition that is responsible for significant morbidity and mortality throughout the world. Over recent decades, its worldwide prevalence has increased. There have been many advances in our understanding of asthma pathophysiology and in therapeutic options during this time as well.

Epidemiology

Prevalence

Prevalence is defined by the total number of cases of a given disease in a specific population at a specific time. Although asthma is present throughout the world, prevalence rates vary greatly, with developed countries having higher values than less affluent nations. Most recent estimates from the 2015 Global Burden of Disease study place worldwide prevalence at approximately 358.2 million people, which is approximately 12.6% higher than in 1990 (GBD 2015). Age-specific asthma prevalence estimates vary tremendously, with ranges of 3 to 38% in children and 2 to 12% in adults (Masoli et al. 2004). A 2002–2003 World Health Survey from the World Health Organization of 177,496 adults from 70 different countries demonstrated that the prevalence of asthma varies greatly among different countries, with an approximate 21-fold difference between the lowest and highest prevalence nations. In this survey, 4.5% of these adults either carried a doctor's diagnosis of asthma or had taken asthma medications in the past year, and approximately 8.6% stated that they had noticed wheezing in the 12 months prior to the survey. Australia, northern and western Europe and Brazil demonstrated the highest prevalence (To et al. 2012). Although the worldwide prevalence of asthma is increasing as a whole, it has stabilized or decreased in some of the highest prevalence countries, such as Australia (Poulos et al. 2005). This stabilization trend is particularly apparent in higher income countries, which may reflect improved asthma control through advanced medication and education (Dharmage et al. 2019).

---

[1] National Jewish Health, 1400 Jackson Street, Denver, Colorado, USA 80206, Email: KatialR@njhealth.org
[2] University of California San Francisco, 400 Parnassus Ave, San Francisco, California, USA 94143. Email: emchoo@gmail.com
* Corresponding author: fclega@gmail.com

Incidence

As opposed to prevalence, incidence is the number of new cases of a given disease in a specific population over a certain time period. The incidence of asthma rates have overall been increasing based on a meta-analysis of European and American studies (Eagan et al. 2005). Data from Rochester, Minnesota (USA) demonstrated that 80% of asthma cases began before the age of 4 years (Yunginger et al. 1992), reflected that incidence rates are highest in the youngest age groups, particularly in boys (Silverstein et al. 1994). By young adulthood, however, women are almost 1.5 times more likely to develop asthma than men, suggesting that sex hormones may play a role (Beckett et al. 2001, Dharmage et al. 2019). Incidence rates decrease during adolescence and young adulthood and then increase later on. Incidence rates between blacks and whites were similar in American studies (Beckett et al. 2001).

Morbidity and mortality

Asthma is associated with significant morbidity, typically measured using data such as quality of life, medication use, hospitalizations, symptom status and lung function. Mortality rates for asthma vary greatly among countries and are difficult to directly compare due to differences in data quality and collection. Nevertheless, in many developed nations, the mortality rate has declined since approximately 1999; in the United States, as of 2004, the mortality rate for patients 5 to 34 years old was approximately 4 per million (CDC 2006). Globally, the mortality rate from asthma decreased by 26.7% from 1990 to 2015, with an estimate of 0.4 million people dying from asthma in 2015 worldwide. The age-standardized death rates decreased by 58.8% over this same time period, with a greater decrease seen in males than females (GBD 2015). Most of the decrease in mortality and hospitalization rates occurred during the 1990s and early 2000s, with steady rates over the past decade (Dharmage et al. 2019).

Risk factors for developing asthma

Lifestyle and environmental variables associated with allergic asthma are reviewed elsewhere in this book. As a brief summary, studies have identified a number of factors associated with the development of asthma, including atopy, diet, obesity, respiratory infections, non-respiratory microbial infections, premature birth, occupational exposures, air pollution (both indoor and outdoor) and tobacco smoke (both primary and secondary). Genetic linkage analysis has also identified a number of genes that have been implicated in asthma, but no direct causative effect from them has yet been proven (Ober and Hoffjan 2006).

Pathophysiology

The pathogenesis of asthma is complex, but the clinical symptoms of wheezing, shortness of breath, chest tightness and a cough are a consequence of airway inflammation, bronchial hyper responsiveness and airflow obstruction. The airway inflammation in asthma involves a multitude of cell types. Studies using flexible bronchoscopy have revealed intense airway infiltration with several immunologic and inflammatory cells: eosinophils are usually predominant, but neutrophils, activated T lymphocytes, alveolar macrophages, dendritic cells, mast cells, innate lymphoid cells and natural killer T cells have also been found. The mediator and cytokine milieu from these cells is then responsible for characteristic changes such as airway mucosa edema, mucus hypersecretion and hyper responsiveness of the airways. Structural changes in asthmatic patients include epithelial damage, subepithelial basement membrane thickening with collagen deposition, airway smooth muscle hyperplasia and vascular tissue changes. Chronic obstruction of the small airways can occur as an outcome of this airway remodeling; eventually, irreversible airflow obstruction may result (Gern and Busse 2008).

There are several genetic and environmental factors associated with asthma, and their complex interaction influences the clinical presentation of the disease. While a review of all of the candidate genes implicated in asthma is beyond the scope of this chapter, polymorphisms have been noted in genes for both airway structure and immunoregulation (Ober 2005). Asthma usually develops early in life, and as described in Chapter 7 of this book, allergen sensitization and infectious causes (e.g., RSV and rhinovirus) impact on the development of childhood asthma. In adulthood, various occupational exposures can also play an important role.

Diagnostic evaluation

Although there is no single diagnostic test for asthma at any age group, careful review of the present and past history, along with a physical examination and selected physiologic tests, can help the clinician support a diagnosis of asthma. In an adult patient, a combination of history, complete pulmonary function testing and bronchial challenges can aid in the correct diagnosis. Diagnostic pulmonary function testing is reviewed elsewhere in this book. Bronchial challenges are most commonly performed using methacholine, mannitol or exercise to induce bronchoconstriction or airway reactivity.

Differential diagnosis

There are multiple conditions that may be similar to asthma; the differential diagnosis of asthma in adults is listed in Table 13.1.

Table 13.1. Differential diagnosis of asthma in adults.

Rhinosinusitis or upper airway cough syndrome (UACS)
Chronic Obstructive Pulmonary Disease (COPD, smoking-induced)
Tracheobronchial narrowing (e.g., tracheobronchomalacia, tumor or stenosis)
Gastroesophageal reflux (GERD)
Foreign body aspiration
Bronchiectasis
Cardiac failure
Pulmonary embolism
Lower respiratory tract infection
Hyperventilation syndrome
Vocal cord dysfunction (VCD)
Cystic fibrosis
Sleep disorders
Mastocytosis
Nonasthmatic eosinophilic bronchitis
Cough due to medications (e.g., Angiotensin-Converting Enzyme inhibitors)
Eosinophilic granulomatosis with polyangiitis (EGPA or Churg-Strauss vasculitis)
Carcinoid tumor
Allergic bronchopulmonary aspergillosis/mycosis (ABPA/ABPM)
Aspirin/NSAID-exacerbated respiratory disease (AERD/NERD)

Modified from Boulet LP. "Approach to adults with asthma". *Middleton's Allergy: Principles & Practice*, 7th edition. Ed. Adkinson, N.F. et al. Elsevier 2009. 1348.

Classification of asthma severity

Three sets of guidelines/consensus statements exist for the classification and management of asthma, one from each of the following organizations: The United States National Asthma Education and Prevention Program (NAEPP), last updated in 2007 (NHLBI 2007); the 2013 joint European Respiratory Society/

American Thoracic Society's Consensus with a focus on severe asthma (Chung et al. 2014), and the Global Initiative for Asthma (GINA) guidelines, updated annually, most recently in 2019 (GINA 2019).

The NAEPP guidelines classify asthma by severity based on impairment (daytime and night time symptom frequency), to include: (1) intermittent asthma, (2) mild persistent asthma, (3) moderate persistent asthma, (4) and severe persistent asthma. The 2007 update of these guidelines demonstrates a paradigm shift toward a focus on asthma control for those patients already on a controller therapy, with severity classification applying only to those patients not yet on a controller (NHLBI 2007).

The GINA classification groups (1) and (2) above as mild asthma and then has separate categories for moderate and severe asthma. The definition of severe asthma is similar in the GINA guidelines and 2013 ERS/ATS guidelines. In both, severe asthma is defined as asthma that can only be controlled with, or remains uncontrolled despite, high dose inhaled corticosteroid (ICS) plus another agent (Long-Acting Beta Agonist (LABA), leukotriene receptor antagonist (LTRA), or theophylline) for a year or systemic corticosteroids for over half of the previous year. This definition assumes that co-morbidities and asthma mimickers have been addressed and that proper adherence and technique have been verified (GINA 2019). The ERS/ATS guidelines add that patients who flare upon weaning their steroids are also defined as severe, even if they do not exactly meet the criteria above (Chung et al. 2014).

Management of chronic asthma with a goal of asthma control

The 2007 update to the NAEPP guidelines outlined recommendations for asthma management, as described below (NHLBI 2007). These broad recommendations are similar to those of GINA, with an emphasis on regular assessment of asthma control and on working together with patients in a partnership to adjust therapy in order to gain control (GINA 2019). The four components of asthma care are described in Table 13.2.

Table 13.2. Four components of asthma care.

1: Assessing and monitoring asthma severity and asthma control
2: Education for a partnership in care
3: Control of environmental factors and comorbid conditions that affect asthma
4: Medications

National Asthma Education and Prevention Program Expert Panel Report 3: Guidelines for the diagnosis and management of asthma[19]

1. Assessing and monitoring asthma severity and control

This first component of asthma care includes initial assessment of asthma severity in patients not yet on controller therapy, followed by regular assessment of asthma control to monitor and adjust therapy with close follow up.

For both guidelines, the primary goals of asthma management are to reduce impairment and risk. Reduction of impairment involves preventing chronic symptoms, minimizing the need for inhaled Short-Acting Beta Agonists (SABA), maintaining normal pulmonary function as much as possible, maintaining normal activity levels and meeting patients' asthma care expectations. Risk reduction includes prevention of recurrent exacerbations, prevention of loss of lung function and optimal pharmacotherapy with minimization of adverse effects. An assessment of asthma control takes all of these factors into consideration. A patient is thought to have 'well-controlled' asthma if they do not require their rescue medication more than twice a week, not having daytime symptoms more than twice a week, not having night time symptoms more than twice a month and not having any activity limitations as a result of their asthma. The NAEPP guidelines also give cutoffs for lung function (Forced Expiratory Volume in 1 second ($FEV1$) or peak flow (PEF) > 80% of predicted or personal best), scores on validated questionnaires (Asthma Control Test (ACT) > 19, Asthma Control Questionnaire (ACQ) $\leq$ 0.75, or Asthma Therapy Assessment Questionnaire (ATAQ) of 0) and rate of exacerbations requiring oral steroids (0–1 per year) when defining 'well-controlled' asthma.

2. Education for a partnership in care

Education of asthma patients includes teaching on self-management measures, such as self-monitoring with peak flow or Piko meters, correct medication use, adherence to prescribed medications and avoidance of exacerbating environmental factors. Development of written asthma action plans has been shown to be more effective in altering patient behavior than simply verbal ones (Gibson et al. 2003). Overall, this education should be integrated into all areas where patients interact with caregivers, including outpatient clinics, hospitals, pharmacies, schools and homes.

3. Control of environmental factors and comorbid conditions that affect asthma

The role of environmental allergens in asthma is discussed in detail elsewhere in this book. Patients should be advised on measures to control exposure to asthma triggers such as allergens, pollutants and irritants. Therefore, testing for aeroallergen sensitivities, avoidance of allergens/tobacco smoke and possibly allergen specific immunotherapy may be appropriate. Comorbid conditions should also be identified and managed; these include entities such as rhinitis, sinusitis, gastroesophageal reflux disease, obesity, obstructive sleep apnea and allergic bronchopulmonary aspergillosis/mycosis. As infections can exacerbate asthma, appropriate vaccinations should be considered in order to minimize respiratory infections. The GINA guidelines recommend inactivated influenza vaccination for all asthma patients over six months old. In the United States, pneumonia vaccination is also recommended for all asthma patients over 19 years old, although the GINA guidelines state that there is insufficient data to make this recommendation (GINA 2019).

4. Medications

The final component of asthma care is pharmacotherapy; please see the Chapter on The Pharmacotherapy of Rhinitis and Asthma for further details. In brief, asthma treatment has been categorized into various tiers (or 'steps') by the National Heart, Lung, and Blood Institute (NHLBI)/NAEPP and by the GINA guidelines. Asthma treatment should be prescribed according to the appropriate corresponding level of asthma severity/control.

Management of acute asthma

Treatment for an acute asthma exacerbation includes bronchodilator therapy and systemic corticosteroids (oral or parenteral). Bronchodilator therapy should be with albuterol or levalbuterol at a dose not more than 10 mg per hour of albuterol or 5 mg per hour of levalbuterol. Recent studies have also demonstrated that albuterol Metered Dose Inhalers (MDIs) used with a spacer device are at least comparable to nebulized delivery (Cates et al. 2006). Anticholinergic therapy with ipratropium bromide used in combination with bronchodilator therapy has been shown to decrease hospitalization rates in children (Qureshis et al. 1997).

The NHLBI Expert Panel Guidelines and the GINA guidelines recommend the prompt initiation of oral corticosteroid therapy for all moderate to severe asthma exacerbations, based on evidence that this can prevent hospital admissions and hasten recovery (NIH 2002, GINA 2019). Additionally oral corticosteroid treatment is preferred and considered equally effective when compared to the parenteral route. Although the exact dose necessary to treat an acute exacerbation has been debated, it remains largely empiric and in the end is left to the clinician. Generally, the dose of prednisone is 1–2 mg/kg/day divided once to twice daily for 4–10 days, with a maximum daily dose of 60–80 mg, although generally less is sufficient.

It is critical that after an acute exacerbation, patients have a follow-up with their primary physician to discuss treatment and potential triggers. Acute asthma exacerbations are also an excellent opportunity to discuss asthma action plans. There is evidence that patients with written asthma plans and PEF monitors are less likely to visit the emergency department, be hospitalized or have low lung function (Gibson et al. 2004).

Asthma heterogeneity

Although asthma was traditionally thought of as one disease, it is now clear that there are different clinical and immunologic manifestations of this condition. Several groups have used large cohorts to help categorize asthma patients into clusters.

The first large-scale attempt at doing so identified five clinical clusters from the United States National Heart Lung and Blood Institute's (NHLBI) Severe Asthma Research Program (SARP). Cluster 1 included patients with early onset atopic asthma with normal lung function and low health care utilization. Cluster 2 included patients with early onset atopic asthma and preserved lung function but increased health care utilization. Cluster 3 included patients with late onset non-atopic asthma with moderately reduced FEV1 and frequent exacerbations requiring oral steroids. Clusters 4 and 5 included the most severe patients, who demonstrate severe airflow obstruction and evidence of bronchodilator responsiveness and have high health care utilization. The age of onset and atopic status is variable in these clusters, although Cluster 4 included more early onset atopic individuals than Cluster 5 (Moore et al. 2010).

More recent cluster analyses have demonstrated phenotypic clustering impacted by gender, atopic status, race, passive smoke exposure for children and aspirin sensitivity for teens and adults. In these clusters, outcomes were worse in nonwhite individuals and aspirin-sensitive patients, who demonstrated decreased quality of life and increased exacerbations (Schatz et al. 2014).

A cluster analysis from the British Thoracic Society (BTS) Severe Refractory Asthma Registry (SRAR) also identified 5 Clusters based on clinical presentation, although these clusters were somewhat different from those identified in the US SARP cohort (Newby et al. 2014). The two sets of clusters are summarized and compared in Table 13.3. Importantly, the molecular, genetic and immunologic features of these phenotypic clusters have yet to be elucidated, in order to move from phenotypic clusters to an understanding of asthma endotypes.

Perhaps the greatest move toward an understanding of asthma endotypes comes from characterization of 'type 2 high' versus 'type 2 low' asthma, which was first described by Wenzel and colleagues in a 1999 study of patients with severe, corticosteroid-dependent asthma. These two groups differed in terms of physiologic and clinical characteristics (Wenzel et al. 1999). Subsequent analysis of sputum from the Belgian Severe Asthma Registry identified eosinophilia in 55% of the subjects. Of the remaining subjects, 21% were identified as neutrophilic, 18% as pauci-granulocytic and 6% as mixed granulocytic (Schleich et al. 2014). In this study, 'type 2 high' asthma was defined as a sputum eosinophil count of $\geq$ 3%, or the presence of both exhaled Nitric Oxide (eNO) $\geq$ 27 ppb and blood eosinophil count $\geq$ 188/μL. The investigators concluded that 57% of the registry's patients had 'type 2 high' or eosinophilic asthma and 43% had asthma characterized as 'type 2 low' or non-eosinophilic (Schleich et al. 2014). Although they do not reveal the full story, sputum eosinophils, blood eosinophils, allergic status and exhaled nitric oxide levels are the currently available biomarkers that can give an idea of the underlying physiology for

Table 13.3. Summary of phenotypic asthma clusters from two studies.

Phenotypic Cluster	NHLBI SARP (Moore 2010)	BTS SRAR (Newby 2014)
1	Atopic, early onset, low healthcare utilization, normal lung function	Atopic, early onset, frequent exacerbations, poor lung function, significant bronchodilator (BD) reversibility
2	Early onset, preserved lung function, increased healthcare utilization	Obese, late onset, frequent exacerbations, near-normal lung function
3	Non-atopic, late onset, moderately reduced lung function, frequent exacerbations	Non-atopic, normal lung function, infrequent exacerbations
4	Variable age of onset, variable atopy, poor lung function, significant BD reversibility, high healthcare utilization	Late onset, high eosinophils, frequent exacerbations
5	Variable age of onset, variable atopy, poor lung function, significant BD reversibility, high healthcare utilization	Lowest lung function but least frequent exacerbations

a given patient's asthma. It is important to realize that the mere presence of eosinophils or allergy does not mean that they are necessarily responsible for asthma pathology in a particular patient. More work is needed to identify better biomarkers that can help tie together clinical presentation with underlying pathophysiology.

Summary

Asthma is a common condition that affects children and adults worldwide and can be associated with significant morbidity and even death. Several variables, the most important of which is atopy, have been implicated as risk factors for the development of asthma. The pathophysiology of asthma is complex but primarily involves airway inflammation, airway hyper responsiveness and variable airflow obstruction; these changes then classically lead to shortness of breath, wheeze, cough and tightness in the chest. As these symptoms can also occur in many other pulmonary conditions, the differential diagnosis of asthma is broad and important to consider when evaluating and treating patients presenting with these symptoms. Management of asthma involves assessing and monitoring asthma severity and control, educating and partnering with the patient, controlling environmental factors and comorbid conditions and using medications. Ultimately, the goal of these interventions is to achieve asthma control, both acutely during an exacerbation, as well as long-term to minimize impairment and risk from asthma.

References

Beckett WS, Jacobs DR, Jr, Yu X, Iribarren C, Williams OD. Asthma is associated with weight gain in females but not males, independent of physical activity. Am J Respir Crit Care Med 2001; 164(11): 2045–2050.

Cates CJ, Crilly JA, Rowe BH. Holding chambers versus nebulizers for beta-agonist treatment of acute asthma. Cochrane Database Sys Rev 2006; 2: CD000052.

Centers for Disease Control and Prevention, National Center for Health Statistics. Compressed Mortality File, CDC Wonder. 2006. Atlanta, GA: Centers for Disease Control and Prevention.

Chung KF, Wenzel SE, Brozek JL, Bush A, Castro M, Sterk PJ, et al. International ERS/ATS guidelines on definition, evaluation, and treatment of severe asthma. Eur Respir J 2014; 43: 343–373.

Dharmage SC, Perret JL, Custovic A. Epidemiology of asthma in children and adults. Frontiers in Pediatrics 2019; 7: 246.

Eagan TM, Brogger JC, Eide GE, Bakke PS. The incidence of adult asthma: a review. Int J Tuberc Lung Dis 2005; 9(6): 603–612.

Gern JE, Busse WW. Contemporary Diagnosis and Management of Allergic Diseases and Asthma, 5th edition. Handbooks in Health Care Co 2008; 102–148.

Gibson PG, Powell H, Coughlan J, Wilson AJ, Abramson M, Haywood P, et al. Self-management education and regular practitioner review for adults with asthma (Cochrane Review). Cochrane Database Syst Rev 2003; CD001117.

Gibson PG, Powell H, Coughlan J, Wilson AJ, Abramson M, Haywood P, et al. Self-management education and regular practitioner review for adults with asthma. Cochrane Database Syst Rev 2004; (1): CD001117.

Global Burden of Disease (GBD) 2015 Chronic Respiratory Disease Collaborators. Global, regional, and national deaths, prevalence, disability-adjusted life years, and years lived with disability for chronic obstructive pulmonary disease and asthma, 1990–2015: a systematic analysis for the Global Burden of Disease Study 2015. The Lancet Respiratory Medicine 2017; 5(9): 691–706.

Global Initiative for Asthma (GINA). Global Strategy for Asthma Management and Prevention 2019. Retrieved from https://ginasthma.org/gina-reports.

Masoli M, Fabian D, Holt S, Beasley R. The global burden of asthma: executive summary of the GINA Dissemination Committee report. Allergy 2004; 59(5): 469–478.

Moore WC, Meyers DA, Wenzel SE, Teague G, Li H, Xingnan Li, et al. Identification of asthma phenotypes using cluster analysis in the severe asthma research program. Am J Respir Crit Care Med 2010; 181(4): 315–23.

National Heart, Lung, and Blood Institute, National Asthma Education and Prevention Program. Expert Panel Report 3: Guidelines for the diagnosis and management of asthma. October 2007.

National Institutes of Health (NIH), National Heart Lung, and Blood Institute. Global initiative for asthma. Global strategy for asthma management and prevention. NIH Pub. No. 02-3659. Bethesda, MD:NIH; 2002.

Newby C, Heaney LG, Menzies-Gow A, Niven RM, Mansur A, Bucknall C, et al. Statistical cluster analysis of the British Thoracic Society Severe refractory Asthma Registry: clinical outcomes and phenotype stability. PLoS One 2014; 9(7): e102987.

Ober C. Perspectives on the past decade of asthma genetics. J Allergy Clin Immunol 2005; 116: 274–278.

Ober C, Hoffjan S. Asthma genetics 2006: the long and winding road to gene discovery. Genes Immun 2006;7(2): 95–100.

Poulos LM, Toelle BG, Marks GB. The burden of asthma in children: an Australian perspective. Paediatr Respir Rev 2005; 6(1): 20–27.

Qureshis F, Zartisky A, Lakkis H. Efficacy of ipratropium in severely asthmatic children. Ann Emerg Med 1997; 29: 205–11.

Schatz M, Hsu JW, Zeiger RS, Chen W, Dorenbaum A, Chipps BE, et al. Phenotypes determined by cluster analysis in severe or difficult-to-treat asthma. J Allergy Clin Immunol 2014; 133(6): 1549–1556.

Schleich F, Brusselle G, Louis R, Vandenplas O, Michils A, Pilette C, et al. Heterogeneity of phenotypes in severeasthmatics. The Belgian Severe Asthma Registry (BSAR). Respir Med 2014; 108(12): 1723–1732.

Silverstein MD, Reed CE, O'Connell EJ, Melton LJ 3rd, O'Fallon WM, Yunginger JW. Long-term survival of a cohort of community residents with asthma. N Engl J Med 1994; 331: 1537–1541.

To T, Stanojevic S, Moores G, Gershon AS, Bateman ED, Cruz AA, et al. Global asthma prevalence in adults: findings from the cross-sectional world health survey. BMC Public Health 2012; 12: 204.

Wenzel SE, Schwartz LB, Langmack EL, Halliday JL, Trudeau JB, Gibbs RL. Evidence that severe asthma canbe divided pathologically into two inflammatory subtypes with distinct physiologicand clinical characteristics. Am J Respir Crit Care Med 1999; 160(3): 1001–1008.

Yunginger JW, Reed CE, O'Connell EJ, Melton LJ 3rd, O'Fallon WM, Silverstein MD. A community-based study of the epidemiology of asthma. Incidence rates, 1964–1983. Am Rev Respir Dis 1992; 146(4): 888–894.

14

The Pharmacotherapy of Rhinitis and Asthma

Amanda Grippen Goddard,* Harold S. Nelson, Rohit Katial and Flavia Hoyte

INTRODUCTION

The available literature on the pharmacotherapy of rhinitis asthma is vast and to a large degree represents publication of studies sponsored by manufacturers with a vested interest in one or a few products. To assist in assessing this literature, we can turn to reviews and meta-analyses, but perhaps the best sources of unbiased information are the national and international guidelines that are evidence-based and written by experts independent of pharmaceutical financial support. Therefore, this chapter of pharmacotherapy will relying largely on the 2008 Update of the ARIA Guidelines (Bousquet et al. 2008), ARIA guidelines-2016 revision (Brozek et al. 2017), the 2008 Diagnosis and management of rhinitis: An updated practice parameter (Wallace and Dykewicz 2008), the 2007 National Asthma Education and Prevention Program (NAEPP)/National Heart, Lung, and Blood Institute (NHLBI) Guidelines for the Diagnosis and Management of Asthma (Expert Panel Report 3 2007) and the 2019 Global Initiative for Asthma (GINA) report (Global Initiative for Asthma 2019).

Rhinitis—Drugs

The available interventions for the treatment of rhinitis are listed in Table 14.1. Avoidance of exposure to allergens and irritants and allergen immunotherapy are discussed in separate chapters in this book and will not be further elaborated here. What remains then is pharmacotherapy, the subject of this chapter.

Corticosteroids

Intranasal corticosteroids

Intranasal corticosteroids are the most effective medication class for controlling symptoms of allergic (Bousquet et al. 2008, Wallace and Dykewicz 2008) and non-allergic rhinitis (Bousquet et al. 2008). They are effective in controlling the four major symptoms of allergic rhinitis: sneezing, itching, rhinorrhea and nasal congestion. They also improve ocular symptoms to some degree (Bousquet et al. 2008). The main mechanism by which they improve symptoms is through their anti-inflammatory activity. For this reason,

---

National Jewish Health, Denver, CO, USA.
 Emails: NelsonH@NJHealth.org; KatialR@NJHealth.org; HoyteF@NJHealth.org
* Corresponding author: aggoddard@allergypartners.com

Table 14.1. Treatment of rhinitis.

I. Allergen Avoidance

II. Pharmacotherapy
    Intranasal corticosteroids
    Antihistamines, oral
    Antihistamines, intranasal
    Decongestants
    Antihistamine/decongestant combinations
    Leukotriene receptor antagonists
    Anticholinergics
    Cromolyn
    Omalizumab
    Dupilumab

III. Allergen Immunotherapy

maximum efficacy may require 2 weeks, although onset of action may be as early as two hours (Bousquet et al. 2008). Despite differences in topical potency, lipid solubility and receptor binding affinity the overall response does not appear to vary among the available products. A meta-analysis of studies that included both an oral antihistamine and an intranasal corticosteroid arm indicated that the intranasal corticosteroids were superior for total and all individual nasal symptoms and equal to oral antihistamines for ocular symptoms (Weiner et al. 1998). In patients with perennial allergic rhinitis, there is evidence to suggest that there is no additional benefit from a combination of an oral antihistamine and intranasal corticosteroid when compared to intranasal corticosteroid alone (Brozek et al. 2017). When given in recommended doses, they are generally not associated with systemic side effects, the one exception being the demonstration of slowing of growth in children with intranasal beclomethasone. This effect has not been observed with fluticasone propionate, budesonide or mometasone (Bousquet et al. 2008).

Nasal steroids may be initiated either prior to or following the onset of symptoms of allergic rhinitis. When they are started after the patient has developed symptoms of seasonal allergic rhinitis, as is the case in the typical pharmaceutically sponsored study, the degree of relief over the first few weeks is only moderate. In one study, in which 291 subjects received intranasal fluticasone propionate 200 mcg/day and 290 received a placebo, the mean reduction in symptoms over the first two weeks with fluticasone, over that with the placebo, was only 19% and over the first four weeks only 23% (Nathan et al. 2005). On the other hand, in a small study in which intranasal corticosteroids were started 3 weeks before the anticipated beginning of the pollen season, nasal symptoms were reduced 55% compared to a placebo in the active treatment group (Pullerits et al. 1999). Studies have compared the regular versus 'as needed' use of intranasal corticosteroids for seasonal allergic rhinitis. In one study, 73% of patients achieved satisfactory control with 'as needed' treatment where as 27% did not (Juniper et al. 1993). In another study, symptoms and quality of life were worse, despite increased use of rescue antihistamines in the 'as needed' group (Juniper et al. 1990). The 'as needed' use of the nasal corticosteroid fluticasone propionate has also been compared to the 'as needed' use of the anti-histamine loratadine for treatment of seasonal allergic rhinitis (Kaszuba et al. 2001). Despite similar frequency of use of each of the treatments, the median nasal symptom score in those using the nasal steroid was only 57% that of the group that used the antihistamine and quality of life was significantly better with the use of the intranasal corticosteroid.

Intranasal corticosteroids have been shown to reduce symptoms in patients who have non-allergic rhinitis as defined by the presence of persistent symptoms and negative prick skin tests to a panel of aeroallergens (Wallace and Dykewicz 2008). This efficacy is independent of the presence or absence of nasal eosinophils (Webb et al. 2002, Scadding et al. 1995).

Oral corticosteroids

Patients with severe symptoms due to seasonal allergic rhinitis may benefit from the rapid relief of a short course of oral steroids (e.g., prednisone 20 mg daily or twice daily for three days). Longer-term use of oral corticosteroids or intramuscular injection should be avoided due to the risks of systemic side effects (Bousquet et al. 2008).

Antihistamines

Oral antihistamines

A number of mediators are released from activated mast cells (e.g., histamine, cysteinyl leukotrienes, prostaglandin D_2) and contribute to the symptoms of allergic rhinitis as indicated by symptom improvement when patients are treated with their antagonists. Nevertheless, histamine by itself can produce all the typical symptoms of itching, rhinorrhea, sneezing and congestion and histamine antagonists are effective in reducing these symptoms. Antihistamines were formerly considered not to reduce nasal congestion (Bousquet et al. 2008), but the second-generation drugs have been shown to have some beneficial effect on this symptom (Bechet 2009). The older, so-called first generation, antihistamines all have a significant potential for sedation, performance impairment and anticholinergic side effects. Therefore, the second-generation antihistamines are to be preferred in most instances (Bousquet et al. 2008, Wallace and Dykewicz 2008). Among the second-generation antihistamines, anticholinergic side effects do not usually occur. Sedation, which is caused by the drug crossing the blood-brain barrier, does not occur with fexofenadine, occurs only with higher than recommended doses of loratadine and desloratadine, but occurs in a subset of patients with approved doses of cetirizine, levocetirizine and the nasal antihistamine azelastine (Wallace and Dykewicz 2008).

The degree of improvement typically achieved with antihistamine therapy is illustrated by results in a study in 722 patients with seasonal allergic rhinitis. Nasal congestion was not included in the symptom score. Fexofenadine 180 mg once daily reduced symptoms 21%, and 10 mg cetirizine once daily reduced symptoms 22% compared to a placebo (Howarth et al. 1999). Similar results were reported in 294 patients with perennial allergic rhinitis due to house dust mites treated with levocetirizine 5 mg once daily (Potter 2003). Over the six weeks of treatment, nasal symptoms not including congestion, were reduced by 23%. On the other hand, 1,179 individuals with perennial allergic rhinitis were treated for 4 weeks with desloratadine 5 mg once daily (Kim et al. 2006). The mean reduction in nasal symptoms, including congestion, was only 4% greater with desloratadine than with a placebo over the 4 weeks. This disparity in results is consistent with the findings of a comparison of studies of levocetirizine and desloratadine for symptoms of allergic rhinitis that concluded: "levocetirizine may be preferred to desloratadine as a treatment option for allergic rhinitis because of its faster onset of action and greater consistency of effect" (Passalacqua and Canonica 2005). However, by adding the decongestant, pseudoephedrine, to desloratadine in a combination treatment, patients with seasonal allergic rhinitis had significantly lower symptom scores including nasal congestion compared to either pseudoephedrine or desloratadine alone. During the 15-day treatment period, the combination of desloratadine and pseudoephedrine reduced the total symptom score by 46.0%, while desloratadine and pseudoephedrine monotherapies reduced the same score by 33.5 and 35.9%, respectively. Nasal congestion was reduced by 37.4% in the combination therapy, but was only reduced by 26.7 and 31.2% with desloratadine and pseudoephedrine, respectively (Grubbe et al. 2009). It should be noted there was no placebo group in this study.

Intranasal antihistamines

Two intranasal antihistamines preparations are available (azelastine and olopatadine). Their onset of action is within 15 to 30 minutes. In comparison studies they have proven of equal or occasionally slightly superior efficacy to the second-generation oral antihistamines (Wallace and Dykewicz 2008). Intranasal antihistamines are equally effective but faster in onset of action as compared with intranasal corticosteroids (Kaliner et al. 2009). In one study comparing intranasal azelastine to intranasal fluticasone, intranasal fluticasone was superior to reducing rhinorrhea, but intranasal azelastine showed comparable efficacy for all other nasal and ocular symptoms. Additionally, compared to baseline ocular symptoms, there was a larger percentage (53.0%) of patients on intranasal azelastine as opposed to intranasal fluticasone (39.6%) that exhibited a 50% reduction in reflective total ocular symptom score by day 14 of treatment (Carr et al. 2012b). The use of intranasal antihistamines in combination with intranasal corticosteroids demonstrates additional symptom reduction and improved quality of life as compared to intranasal antihistamine monotherapy (Brozek et al. 2017). Intranasal antihistamines may have greater efficacy for nasal congestion than oral antihistamines (Brozek et al. 2017). Azelastine is associated with taste perversion and somnolence in some patients (Bousquet et al. 2008), while these symptoms are less frequent with olopatadine (Lieberman et al. 2011).

A combination nasal spray has been approved containing the antihistamine azelastine and the corticosteroid fluticasone propionate. In a meta-analysis of studies in over 3,000 adolescents and adults with seasonal allergic rhinitis, the combination product was significantly superior to each of the individual components and was more rapid in onset of significant relief (Carr et al. 2012a).

Decongestants

Intranasal decongestants

Topical decongestants such as oxymetazoline can be very effective in reducing nasal congestion but do not reduce itching, sneezing or nasal secretions (Wallace and Dykewicz 2008). Due to the development of tolerance and rebound vasodilation with chronic use, termed rhinitis medicamentosa, they are not recommended for long-term treatment (Bousquet et al. 2008, Wallace and Dykewicz 2008).

Oral decongestants

Oral alpha-adrenergic agonists relieve nasal congestion by vasoconstriction of the capacitance vessels in the nasal mucosa. They are most often used in a fixed combination with an antihistamine to reduce symptoms of nasal congestion. In 429 patients with seasonal allergic rhinitis, symptom reduction was 14% with loratadine alone and 21% with the addition of pseudoephedrine to the loratadine (Kaiser et al. 1998). Oral decongestants can cause side effects such as insomnia, irritability and palpitations but they do not cause rhinitis medicamentosa and hence are acceptable for long-term use. Blood pressure should be monitored when they are used in patients with hypertension, and they should be used with caution in patients with arrhythmias, coronary artery disease, glaucoma and bladder neck obstruction (Bousquet et al. 2008, Wallace and Dykewicz 2008).

Leukotriene receptor antagonists

Cysteinyl leukotrienes are released from activated mast cells, and nasal challenge with Leukotriene D4 increases nasal airway resistance. It would be logical, therefore, that Leukotriene Receptor Antagonists (LTRAs) might benefit patients with allergic rhinitis (Bisgaard et al. 1986). A meta-analysis covering eight studies of a leukotriene receptor antagonist in seasonal allergic rhinitis found a mean reduction in rhinitis scores of only 5% compared to a placebo, with results being inferior to both antihistamines and intranasal corticosteroids (Wilson et al. 2004). A similar modest degree of effectiveness has been reported in perennial allergic rhinitis (Patel et al. 2005).

Intranasal anticholinergic agents

Cholinergic stimulation of the nasal mucosa causes increased glandular secretion. In patients with allergic rhinitis, ipratropium bromide nasal spray has been shown to reduce watery anterior nasal discharge but not to reduce post-nasal drainage, sneezing or nasal obstruction (Bousquet et al. 2008). Side effects are minimal (Wallace and Dykewicz 2008).

Intranasal cromolyn sodium

Cromolyn sodium inhibits the degranulation of sensitized mast cells. It acts to prevent symptoms but does not alleviate symptoms once they have occurred (Wallace and Dykewicz 2008) therefore, it is most effective if started prior to the onset of symptoms. In a placebo-controlled study in which treatment was started before the pollen season and the drug was administered 6 times daily for 9 weeks, there was a mean 56% reduction in rhinorrhea, congestion and sneezing compared to a placebo (Handelman et al. 1977). Cromolyn is remarkably free of side effects but must be used multiple times a day in order to achieve clinical benefit.

Immunomodulators

The monoclonal anti-IgE, omalizumab, is approved in the US only for use in patients with severe allergic asthma and chronic idiopathic urticaria, but several studies have confirmed its efficacy in allergic rhinitis either alone or in combination with allergen immunotherapy. Most studies showed a reduction in nasal symptom scores, reduced medication use and improved quality of life scores (Benninger et al. 2010, Wise et al. 2018). When used in combination with allergen immunotherapy, omalizumab significantly reduced symptom load as compared with allergen immunotherapy alone, independent of the allergen (Kopp et al. 2009). The high cost of therapy precludes a widespread use of omalizumab in allergic rhinitis. Dupilumab, an anti-IL-4 receptor α monoclonal antibody which inhibits IL-4 and IL-13 signaling, has been approved for use in patients with eosinophilic or steroid-dependent asthma, atopic dermatitis or nasal polyposis. Although it has been shown to improve allergic rhinitis-associated nasal symptoms in patients with uncontrolled persistent asthma and comorbid perennial allergic rhinitis, its widespread use will also be cost-prohibitive (Weinstein et al. 2018).

Rhinitis—management

Allergic rhinitis

Treatment of allergic rhinitis should be individualized based on the duration and severity of the symptoms, co-morbidities, treatment affordability and patient's preference (Bousquet et al. 2008, Wallace and Dykewicz 2008). The available medications differ in their breadth and degree of effectiveness (Table 14.2).

For mild and intermittent symptoms of allergic rhinitis, second-generation H1 antagonists either orally or intranasally are usually adequate and superior in efficacy to leukotriene receptor antagonists or decongestants (Bousquet et al. 2008). For moderate or severe persistent symptoms, an intranasal corticosteroid is preferred due to its superior efficacy over alternative medications. There is no evidence that the addition of an oral antihistamine (Barnes et al. 2006) or a leukotriene receptor antagonist (Esteitie et al. 2010) increases the response to that achieved with an intranasal corticosteroid alone. Intranasal cromolyn sodium can be used as a pre-medication prior to a known aeroallergen exposure. It also is effective for seasonal allergic rhinitis if started before the season and continued 4 to 6 times daily throughout the season.

Table 14.2. Comparative efficacy of drugs (Modified from Benninger et al. 2010).

Medication Class	Sneezing	Itching	Congestion	Rhinorrhea
Oral Antihistamines	++	++	+/-	++
Intranasal Antihistamines	+++	+++	+++	++
Intranasal corticosteroids	+++	+++	+++	+++
Leukotriene receptor antagonists	+/-	+/-	+/-	+/-
Cromolyn (started before season and given 6 X daily)	++	++	++	++

+++ Most effective, ++ substantial benefit, + modest benefit, +/- little or no benefit

Non-allergic rhinitis

Non-allergic rhinitis is defined by the absence of proven IgE-mediated sensitization to relevant aeroallergens. It represents several entities, some with eosinophilic inflammation and some without. The favorable response to intranasal corticosteroids in patients with non-allergic rhinitis is not different in patients with or without eosinophils in their nasal secretions (Webb et al. 2002, Scadding et al. 1995). While symptoms are generally improved in the first 1 or 2 weeks, there may be further improvement with long-term treatment (Mandl et al. 1997).

Although most forms of non-allergic rhinitis are responsive to intranasal corticosteroids, this does not apply to all forms of this condition. A study of patients with negative skin tests and negative nasal smear for eosinophils, whose symptoms were predominantly triggered by temperature and weather changes showed no response to intranasal corticosteroids (Jacobs et al. 2009).

Decongestants can be used in non-allergic rhinitis to decrease symptoms of stuffiness with the same caveats listed above regarding the frequent occurrence of side effects. Anti-cholinergic nasal sprays can be used in non-allergic rhinitis if watery anterior rhinorrhea is a prominent symptom. There is no data to support the use of oral antihistamines or Cromolyn sodium in non-allergic rhinitis, but azelastine has been approved for use in 'vasomotor rhinitis'.

Conjunctivitis

Allergic rhinitis is often accompanied by allergic conjunctivitis, characterized by findings of conjunctival injection and chemosis and symptoms of itching and tearing (Wallace and Dykewicz 2008). Associated conjunctivitis is very common with seasonal allergic rhinitis due to pollens, while it is less common with perennial allergic rhinitis. Intranasal antihistamines, intranasal corticosteroids, oral antihistamines and leukotriene receptor antagonists have all been reported to significantly improve ocular symptoms, but the effect of each is inferior to that achievable with topical ocular treatment (Wallace and Dykewicz 2008, Bielory et al. 2007).

The various medications available for topical treatment of ocular allergy are covered in Chapter 10: Allergic Diseases of the Eye.

Bronchial asthma—drugs

The classes of drugs used for treating bronchial asthma are listed in Table 14.3. They are classified, according to their role in asthma management, as either quick-relief or long-term-control medications (Expert Panel Report 3 2007, Global Initiative for Asthma 2019a, Assaf and Hanania 2019).

Quick-relief medications

Short-acting beta$_2$-adrenergic agonists (SABAs)

These drugs relax airway smooth muscle through stimulation of the beta-2 adrenergic receptors. Inhaled, they are the drugs of choice for rapid relief of asthma symptoms and for prevention of broncho constriction induced by exercise (EIB). Except for the prevention of EIB, regular use of SABAs is not recommended, and 'as needed' use more than twice weekly (except for EIB prevention) is a marker of inadequately controlled asthma.

Although the inhaled route is generally preferred and adequately effective, in cases of severe bronchoconstriction, injection of epinephrine or terbutaline may be considered. Oral administration of SABAs, while common in the past, is no longer recommended (Expert Panel Report 3 2007).

Short acting inhaled anti-cholinergic agents

Drugs of this class (e.g., Ipratropium) inhibit muscarinic cholinergic receptors and reduce intrinsic vagal tone of the airway. They provide additive benefit to SABAs in moderate or severe exacerbations in an emergency care setting. They may be used for relief of asthma symptoms in patients not tolerating SABAs, but are slower in onset and generally less effective than SABAs (Expert Panel Report 3 2007).

Table 14.3. Drugs for treatment of bronchial asthma.

Reliever Inhaled short-acting beta-adrenergic agonists Injected adrenergic agonists Inhaled anticholinergic agents Systemic corticosteroids

Controller
Corticosteroids
       Inhaled
       Oral
       Injectable
Long acting beta-adrenergic agonists (used in combination with inhaled corticosteroids)
Long-acting anticholinergic agents
Methylxanthine
       Theophylline
Leukotriene pathway modifying agents
       Cysteinyl leukotriene receptor antagonists
       5-Lipoxygenase inhibitors
Cromolyn/nedocromil
Immunomodulators
       Omalizumab
       Mepolizumab
       Resilizumab
       Benralizumab
       Dupilumab

Systemic corticosteroids

Oral or intravenous corticosteroids are used for moderate and severe exacerbations of asthma to speed recovery and prevent recurrence of exacerbations. A recent systematic literature review investigated the real-world extent and burden of oral corticosteroid (OCS) use in asthma and found that increased used of OCS was associated with increased health care costs, resource utilization and adverse events (Bleecker et al. 2019). The increased health care costs utilization may be due to the OCS themselves or disease severity. Compared to no OCS use, both short- and long-term OCS use were associated with risk of acute and chronic corticosteroid-related complications. Acute complications from OCS include infections and gastrointestinal complications such as bleeding and reflux. Chronic complications of OCS were more diverse and included osteoporosis, bone fractures, hypertension, coronary artery disease, heart failure, anxiety, cataracts, chronic kidney disease and sleep disorders (Bleecker et al. 2019).

Long-term-control medications

Corticosteroids

This class of drug has broad anti-inflammatory activity and is the most effective long-term control medication for most patients with asthma. In general, Inhaled Corticosteroids (ICSs) are well tolerated and safe at the recommended doses. For most patients, the benefits are achieved at low to medium doses without the need to escalate to high doses, which are more likely to lead in the long term to systemic side effects (Expert Panel Report 3 2007). Use of intermittent ICSs compared to controller use of ICSs has been studied in asthmatics older than 12 years with persistent but not severe asthma, but no significant differences were found between the two approaches to therapy (Sobieraj et al. 2018). Systemic corticosteroids for maintenance therapy of asthma are required by only a small number of patients and are to be avoided, if possible due to long-term development of systemic side effects.

Long-acting beta$_2$-adrenergic agonists (LABAs)

LABAs provide prolonged bronchodilation that allows dosing once or twice daily with sustained effect. While they can reduce symptoms, they do not provide treatment for the underlying inflammation; therefore, they should only be used in conjunction with inhaled corticosteroid for maintenance treatment of asthma. However, using combination ICS/LABA therapy as both controller and quick relief therapy may be more effective at preventing exacerbations than using ICS, with or without a LABA, as controller therapy with only SABA added for quick relief (Sobieraj et al. 2018).

Long-acting anti-cholinergic agents

Tiotropium, a once daily anti-muscarinic agent, is now approved in the US for treatment of asthma. It can be used as add-on therapy to ICS or the combination of ICS/LABA. Current evidence does not suggest a clinical difference between adding Tiotropium or a LABA to ICS therapy (Global Initiative for Asthma 2019a, Peters et al. 2010).

Methylxanthines

Theophylline has moderate bronchodilator properties but a narrow therapeutic/toxic ratio and need for serum level monitoring severely limits its use. Theophylline at low doses (e.g., 400 mg/day) has been found to induce histone deacetylase activity that could enhance the anti-inflammatory properties of corticosteroids (Cosio and Soriano 2009).

Leukotriene pathway modifying agents

The arachidonic acid pathway can be interrupted by inhibition of the enzyme 5-lipoxygenase (5-LO) using zileuton or by inhibition of the cysteinyl leukotriene receptor (LTRA) using zafirlukast or montelukast. 5-LO inhibition provides broader interruption of the pathway, decreasing production of the chemoattractant leukotriene B4, as well as the cysteinyl leukotrienes; however zileuton induces significant elevations of liver enzymes in about 2% of recipients and therefore requires liver function monitoring (Nelson et al. 2007). The LTRAs, are well tolerated without need for laboratory monitoring. They moderately improve asthma as monotherapy, but are thought to be inferior to ICS monotherapy (Ducharme 2003). They have modest efficacy when added to an ICS, but in most patients are inferior to adding a LABA (Nelson et al. 2000) or increasing the dose of ICS (Ducharme 2002).

Cromolyn/nedocromil

These drugs stabilize mast cells, preventing mediator release. The dose required is large, and difficulty formulating this dose into a convenient delivery system has limited their use. They are not as effective as ICSs. Persisting roles for cromolyn are as premedication prior to a known allergen exposure and to prevent EIB (Expert Panel Report 3 2007).

Immunomodulators

There are now five approved drugs in this category. The monoclonal anti-IgE antibody, omalizumab, was the first immunomodulator approved for allergic asthma in 2003. Omalizumabreduces levels of free-IgE, resulting in a marked reduction in the number of IgE receptors on cell surfaces and a reduction in airway inflammation (Djukanovic et al. 2004). There is a small risk for anaphylactic reactions to omalizumab (Lin et al. 2009).

Since 2015, there have been three anti-IL-5 therapies (mepolizumab, reslizumab and benralizumab) approved for add-on maintenance treatment for patients with severe eosinophilic asthma. Mepolizumab is a recombinant, humanized IgG1κ monoclonal antibody against IL-5 that inhibits IL-5 from binding to the α-subunit of the IL-5 receptor complex expressed on the eosinophil cell surface. There is a small risk for hypersensitivity reactions and herpes zoster infections with mepolizumab. Reslizumab is a humanized IgG4κ monoclonal anti-IL-5 antibody that also inhibits binding of IL-5 to its receptor. As opposed to mepolizumab that is given subcutaneously, reslizumab is given intravenously. There are small risks for developing anaphylaxis and elevated creatinine phosphokinase levels with reslizumab. Both mepolizumab and reslizumab inhibit the growth, differentiation, recruitment, activation and survival of eosinophils. Benralizumab is a humanized afucosylated recombinant IgG1κ monoclonal antibody that binds with high affinity to the α-subunit of the IL-5 receptor. By doing so, benralizumab inhibits the proliferation and activation of eosinophils by blocking the same IL-5-mediated eosinophil properties that are blocked by mepolizumab and reslizumab. In addition, the Fc portion of benralizumab binds to Fc receptors on immune effector cells, such as natural killer cells, which then deplete existing eosinophils and precursors in the bone marrow by inducing apoptosis through antibody-dependent cell-mediated cytotoxicity (Assaf and Hanania 2019, Katial et al. 2017).

Dupilumab is indicated for add-on maintenance treatment of patients with moderate to severe asthma with an eosinophilic phenotype or oral-corticosteroid dependent asthma. It is a fully human monoclonal antibody to the IL-4 receptor alpha subunit, a heterodimeric receptor complex for both IL-4 and IL-13. Blocking this receptor with dupilumab simultaneously inhibits IL-4 and IL-13 signaling. Dupilumab is effective by halting differentiation of CD4 positive lymphocytes, decreasing IgE production, decreasing fractional exhaled nitric oxide levels and decreasing airway hyper responsiveness and remodeling (Assaf and Hanania 2019). This drug should be used with caution in patients with extremely elevated baseline eosinophil counts due to the potential for a further rise in eosinophil counts (Katial et al. 2017).

The immunomodulators have been shown to decrease symptoms and exacerbation rates as well as to improve quality of life, overall asthma control and to a smaller degree lung function. Several of them have also demonstrated the ability to decrease the daily systemic steroid requirement in oral steroid-dependent patients. Given the high cost of these medications, they are reserved for severe persistent patients who remain poorly controlled despite regular use of ICS therapy in conjunction with another controller. Choosing the correct immunomodulator for a given patient relies on the use of currently available biomarkers such as circulating eosinophils, total IgE levels, fractional exhaled nitric oxide levels and atopy testing.

Management of bronchial asthma

The 2007 NAEPP/NHLBI Guidelines for the Diagnosis and Management of Asthma categorize asthma severity into intermittent and persistent; the latter divided into mild, moderate and severe (Fig. 14.1). The classification of the severity of a patient's asthma is used to determine the appropriate treatment only when the patient is not receiving any long-term control therapy. Once a patient is receiving controller therapy, further decisions regarding changes in treatment are dictated by the degree of asthma control they have achieved in their current therapy (Fig. 14.2). The categories of management are well-controlled, not well-controlled and very poorly controlled.

The previous iterations of the NAEPP/NHLBI guidelines had outlined the goals of asthma therapy which were to: prevent chronic symptoms, maintain normal activity levels, maintain normal lung function and prevent exacerbations of asthma, while incurring minimal or no adverse effects of treatment. Random telephone surveys conducted in America, Europe and Asia suggested that very few asthmatics were achieving these goals (Rabe et al. 2004). To determine whether most asthmatics could achieve control with the currently available therapies, an international study was conducted in roughly 3,500 individuals with current asthma not fully controlled on no-, low- or medium-dose inhaled corticosteroids (Bateman et al. 2004). In this year-long study, subjects received escalating doses of fluticasone propionate to a maximum of 500-mcg twice daily. Half of the subjects were randomized to receive salmeterol 50 mcg twice daily in addition to the fluticasone propionate. Using a definition of 'well controlled' similar to that used in the 2007 NAEPP/NHLBI guidelines, 50% of participants achieved control with fluticasone propionate alone and 65% with fluticasone plus salmeterol. The positive findings encouraged the Expert

CLASSIFYING ASTHMA SEVERITY AND INITIATING TREATMENT IN YOUTHS ≥12 YEARS OF AGE AND ADULTS

Assessing severity and initiating treatment for patients who are not currently taking long-term control medications

Components of Severity		Classification of Asthma Severity ≥12 years of age			
		Intermittent	Persistent Mild	Persistent Moderate	Persistent Severe
Impairment Normal FEV_1/FVC: 8–19 yr 85% 20–39 yr 80% 40–59 yr 75% 60–80 yr 70%	Symptoms	≤2 days/week	>2 days/week but not daily	Daily	Throughout the day
	Nighttime awakenings	≤2x/month	3–4x/month	>1x/week but not nightly	Often 7x/week
	Short-acting $beta_2$-agonist use for symptom control (not prevention of EIB)	≤2 days/week	>2 days/week but not daily, and not more than 1x on any day	Daily	Several times per day
	Interference with normal activity	None	Minor limitation	Some limitation	Extremely limited
	Lung function	• Normal FEV_1 between exacerbations • FEV_1 >80% predicted • FEV_1/FVC normal	• FEV_1 >80% predicted • FEV_1/FVC normal	• FEV_1 >60% but <80% predicted • FEV_1/FVC reduced 5%	• FEV_1 <60% predicted • FEV_1/FVC reduced >5%
Risk	Exacerbations requiring oral systemic corticosteroids	0–1/year (see note)	≥2/year (see note) Consider severity and interval since last exacerbation. Frequency and severity may fluctuate over time for patients in any severity category. Relative annual risk of exacerbations may be related to FEV_1.		
Recommended Step for Initiating Treatment (See figure 4–5 for treatment steps.)		Step 1	Step 2	Step 3	Step 4 or 5 and consider short course of oral systemic corticosteroids
		In 2–6 weeks, evaluate level of asthma control that is achieved and adjust therapy accordingly.			

Key: FEV_1, forced expiratory volume in 1 second; FVC, forced vital capacity; ICU, intensive care unit

Figure 14.1. Classifying asthma severity and initiating treatment in youths ≥ 12 years of age and adults.

Panel that drew up the 2007 NAEPP/NHLBI guidelines to make 'well controlled' the goal of asthma therapy (Expert Panel Report 3 2007).

In the 2007 NAEPP/NHLBI guidelines, asthma control is regarded as having two domains, current burden or impairment (daytime symptoms, night time awakenings, interference with normal activity, need for rescue medication, and impaired pulmonary function) and future risk (asthma exacerbations, development of fixed airflow obstruction and side effects from asthma medication) (Expert Panel Report 3 2007). In addition to the five listed elements of impairment, Fig. 14.2 includes values for three questionnaires that have been validated as being responsive to changes in an individual's asthma control. The criterion in Fig. 14. 2 for 'well controlled' status are essentially those that define intermittent asthma in Fig. 14.1. Although the three components of future risk are listed, only the frequency of exacerbations requiring oral or systemic corticosteroids is used to assess control. For each level of control, a therapeutic course is recommended: maintaining the current step of therapy if the patient is 'well controlled', stepping up one step if the patient is 'not well controlled', and considering a short course of oral corticosteroids and stepping up one or two steps if the patient is 'very poorly controlled'. For each intervention, there is also a recommendation for follow-up; in 1–6 months if no change in treatment is made, but sooner if there is an increase in the step-level of therapy. This recommendation for scheduled follow-up is based on the rationale that patients must be seen for follow-up so that the effectiveness of treatment interventions can be evaluated and the level of control are re-assessed. This cannot be done if they are only told to return when having difficulty with their asthma.

Except for the initiation of long-term control therapy, the levels of step therapy are no longer dictated by the underlying severity of the individual's asthma. Instead patients are moved up and down the steps

ASSESSING ASTHMA CONTROL AND ADJUSTING THERAPY IN YOUTHS ≥12 YEARS OF AGE AND ADULTS

Components of Control		Classification of Asthma Control (≥12 years of age)		
		Well Controlled	Not Well Controlled	Very Poorly Controlled
Impairment	Symptoms	≤2 days/week	>2 days/week	Throughout the day
	Nighttime awakenings	≤2x/month	1–3x/week	≥4x/week
	Interference with normal activity	None	Some limitation	Extremely limited
	Short-acting beta₂-agonist use for symptom control (not prevention of EIB)	≤2 days/week	>2 days/week	Several times per day
	FEV_1 or peak flow	>80% predicted/ personal best	60–80% predicted/ personal best	<60% predicted/ personal best
	Validated questionnaires ATAQ ACQ ACT	0 ≤0.75* ≥20	1–2 ≥1.5 16–19	3–4 N/A ≤15
Risk	Exacerbations requiring oral systemic corticosteroids	0–1/year	≥2/year (see note)	
		Consider severity and interval since last exacerbation		
	Progressive loss of lung function	Evaluation requires long-term followup care		
	Treatment-related adverse effects	Medication side effects can vary in intensity from none to very troublesome and worrisome. The level of intensity does not correlate to specific levels of control but should be considered in the overall assessment of risk.		
Recommended Action for Treatment (see figure 4–5 for treatment steps)		• Maintain current step. • Regular followups every 1–6 months to maintain control. • Consider step down if well controlled for at least 3 months.	• Step up 1 step and • Reevaluate in 2–6 weeks. • For side effects, consider alternative treatment options.	• Consider short course of oral systemic corticosteroids. • Step up 1–2 steps, and • Reevaluate in 2 weeks. • For side effects, consider alternative treatment options.

*ACQ values of 0.76–1.4 are indeterminate regarding well-controlled asthma.
Key: EIB, exercise-induced bronchospasm; ICU, intensive care unit

Figure 14.2. Assessing asthma control and adjusting therapy in youths ≥ 12 years of age and adults.

of therapy shown in Fig. 14.3 as needed to achieve control and maintain this control with the minimum quantity of medication deemed necessary.

According to the 2007 NAEPP/NHLBI guidelines, step 1 reflects the feeling that patients who are exhibiting symptoms and the need for rescue medication only two days a week or less, awakening with asthma two nights a month or less, having no interference with their normal activities and who have normal pulmonary function when not having symptoms are adequately managed with just a rescue inhaler.

Step 2 is the lowest level of therapy with a long-term controller medication. Inhaled corticosteroids have been shown repeatedly to be superior to the other modalities, LTRAs, theophylline and cromolyn/nedocromil (Expert Panel Report 3 2007). In low doses they are generally free of systemic side effects with the one exception of some slowing of the rate of growth in children (The Childhood Asthma Management Program Research Group 2000, Guilbert et al. 2006). Furthermore, there is no evidence that there is any benefit from additional therapy in these mild patients. In a study of 698 steroid-naïve patients with mild persistent asthma, budesonide 100 mcg twice daily was superior to a placebo for all outcomes, the addition of formoterol to the budesonide improved lung function but did not improve symptoms or reduce the frequency of asthma exacerbations over what was achieved with the ICS alone (O'Byrne et al. 2001).

Step 3, for patients not well controlled on a low-dose of inhaled corticosteroids, offers two equally recommended regimens, increasing from low to medium dose inhaled corticosteroid or adding a LABA to the low-dose ICS. The GOAL study had shown that many asthmatics can become 'well controlled' with an ICS alone. It also showed, however, that more patients became 'well controlled' if they received a LABA in addition to the ICS and that this allowed asthma control at lower doses of ICS (Bateman et al. 2007). Even more impressive were the findings in the FACET study in which the combination of budesonide 100 mcg and formoterol twice daily was superior to budesonide 400 mcg twice daily for all outcomes reflecting the burden of asthma (Pauwels et al. 1997). The only outcome that was superior with the high dose budesonide was reduction in severe asthma exacerbations, but these too were reduced by

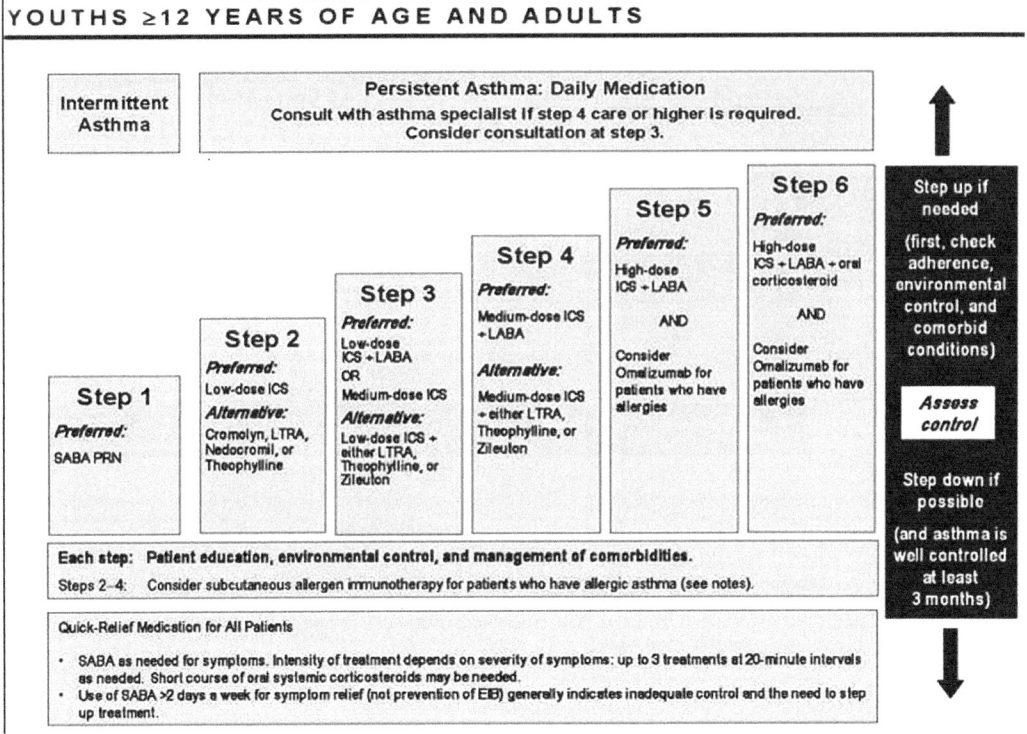

STEPWISE APPROACH FOR MANAGING ASTHMA IN YOUTHS ≥12 YEARS OF AGE AND ADULTS

Intermittent Asthma

Persistent Asthma: Daily Medication
Consult with asthma specialist if step 4 care or higher is required.
Consider consultation at step 3.

Step 1
Preferred:
SABA PRN

Step 2
Preferred:
Low-dose ICS
Alternative:
Cromolyn, LTRA, Nedocromil, or Theophylline

Step 3
Preferred:
Low-dose ICS + LABA
OR
Medium-dose ICS
Alternative:
Low-dose ICS + either LTRA, Theophylline, or Zileuton

Step 4
Preferred:
Medium-dose ICS + LABA
Alternative:
Medium-dose ICS + either LTRA, Theophylline, or Zileuton

Step 5
Preferred:
High-dose ICS + LABA
AND
Consider Omalizumab for patients who have allergies

Step 6
Preferred:
High-dose ICS + LABA + oral corticosteroid
AND
Consider Omalizumab for patients who have allergies

Step up if needed
(first, check adherence, environmental control, and comorbid conditions)

Assess control

Step down if possible
(and asthma is well controlled at least 3 months)

Each step: Patient education, environmental control, and management of comorbidities.
Steps 2–4: Consider subcutaneous allergen immunotherapy for patients who have allergic asthma (see notes).

Quick-Relief Medication for All Patients
- SABA as needed for symptoms. Intensity of treatment depends on severity of symptoms: up to 3 treatments at 20-minute intervals as needed. Short course of oral systemic corticosteroids may be needed.
- Use of SABA >2 days a week for symptom relief (not prevention of EIB) generally indicates inadequate control and the need to step up treatment.

Figure 14.3. Stepwise approach for managing asthma in youths ≥ 12 years of age and adults.

the addition of formoterol to either dose of budesonide. With such strong evidence for the superiority of the combination of an ICS and LABA over a higher dose of ICS, why is there an ambiguity? The answer lies in the results of two studies of LABAs in which many of the participants were not using ICSs (Nelson et al. 2006, Castle et al. 1993). In both studies there were increased deaths in subjects receiving salmeterol. In those studies, subjects who had reported using ICSs at randomization had not experienced the significant increase in asthma deaths seen in those not taking ICSs. Because of the increased adverse events seen in patients taking combination ICS and LABA, the FDA placed a black box warning on these combination drugs in 2003. To further address this issue, the FDA mandated five prospective trials be conducted to assess the safety and efficacy of combination ICS/LABA inhalers. In 2018, a New England Journal of Medicine publication showed that the combined analysis of these safety trials of LABAs did not show increased risk of serious asthma-related events in the combination therapy group compared to ICS alone. The black box warning on ICS/LABA combination inhalers was removed by the FDA in December 2017 based on the results of these prospective trials (Busse et al. 2018).

Step 4 addresses the failures of Step 3. In this step, all subjects receive a LABA and a medium dose ICS. The alternative strategies of adding theophylline or a LTRA have shown a moderate benefit, but inferiority to adding a LABA.

Step 5 incorporates the highest approved dose of an ICS plus a LABA. Failure to achieve control with this combination is an indication to consider the use of immunomodulators. At the time when these guidelines were published, the only available immunomodulator was omalizumab. In 419 patients uncontrolled on high-dose ICS and LABA and with a recent history of a significant asthma exacerbation, the addition of omalizumab to their treatment reduced severe asthma exacerbations by 50% as well as reducing rescue medication use and improving in their AQLQ score by an average of 0.45 (0.5 being a clinically important change) (Humbert et al. 2005). Currently omalizumab is approved only for patients with allergic asthma, defined by the presence of a positive skin test or elevated serum specific IgE level to a perennial allergen as well as a total IgE level of 30 or greater. Omalizumab is given by injection and must be administered in a health care facility due to the rare occurrence of anaphylaxis following its administration. Its dosing is based on weight and total IgE level.

Step 6 differs from Step 5 only in the addition of chronic oral corticosteroid therapy.

As opposed the 2007 NAEPP/NHLBI Asthma Guidelines that have not been updated since 2007, the GINA report is updated annually, most recently in 2019. The GINA report is not a guideline, but an integrated evidenced-based strategy focusing on translation into clinical practice (Global Initiative for Asthma 2019a). The GINA goals are to prevent asthma deaths and exacerbations, as well as improve symptom control. The report points out that mild asthma has been previously shown to make up 30–37% of adults with acute asthma, 16% of patients with near-fatal asthma and 15–20% of adults dying of asthma (Dusser et al. 2007). Regular and frequent use of SABAs is associated with increased risk for asthma exacerbations. Another paper showed that dispensing more than three canisters of SABA per year is associated with higher risk of emergency department presentations (Stanford et al. 2012).

Because of these safety risks, GINA no longer recommends SABA-only treatment for Step 1, and it is now recommended that all adults and adolescents with asthma should receive symptom-driven or regular low dose ICS-containing controller treatment, to reduce the risk of serious exacerbations. Additionally, the preferred controller is as needed low dose ICS-formoterol (Fig. 14.4) (Global Initiative for Asthma 2019b).

Step 2 in the GINA report suggests using daily low dose ICS with as needed SABA or as needed low dose ICS-formoterol for preferred controller treatment. The preferred reliever treatment for both Step 1 and Step 2 is as needed low dose ICS-formoterol.

For Step 3 treatment, GINA recommends low dose ICS-LABA as the preferred controller. House dust mite sublingual immunotherapy should be considered for add-on therapy for patients with allergic rhinitis, HDM sensitization and an FEV1 > 70% predicted.

Step 4 treatment is medium dose ICS-LABA as the preferred controller therapy. Alternate controller options also include high dose ICS, add-on tiotropium or add-on LTRA. House dust mite sublingual immunotherapy should again be considered for the same patients as in Step 3.

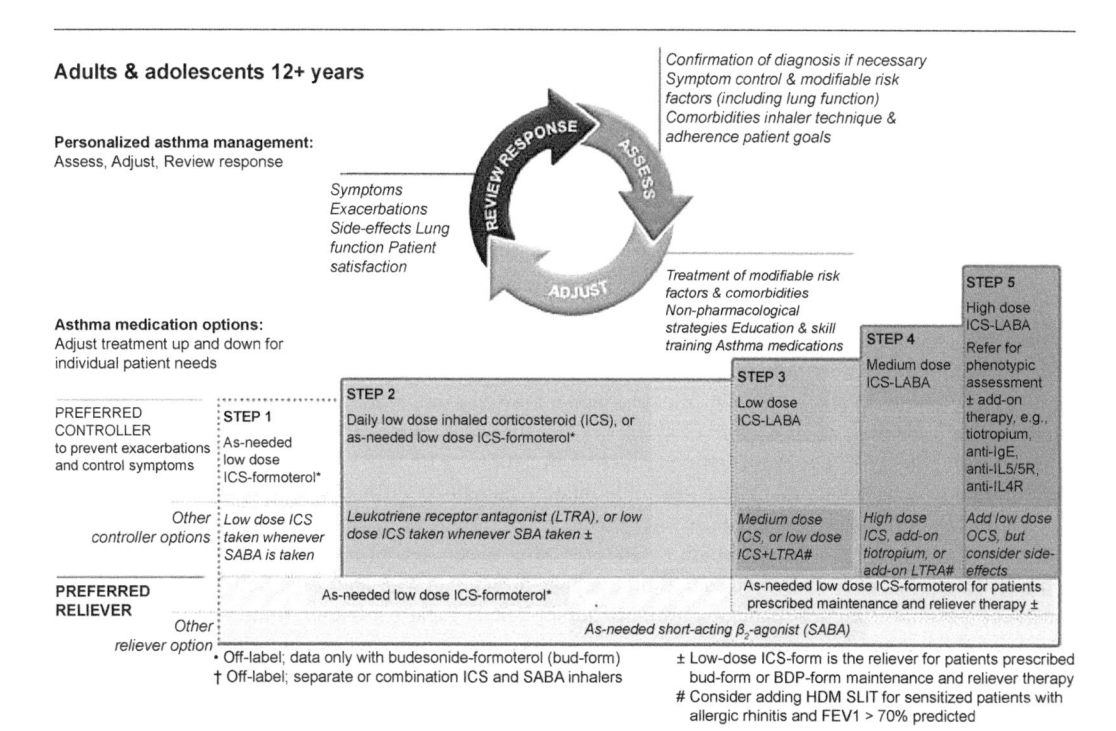

Figure 14.4. Personalized management for adults and adolescents to control symptoms and minimize future risk. ©2019 Global Initiative for Asthma, available from www.ginasthma.org, reprinted with permission.

Step 5 treatment is high dose ICS-LABA as the preferred controller therapy. Based on phenotypic assessment, add-on tiotropium, anti-IgE, anti-IL5/5R or anti IL-4R monoclonal antibodies can also be used in this step.

The preferred reliever treatment for Steps 3–5 is as needed low dose ICS-formoterol (Global Initiative for Asthma 2019b).

Special considerations

There are other considerations, in addition to pharmacotherapy, in achieving asthma control. The box on the far right in Fig. 14.3 lists some of these. An important cause for patients not being able to achieve control of their asthma with ICS and other controller medication is failure to take the medicine correctly, regularly or even at all. In a retrospective survey of over 5,000 individuals who were placed on combination therapy with an ICS and a LABA, adherence fell to 13% for the ICS and 11% for the LABA by the end of one year following the initial prescription (Marceau et al. 2006). As such, verifying proper technique and adherence is important at each visit. Other recommendations prior to increasing pharmacotherapy are to see if environmental controls for allergens and irritants such as exposure to tobacco smoke are being followed and to enquire if any co-morbid conditions, such as gastrointestinal reflux, vocal cord dysfunction, sinusitis, and rhinitis are adequately controlled.

Patients with asthma tend to have their dose of medication increased when they experience aggravation, but often the medication is not reduced after the cause of the exacerbation is gone. Thus, patients who are doing well often are receiving higher doses of medication than they currently require for asthma control. For this reason, the guidelines recommend that if asthma has been well controlled for at least 3 months, a step-down in therapy be considered.

Asthma is a heterogenous disease that can be broken down into various phenotypes and endotypes. Using these subgroups, asthmatics can be categorized as having Th2-high inflammation or Th2-low inflammation (McDowell and Heaney 2019). Th2-high patients have predominantly eosinophilic inflammation and respond to glucocorticoids as opposed to Th2-low patients that have predominantly neutrophilic or pauci-cellular inflammation and lack a response to glucocorticoids. Th2-low patients frequently have lower blood eosinophil counts and Fractional exhaled Nitric Oxide (FeNO) levels as compared to their Th2-high counterparts (McDowell and Heaney 2019, Robinson et al. 2016).

Since most of the Th2-low patients have a poor response to oral steroids, other pharmacologic therapies have shown promise in reducing exacerbations and improving symptoms. Azithromycin used as add-on therapy in patients with uncontrolled, persistent asthma on medium-to-high ICS plus LABA has shown significant reductions in asthma exacerbations and improved asthma-related quality of life compared to a placebo (Gibson et al. 2017). Tiotropium and bronchial thermoplasty can provide benefit for asthma patients, regardless of the type of inflammation driving their disease. Other interventions targeting non-type-2 inflammation in asthma including IL-17 and CXCR2 have been disappointing in clinical trials (Busse et al. 2013, O'Byrne et al. 2016). IL-6 and CRP have been shown to be elevated in Th2-low asthmatics, particularly those with obesity. There have been promising reductions in neutrophil recruiting cytokines/chemokines and allergen-induced airway inflammation in mice using antibody-mediated neutralization of IL-6 (Chu et al. 2015). Tezepelumab (anti-TSLP monoclonal antibody) has shown, small but significant exacerbation reduction in patients with low FeNO in phase 2 clinical trials suggesting it may be beneficial in Th2-low inflammation patients (Corren et al. 2017).

Figure 14.3 and the updated GINA report as a reminder that patient education, environmental control and management of co-morbidities are critical at every step of asthma management. Allergen immunotherapy has been evaluated as add-on therapy for patients who have allergic rhinitis and poorly controlled asthma. Both subcutaneous immunotherapy (SCIT) and sublingual immunotherapy (SLIT) have been shown to reduce asthma symptoms and asthma medication use in comparison to a placebo or usual care as a primary outcome in a meta-analysis of double-blind randomized controlled trials (Dhami et al. 2017, Demoly et al. 2017). In reviewing post-hoc results from a randomized trial, house dust mite SLIT was found to be an effective steroid sparing treatment (de Blay et al. 2014). House dust mite SLIT has also been effective at reducing asthma exacerbation rates in adults with house dust mite allergy-related asthma (Virchow et al. 2016).

Summary statements

1. Intranasal corticosteroids are the most effective medication class for controlling symptoms of allergic and non-allergic rhinitis.
2. The response of seasonal allergic rhinitis to nasal corticosteroids is better if treatment is initiated prior to the onset of the season, rather than after symptoms have developed.
3. In the treatment of seasonal allergic rhinitis 'as needed' intranasal fluticasone was more effective than 'as needed' loratadine for controlled symptoms and improving the quality of life.
4. A combination of the intranasal antihistamine azelastine and the intranasal corticosteroid fluticasone propionate is more effective and has more rapid onset than either component alone.
5. Oral antihistamines, intranasal antihistamines and intranasal corticosteroids moderately reduce ocular symptoms in patients with allergic conjunctivitis.
6. The most effective treatment for allergic conjunctivitis is ocular drops combining antihistaminic and mast cell stabilizing properties.
7. Treatment of bronchial asthma is directed toward achieving and maintaining asthma control.
8. In seeking asthma control, attention should be directed towards both reducing the current burden of asthma and preventing asthma exacerbations.
9. Inhaled corticosteroids are the most effective treatment for most patients with bronchial asthma.
10. If inhaled corticosteroids alone are not adequate, the most effective strategy is the addition of a long acting beta agonist.
11. Long-acting beta agonists should not be used without an accompanying corticosteroid.
12. In patients whose asthma has been well controlled for at least 3 months, a step-down in controller therapy should be considered.
13. In all patients with asthma, attention should be directed towards ensuring adherence to medication, environmental controls and control of co-morbid conditions.
14. Patients with refractory asthma should be phenotyped to determine if an immunomodulator can be used as an add-on therapy.
15. Currently available immunomodulators target inflammation mediated by IgE, IL-5, and IL-4/IL-13, but research is underway to investigate various other inflammatory targets.
16. Allergen immunotherapy should be considered in patients with stable asthma that have significant allergic triggers.

References

Assaf SM, Hanania NA. Biologic treatments for severe asthma. Curr Opin Allergy Clin Immunol 2019; 19: 379–386.
Barnes ML, Ward JH, Fardon TC, Lipworth BJ. Effects of levocetirizine as add-on therapy to fluticasone in seasonal allergic rhinitis. Clin Exp Allergy 2006; 36: 67–84.
Bateman ED, Boushey HA, Bousquet J, Busse WW, Pauwels RA, Pedersen SE, et al. Can guideline-defined asthma control be achieved? The gaining optimal asthma control study. Am J Respir Crit Care Med 2004; 170: 836–44.
Bateman ED, Bousquet J, Keech ML, Busse WW, Clark TJ, Pedersen SE. The correlation between asthma control and health status: the GOAL study. Eur Respir J 2007; 29: 56–62.
Bechet C. A review of the efficacy of desloratadine, fexofenadine, and levocetirizine in the treatment of nasal congestion in patients with allergic rhinitis. Clin Ther 2009; 31: 921–44.
Benninger M, Farrar JR, Blaiss M, Chipps B, Ferguson B, Krouse J, et al. Evaluating approved medications to treat allergic rhinitis in the United States: an evidence-based review of efficacy for nasal symptoms by class. Ann Allergy, Asthma and Immunol 2010; 104: 13–29.
Bielory L, Katelaris CH, Lightman S, Naclerio RM. Treating the ocular component of allergic rhinoconjunctivitis and related eye disorders. Med Gen Med 2007; 9: 35–49.

Bisgaard H, Olsson P, Bende M. Effect of leukotriene D4 on nasal mucosal blood flow, nasal airway resistance and nasal secretions in humans. Clin Allergy 1986; 16: 289–97.

Bleecker ER, Menzies-Gow AN, Price DB, Bourdin A, Sweet S, Martin AL, et al. Systemic literature review of systematic corticosteroid use for asthma management. Am J Respir Crit Care Med 2019; Epub ahead of print.

Bousquet J, Khaltaev N, Cruz AA, Dengurg J, Fokkens WJ, Togias A, et al. Allergic Rhinitis and its Impact on Asthma (ARIA) 2008 update (in collaboration with the World Health Organization, GA(2)LEN and Aller Gen). Allergy 2008 Apr; 63(Suppl 86): 8–160. 23.

Brozek J, Bousquet J, Agache I, Agarwal A, Bachert C, Bosnic-Anticevich S, et al. Allergic Rhinitis and its Impact on Asthma (ARIA) guidelines-2016 revision. J Allergy Clin Immunol 2017; 140: 950–958.

Busse WW, Holgate S, Kerwin E, Chon Y, Feng J, Lin J, et al. Randomized, double-blind, placebo-controlled study of brodalumab, a human Anti–IL-17 receptor monoclonal antibody, in moderate to severe asthma. Am J Respir Crit Care Med 2013; 188: 1294–1302.

Busse WW, Bateman ED, Caplan AL, Kelly HW, O'Byrne PM, Rabe KF, et al. Combined analysis of asthma safety trials of long-acting B2-Agonists. New England J Med 2018; 378: 2497–2505.

Carr W, Bernstein J, Lieberman P, Meltzer E, Bachert C, Price D, et al. A novel intranasal therapy of Azelastine with fluticasone for the treatment of allergic rhinitis. J Allergy Clin Immunol 2012a; 129: 1282–9.

Carr WW, Ratner P, Munzel U, Murray R, Price D, Canonica GW, et al. Comparison of intranasal azelastine to intranasal fluticasone propionate for symptom control in moderate-to-severe seasonal allergic rhinitis. Allergy Asthma Proc. 2012b; 33: 450–8.

Castle W, Fuller R, Hall J, Palmer J. Serevent nationwide surveillance study: comparison of salmeterol with salbutamol in asthmatic patients who require regular bronchodilator treatment. BMJ 1993; 306: 1034–7.

Chu DK, Al-Garawi A, Llop-Guevara A, Pillai RA, Radford K, Shen P, et al. Therapeutic potential of anti-IL-6 therapies for granulocytic airway inflammation in asthma. Allergy Asthma Clin Immunol 2015; 11: 14.

Corren J, Parnes JR, Wang L, Mo M, Roseti SL, Griffiths JM, et al. Tezepelumab in adults with un-controlled asthma. N Engl J Med 2017; 377: 936–946.

Cosio BG, Soriano JB. Theophylline again? Reasons for believing. Eur Respir J 2009; 34: 5–6.

de Blay F, Kuna P, Prieto L, Ginko T, Seitzberg D, Riis B, et al. SQ HDM SLIT-tablet (ALK) in treatment of asthma—post hoc results from a randomized trial. Respir Med 2014; 108: 1430–37.

Demoly P, Makatsori M, Casale TB, Calderon MA. The potential role of allergen immunotherapy in stepping down asthma treatment. J Allergy Clin Immunol Pract 2017; 5: 640–648.

Dhami S, Kakourou A, Asamoah F, Agache I, Lau S, Jutel M, et al. Allergen immunotherapy for allergic asthma: A systematic review and meta-analysis. Allergy 2017; 72: 1825–1848.

Djukanovic R, Wilson SJ, Kraft M, Jarjour NN, Steel M, Chung KF, et al. Effects of treatment with anti-immunoglobulin E antibody Omalizumab on airway inflammation in allergic asthma. Am J Respir Crit Care Med 2004; 170: 583–93.

Ducharme FM. Anti-leukotrienes as add-on therapy to inhaled glucocorticoids in patients with asthma: systematic review of current evidence. BMJ 2002; 324: 154–8.

Ducharme FM. Inhaled glucocorticoids versus leukotriene receptor antagonists as single agent asthma treatment: systematic review of current evidence. BMJ 2003; 326: 621–3.

Dusser D, Montani D, Chanez P, de Blic J, Delacourt C, Deschildre A, et al. Mild asthma: an expert review on epidemiology, clinical characteristics and treatment recommendations. Allergy 2007; 62: 591–604.

Esteitie R, deTineo M, Naclerio RM, Baroody FM. Effect of the addition of montelukast to fluticasone propionate for the treatment of perennial allergic rhinitis. Ann Allergy Asthma Immunol 2010; 105: 155–61.

Expert Panel Report 3 (EPR-3). Guidelines for the diagnosis and management of asthma: summary report 2007. J Allergy Clin Immunol 2007; 120(5 Suppl): S94–S138. The entire EPR3 Report is available online (http://www.nhlbi.nih.gov/guidelines/asthma/asthgdln.htm).

Gibson PG, Yang IA, Upham JW, Reynolds PN, Hodge S, James AL, et al. Effect of azithromycin on asthma exacerbations and quality of life in adults with persistent uncontrolled asthma (AMAZES): a randomized, double-blind, placebo-controlled trial. Lancet. 2017; 390: 659–668. Global Initiative for Asthma (GINA). Global Strategy for Asthma Management and Prevention 2019a. Retrieved from https://ginasthma.org/gina-reports.

Global Initiative for Asthma (GINA). Global Strategy for Asthma Management and Prevention 2019b.© Global Initiative for Asthma, available from www.ginaasthma.org, reprinted with permission.

Grubbe RE, Lumry WR, Anolik R. Efficacy and safety of desloratadine/pseudoephedrine combination vs its components in seasonal allergic rhinitis. J Investig Allergol Clin Immunol 2009; 19: 117–24.

Guilbert TW, Morgan WJ, Zeiger RS, Mauger DT, Boehmer SJ, Szefler SJ, et al. Long-term inhaled corticosteroids in preschool children at high risk for asthma. N Engl J Med 2006; 354: 1985–97.

Handelman NL, Friday GA, Schwartz HJ, Kuhn FS, Lindsay DE, Koors PG, et al. Cromolyn sodium nasal solution in the prophylactic treatment of pollen-induced seasonal allergic rhinitis. J Allergy Clin Immunol 1977; 59: 237–42.

Howarth PH, Stern MA, Roi L, Reynolds R, Bousquet J. Double-blind, placebo-controlled study comparing their efficacy and safety of fexofenadine hydrochloride (120 and 180 mg once daily) and cetirizine in seasonal allergic rhinitis. J Allergy Clin Immunol 1999; 104: 927–33.

Humbert M, Beasley R, Ayres J, Slavin R, Hebert J, Bousquet J, et al. Benefits of omalizumab as add-on therapy in patients with severe persistent asthma who are inadequately controlled in spite of best available therapy (GINA 2002, Step 4). INNOVATE. Allergy 2005; 60: 309–16.

Jacobs R, Lieberman P, Kent E, Silvey MJ, Locantore N, Philpot EE. Weather/temperature-sensitive vasomotor rhinitis may be refractory to intranasal corticosteroid treatment. Allergy Asthma Proc 2009; 30: 120–7.

Juniper EF, Guyatt GH, O'Byrne PM, Viveiros M. Aqueous beclomethasone dipropionate nasal spray: regular versus "as required" use in the treatment of seasonal allergic rhinitis. J Allergy Clin Immunol 1990; 86: 380–6.

Juniper EF, Guyatt GH, Archer B, Ferrrie PJ. Aqueous beclomethasone dipropionate in the treatment of ragweed pollen-induced rhinitis: further exploration of "as needed" use. J Allergy Clin Immunol 1993; 92: 66–72.

Kaiser HB, Banov CH, Berkowitz RR, Bernstein DI, Bronsky EA, Georgitis JW, et al. Comparative efficacy and safety of once-daily versus twice-daily loratadine-pseudoephedrine combinations versus placebo in seasonal allergic rhinitis. Am J Ther 1998; 5: 245–51.

Kaliner MA, Storms W, Tilles S, Spector S, Tan R, LaForce C, et al. Comparison of olopatadine 0.6% nasal spray versus fluticasone propionate 50 microg in the treatment of seasonal allergic rhinitis. Allergy Asthma Proc 2009; 30: 255–62.

Kaszuba SM, Baroody FM, deTineo M, Haney L, Blair C, Naclerio RM. Superiority of an intranasal corticosteroid compared with an oral antihistamine in the as needed treatment of seasonal allergic rhinitis. Arch Intern Med 2001; 161: 2581–7.

Katial RK, Bensch GW, Busse WW, Chipps BE, Denson JL, Gerber AN, et al. Changing paradigms in the treatment of severe asthma: the role of biologic therapies. J Allergy Clin Immunol Pract 2017; 5: S1–S14.

Kim K, Sussman G, Hebert J, Lumry W, Lutsky B, Gates D. Desloratadine therapy for symptoms associated with perennial allergic rhinitis. Ann Allergy Asthma Immunol 2006; 96: 460–5.

Kopp MV, Hamelmann E, Zielen S, Kamin W, Bergmann KC, Sieder C, et al. Combination of omalizumab and specific immunotherapy is superior to immunotherapy in patients with seasonal allergic rhinoconjunctivitis and comorbid seasonal allergic asthma. Clin Exp Allergy 2009; 39: 271–279.

Lieberman P, Meltzer EO, LaForce CF, Darter AL, Tort MJ. Two-week comparison study of olopatadine hydrochloride nasal spray 0.6% versus Azelastine hydrochloride nasal spray 0.1% in patients with vasomotor rhinitis. Allergy Asthma Proc 2011; 32: 151–8.

Lin RY, Rodriquez-Baez G, Bhargave GA. Omalizumab-associated anaphylactic reactions reported between January 2007 and June 2008. Ann Allergy Asthma Immunol 2009; 103: 442–8.

Mandl M, Nolop K, Lutsky BN. Comparison of once daily mometasone furoate (Nasonex) and fluticasone propionate aqueous nasal sprays for the treatment of perennial rhinitis. Ann Allergy Asthma Immunol 1997; 79: 370–8.

Marceau C, Lemiere C, Berbiche D, Perreault S, Blais I. Persistence, adherence and effectiveness of combination therapy among adult patients with asthma. J Allergy Clin Immunol 2006; 118: 574–581.

McDowell PJ and Heaney LG. Different endotypes and phenotypes drive the heterogeneity in severe asthma. Allergy 2019; 00: 1–9.

Nathan RA, Yancey SW, Waitkus-Edwards K, Prillaman BA, Stauffer JL, Philpot E, et al. Fluticasone propionate nasal spray is superior to montelukast for allergic rhinitis while neither affects overall asthma control. Chest 2005; 128: 1910–20.

Nelson HS, Busse WW, Kerwin E, Church N, Emmett A, Rickard K, et al. Fluticasone propionate/salmeterol combination provides more effective asthma control than low-dose inhaled corticosteroid plus montelukast. J Allergy Clin Immunol 2000; 106: 1088–1095.

Nelson HS, Weiss ST, Bleecker ER, Yancey SW, Dorinsky PM. The salmeterol multicenter asthma research trial: A comparison of usual pharmacotherapy for asthma or usual pharmacotherapy plus salmeterol. Chest 2006; 129: 15–26.

Nelson H, Kemp J, Berger W, Corren J, Casale T, Dube L, et al. Efficacy of Zileuton controlled-release tablets administered twice daily in the treatment of moderate persistent asthma: a 3-month randomized controlled study. Ann Allergy Asthma Immunol 2007; 99: 178–84.

O'Byrne PM, Barnes PJ, Rodriquez-Rolisin R, Runnerstrom E, Sanstrom T, Svensson K, et al. Low dose budesonide and formoterol in mild persistent asthma: the OPTIMA randomized trial. Am J Respir Crit Care Med 2001; 164: 1392–7.

O'Byrne PM, Metev H, Puu M, Richter K, Keen C, Uddin M, et al. Efficacy and safety of a CXCR2 antagonist, AZD5069, in patients with uncontrolled persistent asthma: a randomized, double-blind, placebo-controlled trial. Lancet Respir Med 2016; 4: 797–806.

Passalacqua G, Canonica GW. A review of the evidence from comparative studies of levocetirizine and desloratadine for the symptoms of allergic rhinitis. Clin Ther 2005; 27: 979–92.

Patel P, Philip G, Yang W, Call R, Horak F, La Force C, et al. Randomized, double-blind, placebo-controlled study of montelukast for treating perennial allergic rhinitis. Ann Allergy Asthma Immunol 2005; 95: 551–7.

Pauwels RA, Lofdahl CG, Postma DS, Tattersfield AE, O'Byrne P, Barnes PJ, et al. Effect of inhaled formoterol and budesonide on exacerbations of asthma. Formoterol and Corticosteroids Establishing Therapy (FACET) International Study Group. N Engl J Med 1997; 337: 1405–1411.

Peters SP, Kunselman SJ, Icitovic N, Moore WC, Pascual R, Ameredes BT, et al. Tiotropium bromide step-up therapy for adults with uncontrolled asthma. New England J Med 2010; 126: 225–31.

Potter PC. Levocetirizine is effective for symptom relief including nasal congestion in adolescent and adult (PAR) sensitized to house dust mites. Allergy 2003; 58: 893–9.

Pullerits T, Praks L, Skoogh B-E, Ani R, Lotvall J. Randomized placebo-controlled study comparing a leukotriene receptor antagonist and a nasal glucocorticoid in seasonal allergic rhinitis. Am J Respir Crit Care Med 1999; 159: 1814–8.

Rabe K, Adachi M, Lai CK, Soriano JB, Vermeire PA, Weiss KB, et al. Worldwide severity and control of asthma in children and adults: the global asthma insights and reality surveys. J Allergy Clin Immunol 2004; 114: 40–7.

Robinson D, Humbert M, Buhl R, Cruz AA, Inoue H, Korom S, et al. Revisiting Type-2 high and Type-2 low airway inflammation in asthma: current knowledge and therapeutic implications. Clin Exp Allergy; 47: 161–75.

Scadding GK, Lund VJ, Jacques LA, Richards DH. A placebo-controlled study of fluticasone propionate aqueous nasal spray and beclomethasone dipropionate in perennial rhinitis: efficacy in allergic and non-allergic perennial rhinitis. Clin Exp Allergy 1995; 25: 737–3.

Sobieraj DM, Weeda ER, Nguyen E, Coleman CI, White CM, Lazarus, et al. Association of inhaled corticosteroids and long-acting β-Agonists as controller and quick relief therapy with exacerbations and symptom control in persistent asthma: a systematic review and meta-analysis. J American Med Assoc 2018; 319(14): 1485–1496.

Stanford RH, Shah MB, D'Souza AO, Dhamane AD, Schatz M. Short-acting β-agonist use and its ability to predict future asthma-related outcomes. Ann Allergy Asthma Immunol 2012; 109: 403–407.

The Childhood Asthma Management Program Research Group. Long-term effects of budesonide or nedocromil in children with asthma. N Engl J Med 2000; 343: 1054–63.

Virchow JC, Backer V, Kuna P, Prieto L, Nolte H, Villesen HH, et al. Efficacy of a house dust mite sublingual allergen immunotherapy tablet in adults with allergic asthma: a randomized clinical trial. JAMA 2016; 315: 1715–25.

Wallace DV, Dykewicz MS. The diagnosis and management of rhinitis: An updated practice parameter. J Allergy Clin Immunol 2008; 122: S1–84.

Webb RD, Meltzer EO, Finn AF Jr, Rickard KA, Pepsin PJ, Westlund R, et al. Intranasal fluticasone propionate is effective for perennial nonallergic rhinitis with or without eosinophilia. Ann Allergy Asthma Immunol 2002; 88: 385–90.

Weiner JM, Abramson MJ, Puy RM. Intranasal corticosteroids versus oral H1 receptor antagonists in allergic rhinitis: systematic review of randomized controlled trials. BMJ 1998; 317: 1624–9.

Weinstein SF, Katial R, Jayawardena S, Pirozzi G, Staudinger H, Eckert L, et al. Efficacy and safety of dupilumab in perennial allergic rhinitis and comorbid asthma. J Allergy Clin Immunol 2018; 142: 171–177.

Wilson AM, O'Byrne PM, Parameswaran K. Leukotriene receptor antagonists for allergic rhinitis; a systematic review and meta-analysis. Am J Med 2004; 116: 338–44.

Wise SK, Lin SY, Toskala E, Orlandi RR, Akdis CA, Alt JA, et al. International consensus statement on allergy and rhinology: allergic rhinitis. Int Forum Allergy Rhinol 2018; 8: 108–352.

15

Allergen Immunotherapy

Harold S Nelson

INTRODUCTION

Allergy immunotherapy (AIT), much as it is practiced today, was introduced in 1911 by the reports of Leonard Noon (Noon 1911) and John Freeman (Freeman 1911) on their injection of increasing doses of timothy pollen extract to patients with a history of hay fever. However, controlled studies confirming the effectiveness of immunotherapy in allergic rhinitis (Frankland and Augustin 1954, Lowell and Franklin 1965, Franklin and Lowell 1967) and bronchial asthma (Johnstone and Dutton 1968) were not conducted until some 40 years after its introduction. Understanding the mechanism behind the improvement came even later (Hamid et al. 1997, Jutel et al. 2003) and even now, the relative contribution of the observed immunologic changes in producing the improvement in symptoms and the persisting benefit after discontinuation is not well understood. With the demonstration that immunotherapy is the only truly disease modifying treatment for the allergic diseases there is currently a high degree of enthusiasm among allergy/immunology specialists for immunotherapy, but this has not been translated into increased use in suitable patients. There are two main reasons for this is, one is the availability of reasonably effective symptomatic treatment, the other, the investment in time, the expense and the risks of adverse reactions that are associated with immunotherapy by the current subcutaneous route (SCIT). For this reason, alternative routes of administration or modifications in the allergen extracts are being explored to enhance the safety and reduce the inconvenience of this form of treatment. The approach that has achieved widespread use is sublingual administration of the allergen (SLIT). While SLIT does not carry the risk of near fatal or fatal systemic reactions, it still is expensive and requires the same long duration of treatment to achieve lasting benefit.

Indications

The use of immunotherapy by injection for treatment of allergic rhinitis (Calderon et al. 2007) and allergic asthma (Abramson et al. 2010) is supported by meta-analyses of randomized, controlled clinical studies. Injection immunotherapy with hymenoptera venom and with the whole body extracts of some ants (e.g., imported fire ant in the United States) is well established. There are a few studies that suggest that patients with atopic dermatitis who are sensitive to inhalant allergens may benefit, although this indication requires more investigation. Injection immunotherapy for food allergy, on the other hand, has been found to be associated with too frequent systemic reactions to be considered appropriate (Nelson et al. 1997) leading to current interest in oral administration to achieve improved tolerance.

National Jewish Health, Denver. Colorado. USA, Email: nelsonh@njhealth.org

The effectiveness of immunotherapy with pollen, house dust mite and animal dander extracts is well established. For the most part these extracts are standardized or in the case of pollens, produced from a highly concentrated source material ensuring a potent extract. The one exception among these extracts is the dog, which in the United States is not standardized and is generally of very low potency. There is only one exception among the U.S. dog extracts and that is an acetone precipitated extract (A.P. Dog) that is about 35 times more potent than the usual dog extract (Meiser and Nelson 2001). There are controlled studies showing clinical efficacy with extracts of Cladosporium (Malling et al. 1986) and Alternaria (Kuna et al. 2011). These were conducted with high quality extracts that probably exceed in potency the usual commercial fungal extracts in the U.S. (Vailes et al. 2001). Cockroach extracts are also of low and very variable potency (Slater et al. 2007). Therefore, the ability to achieve effective doses with currently available fungal and cockroach extracts is uncertain.

Mechanisms of action

Noon's original publication reported that immunotherapy induced an increasing resistance of the conjunctiva to instillation of timothy pollen extract (Noon 1911). Cooke demonstrated the generation of 'blocking antibody' (Cooke et al. 1935) that was later found to be predominantly in the IgG_4 subclass. After the discovery of IgE, *in vitro* studies showed that the initial response to immunotherapy was a rise in titer of allergen-specific IgE, followed after a period of months or years, by a gradual fall (Gleich et al. 1982). Neither of these immunoglobulin responses correlated with clinical improvement, however a functional assay of IgE-blocking by IgG has shown a low, but significant correlation with symptom/medication scores (Shamji et al. 2012). Examination of another arm of the immune system, the T-lymphocytes, showed that AIT induced regulatory T-cells (Jutel et al. 2003). Studies in patients who had been on immunotherapy for a number of years demonstrated, at the site of the late cutaneous response, increased numbers of cells producing IL-12 and interferon-gamma (INF-g) while cells producing IL-4 were decreased (Hamid et al. 1997). It appears likely that the regulatory T cell response occurs early, but then wanes and the immune deviation response predominates later in the treatment (Bohle et al. 2007).

Disease modification

Immunotherapy restores the response to allergens to a pattern similar to that seen in non-allergic individuals (Jutel et al. 2003). A number of observations in allergic individuals treated with immunotherapy suggest that immunotherapy modifies the underlying disease process; these observations include the reduction in new sensitivities in monosensitized individuals (Pajno et al. 2001), the blocking of the development of asthma in children who only have allergic rhinitis (Valovirta et al. 2018) and the persistence of improvement after cessation of treatment of several years duration (Durham et al. 1999).

Safety

SCIT causes local reactions at the site of injection and systemic reactions which may be only urticaria or nasal congestion, but can be severe and even fatal bronchospasm or anaphylaxis. The incidence of local and systemic reactions varies with the highest dose of extract administered. Systemic reactions are more common during the build-up and among the most sensitive patients (Lin et al. 1993). They do not appear to increase during the pollen season in subjects receiving pollen immunotherapy (Lin et al. 1993, Wong et al. 2017) and they are not predicted by the prior occurrence of large local reactions (Tankersley et al. 2000). In patients with asthma undergoing rush immunotherapy to house dust mites, the most common systemic reaction was bronchoconstriction and it occurred with increasing frequency as the baseline FEV1 was below 80% of the predicted (Bousquet et al. 1990). Between 1985 and 2001, information on 33 deaths following allergen injections and one following skin testing that occurred in the U.S. was collected by the immunotherapy committee of the American Academy of Allergy, Asthma and Immunology (Reid et al. 1993, Bernstein et al. 2004). Significant risk factors for fatal reactions identified in these reports were: (1) 88% occurred in patients with asthma; (2) the asthma was usually severe or uncontrolled, (3) 21% occurred with the first injection from a new vial of extract, and (4) 15% followed dosing errors.

Patient selection

Suitable candidates for SCIT with inhalant allergens should have allergic rhinitis or allergic asthma. The use in atopic dermatitis, though the few reports are encouraging, must still be considered outside usual practice. The patient should have demonstrated sensitivity (preferably by a prick skin testing) to the allergens under consideration. There should be evidence that the allergens are present in sufficient concentrations in the patient's environment and the patient's pattern of symptoms should be consistent with the pattern of exposure to the aeroallergen. Finally, the degree of symptoms must be of sufficient severity and duration to warrant the risk, expense and inconvenience of injection immunotherapy. Since only immunotherapy can modify the underlying disease and produce improvement that persists for years after it is discontinued, it is not necessary that the patient's symptoms be uncontrollable by symptomatic therapy.

There is no absolute lower age limit for treatment with subcutaneous immunotherapy. Arguments have been made that it should not be administered to children less than 6 years of age because of difficulty in recognizing a systemic reaction in young children and because of the traumatic effect on the child of repeated injections. However, in the study of immunotherapy for children with asthma by Johnstone (Johnstone and Dutton 1968) nine of the children were less than 2 years and 53 more were between 2 and 5 years of age. In a study that demonstrated the prevention by subcutaneous immunotherapy of the development of new sensitivities in monosensitized children, all the subjects were less than 6 years of age (Des Roches et al. 1997). In neither study were problems reported related to the children's ages. The results of 6,689 injections in 239 children aged 1 to 5 years have been reported (Rodriquez et al. 2006). There was only one systemic reaction and it responded rapidly to treatment. The ability of immunotherapy to prevent the development of additional sensitivities and the progression from rhinitis to asthma has encouraged rethinking of the age at which immunotherapy may be introduced.

Preparation of allergen extracts for subcutaneous immunotherapy

There are three considerations in preparing an allergen extract for SCIT: using adequate doses, considering cross-reactivity in choosing which extracts to include and avoiding mixing extracts with strong proteolytic activity with extracts containing allergens susceptible to proteolytic activity.

Adequate doses of each allergen

There is a large placebo effect with immunotherapy. Therefore, what constitutes an adequate dose can only be determined in a randomized, Double-Blind, Placebo-Controlled (DBPC) trial. It is helpful if the trial contains more than one dose so that the ineffective, effective and excessive doses can be determined. Unfortunately, such a dose response has only rarely been studied (Haugaard et al. 1993, Frew et al. 2006, Ewbank et al. 2003, Nanda et al. 2004, Lent et al. 2006). A second problem in applying the information from the DBPC studies is the varying units in which the dose is expressed. Many of the studies were performed in Europe, where each extract company has its own internal measure of potency. The only universally intelligible measure of dosing and potency is the amount of major allergen contained in the extract and administered as a maintenance dose. The tables below list the effective and when available ineffective doses from DBPC studies (Table 15.1), the average content of major allergens that has been found by examining a number of U.S. commercial and FDA Standardized extracts (Table 15.2), and finally, recommendations for dosing expressed in the U.S. nomenclature derived from the information given in Tables 15. 1 and 15.2 (Table 15.3). This formulation assumes a maintenance injection of 0.5 mL.

There are no studies that have compared dosing in children and adults for SCIT. In general, the same strength of extract is used for children as for adults. Sometimes, however, the maintenance dose in young children is reduced in volume to about half that of the adult dose.

Table 15.1. Effective and less effective maintenance doses for subcutaneous immunotherapy based on double-blind, placebo-controlled studies.

Allergen Extract	Major Allergen	Effective Doses	Less Effective or Ineffective Doses
Timothy grass	Phl p 5	20 mcg (33)	2 mcg (33)
Short ragweed	Amb a 1	6 mcg (37)–12.4 mcg (38)	2 mcg (39)
Birch	Bet v 1	3.28 mcg (40)–12 mcg (41)	Not determined
Dermatophagoides pteronyssinus Farinae	Der p 1 Der f 1	7 mcg (32) 10 mcg (42)	0.7 mcg (32) Not determined
Cat Dander	Fel d 1	15 mcg (34,35)	3 mcg (34,35)
Dog Dander	Can f 1	15 mcg (36)	3 mcg (36)

Table 15.2. Average major allergen content of some U.S. standardized and non-standardized extracts.

Allergen Extract	Listed Potency	Major Allergen	Mean Content of Major Allergen
Standardized			
Short ragweed	1:10 w/v or 100,000 AU/mL	Amb a 1	520 mcg/mL
Timothy grass	100,000 BAU/mL	Phl p 5	660 mcg/mL
Kentucky blue grass (June)	100,000 BAU/mL	Poa p 5	300 mcg/mL
Orchard grass	100,000 BAU/mL	Dac g 5	740 mcg/mL
Bermuda grass	10,000 BAU/mL	Cyn d 1	225 mcg/mL
Dermatophygoides Pteronyssinus farinae	10,000 AU/mL 10,000 AU/mL	Der p 1 Der f 1	67 mcg/mL 65 mcg/mL
Cat dander	10,000 BAU/mL	Fel d 1	40 mcg/mL
A.P. Dog dander	1:100 w/v	Can f 1	140 mcg/mL
Unstandardized			
Dog dander	1:10 w/v	Can f 1	5 mcg/mL
Birch	1:10 w/v	Bet v 1	390 mcg/mL
Olive	1:10 w/v	Ole e 1	430 mcg/mL
Sagebrush	1:10 w/v	Art v 1	1300 mcg/mL
Alternaria alternata	1:20 w/v (glycerin)	Alt a 1	< 0.01 to 6.1 mcg/mL (16)
Aspergillus fumigatus	1:20 w/v (glycerin)	Asp f 1	< 0.01 to 64 mcg/mL (16)
German cockroach	1:20 w/v (glycerin)	Bla g 2	8 to 66 mcg/mL (17)

Except where referenced, data provided by Greg Plunket PhD, ALK-Abello', Round Rock, Texas. Values represent averages of multiple U.S. commercial and FDA extracts.

Consideration of cross-reacting allergens

The botanical considerations are discussed at length in Chapter 6. Important cross-allergenicity can be handled in two ways. If multiple members of the cross-reacting group are locally important (e.g., several northern grasses or several varieties of ragweed) a mixture of these extracts can be prepared and added in the amount that would be appropriate for a single extract. Alternatively, if only one of the group is locally important, or if the degree of cross-reactivity is very high (e.g., cottonwood, poplar and aspen in the genus *populus* or members of the Family *Artemisia*) than the allergen that is most prevalent locally can be used.

Table 15.3. Recommended dosing of U.S. standardized and non-standardized extracts for subcutaneous immunotherapy (Cox et al. 2011).

Allergen Extract	Potencies Available	Recommended Doses
Short ragweed	1:10 w/v (100,000 AU/mL)	1,000 to 4,000 AU
Timothy grass	100,000 BAU/mL	1,000 to 4,000 BAU
Bermuda grass	10,000 BAU/mL	300 to 1,500 BAU
Cat hair or pelt	5,000 and 10,000 BAU/mL	1,000 to 4,000 BAU
Dermatophagoides Pteronyssinus Farinae	3,000, 5,000, 10,000 & 30,000 AU/mL	500 to 2,000 AU
Acetone Precipitated Dog	1:100 w/v	0.04 to 0.19 mL 1:100 w/v
Non-standardized Pollen extracts	1:10 to 1:40 w/v and 10,000 to 40,000 PNU	0.5 mL 1:100 w/v non glycerinated or 1:200 w/v glycerinated
Cockroach and Fungal extracts	1:10 to 1:40 w/v and 10,000 to 40,000 PNU	Highest tolerated dose (use only glycerinated extracts)

Avoidance of proteolysis of allergens

Extracts of fungi and cockroach contain enzymes that are capable of degrading allergens in other extracts. House Dust Mites (HDM) extracts manufactured in the US, but not some of the European HDM extracts, do not have significant proteolytic activity. Virtually all pollen, dander and house dust mite extracts are potentially susceptible to this action (Nelson et al. 1996, Grier et al. 2007). The best rule is to not mix any fungal or cockroach extracts with these susceptible extracts. It is also important to only use glycerinated extracts for fungi and cockroach, so that as far as possible of their own allergenicity is retained.

Use of multiple allergens in a treatment extract

Most patients are sensitized to multiple aeroallergens and in the U.S. most patients appear to have multiple clinically relevant sensitivities. It is a common practice in the U.S. for allergists to prescribe extracts for treatment containing a number of unrelated allergen extracts. Although the clinical effectiveness of these multiple allergen mixes has not been compared directly with that of monotherapy with the same doses, there are studies that report good clinical responses in both allergic rhinitis (Lowell and Franklin 1965, Franklin and Lowell 1967) and allergic asthma (Johnstone and Dutton 1968).

Writing the allergen extract prescription

In writing a prescription for an allergen extract to be administered by SCIT the directions should be made in writing so that it is easily understood and reproducible by other physicians. An example of such a prescription is given in Table 15.4. Except for cross-reacting allergen extracts, mixes should not be used to prepare an extract for immunotherapy since they result in dilution of the clinically relevant allergens. It is important that at least two identifiers for the patient, such as their name and birth date, be included in the prescription and carried over onto the label on the extract vial. It is also important that the maintenance and dilution vials have different colored caps preferably using the color-coding recommended by the Immunotherapy Practice Parameters (Table 15.6) (Cox et al. 2011).

Allergen extract injection schedules

Allergen extracts may be administered by rush, cluster or conventional schedules. Rush immunotherapy involves multiple injections on a single day or consecutive days. It is associated with an increased risk of systemic reactions, even with the use of pre-medication (Portnoy et al. 1994). Cluster schedules usually

Table 15.4. Representative prescription for an extract for subcutaneous immunotherapy.

Name: Medical Record Number
Address
Phone Date of Birth

Extract #1	Volume	Concentration	Expiration Date (to be completed by compounder)
Timothy	0.6 mL	100,000 BAU/mL	
Short ragweed	0.5 mL	1:10 w/v or 100,000 AU/mL	
Cottonwood	1.0 mL	1:10 w/v	
Common Sagebrush	1.0 mL	1:10 w/v	
Diluent (to make 10 mL)	6.9 mL		
Extract # 2	**Volume**	**Concentration**	**Expiration Date (to be completed by compounder)**
D. pteronyssinus	2.1 mL	10,000 AU/mL	
Cat hair & dander	7.5 mL	10,000 AU/mL	
Diluent (to make 10 mL)	0.4 mL		

involve two or three injections per day, but not on consecutive days. Cluster dosing has been shown to be not associated with an increased risk of reactions (Tabar et al. 2005) and further has the advantage of achieving a clinical response more rapidly than conventional dosing (Tabar et al. 2005). A representative schedule for cluster dosing is given in Table 15.5.

Conventionally subcutaneous immunotherapy is administered weekly or twice weekly during a build-up phase that lasts several months. Once the maintenance dose is achieved, the frequency of injections is gradually reduced until injections are given at monthly intervals. An example of a conventional schedule for injection immunotherapy is given in Table 15.6.

Table 15.5. Representative schedule for cluster dosing of subcutaneous immunotherapy.

Visit (weekly to three times per week)	Extract Dose	Extract Concentration
1	0.10 mL 0.40 mL 0.10 mL	1:1,000 v/v 1:1,000 v/v 1:100 v/v
2	0.20 mL 0.40 mL 0.07 mL	1:100 v/v 1:100 v/v 1:10 v/v
3	0.10 mL 0.15 mL 0.25 mL	1:10 v/v 1:10 v/v 1:10 v/v
4	0.35 mL 0.50 mL	1:10 v/v 1:10 v/v
5	0.07 mL 0.10 mL	1:1 v/v 1:1 v/v
6	0.15 mL 0.20 mL	1:1 v/v 1:1 v/v
7	0.30 mL 0.40 mL	1:1 v/v 1:1 v/v
8	0.5 mL (1st maintenance dose)	1:1 v/v

Table 15.6. Representative conventional schedule for subcutaneous immunotherapy. Vial # 5 used for highly sensitive patients. Otherwise begin with Vial #4.

10,000-fold dilution Vial # 5 (Silver Cap)	1,000-fold dilution Vial #4 (Blue Cap)	100-fold dilution Vial #3 (Green Cap)	10-fold dilution Vial #2 (Gold Cap)	Maintenance Concentration Vial #1 (Red Cap)
0.05 mL 0.10 mL 0.20 mL 0.40 mL	0.05 mL 0.10 mL 0.20 mL 0.40 mL	0.05 mL 0.10 mL 0.20 mL 0.40 mL	0.05 mL 0.07 mL 0.10 mL 0.15 mL 0.25 mL 0.35 mL 0.50 mL	0.05 mL 0.07 mL 0.10 mL 0.15 mL 0.20 mL 0.30 mL 0.40 mL 0.50 mL

Special considerations in administering subcutaneous immunotherapy

Premedication

With rush immunotherapy it has become customary to administered multi-drug premedication to reduce the incidence of systemic reactions (Portnoy et al. 1994). Although premedication for cluster and conventional subcutaneous immunotherapy is not routinely practiced, there are well-controlled studies that show that antihistamines, administered 2 hours prior to the injections, reduce both local and systemic reactions during cluster (Nielsen et al. 1996) and conventional (Yoshihiro et al. 2006) immunotherapy. The monoclonal antibody, omalizumab, when administered for several months before initiation of immunotherapy has been shown to reduce systemic reactions during rush, cluster and conventional subcutaneous immunotherapy (Casale et al. 2006, Massanari et al. 2010).

Patients with asthma

Reported fatal reactions to subcutaneous immunotherapy have occurred particularly in patients with asthma and often there was evidence that the patient's asthma was severe and more importantly poorly controlled at the time of the fatal reaction (Reid et al. 1993, Bernstein et al. 2004). This points to the importance of assessing the status of the patient's asthma, if present, prior to administering the allergen extract. This can be done by careful questioning for recent night time awakenings or use of rescue inhalers. Perhaps even better is to have documented the patient's peak expiratory flow when their asthma was well controlled and to recheck it at each clinic visit prior to giving the immunotherapy injection. If the reading is 15% below the level obtained when their asthma was well controlled, immunotherapy should not be given.

Duration of immunotherapy

If immunotherapy has not been of clear benefit after one year on maintenance it should be discontinued. Successful immunotherapy can be stopped after an adequate period of treatment with the expectation that most patients will continue to benefit for a number of years after its discontinuation. While there is a need for considering the individual circumstances, studies suggest that for many patients three years of treatment is adequate both for pollens (Durham et al. 1999) and for HDMs (Greer Labs, unpublished).

Site and administration of subcutaneous immunotherapy

Because of the possibility of a serious and even fatal reaction to SCIT it should only be administered in a medical facility with the presence of personnel trained in emergency treatment and the medications needed to treat anaphylaxis and severe bronchoconstriction. The person administering the injection should obtain an interval history of reactions to the earlier injection and changes in health status or medications.

The identity of the patient should be confirmed by at least two identifying items (e.g., full name and birth date). The injections should be administered into the subcutaneous tissue of the lateral or posterior middle portion of the asthma. The patient should wait under observation at the medical facility for 30 minutes following the injection. If a systemic reaction occurs, the first treatment should be epinephrine 1:1,000, 0.2 to 0.5 mL for adults and children over the age of 6 years. Uptake of epinephrine is slow from the subcutaneous tissue therefore for all severe reactions the epinephrine should be administered intramuscularly in the thigh (Cox et al. 2011).

Maintenance of extract potency

Allergen extracts lose potency over time, some such as grass, more rapidly than others. Loss of potency is retarded by keeping extracts refrigerated at 4 degrees centigrade at all times when not in use. Dilutions should be prepared using saline with 0.03% t human serum albumin to provide further stability. If there is an objection to the use of a human blood product, 10% glycerin will provide a similar stability. Extracts in 50% glycerin are by far the most stable, but the pain associated with their injection make a lesser concentration of glycerin desirable (Cox et al. 2011). Maintenance extracts and extracts in 50% glycerin generally retain their potency for a year. Dilutions of the maintenance extracts tend to lose potency more rapidly as the dilution is increased. There are no adequate studies to address the rate of loss of potency but a safe rule may be to consider dilutions of 1:10 and 1:100 usable for 6 months and dilutions of 1:1000 usable for one month.

Dosing adjustments

Since extracts tend to lose potency with time and even standardized extracts from the same manufacturer will vary somewhat in potency from lot to lot, it is appropriate to reduce the dose of extract when a new treatment vial is prepared. If there have been no changes in the source of the components, a 50% reduction, with buildup to the maintenance dose over a period of several injections is adequate. If there is a new source for a standardized or pollen extract a reduction of one 10-fold dilution would be indicated, while if there is a new source for a fungal or cockroach extract two 10-fold reductions would be indicated. If a new extract is to be administered, it should be given as a separate injection, built up according to the conventional schedule, and added to the treatment extracts after maintenance has been reached.

There are no studies that determine the necessary adjustment for missed doses. Recommendations from the Immunotherapy Practice Parameters (Cox et al. 2011) for the build-up phase are given in Table 15.7. A recommendation for adjustments during maintenance treatment is if the injections are 2–4 weeks late the dose should be reduced by 75%; if the missed time is greater than 4 weeks the dose should be reduced by one or more dilutions depending on the length of time and patient's sensitivity (Greer Labs, unpublished).

The dose of extract should be reduced after a patient experiences a systemic reaction. Usually the dose is reduced to the previously tolerated dose or to the next lower dose on the build-up schedule if the patient is on maintenance injections. In the case of very severe systemic reactions, the prescribing physician should re-evaluate the patient to determine if the risk/benefit assessment justifies continuing with the treatment (Cox et al. 2011).

Table 15.7. Dose adjustments for missed doses during the build-up phase (Cox et al. 2011).

Up to 7 days late	Continue build-up as scheduled
8 to 13 days late	Repeat previous dose
14 to 21 days late	Reduce dose by 25%
21 to 28 days late	Reduce dose by 50%

Use of alternative routes of administering allergen extracts

Because of the inconvenience and risks for serious reactions with SCIT different approaches are being used to overcome these problems. The alternative approach that has been studied the most and has gained the greatest acceptance is SLIT. In a number of European countries this is the most common form of immunotherapy. Many aspects of SLIT are the same as for SCIT so only areas where they differ will be discussed.

Although local side effects (itching and swelling in the mouth) are common for a few days after initiation of SLIT, systemic reactions are uncommon and severe life threatening or fatal reactions have not been reported (Canonica et al. 2009). Due to its record of safety, it is customary, after the first dose is taken in the physician's office, for subsequent doses to be administered by the patient at home, thus reducing the expense and inconvenience of regular visits to a medical center to receive injections. Furthermore, the maintenance dose is administered without build-up of dosing.

SLIT tablets are available in the US for grasses, short ragweed and HDMs, while tablets for birch and Japanese cedar are under development. There are also approved liquid SLIT products in Europe, but in the US liquid dosing is administered with extracts approved for SCIT, but unstudied and unapproved for use by SCIT. SLIT dose-finding studies with US liquid allergen extracts are lacking and currently in Europe a wide range of doses are being reported as effective with sublingual administration (Larenas-Linnemann and Mosqes 2016).

The optimal duration of treatment with SLIT appears to be similar to with subcutaneous immunotherapy (Marogna et al. 2010) and persisting benefit has been reported for a number of years after its discontinuation (Marogna et al. 2010). The relative effectiveness of SCIT and SLIT is still debated, however two studies with approved dosing of timothy by SCIT and SLIT revealed significantly better results with SCIT compared to SLIT, at least in the first year of treatment (Aasbjerg et al. 2014, Scadding et al. 2017). One further possible advantage of SCIT over SLIT is that with the former, as previously discussed, there are several studies supporting the efficacy of the administration of multiple unrelated allergens in the same injection (Lowell and Franklin 1965, Franklin and Lowell 1967, Johnstone and Dutton 1968). With SLIT, on the other hand, only simultaneous administration of two different allergens has been shown to be clinically effective. One study that examined the response to timothy alone or the same dose of timothy mixed with nine other pollen extracts, suggested that the response to monotherapy was much more robust than that to timothy in a multi-allergen mixture (Amar et al. 2009).

Two other alternative routes of allergen extract administration have been reported. Three injections of allergen extract into an inguinal lymph node, given at monthly intervals, produced symptom improvement three years later that was equivalent to what was obtained with a three year course of subcutaneous injections; with a total allergen extract dose of < 1/1000th of the latter (Senti et al. 2008). Another route is transcutaneous application of the extract on a patch (Senti et al. 2015). In three studies patches were applied weekly for 6 weeks to 3 months and with various doses and durations of application. Side effects varied, but with each trial there was a good reduction in symptoms compared to a placebo that persisted a second season without further treatment in one of the studies. Both of these approaches appear promising, but further studies are required before they can be accepted as standard therapy.

Use of modified allergen extracts for subcutaneous immunotherapy

Modifications in the allergen extract are designed to increase the safety and convenience of SCIT. The structure of the allergen molecules can be altered by treatment with gluteraldehyde or formalin. This reduces the IgE binding epitopes making the treatment safer and allowing more rapid build-up. Many of these modified allergens, known as allergoids, are in commercial use in Europe. Although many of them appear to be clinically effective, studies suggest that in some there is not only a reduction in IgE-binding, but also in T-cell responses (Henmar et al. 2008). The latter would reduce their clinical efficacy. Use of allergoids should be limited to preparations that have proven efficacy in RDBPC trials.

Allergenic proteins can be generated by recombinant technology either in their natural form, or in a mutated form that has reduced reactivity with IgE. Alternatively, T-cell epitopes can be identified within the allergen molecule and peptides can be generated that react with these T-cell epitopes but are too small to react with specific IgE. All of these approaches using recombinant technology are under active investigation, particularly in Europe.

Another approach is to covalently bind the allergen to a molecule that reacts with the Toll-Like Receptors (TLR) on antigen presenting cells. This presentation tends to direct the response towards Th1 and regulatory T cells. Studies are presently underway in the US with one such product containing monophosphoryl lipid A that reacts with TLR-4 (65).

Summary

1) SCIT with inhalant allergens is indicated for patients with allergic rhinitis or allergic asthma whose symptoms warrant the risk and inconvenience of the treatment. Since immunotherapy is the only disease modifying treatment available for allergic diseases, its use should not be limited to patients who cannot obtain relief with symptomatic treatment.

2) Treatment extracts for SCIT should contain doses of each allergen that have been demonstrated to be effective in DBPC trials. In prescribing an extract for treatment consideration should be given to cross-reactivity among allergens and to not mixing extracts with protease activity with extracts whose allergens are susceptible to this action. Mixtures containing multiple allergen extracts have been shown to be effective as long as the individual allergens are not diluted below an effective dose.

3) Allergen extracts for subcutaneous immunotherapy may be administered by rush, cluster or conventional schedules. Rush is not advocated due to the high rate of systemic reactions, even with premedication. Use of premedication with antihistamines is recommended at least during the build-up phase of cluster immunotherapy.

4) Patients should have their identity confirmed in at least two ways before they receive their injection.

5) Patients with asthma should receive immunotherapy only if their asthma is well controlled.

6) Doses should be reduced for new vials, for missed injection visits and for systemic reactions. Large local reactions do not predict systemic reactions, so reductions in a dose should only be made for the sake of patient comfort.

7) SLIT has become an accepted alternative to SCIT. The indications, mechanisms, duration and disease modifying potential of SLIT are the same as for SCIT. They differ in SLIT being safer and able to be administered at home after the first dose, while SCIT appears to be more effective, at least in the first year and has proven efficacy for treatment with multi-allergen mixes.

8) Future directions for immunotherapy include administering the current extracts by alternative routes including Intralymphatic and Epicutaneous. Other approaches involve modification of the allergen extracts through reacting with aldehydes to produce allergoids, recombinant technology to produce mutated allergens or T-cell directed peptides or by linking the allergens to molecules that react with the TLRs of the antigen presenting cells, thus biasing towards Th1 or T-regulatory response.

References

Aasbjerg K, Backer V, Lund G, Holm J, Nielsen NC, Holse M, et al. Immunological comparison of allergen immunotherapy against grass allergy. Clin Exp Allergy 2014; 44: 417–28.

Abramson MJ, Puy RM, Weiner JM. Injection allergen immunotherapy for asthma. Cochrane Database Syst Rev 2010 Aug 4;8: CD001186.

Amar S, Harbeck RJ, Sills M, Silveira LJ, O'Brien H, Nelson HS. Response to sublingual immunotherapy with grass pollen extract: monotherapy versus combination in a multiallergen extract. J Allergy Clin Immunol 2009; 124: 150–156.

Bernstein DI, Wanner M, Borish L, Liss GM. Twelve-year survey of fatal reactions to allergen injections and skin testing 1990–2001. J Allergy Clin Immunol 2004; 113: 1129–36.

Bohle, B, Kinaciyan T, Gerstmayr M, Radakovics A, Jahn-Schmid B, Ebner C. Sublingual immunotherapy induces IL-10-producing T regulatory cells, allergen-specific T-cell tolerance, and immune deviation. J Allergy Clin Immunol 2007; 120: 707–13.
Bousquet J, Hejjaoui A, Michel FB. Specific immunotherapy in asthma. J Allergy Clin Immunol 1990; 86: 292–305.
Calderon MA, Alves B, Jacobson M, Hurwitz B, Sheikh A, Durham S. Allergen injection immunotherapy for seasonal allergic rhinitis. Cochrane Database Syst Rev 2007; (1): CD001936.
Canonica GW, Bousquet J, Casale T, Lockey R, Baena-Cagnani C, Pawankar R, et al. Sub-lingual immunotherapy: World Allergy Organization Position Paper 2009.Allergy 2009; 64(Suppl 91): 1.59.
Casale TB, Busse WW, Kline JN, Ballas ZK, Moss MH, Townley RG, et al. Omalizumab pretreatment decreases acute reactions after rush immunotherapy for ragweed-induced seasonal allergic rhinitis. J Allergy Clin Immunol 2006; 117: 134–40.
Cooke RA, Barnard JH, Hebald S, Stull A. Serological evidence of immunity with coexisting sensitization in a type of human allergy (hay fever). J Exp Med 1935; 62: 733–50.
Cox L, Nelson H, Lockey R. Allergen immunotherapy: A Practice Parameter. Third Update. J Allergy Clin Immunol 2011; 127: S1–S55.
Creticos PS, Adkinson NF Jr, Kagey-Sobotka A Proud D, Meier HL, Naclerio RM, et al. Nasal challenge with ragweed pollen in hay fever patients: Effect of immunotherapy. J Clin Invest 1989a; 76: 2247–53.
Creticos PS, Marsh DG, Proud D, Kagey-Sobotka A, Adkinson NF, Jr, Friedhoff L, et al. Responses to ragweed-pollen nasal challenge before and after immunotherapy. J Allergy Clin Immunol 1989b; 84: 197–205.
Creticos PS, Schroeder JT, Hamilton RG, Balcer-Whaley SL, Khattignavong AP, Lindblad R, et al. Immunotherapy with a ragweed toll-like receptor 9 agonist vaccine for allergic rhinitis. N Engl J Med 2006; 355: 1445–55.
Des Roches A, Paradis L, Menardo JL, Bouges S, Daures JP, Bousquet J. Immunotherapy with a standardized *Dermatophagoides pteronyssinus* extract. VI. Specific immunotherapy prevents the onset of new sensitization in children. J Allergy Clin Immunol 1997; 99: 450–3.
Didier A, Malling HJ, Worm M, Horak F, Jäger S, Montagut A, et al. Optimal dose, efficacy, and safety of once-daily sublingual immunotherapy with a 5-grass pollen tablet for seasonal allergic rhinitis. J Allergy Clin Immunol 2007; 120: 1338–45.
Drachenberg KJ, Wheeler AW, Stuebner P, Horak F. A well-tolerated grass pollen-specific allergy vaccine containing novel adjuvant, monophosphoryl lipid A, reduces allergic symptoms after only four preseasonal injections. Allergy 2001; 56: 498–505.
Durham SR, Walker SM, Varga E-M, Jacobson MR, O'Brien F, Noble W, et al. Long-term clinical efficacy of grass pollen immunotherapy. N. Engl J Med 1999; 341: 468–75.
Ewbank PA, Murray J, Sanders K, Curran-Everett D, Dreskin S, Nelson HS. A double-blind, placebo-controlled immunotherapy dose-response study with standardized cat extract. J Allergy Clin Immunol 2003; 111: 155–61.
Frankland AW, Augustin R. Prophylaxis of summer hay-fever and asthma: A controlled trial comparing crude grass-pollen extracts with the isolated main protein component. Lancet 1954; i: 1055–7.
Franklin W and Lowell FC. Comparison of two dosages of ragweed extract in the treatment of pollinosis. JAMA 1967; 201: 915–7.
Freeman J. Further observations on the treatment of hay fever by hypodermic inoculations of pollen vaccine. Lancet 1911; iiL814–7.
Frew AJ, Powell RJ, Corrigan CJ, Durham SR. Efficacy and safety of specific immunotherapy with SQ allergen extract in treatment-resistant seasonal allergic rhinoconjunctivitis. J Allergy Clin Immunol 2006; 117: 319–28.
Furin MJ, Norman PS, Creticos PS, Proud D, Kagey-Sobotka A, Lichtenstein LM, et al. Immunotherapy decreases antigen-induced eosinophil cell migration into the nasal cavity. J Allergy Clin Immunol 1991; 88: 27–32.
Gleich GJ, Zimmermann EM, Henderson LL, Yunginger JW. Effect of immunotherapy on immunoglobulin E and immunoglobulin G antibodies to ragweed antigens: a six-year prospective study. J Allergy Clin Immunol 1982; 70: 261–71.
Greer Labs, Allergenic extracts, Standardized Cat Hair Extract. www.greerlabs.com.
Grier TJ, LeFevre DM, Duncan EA, Esch RE. Stability of standardized grass, dust mite, cat and short ragweed allergens after mixing with mold or cockroach extracts. Ann Allergy Asthma Immunol 2007; 99: 151–160.
Hamid QA, Schotman E, Jacobson MR, Walker SM, Durham SR. Increases in IL-12 messenger RNA+ cells accompany inhibition of allergen-induced late skin responses after successful grass pollen immunotherapy. J Allergy Clin Immunol 1997; 99: 254–60.
Haugaard L, Dahl R, Jacobsen L. A controlled dose-response study of immunotherapy with standardized, partially purified extract of house dust mite: clinical efficacy and side effects. J Allergy Clin Immunol 1993; 91: 709–22.
Henmar H, Lund G, Lund L, Petersen A, Wurtzen PA. Allergenicity, immunogenicity and dose-relationship of three intact allergen vaccines and four allergoid vaccines of subcutaneous grass pollen immunotherapy. Clin Exp Immunol 2008; 153: 316–23.
Johnstone DA and Dutton DA. The value of hyposensitization therapy for bronchial asthma in children: A 14-year study. Pediatrics 1968; 42: 793–802.
Jutel M, Akdis M, Budak F, Aebischer-Casaulta C, Wrzyszcz M, Blaser K, et al. IL-10 and TGF-bcooperate in the regulatory T cell response to mucosal allergens in normal immunity and specific immunotherapy. Eur J Immunol 2003; 33: 1205–14.

Khinchi MS, Poulsen LK, Carat F, Andre C, Hansen AB, Malling HJ. Clinical efficacy of sublingual and subcutaneous birch pollen allergen specific immunotherapy: a randomized, placebo-controlled, double-blind, double-dummy study. Allergy 2004; 59: 45–53.

Kuna P, Kaczmarek J, Kupczyk M. Efficacy and safety of immunotherapy for allergies to Alternaria alternata in children. J Allergy Clin Immunol 2011; 127: 502–8.

Larenas-Linnemann DE, Mosqes R. Dosing of European sublingual immunotherapy maintenance solutions relative to monthly recommended dosing of subcutaneous immunotherapy. Allergy Asthma Proc 2016; 37: 50–6.

Lent A, Harbeck R, Strand M, Sills M, Schmidt K, Efaw B, et al. Immunological response to administration of standardized dog allergen extract at differing doses. J Allergy Clin Immunol 2006; 118: 1249–56.

Lin MS, Tanner E, Lynn J, Friday GA, Jr. Nonfatal systemic allergic reactions induced by skin testing and immunotherapy. Ann Allergy 1993; 71: 557–62.

Lowell FC, Franklin W. A double-blind study of the effectiveness and specificity of injection therapy in ragweed hay fever. N Engl J Med 1965; 273: 675–9.

Malling H-J, Dreborg S, Weeke B. Diagnosis and immunotherapy of mould allergy V. Clinical efficacy and side effects of immunotherapy with *Cladosporium herbarum*. Allergy 1986; 41: 507–19.

Marogna M, Spadolini L, Massolo A, Zanon P, Berra D, Chiodini E, et al. Effects of sublingual immunotherapy for multiple or single allergens in polysensitized patients. Ann Allergy Asthma Immunol 2007; 98: 274–80.

Marogna M, Spadolini L, Massolo A, Canonica GW, Passalacqua G. Long-lasting effects of sublingual immunotherapy according to its duration: A 15-year prospective study. J Allergy Clin Immunol 2010; 1126: 969–75.

Massanari M, Nelson H, Casale T, Busse W, Kianifard F, Geba GP, Zeldin RK. Effect of pretreatment with omalizumab on the tolerability of specific immunotherapy in allergic asthma. J Allergy Clin Immunol 2010; 125: 383–9.

Meiser JB, Nelson HS. Comparing conventional and acetone-precipitated dog allergen extract skin testing. J Allergy Clin Immunol 2001;107:744-5

Nanda A, O'Connor M, Anand M, Dreskin SC, Zhang L, Hines B, et al. Dose dependence and time course of he immunologic response to administration of standardized cat allergen extract. J Allergy Clin Immunol 2004; 114: 1339–44.

Nelson HS, Ikle D, Buchmeier A. Studies of allergen extract stability: the effects of dilution and mixing. J Allergy Clin Immunol 1996; 98: 382–8.

Nelson HS, Lahr J, Rule R, Bock A, Leung D. Treatment of anaphylactic sensitivity to peanuts by immunotherapy with injections of aqueous peanut extract. J Allergy Clin Immunol 1997; 99: 44–51.

Nielsen L, Johnsen CR, Mosbech H, Poulsen LK, Mallin HJ. Antihistamine premedication in specific cluster immunotherapy: A double-blind, placebo-controlled study. J Allergy Clin Immunol 1996; 97: 1207–13.

Noon L. Prophylactic inoculation against hay fever. Lancet 1911; i: 1572–3.

Olsen OT, Larsen KR, Jacobsen L, Svendsen UG. A 1-year, placebo-controlled, double-blind house dust mite immunotherapy studying asthmatic adults. Allergy 1997; 52: 853–9.

Pajno GB, Barberio G, De Luca Fr. Morabito L, Parmiani S. Prevention of new sensitizations in asthmatic children monosensitized to house dust mite by specific immunotherapy. A six-year follow-up study. Clin Exp Allergy 2001; 312: 1392–7.

Portnoy J, Bagstad K, Kanarek H, Pacheco F, Fall B, Barnes C. Premedication reduces the incidence of systemic reactions during inhalant rush immunotherapy with mixtures of allergenic extracts. An Allergy 1994; 73: 409–18.

Rak S, Heinrich C, Schevnius A. Comparison of nasal immunopathology in patients with seasonal rhinoconjunctivitis treated with topical steroids or specific allergen immunotherapy. Allergy 2006; 60: 643–9.

Reid MJ, Lockey RF, Turkeltaub PC, Platts-Mills TAE. Survey of fatalities from skin testing and immunotherapy 1985–9. J Allergy Clin Immunol 1993; 92: 6–15.

Rodriquez Perez N, Ambriz Moreno MJ. Safety of immunotherapy and skin tests with allergens in children younger than 5 years. Rev AlergMex 2006; 53: 47–51.

Scadding GW, Calderon MA, Shamji HM, Eifan AO, Penagos M, Dimitru F, et al. Effect of 2 years of treatment with sublingual grass pollen immunotherapy on nasal response to allergen challenge at 3 years among patients with moderate to severe seasonal allergic rhinitis: the GRASS randomized clinical trial. JAMA 2017; 317: 615–625.

Senti G, Vavricka P, Erdmann I, Diaz MI, Markus R, McCormack SJ, et al. Intralymphatic allergen administration renders specific immunotherapy faster and safer: A randomized controlled trial. Proc Nat AcadSci 2008; 105: 17908–12.

Senti G, von Moos S, Tay F, Graf N, Johansen P, Kündig TM et al. Determinants of efficacy and safety in epicutaneous allergen immunotherapy: summary of three clinical trials. Allergy 2015; 70: 707–10.

Shamji MH, Liorring C, Francis JN, Calderon MA, Larché M, Kimber I et al. Functional rather than immunoreactive levels of IgG4 correlate closely with clinical response to grass pollen immunotherapy. Allergy 2012; 67: 217–26.

Slater JE, James R, Pongracic JA, Liu AH, Sarpong S, Sampson HA, et al. Biological potency of German cockroach allergen extracts determined in an inner city population. Clin Exp Allergy 2007; 37: 1033–9.

Tabar AI, Echechipia S, Garcia BE, Olaguibel JM, Lizaso MT, Gómez B, et al. Double-blind comparative study of cluster and conventional immunotherapy schedules and *Dermatophagoides pteronyssinus*. J Allergy Clin Immunol 2005; 116: 109–18.

Tabar AI, Aarroabarren E, Echechipia S, Garcia BE, Martin S, Alvarez-Puebla J. Three years of specific immunotherapy may be sufficient in house dust mite respiratory allergy. J Allergy Clin Immunol 2011; 127: 57–63.

Tankersley MS, Butler KK, Butler WK, Goetz DW. Local reactions during allergen immunotherapy do not require dose adjustment. J Allergy Clin Immunol 2000; 106: 840–843.

Vailes L, Sridhara S, Cromwell O, Weber B, Breitenbach M, Chapman M. Quantitation of the major fungal allergens, Alt a 1 and Asp f 1, in commercial allergenic products. J Allergy Clin Immunol 2001; 107: 641–6.

Valovirta E, Petersen TH, Piotrowska T, Laursen MK, Andersen JS, Sørensen HF, et al. Results from the 5-year SQ grass sublingual immunotherapy tablet asthma prevention (GAP) trial in children with grass pollen allergy. J Allergy Clin Immunol 2018; 141: 529–538.

Wong PH, Quinn JM, Gomez RA, Webb CN. Systemic reactions to immunotherapy during mountain cedar season: implications for seasonal dose adjustment. J Allergy Clin Immunol Pract 2017; 5: 1438–1439.

Yoshihiro O, Yoshinon N, Kiyotaka M. Effect of premedication with fexofenadine on the safety of immunotherapy in patients with allergic rhinitis. Ann Allergy Asthma Immunol 2006; 96: 600–5.

16

Pulmonary Function Testing

Ekta Kakkar,[1,][*] *Flavia CL Hoyte,*[1] *Devasahayam J Christopher*[2] *and Rohit K Katial*[1]

INTRODUCTION

Pulmonary Function Tests (PFTs) are important in the assessment of patients presenting with respiratory complaints. PFTs are readily available and noninvasive tests that aid in the diagnosis of pulmonary conditions. They can often help in distinguishing between various conditions that can appear quite similar. As such, these tests can be used to guide decisions regarding changes to therapy. Pulmonary function is also frequently assessed pre-operatively to assess safety before a patient undergoes an invasive procedure.

Methods of pulmonary function testing

Peak flow measurement is a quick, inexpensive way to measure the maximal flow rate achieved during forced expiration following a full inspiration. It is a portable, hand-held device in which patients blow forcefully into the mouthpiece. It is important to note that peak flows can be variable between devices. Therefore, patients should monitor their peak flow using the same device to guide management (DeVrieze et al. 2019).

Impulse oscillometry measures the resistance and reactance of the airways to small pressure oscillations which are applied at the mouth and transmitted to the lungs. Resistance is the energy required to propagate the oscillation through the lungs, and reactance is the amount of recoil generated against the pressure wave (Komarow et al. 2011). This method of pulmonary function testing is noninvasive and requires only passive patient cooperation. For this reason, it is useful in both adults and young children to diagnose and manage chronic lung diseases such as asthma (Komarow et al. 2011).

Other ways to measure pulmonary function are spirometry and plethysmography which provide more information about lung volumes and capacities. Spirometry is a common test that can be done in the clinic and measures the volume of air a patient inhales and exhales and the time it takes the patient to do so. It can also be helpful in diagnosing a pulmonary condition and in monitoring disease progression. Lung plethysmography measures lung volumes and provides more information than spirometry for diagnosis and management. This test requires a patient to sit or stand in a closed, air-tight chamber and provides data about the absolute volumes and capacities of air in the lungs with different breathing maneuvers.

---

[1] National Jewish Health, Denver, Colorado USA, Emails: fciega@gmail.com; katialR@njhealth.org
[2] Christian Medical College Hospital, Vellore, TN INDIA, Email: djchris@cmcvellore.ac.in
* Corresponding author: kakkarekta@njhealth.org

Validity of testing

A few factors are used to assess the validity of pulmonary function testing. First, the volume-time curve that is output during PFTs must demonstrate a normal plateau that is reached during expiration and each expiration must last at least 6 seconds (Fig. 16.1).

Second, the results of the two best Forced Vital Capacity (FVC) and Forced Expiratory Volume in 1 second (FEV1) efforts on PFTs must be within 0.2 L of each other. This ensures a patient's results are reproducible. Finally, the flow-volume loop, which is discussed next, should not contain abnormalities or artifacts (Johnson et al. 2014). In addition, the back extrapolation, which is a measure of hesitation at the start of an effort, must be less than 5% or 150 mL, whichever is greater, if the FVC is ≤ 3 L (McKibben et al. 2011).

For peak flow, patients must be taught how to perform accurate measurements, and this must continually be monitored at follow up since results are effort dependent. Like spirometry, normal values for peak flow depend on the patient's age, sex and height. For example, the predicted peak flow for a 40 year-old healthy adult with a height of 70 inches is 611 liters/minute (Hankinson et al. 1999). Diurnal variation in peak flow values is also common, with the morning values being slightly lower than afternoon measurements (Reddel et al. 1999). Therefore it is important to tell patients to monitor peak flows at the same time each day.

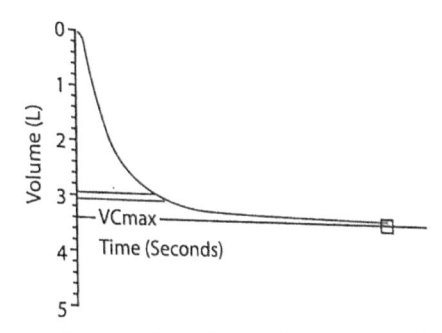

Figure 16.1. Normal volume-time curve demonstrating a plateau of the volume of air expired and an expiration of at least 6 seconds.

Types of lung disease

Pulmonary function testing helps to differentiate between obstructive and restrictive lung disease. Obstructive lung disease is characterized by obstruction or narrowing of the airways. This is often due to excessive smooth muscle contraction. Examples of obstructive lung disease include asthma, Chronic Obstructive Pulmonary Disease (COPD) and bronchiectasis. Restrictive lung disease is characterized by the inability to fully expand the lungs. This results in decreased lung volume and increased work of breathing. Restrictive lung disease can be due to occupational exposures, medications, neuromuscular disorders or pulmonary fibrosis. Extrinsic diseases can also restrict expansion of the lung. For a comprehensive list of etiologies of restrictive lung disease see Table 16.1 (Johnson et al. 2014).

An effective way to differentiate between obstructive and restrictive lung disease is through interpretation of the flow-volume loop. The flow-volume loop is a plot of inspiratory and expiratory flow against volume during pulmonary function testing depicted in Fig. 16.2.

A flow-volume loop is the output during both spirometry and plethysmography. Analysis of specific lung volumes can also help differentiate between obstructive and restrictive lung disease. These volumes will be discussed in detail later in the chapter.

Components of pulmonary function tests

Pulmonary function testing measures Tidal Volume (TV), Vital Capacity (VC), Inspiratory Capacity (IC), Functional Residual Capacity (FRC), Residual Volume (RV), Total Lung Capacity (TLC), Forced

180 *Textbook of Allergy for the Clinician*

Table 16.1. Common causes of restrictive lung disease.

Chest Wall(Extrinsic)	Medications
Ankylosing spondylitis	Amiodarone
Kyphosis	Methotrexate
Morbid obesity	Nitrofurantoin
Scoliosis	Radiation therapy
Neuromuscular Disorders	**Interstitial Lung Disease**
Amyotrophic lateral sclerosis	Asbestosis
Guillain-Barre syndrome	Berylliosis
Myasthenia gravis	Silicosis
Muscular dystrophy	Hypersensitivity pneumonitis
	Eosinophilic pneumonia
	Idiopathic pulmonary fibrosis
	Sarcoidosis

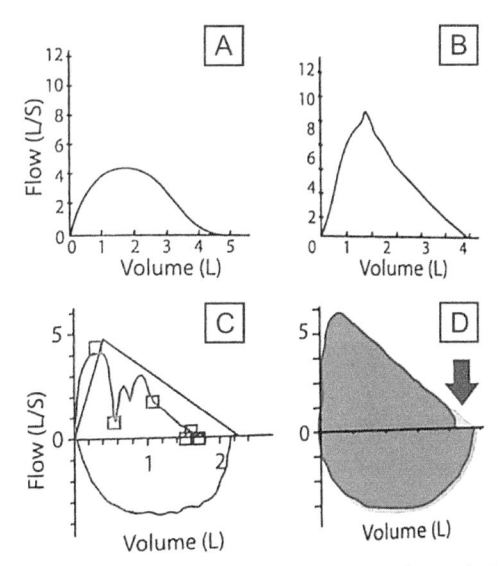

Figure 16.2. Flow-volume loops. The upper panel shows a normal flow-volume loop. The blue line is before bronchodilator therapy and the red line demonstrates post-bronchodilator spirometry. The bottom panel demonstrates changes in the flow-volume loops seen in A) reversible obstructive disease such as asthma, B) obstructive disease without reversibility such as Chronic Obstructive Pulmonary Disease or COPD and C) restrictive disease.

Vital Capacity (FVC), Forced Expiratory Volume (FEV), Expiratory Reserve Volume (ERV), Inspiratory Reserve Volume (IRV), Forced Expiratory Flow (FEF) and Peak Expiratory Flow Rate (PEFR). Capacities are the sum of two or more volumes. An illustration of this data is depicted in Fig. 16.3.

Normal values for each lung volume will vary from person to person. The values in PFTs are compared to the average for someone of the same age, sex and height for each patient, and these data are recorded as a percentage.

Tidal Volume (TV)

TV is a measure of the amount of air a person inhales during a normal breath. In a healthy, young adult, TV is approximately 7 mL/kg of body mass (Ricard 2003). TV plays a significant role in mechanical ventilation and can be adjusted to ensure adequate ventilation without causing lung injury. Lower tidal volumes on a ventilator are preferred in patients with pre-existing lung disease or acute respiratory distress syndrome (Hallett et al. 2019). TV is also essential in calculating a patient's minute ventilation or the volume of gas exchanged by a person's lungs per minute. Minute ventilation is calculated by multiplying

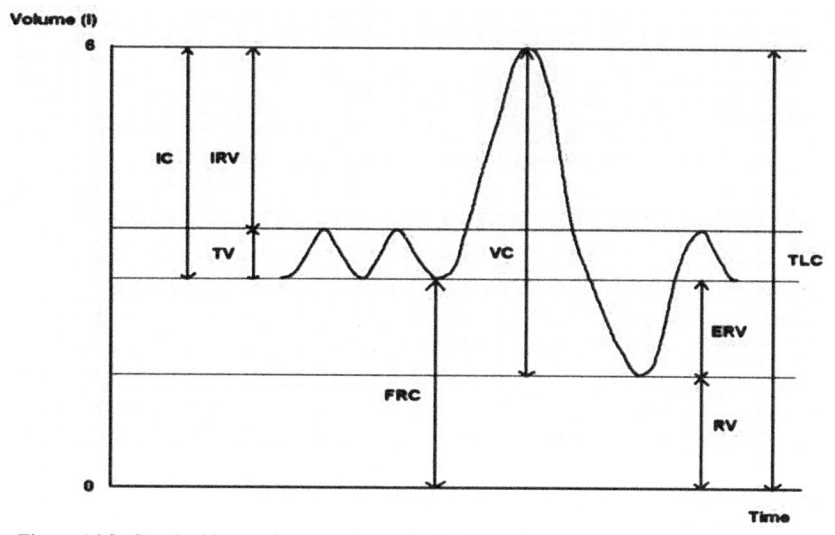

Figure 16.3. Standard lung volumes and capacities that can be measured with plethysmography.

the TV and respiratory rate. During exercise, the minute ventilation increases due to physiological demands for increased oxygenation.

Vital Capacity (VC)

VC is the maximum amount of air a person can expire from the lungs after a maximum inhalation. It is also the sum of the tidal volume and inspiratory and expiratory reserve volumes (i.e., VC = TV + IRV + ERV). VC is used in neuromuscular diseases like Guillain-Barre Syndrome and myasthenia gravis to determine the severity of respiratory muscle involvement. A normal, healthy adult has a vital capacity between 3 and 5 liters (David et al. 2019). VC is decreased in restrictive diseases. In obstructive lung disease, VC can be normal or slightly decreased (David et al. 2019).

Inspiratory Capacity (IC) and Inspiratory Reserve Volume (IRV)

IC is the volume of air that can be inspired following a normal expiration. IC is equivalent to the sum of the TV and the Inspiratory Reserve Volume (IRV). The IRV is the additional volume of air, above tidal volume, that can be inhaled during maximal inspiration. In a healthy adult male, the IRV is approximately 3,100 mL (Tortora 2016).

Functional Residual Capacity (FRC), Residual Volume (RV) and Expiratory Reserve Volume (ERV)

FRC is the volume of air in the lungs after a normal expiration. It is the point at which the forces of the chest wall, which expands outward and the lungs, which collapse inward, are at equilibrium (Hopkins et al. 2019). The Residual Volume (RV) is the amount of air in the lungs that an individual cannot physiologically expire, or the air that remains in the lung after maximal expiration. Without this RV, the lungs would collapse. RV can only be obtained from plethysmography. ERV is the additional amount of air that can be expired forcefully after a normal expiration. FRC is the sum of RV and ERV.

Total Lung Capacity (TLC)

TLC refers to the total amount of air in the lungs after a maximal inspiration. Patients with obstructive disease and air trapping leading to hyperinflation of the lungs may have an increase in TLC. On the other hand, in restrictive disease, the TLC is decreased. TLC is measured through body plethysmography. In healthy adults, the TLC is about 6 L (Delgado et al. 2019).

Peak Expiratory Flow Rate (PEFR)

PEFR is the maximum flow rate generated during a forced expiration. It is measured in liters per minute and is dependent on a patient's effort. A low PEFR could be indicative of airflow obstruction or of poor patient effort. If effort and technique are adequate, a PEFR percent predicted correlates with the percent predicted value for FEV1 (Choi et al. 2002). Peak flow measurements are commonly used to detect changes or trends in a patient's asthma control. PEFR is sensitive for asthma and COPD. However, it can underestimate the degree of airflow limitation in both conditions, and spirometry or plethysmography is a more reliable method to diagnose and treat patients (Choi et al. 2002). PEFR is a useful tool in patients that have poor perception of their bronchoconstriction since it provides an objective measurement of lung function and can be performed by the patient at home. Serial peak flow measurements at work and away from work can also be used as a screening method in patients who may be affected with occupational asthma.

Forced Expiratory Volume (FEV)

FEV measures the amount of air a person can exhale during forced expiration following a deep inhalation. It can be broken down further into the amount of air exhaled in the first second of expiration, or FEV1. Changes in FEV in response to bronchodilator guide management and diagnosis of obstructive lung disease (Dales et al. 1988). For example, a significant improvement in FEV1 or forced vital capacity (FVC) by 12% and 200 mL following bronchodilator administration is consistent with asthma per the American Thoracic Society. On the other hand, COPD is characterized by fixed airway obstruction and lack of reversibility with bronchodilator.

Forced Vital Capacity (FVC)

FVC is the total amount of air exhaled during forced expiration following a deep inhalation. If it is normal, this is an indication that the respiratory muscle strength is intact. In lung function testing, the ratio of FEV1/FVC is used to differentiate between obstructive and restrictive lung disease. Patients with obstructive defects have a disproportionate decrease in FEV1 compared to FVC. This results in a low FEV1/FVC ratio. The American Thoracic Society (ATS) guidelines outline that a FEV1/FVC ratio lower than 70 or 65% in patients over the age of 65, is consistent with obstructive disease. More recent updates consider a FEV1/FVC ratio below the lower limit of normal as diagnostic of obstruction where the lower limit of normal is equal to the 5th percentile in normal, healthy adults (Swanney et al. 2008). In restrictive disease, on the other hand, both FEV1 and FVC are reduced, resulting in a normal or even elevated FEV1/FVC ratio. Restrictive defects cannot be diagnosed by spirometry alone; decreased lung volumes, particularly TLC on a body plethysmography test would be needed to confirm the diagnosis. Table 16.2 below outlines the ways in which PFTs can aid in differentiating between obstructive and restrictive lung disease (Dweik 2011). It is important to note that a patient can have a mixed pattern of both obstruction and restriction.

Table 16.2. Patterns of lung volumes in obstructive and restrictive lung disease.

Measures	Obstructive Disorders	Restrictive Disorders	Mixed Disorders
FEV1/FVC	Decreased	Normal or Increased	Decreased
FEV1	Decreased	Decreased	Decreased
FVC	Normal or Decreased	Decreased	Decreased
TLC	Normal or Increased	Decreased	Decreased, Normal, or Increased
RV	Normal or Increased	Decreased	Decreased, Normal, or Increased

Forced Expiratory Flow (FEF)

FEF is the speed of air flow during the middle of forced expiration. It is usually recorded as a mean of 25 to 75% of the FVC or as FEF25–75%. Prior studies suggested this mean may be more accurate than FEV1 in detecting small airway obstruction. However, more recent data has shown that FEF25–75% lacks reproducibility and is not specific for small airway obstruction (Quanjer et al. 2014). Current practice guidelines continue to recommend using FEV1 and the FEV1/FVC ratio to evaluate the degree of obstruction. However, FEF25–75% may be useful in predicting the presence of clinically relevant asthma in children with a normal FEV1 and has been shown to correlate with bronchodilator responsiveness in this population (Simon et al. 2010).

Diffusion capacity

Diffusion capacity provides information about gas exchange in the lung. It measures how well the oxygen gets from the air in the lungs to the red blood cells in the vessels. PFTs measure the diffusing capacity of the lung for carbon monoxide or DLCO. Carbon monoxide is used in this test because it binds to hemoglobin with a higher affinity than oxygen. DLCO must be obtained in a closed air-tight chamber. It is measured by having a patient exhale completely to RV then maximally inhale air from a chamber containing a mixture of carbon monoxide and helium. The patient then holds his or her breath for 10 seconds and exhales into a chamber without carbon monoxide. The exhaled air is then analyzed by the machine for carbon monoxide content. Diffusion capacity is affected by altitude, the amount of surface area over which diffusion can occur, the volume of blood in pulmonary capillaries, the hemoglobin concentration in the blood, the thickness of the membrane between the lungs and capillaries and the presence of fluid in the airways (Mehra et al. 2009). Table 16.3 shows the effects of different pulmonary conditions on the DLCO (Weinberger et al. 2013).

A normal DLCO is between 80–120%. Diffusion capacity is corrected for gender, age, altitude and hemoglobin level. It can be expressed as DLCO alone or as DLCO/VA, which is DLCO corrected for alveolar volume.

Table 16.3. Pulmonary conditions associated with a decreased, normal or increased DLCO.

DLCO Decreased	DLCO Normal	DLCO Increased
Emphysema Interstitial Lung Disease Pulmonary Vasculitis Anemia Pulmonary Embolism	Asthma (or increased) Bronchitis	Obesity Polycythemia Vera Intracardiac Shunts Asthma (or normal)

Summary

This chapter has reviewed the data available through pulmonary function testing and its utility in management of pulmonary conditions. Spirometry is often completed in-office as providers monitor the progression of chronic lung diseases. Lung plethysmography and diffusion capacity testing must be completed in an air-tight chamber but can provide additional information to help physicians make diagnostic and treatment decisions. The data obtained from PFTs can help differentiate between lung diseases, including obstructive and restrictive disease and can be used to assess safety before surgical procedures.

References

Choi IS, Koh YI, Lim H. Peak expiratory flow rate underestimates severity of airflow obstruction in acute asthma. Korean J Int Med 2002; 17(3): 174.

Dales RE, Spitzer WO, Tousignant P, Suissa S. Clinical interpretation of airway response to a bronchodilator. Epidemiologic considerations. Am Rev Respir Dis 1988 Aug; 138(2): 317–20.

David S, Sharma S. Vital Capacity. [Updated 2019 Feb 2]. In: StatPearls [Internet]. Treasure Island (FL): StatPearls Publishing; 2019 Jan.

Delgado BJ, Bajaj T. Physiology, lung capacity. [Updated 2019 Apr 16]. In: StatPearls [Internet]. Treasure Island (FL): StatPearls Publishing; 2019 Jan.

DeVrieze BW, Giwa AO. Peak flow rate measurement [Updated 2019 Mar 26]. In: StatPearls [Internet]. Treasure Island (FL): StatPearls Publishing; 2019 Jan.

Dweik RA. Interpretation of Common Lung Function Tests. Cleveland Clinic. 2011. Web. 2019 Oct.

Hallett S. Ashurst JV. Physiology, tidal volume. [Updated 2019 Feb 2]. In: StatPearls [Internet]. Treasure Island (FL): StatPearls Publishing; 2019 Jan.

Hankinson JL, Odencrantz JR, Fedan KB. Spirometric reference values from a sample of the general U.S. population. Am J Respir Crit Care Med 1999; 159(1): 179.

Hopkins E, Sharma S. Physiology, functional residual capacity. [Updated 2019 Mar 14]. In: StatPearls [Internet]. Treasure Island (FL): StatPearls Publishing; 2019 Jan.

Johnson SD, Theurer WM. A stepwise approach to the interpretation of pulmonary function tests. Am Fam Physician 2014 Mar 1; 89(5): 359–66.

Komarow HD, Myles IA, Uzzaman A, Metcalfe DD. Impulse oscillometry in the evaluation of diseases of the airways in children. Ann Allergy Asthma Immunol 2011 Mar; 106(3): 191–9.

McKibben JM, McKay RT, Freeman AG, Levin LS, Pinney SM, Alshaikh E. Redefining spirometry hesitating criteria based on the ratio of extrapolated volume to timed FEVs. Chest 2011 Jul; 140(1): 164–9.

Mehra R, Strohl KP. Chapter 14—Evaluation and monitoring of respiratory function. Sleep Disorders Medicine (Third Edition). Published online 2009 Oct: 188–97.

Quanjer PH, Weiner DJ, Pretto JJ, Brazzale DJ, Boros PW. Measurement of FEF25–75% and FEF75% Does Not Contribute to Clinical Decision Making. Eur Resp J 2014; 43: 1051–8.

Reddel H, Jenkins C, Woolcock A. Diurnal variability—time to change asthma guidelines? Br Med J 1999; 319: 45.

Ricard JD. Are we really reducing tidal volume-should we? Am J Respir Crit Care Med 2003 May; 167(10): 1297–8.

Simon MR, Chinchilli VM, Phillips BR, Sorkness CA, Lemanske RF, Szefler SJ, et al. Forced expiratory flow between 25% and 75% of vital capacity and FEV1/Forced vital capacity ratio in relation to clinical and physiological parameters in asthmatic children with normal FEV1 Values. J Allergy Clin Immunol 2010 Sep; 126(3): 527–34.

Swanney MP, Ruppel G, Enright PL, Pederson OF, Crapo RO, Miller MR, et al. Using the lower limit of normal for the FEV1/FVC ratio reduces the misclassification of airway obstruction. Thorax 2008; 63: 1046–51.

Tortora, GJ. Principles of Anatomy and Physiology. Derrickson, Bryan, (15th ed.); 2016. Hoboken, NJ. p. 874.

Weinberger SE, Cockrill BA, Mandel J. Chapter 3—Evaluation of the patient with pulmonary disease. Principles of Pulmonary Medicine (Sixth Edition). Published online 2013 May 30–63.

17

Common Office Tests and Procedures for the Allergist

Vinay Mehta

INTRODUCTION

The purpose of this chapter is to provide an overview of the common tests and procedures that are performed in the allergist's office. Topics that are discussed include spirometry, fractional exhaled nitric oxide measurement, exercise challenge, eucapnic voluntary hyperventlilation test, methacholine challenge, skin prick testing, intradermal testing, local anesthetic testing, penicillin testing, venom testing, patch testing, atopy patch testing, allergen immunotherapy administration, oral food challenge, aspirin desensitization, nebulizer administration and rhinoscopy. In addition to describing the methodology, information on procedure setup, suitable equipment and appropriate documentation is also discussed.

Many of the topics covered here will be discussed more exhaustively in other chapters of this book. The purpose of this chapter is only to serve as a quick reference guide for the busy clinician.

Pulmonary function testing

Spirometry

Spirometry is a basic pulmonary function test which measures the volume of air inspired or expired as a function of time. It allows easy and direct measurement of FEV_1, FVC and FEV_1/FVC ratio. Spirometry cannot, however, measure lung volumes. Thus, information about FRC and lung volumes computed from FRC, such as total lung capacity and residual volume, require body plethysmography or gas dilution. The *youngest age* to perform *spirometry* with reproducible results varies between 5 and 7 years.

Healthy young children may reach FVC in a few seconds, but it can take older patients much longer, especially those with airflow obstruction. In such cases, sustaining a maximal expiratory effort until achieving FVC may cause lightheadedness. In adults, FEV_6 has been shown to be equivalent to FVC for identifying obstructive and restrictive patterns.

Procedures. Calibration with a 3 L syringe should be performed each day of testing. Calibration should be repeated when the room temperature changes, when the equipment is disassembled and reassembled or when the equipment has been performing frequent tests for 4 hours. American Thoracic Society (ATS) standards state that calibration should be performed by discharging the calibration syringe at least three

---

Allergy, Asthma & Immunology Associates, P.C, Lincoln, NE, USA, Email: drvinaymehta@gmail.com

times with a low, medium and high flow varying between 0.5 and 12 L/s. If the calibration is not within ± 3.5% of the syringe volume, it should be repeated.

All patients undergoing spirometry should be given instructions prior to the test. The patient should be reminded to maintain a good posture during the test, remaining upright until the test is completed. For safety reasons, the ATS recommends that patients be allowed to sit during the procedure (Miller et al. 2005a). If you choose to have patients stand, it is a good idea to have a chair behind them so that they may sit during the test if they begin to feel lightheaded. Regardless of the position you choose, it is important that the position remain consistent from test to test and visit to visit, as patients may have slightly lower lung functions when sitting than they would when standing.

There are two techniques for performing the FVC test: the open method and the closed method. In the open method, the patient begins by inhaling completely. The patient places the mouthpiece in his or her mouth and immediately exhales forcefully and rapidly. The patient continues to exhale until no more air can be expelled, followed by a full inspiratory effort. This maneuver is repeated at least three times, with a maximum of eight attempts to meet the reproducibility and acceptability criteria.

In the closed-technique, the patient first places the mouthpiece in the mouth, ensuring a good seal. He or she then inhales completely and rapidly, and immediately exhales forcefully and rapidly until no more air can be expelled, followed by a full inspiratory effort. This maneuver is repeated at least three times, with a maximum of eight attempts to meet the reproducibility and acceptability criteria. Depending on the particular software that you are using, the patient may be required to breathe tidally into the spirometer prior to taking the initial forceful inhalation.

Reversibility is the process of determining the patient's response to a bronchodilator. It is technically defined by an increase in FEV_1 of at least 12% compared to baseline and a 200 mL improvement in FEV_1. Current ATS guidelines recommend administering four puffs of albuterol MDI (90 μg/puff) at 30 second intervals via a spacer device (Miller et al. 2005b). When evaluating reversibility, the ATS recommends that the patient abstain from short-acting β2-agonists for four hours before the test, and from long-acting β2-agonists for 12 hours prior to testing. Smoking should be avoided for one hour prior to the test.

Acceptability of a test

Any of following criteria makes a spirometry effort unacceptable:

- Poor start
- Poor end
- Cough during the first second
- A Valsalva maneuver or hesitation
- An air leak at the mouth
- Obstruction of the mouthpiece

A poor start occurs when the patient hesitates between maximal inhalation and exhalation. The delay before maximal exhalation may be calculated into the FEV_1 and result in an inaccurate measurement. A poor end occurs when the patient does not blow long enough, resulting in a falsely low FVC. Technicians should instruct patients to completely exhale through energetic coaching. The ATS recommends an exhalation time of six seconds. However, some patients may not be able to meet this criterion in spite of multiple attempts. For these patients, an obvious plateau on the time/volume graph will demonstrate an acceptable end.

A cough during the first second of an effort will result in an unacceptable effort because of the potential effect on the FEV_1. A Valsalva maneuver prematurely stops airflow, influencing FEV_1 or FVC. A good seal around the mouthpiece is needed to prevent air leaks during the procedure. If a patient is breathing through his or her nose during the test, nose clips can be used to obstruct the nasal passages. The mouthpiece should be clear of obstruction. Technicians should instruct patients not to occlude the mouthpiece with their tongue or teeth, and chewing gum should be discarded prior to testing.

Spirometry efforts are considered acceptable only if they meet <u>all</u> of the following criteria:

- They are free of artifact
- There is a rapid start
- There is an acceptable end (6 seconds or an obvious plateau)
- The two highest FVC values are within 0.15 L of each other
- The two highest FEV_1 values are within 0.15 L of each other.

Documentation. When performing spirometry, proper documentation of the equipment should be kept. This documentation should include calibration procedures.

According to the National Heart, Lung, and Blood Institute (NHLBI) asthma guidelines, a spirometry is recommended at the initial assessment and after treatment is initiated and symptoms have stabilized (National Heart, Lung, and Blood Institute 2007). It is also recommended during a period of progressive or prolonged loss of asthma control. Finally, spirometric assessment is recommended at least every 1–2 years to assess the maintenance of the lung function. These spirometry measures should be followed over the patient's lifetime to detect potential for decline and rate of decline of pulmonary function over time.

Equipment. There are many available choices of spirometry equipment, and no one system is best for everyone. When deciding what system to invest in, consider the set-up of your office and how you would like to utilize the equipment. Do you want to have a hand-held unit that can go into patient rooms or will you have an exclusive procedure room?

Built-in quality control aids can be helpful in obtaining good spirometry results. The use of incentives can encourage patients, particularly children, to blow out longer and faster than they otherwise would. Alerts can be helpful in detecting potential errors in technique and pointing them out to the technician. Finally, a reminder message from the equipment if calibration has not been performed will help ensure that test results are reliable.

Exercise challenge

The exercise challenge is used to evaluate for exercise-induced bronchoconstriction, both for the purpose of diagnosis and to evaluate the effectiveness of treatment. Exercise challenge testing can also be used to rule out other causes of exercise-induced shortness of breath, such as vocal cord dysfunction (Crapo et al. 2000). The ATS recommendations for performing exercise challenges are summarized here. Contraindications for this test include unstable cardiac conditions and orthopedic limitations.

Procedures. The patient should be instructed to wear comfortable running clothes. If possible, medication that can alter bronchial responsiveness should be withheld (see Table 17.1). In addition, prior exercise should be avoided for at least 4 hours before testing, as it can exert a protective effect. A baseline spirometry should be performed immediately prior to exercise for comparison to post test results.

The treadmill is the preferred method for performing the exercise challenge. The patient's heart rate should be monitored by EKG. Alternatively, a pulse oximeter may be used. Testing should be done at a temperature < 25°C and a relative humidity < 50%.

The exercise portion of the procedure consists of exercising vigorously to quickly achieve a target heart rate between 80 and 90% of the patient's maximum predicted heart rate, which is calculated with the following equation:

Maximum predicted heart rate = 220 - age in years

Once the target heart rate is reached, the patient should maintain that heart rate for 4–6 minutes. The test is concluded when the patient has completed at least 4 minutes of exercise at the target heart rate, or when the patient becomes too symptomatic to continue. Alternatively, ventilation rather than heart rate can be used to monitor exercise intensity. Ventilation should reach 40–60% of the predicted Maximum Voluntary Ventilation (MVV), calculated as $FEV_1 \times 35$. Although not always accurate during exercise, estimation of arterial O_2 saturation by pulse oximetry is recommended both during and after exercise.

Table 17.1. Factors that decrease bronchial responsiveness.

Second generation antihistamines	72 hours
Short-acting bronchodilators	8 hours
Ipratropium	24 hours
Long-acting bronchodilators	48 hours
Theophylline	12–48 hours
Cromolyn sodium	8 hours
Leukotriene modifiers	24 hours
Caffeine	Day of the test

Source: Crapo et al. 2000

Serial spirometries are performed at 5, 10, 15, 20, and 30 minutes after cessation of exercise. At least two acceptable tests should be obtained at each time interval. A decrease in $FEV_1 \geq 10\%$ is considered to be a positive challenge, although some authors suggest a value of 15%. A significant decline in FEV_1 can also be seen in VCD, but it is usually associated with flattening of the inspiratory phase of the flow-volume curve.

Technician Training. The technician performing the exercise challenge should be skilled in pulmonary function testing and be able to recognize signs of respiratory and cardiac distress. For high risk patients, it is recommended that the physician personally monitor the entire procedure.

Equipment. Necessary equipment to perform an exercise challenge includes:

- Crash cart
- Pulse oximeter
- Sphygmomanometer
- Treadmill or exercise bicycle
- Air temperature and humidity monitor

Documentation. All documentation recommended in the spirometry section of this chapter also applies to the exercise challenge. In addition, a log should be kept detailing the temperature and humidity of the testing room.

Eucapnic Voluntary Hyperpnea (EVH)

A number of surrogates for exercise testing have been developed that may be easier to implement than an exercise challenge. These include Eucapnic Voluntary Hyperpnea (EVH) of dry air and inhalation of hyperosmolar aerosols, such as 4.5% saline or dry powder mannitol. Of these, the most widely recognized is EVH. In fact, EVH is now the gold standard of the International Olympic Committee to identify athletes with exercise-induced asthma who may legitimately be allowed to take bronchodilators before a competition. With EVH, the patient voluntarily, without exercising, rapidly breathes dry air enriched with 5% CO_2 for 6 minutes. As with exercise, a $\geq 10\%$ decline in FEV_1 from the pre-challenge value following EVH is consistent with a diagnosis of exercise-induced bronchoconstriction.

Methacholine challenge

Methacholine challenge testing is often performed when asthma is a diagnostic possibility but traditional methods such as pre- and post-bronchodilator spirometry and fractional exhaled nitric oxide measurement are inconclusive. The test is more suited to rule out the diagnosis of asthma due to its high sensitivity and high negative predictive value. It is less well suited to confirm the diagnosis of asthma because of its moderate specificity and low positive predictive value. Indeed, increased bronchial hyper responsiveness can also be seen in COPD, congestive heart failure, cystic fibrosis, bronchitis and allergic rhinitis. Contraindications for testing are listed in Table 17.2.

Table 17.2. Contraindications for methacholine challenge testing.

Absolute:	
	Severe airflow limitation (FEV_1 <50% predicted or <1.0 L)
	Heart attack or stroke in the last 3 months
	Uncontrolled hypertension, systolic BP >200 mm Hg or diastolic BP >100 mm Hg
	Known aortic aneurysm
Relative:	
	Moderate airflow limitation (FEV_1 <60% predicted or <1.5 L)
	Inability to perform acceptable-quality spirometry
	Pregnancy
	Nursing mothers
	Cholinesterase inhibitors (for myasthenia gravis)

Source: Crapo et al. 2000

Drugs that may decrease bronchial responsiveness should ideally be withheld prior to testing (see Table 17.1). In addition, coffee, tea, cola drinks and chocolate should also be withheld the day of the study. Finally, patients should be free of respiratory tract infections prior to testing, as they may increase bronchial responsiveness.

Technician Training. The technician performing the test should:

- Be familiar with the guidelines and be knowledgeable about specific test procedures
- Be capable of managing the equipment, including set-up, verification of proper function, maintenance and cleaning
- Be proficient at spirometry
- Know the contraindications to methacholine challenge testing
- Be familiar with safety and emergency procedures
- Know when to abort testing
- Be proficient in the administration of bronchodilators and evaluation of the response to them.

Inhaled methacholine causes bronchoconstriction. Technicians with asthma are at increased risk of bronchospasm during testing and should take extra precautions to minimize their exposure to the aerosolized methacholine.

Procedure. Methacholine is the agent of choice for nonspecific bronchoprovocation challenge testing. It is FDA-approved and available in 100 mg vials as a dry powder. Normal saline is the recommended diluent. There are different published dilution schemes that depend on the dosing protocol used. Both two-minute tidal breathing and five-breath dosimeter protocols are available. The reader is referred to the ATS guidelines for specifics on dilutions and dosing schemes (Crapo et al. 2000). In general, a baseline spirometry is obtained. If the baseline FEV_1 is < 60%, albuterol is administered and the spirometry is repeated. The first dose of methacholine is given, followed by spirometry at the appropriate time interval. If the drop in FEV_1 is < 20% from the baseline, the testing proceeds to the next dose. If at any point the change in FEV_1 is > 20% from baseline, testing is stopped, signs and symptoms are recorded, albuterol is given and spirometry is performed 10 minutes later. If the highest dose of methacholine is given and the decline in FEV_1 is < 20% from baseline, the test is complete. A sample methacholine challenge test report form is available in Appendix C of the ATS guidelines (Crapo et al. 2000).

Fractional exhaled nitric oxide measurement

Measurement of fractional nitric oxide in exhaled breath (FENO) is a noninvasive, simple and safe method of measuring eosinophilic airway inflammation. The ATS recently released a clinical practice guideline regarding the interpretation of FENO in the clinical setting (Dweik et al. 2011). Unlike conventional spirometry or methacholine challenge, FENO offers added advantages, including (1) detecting eosinophilic airway inflammation, (2) determining the likelihood of corticosteroid responsiveness, (3) monitoring airway inflammation and (4) monitoring adherence to corticosteroid therapy.

Procedure. As opposed to pulmonary function testing, the exhalation maneuver for FENO is slow and steady, with a desired optimal flow rate of 50 mL/s over 6 seconds. A mouthpiece filter is used to provide enough resistance to close the soft palate on exhalation and prevent contamination of exhaled nitric oxide from the nasal passages.

Spirometry may transiently affect FENO results; therefore, it is more accurate to assess FENO before the spirometry. Patients should avoid nitrate-rich foods one hour before FENO testing. Likewise, alcohol may alter FENO levels and should be avoided. Smoking may reduce FENO levels, and therefore patients should not smoke for 1hour earlier. Finally, URIs can increase FENO levels and such infections should be documented along with the test.

Calibration of the machine varies by the manufacturer. Some require daily calibration by a healthy control volunteer. Others use bottled nitrous oxide of a known quantity. Familiarity with calibration and control measures is important for accurate results.

FENO is an indirect measure of eosinophilic inflammation. Interpretation of findings is beyond the scope of this chapter. Cut-off values have recently been published (Dweik et al. 2011) to help determine which patients will likely respond to inhaled corticosteroids (> 50 ppb in adults and > 35 ppb in children) and those who are less likely to respond (< 25 ppb in adults and < 20 ppb in children). Following values longitudinally in an individual can also help fine-tune their dose of inhaled corticosteroid and monitor for adherence.

Technician Training. Staff should be educated on the correct FENO technique. The test is less dependent on patient effort than spirometry. An effort will be deemed either adequate or inadequate by the machine with little need for interpretation by staff. If calibration is required by a healthy control, staff volunteers should be taught the proper methods. Having more than one healthy control may be advantageous to avoid problems if a single control is absent.

Documentation. When performing FENO in your office, proper documentation of the equipment should be kept. Manuals should be easily accessible to staff in case of error codes or malfunction. Calibration logs, if necessary, should be kept as well. FENO measurements should be recorded for each patient in a manner that can be easily tracked over time.

Equipment. There is currently at least one portable FENO measurement device available (NIOX VERO, Circassia), along with a full-sized device that is more appropriate for research and academic centers. These devices are better utilized if kept in a central location rather than moving them from room to room. When deciding which device to purchase, consider how many tests you will likely perform in a month, as the sensors for each device expire after a certain number of tests or a specified time period. Consider the cost per test for disposable equipment. Does the machine itself need to be replaced after a set number of tests? What control measures are needed? Does the machine lock you out if you do not perform controls? Does the software interface with your electronic medical record system? These questions should be considered before deciding on a particular device.

Allergen skin testing

Skin testing is a bioassay which detects the presence of allergen-specific IgE on a patient's mast cells. When an allergen is introduced into the skin of a patient during skin testing, it comes into contact with cutaneous mast cells. Binding of the allergen occurs if the patient's mast cells are coated with IgE to the specific allergen. If both IgE and allergen are present in sufficient quantities, adjacent allergen-specific IgE molecules become cross-linked on the mast cell surface and trigger mast cell degranulation.

The clinical result is a transient 'wheal-and-flare' reaction consisting of a localized central area of skin edema (wheal) surrounded by erythema (flare). This pruritic reaction represents the immediate phase of the allergic reaction.

Skin testing is useful in the diagnosis of a variety of allergic disorders that involve IgE-mediated immediate reactions, including allergic rhinitis, allergic conjunctivitis, allergic asthma, food allergy, venom allergy, latex allergy and to a limited extent, drug allergy (Bernstein et al. 2008).

Skin testing vs. in vitro testing

The presence of specific IgE antibodies can be determined by either allergen skin testing or *in vitro* tests. Both skin tests and *in vitro* tests can be performed with standardized and stable materials. The advantage of skin testing is that it is more rapid, sensitive and cost-effective. Furthermore, extracts for skin testing can be made from a wide variety of allergenic inhalants, foods and medications, whereas commercial *in vitro* tests are available for a more limited number of allergens. On the other hand, skin testing can be influenced by medications and the results may be challenging to interpret in the presence of dermatographia or extensive dermatitis.

Procedure

There are several published practice parameters for allergen skin testing. Skin testing for the diagnosis of immediate hypersensitivity is performed by one of two methods: percutaneous (prick/puncture) or intradermal. Both methods yield similar information. The intradermal method is more sensitive and reproducible, whereas the percutaneous method is more rapidly performed, less painful and associated with fewer systemic reactions. Consequently, percutaneous testing is usually the preferred initial procedure.

To prepare for skin prick testing, you will need to assemble a tray of antigens for testing purposes. There are commercially available products with wells that can be filled with antigens. An alternative is small dropper bottles that can be used to apply the antigen to the patient's skin. The testing procedure will be most efficient if the tray is arranged in such a way that the bottles of antigen stay in the correct order. This will allow the technician to anticipate the order of the bottles and quickly find the antigen.

The number of skin tests and the allergens selected should be based on the patient's age and clinical history, and should take into consideration local aerobiologic data and pollen cross-allergenicity. The indiscriminate use of a large number of skin tests is cost-inefficient and strongly discouraged.

Prior to skin testing, assess whether the patient has inadvertently taken medications that may suppress wheal-and-flare responses. In the affirmative, one can check a histamine control and still proceed with skin testing if it is adequately positive. A list of common medications and their recommended withhold periods is found in Table 17.3.

The first step is to gather supplies and prepare the patient. Skin testing can be performed on the patient's upper back or the volar surface of the forearm. The back is generally preferred because it is more reactive than the forearm and offers a greater surface area to work with. Skin testing should not be performed in areas of active dermatitis or if dermatographia is present.

Begin by cleaning the skin with an alcohol wipe and allowing the area to dry. Using a washable marker, designate the areas for each antigen. This can be done in a code that is standardized for your clinic. For example, the code may be the first letter of the antigen in a standardized order. For a group of similar antigens such as molds, an 'M' can be put above a series of dots or numbers to keep track of the antigen to be placed in the designated area. Rows of antigens should be at least 2 inches apart and 2 inches lateral from the spine.

Prior to skin testing, a positive and a negative control should be placed. Some offices choose to check the controls prior to skin testing, whereas others perform allergen testing concurrently with the controls. For the positive control, a 10 mg/mL histamine dihydrochloride control is placed on the skin and pricked with a needle. The positive histamine control must have a wheal ≥ 3 mm surrounded by erythema for it to be considered valid. A 50% glycerinated human serum albumin–saline solution is generally used for the negative control.

Place a small drop of each antigen on the patient's skin. Using a small needle, lightly prick the skin at a 45 to 60-degree angle. The skin is then gently lifted, creating a small break in the epidermis through

Table 17.3. Recommended withhold period prior to skin prick testing.

Medication	Recommended Withhold Period
First-generation H_1-blockers	2–3 days
Second-generation H_1-blockers	3–5 days
H_2-blockers	0–2 days
Tricyclic antidepressants	5–7 days
Benzodiazepines	5–7 days
Atypical antidepressants/sedatives	
Mirtazapine	5–7 days
Quetiapine	5–7 days
Bupropion	0–3 days
Eszopiclone	0–3 days
Trazodone	0–3 days
Zolpidem	0–3 days
Topical corticosteroids (at site of skin testing)	2–3 weeks

Source: Shah et al. 2010

which the allergen solution penetrates. The prick does not need to be deep and should not cause bleeding. To avoid cross-contamination of the testing sites, the needle should be cleaned between pricks. This can be done by wiping the needle with a 2-inch ´2-inch gauze pad containing alcohol. Once all of the antigens have been placed and pricked, wait for 15 minutes before assessing reactivity.

To read the tests, use a small ruler with millimeter markings. Using a cotton ball, wipe off each antigen individually. The size of both the wheal and flare should be recorded. This method enables objective interpretation of the results and easier comparison among physicians. Moreover, specific cutoff levels may obviate the necessity for confirmatory challenge tests to certain foods. The old qualitative scoring (0 to 4) method is discouraged because of inter-physician variability. A positive skin test is defined as a wheal > 3 mm in diameter compared to the negative control, and accompanied by surrounding erythema.

After the tests have been read, thoroughly wipe the testing site. If desired by the patient, apply a topical corticosteroid or other anti-itch cream. An oral antihistamine can also be administered. Prepare the patient to see the physician by instructing him or her to get dressed.

The **Duotip-Test**, **Duotip-Test II**, **Unitest PC and Pick** devices come with wells that can be filled with antigen. The patient is prepared in the same manner as with the single needle except that the testing device will already have antigen on it, and the prick will cause that antigen to be introduced to the skin.

If using a **Multi-Test, Multi-Test II, Multi-Test PC, Skintestor-OMNI, QUINTEST** or **ComforTen** skin test system, the procedure is very similar. After cleaning the skin, the antigen-loaded testing device is placed on the patient's back. Use a slight rocking motion to ensure that each antigen has penetrated the skin. On removal of the device, the pattern of the device should be seen. The device is then discarded in a sharps disposal container. After 15 minutes, the test results are measured and recorded in the same manner as described earlier.

Technician Training. To ensure quality control, it is suggested that skin test proficiency be periodically assessed. The target Coefficient Variation (CV) should be less than 30%. The reader is referred to Table 3 of the Allergy Diagnostic Testing Practice Parameter (Bernstein et al. 2008) for more details.

Equipment. Equipment needed to perform skin prick testing will vary depending on the device chosen. In addition, you will need to determine what antigens you will be testing after carefully considering your geographic location.

Cotton balls or 2-inch´2-inch pads, alcohol wipes and a marker are also required. It is also necessary to have the appropriate emergency medications on hand in the rare event of a systemic reaction. You will also need a refrigerator to store the antigens when not in use.

Documentation. Results of skin prick testing must be appropriately documented in the patient's medical record. Office-specific information, such as location and the antigens that you commonly use, can be added to the template.

Intradermal testing

Intradermal (ID) tests are generally done when increased sensitivity is needed (i.e., when the prick test is negative despite a very convincing history). In addition, sensitivity to low-potency allergenic extracts may best be evaluated by this method. ID tests are especially useful in the diagnosis of drug and venom sensitivity. However, because of very high false-positive rates and potential risks for anaphylaxis, ID testing to foods is not recommended (Boyce et al. 2010).

Procedure. ID testing is performed by injecting a small amount of diluted antigen into the intradermal space. ID testing should be performed using disposable 0.5 or 1.0 mL syringes. Begin by cleaning the forearms and marking the testing locations. Always wear gloves while performing ID testing. To perform an ID test, hold the skin taut. With the bevel of the needle up, insert the needle almost parallel to the skin. When the bevel is just into the skin, inject 0.02–0.05 mL of diluted antigen, forming a small wheal on the skin. Both positive and negative controls should also be placed. The tests are read 15–20 minutes after injection, and both wheal and flare (in millimeters) should be recorded.

Unlike the interpretation of skin prick tests, there is no consensus as to what constitutes a positive intradermal test. Most allergists, however, use the criterion of 3 mm above the negative control as a threshold for a positive ID test result.

After the tests have been read, thoroughly wipe the testing site. If desired by the patient, apply a topical steroid or other anti-itch cream. An oral antihistamine can also be administered. Prepare the patient to see the physician by instructing him or her to get dressed.

Technician Training. All considerations for skin prick testing also apply to ID testing. It is important that the technician be well trained in the correct technique so that antigens are not accidentally injected into the subcutaneous tissue or muscle.

Equipment. An ID testing tray should be available. The antigens used for ID testing should be 500- to 1000-fold more dilute than the concentration used for prick testing. The histamine control dilution should be 0.1 mg/mL. The technician should always wear gloves to minimize the risk of contact with body fluids. Emergency medications should be readily available, as systemic reactions are more common with ID tests.

Documentation. Results of ID testing should be documented on the allergy testing record and placed in the patient's medical record.

Local anesthetic testing

Most adverse reactions to local anesthetics are not due to IgE-mediated mechanisms but rather nonallergic factors such as vasovagal responses, anxiety or toxic reactions related to epinephrine. Nonetheless, to exclude the rare possibility of an IgE-mediated reaction to local anesthetics, skin testing and graded challenge can be performed in patients with a convincing history (Trautmann et al. 2018).

Local anesthetics are divided into two groups based upon their chemical structure:

- [?] Group I: The benzoic acid ester agents, which include benzocaine, procaine and tetracaine
- [?] Group II: The amide agents, which include bupivacaine, lidocaine and mepivacaine

There is evidence for cross-reactivity among group II agents and a lack of cross-reactivity between group I and II agents.

Procedure. Skin prick tests are first performed with the undiluted anesthetic. The anesthetic should not contain epinephrine to avoid vasoconstriction. If the result is negative, successive subcutaneous injections of 0.1 mL at 1:100, 1:10 and full-strength solutions are given at 15 minute intervals. If no reactions are encountered, 0.5 to 1 mL of full-strength anesthetic is injected subcutaneously.

Penicillin testing

Skin testing is the most rapid, sensitive, and cost-effective testing modality for evaluating both adults and children with suspected penicillin allergy (Fox and Park 2014). However, it has no role in the diagnosis of exfoliative skin reactions, such as Stevens-Johnson syndrome or toxic epidermal necrolysis.

Procedure. Penicillin skin testing involves at least two steps. Skin prick test should be performed first, and, if negative, intradermal tests should follow. Skin testing should not be performed for at least four weeks following anaphylaxis to allow enough time for the cutaneous mast cell population to replenish.

Penicillin skin testing is performed with the following reagents:

- The major determinant: penicilloyl-polylysine (Pre-Pen)
- The minor determinant: penicillin G (10,000 units/mL)
- Ampicillin (2.5 mg/mL) and/or amoxicillin (3 mg/mL) if relevant to the patient's situation

Aminopenicillins, such as amoxicillin and ampicillin, should be included in patients who report an immediate systemic reaction to these drugs. These patients can form IgE antibodies to the R-group side chain rather than the penicilloyl determinant. Therefore, they would not necessarily react to Pre-Pen or penicillin G.

Each test solution may be applied single or in duplicate. However, if a single intradermal test result is equivocal, it should be repeated in duplicate. Furthermore, both a positive and negative control should be applied to verify that the patient's skin is normally responsive.

Interpretation of results

Skin prick tests are read 15 minutes after application.

- A positive response is a wheal that is 3 mm or greater in mean diameter than the negative control.
- A negative response is no reaction at the prick site or erythema alone without a wheal.

Intradermal skin tests are read 15–20 minutes after application:

- A positive response is a wheal that has increased in size from the original bleb and is 3 mm or greater in mean diameter than the negative control.
- A negative response is no increase in the size of the original bleb and no wheal greater than the control site.

Confirmatory challenge

The negative predictive value for penicillin skin testing with a combination of Pre-Pen and penicillin G is high, but not 100%. For this reason, negative testing should be confirmed by an oral challenge followed by a two-hour observational period. If possible, the patient should be challenged to the same specific penicillin to which he or she reacted. For inpatients with a current need for a particular penicillin product, the challenge procedure can be incorporated into the first parenteral dose by administering one-tenth the normal dose, observing for one hour then if there is no adverse reaction, administering the remaining nine-tenths of the dose and observing for another hour.

Hymenoptera venom testing

Patients older than 16 years of age who have experienced a systemic reaction to a suspected hymenoptera insect should be venom tested, as they are potential candidates for venom immunotherapy (Golden et al. 2017). This includes older adults in whom the stinging event and systemic reaction occurred decades earlier, because the risk of another reaction can persist. On the other hand, skin testing is generally not indicated in patients younger than 16 years of age who have had systemic reactions limited to the skin (i.e. urticaria/angioedema), as these patients have only a 10% chance of a future systemic reaction.

Timing of testing

If the sting event was recent, wait at least four weeks before skin testing to allow enough time for the cutaneous mast cell population to replenish.

Choice of venoms

In the United States, purified, standardized venom extracts exist for honeybee, yellow jacket, yellow hornet, white-faced hornet and wasp. Due to the difficulty in correctly identifying the insect that caused the sting, testing is generally performed with all five venoms. In addition, clinicians in areas inhabited by imported red fire ants should consider fire ant venom testing.

Procedure. In patients who have experienced severe anaphylaxis, start with a skin prick test at a concentration of 0.1 mg/ml. Otherwise, proceed directly to intradermal testing. The recommended starting concentration is either 0.001 or 0.01 mg/ml (depending on the likelihood of a positive test). The concentration is subsequently increased by 10-fold increments until a positive skin test response occurs or a maximum concentration of 1.0 mg/mL is reached.

For imported red fire ant venom testing, whole-body extract is used, available as 1:10 weight/volume stock solution. Start with a skin prick test at a concentration of 1:100 w/v, followed by intradermal testing at a concentration of 1:1,000,000 w/v. The concentration is then increased in 10-fold increments until a positive skin test response occurs or a maximum concentration of 1:500 or 1:1000 w/v is reached.

Patch testing

Patch testing is the gold standard for identification of a contact allergen. Although many contact allergens have been identified and reported, fewer than 40 allergens are responsible for the majority of cases of allergic contact dermatitis. The T.R.U.E. TEST® is an FDA-approved test to screen for contactant allergens. The test is preloaded with 35 common contactants and a negative vehicle control. In certain situations, supplementary patch test series may be required based on specific occupations (e.g., hairdressers, machinists) or exposures (e.g., shoes, plants, photoallergens).

Procedure. Before patch testing, verify that the skin site where the patch tests will be placed has been free of topical corticosteroids and calcineurin inhibitors (tacrolimus or pimecrolimus) for at least 7 days prior to testing. Also, note that oral corticosteroids in moderate doses (> 20 mg/d of prednisone or its equivalent) may result in diminished reactivity, although lower doses are generally safe. Oral antihistamines and leukotriene modifiers do not interfere with patch test reactivity. Patch testing a patient with significant atopic dermatitis can result in an 'angry back' reaction, resulting in a false-positive reading.

The T.R.U.E. TEST is composed of three panels. Peel open the foil sleeve and remove the first test panel from its protective plastic cover, being careful not to touch the test substances. Position the panel on the patient's upper back, approximately 2.5 cm lateral to the mid-spine. Select an area that is rash-free. The panel should be smoothed out from the center to ensure that each of the allergen windows is in contact with the skin. While the panel is in place, a marker can be used to mark the test location at the notches found on the panel. Repeat the above steps for the second and third panels. Once completed, secure the edges of the panels with adhesive tape to ensure that they remain firmly on the patient's back. Instruct the patient to keep the back dry until the patches are removed. Showering, bathing (except for sponge baths) and swimming should be avoided. If any of the patches begins to peel loose, ask the patient to reinforce them with adhesive tape.

Patch tests should be kept in place for 48 hours, then removed for interpretation. After the first reading (at 48 hours), an additional reading at 72–96 hours is recommended to reduce false-positives (i.e., positive at first reading but negative at second reading) and false negatives (i.e., negative at first reading but positive at second reading). Approximately 30% of relevant allergens that are negative at the 48 hour reading become positive at 72–96 hours. Conversely, irritant reactions at 48 hours tend to disappear by 72–96 hours. For weak sensitizers such as neomycin or *p*-phenylenediamine, additional readings at 5–7 days may be necessary.

Interpretation. Tests may need to be read 30 minutes after removal of the patches to allow resolution of erythema due to occluding pressure. Interpret reactions using the descriptive scale developed and validated by the International Contact Dermatitis Research Group (Table 17.4).

With positive reactions of clinical relevance, counsel patients on avoidance. A patient education handout on each contactant is available from the manufacturer.

Table 17.4. Descriptive interpretation scale recommended by the International Contact Dermatitis Research Group, visual key, instruction sheet for patients, and standard patch test record from.

No.	Grade	Meaning/appearance	Clinical relevance*
1	-	Negative reaction	Excludes ACD. If ACD is still suspected, recheck technique or do ROAT.
2	R	Irritant reaction	Controls show similar response or these was an excited skin response.
3	± + or ?	Doubtful reaction	Negative test result. Repea treadings at 3, 4 and 7 days after patch removed. If ACD still suspected, recheck technique or do ROAT.
4	1+	Light erythema, nonvesicular	Equivocal test result. Could either be negative or indicative of waning prior sensitization. False-positive test result or excited skin syndrome must be ruled out by test in control subject. Repeat steps in 3.
5	2+	Edema, erythema, discrete vesicles	Positive test result. Indicative of prior or current sensitization. Should correlate with history and physical finding. False-positive test result or excited skin syndrome must be ruled out by test in control subject.
6	3+	Coalescing vesiculobullous papules	Strongly positive result. Same condition in 5 apply.

Abbreviations: ACD, allergic contact dermatitis; ROAT, repeat open application test.
− Negative reaction; ?+ Doubtful reaction; faint erythema only; + Weak positive reaction; non-vesicular erythema, infiltration, possibly papules; ++ Strong positive reaction; vesicular erythema, infiltration, papules; +++ Extreme positive reaction; intense erythema and infiltration and coalescing vesicles; IR Irritant reaction; NT Not tested
* Clinical relevance is based on the Joint Task Force's appraisal of current literature.
Source: Wilkinson et al. 1970

Atopy patch testing

Atopy Patch Testing (APT) is a variant of traditional patch testing used for the diagnosis of non-IgE cell-mediated immune responses. In the United States, it has been used primarily as an adjuvant to skin prick tests in the investigation of food sensitivities associated with eosinophilic esophagitis. However, the lack of standardized test materials and methodology is an important limitation. Reimbursement by insurance may also be problematic, as most carriers consider it to be investigational.

Procedure. APTs for foods are usually prepared with 2 g of dried foods mixed with 2 mL of isotonic saline. The mixtures are placed in 8 or 12 mm Finn Chambers® mounted on Scanpor® tape, and placed on the patient's back. Undiluted samples of commercially prepared single-ingredient foods may be placed directly in the Finn Chambers. The patches are removed at 48 hours but interpreted at 72 hours.

Allergen immunotherapy

Allergen immunotherapy is a cornerstone of the allergist's practice. The focus here will be on subcutaneous allergen immunotherapy. Although an increasing number of studies have demonstrated the efficacy of sublingual immunotherapy (SLIT), FDA-approved products are limited to only three antigens: dust mite, grass pollen and ragweed. Therefore, SLIT will not be discussed. Similarly, oral immunotherapy (OIT) for food allergy is considered investigational at this juncture, and will not be discussed either.

Subcutaneous allergen immunotherapy is a method of employing subcutaneous injections of gradually increasing doses of antigenic materials for the purpose of inducing immune tolerance in allergic patients. This chapter will focus on immunotherapy administration. The principles behind allergen immunotherapy and the preparation of allergen extract are discussed in Chapter 15.

Procedures

Injection Procedure. The medical assistant completes the following steps when administering immunotherapy:

1. The patient shot record is compared with the check-in slip to verify full name and date of birth.
2. The date of last immunotherapy injection is noted. If it does not fall within the normal dosing schedule, a dose adjustment is made according to a standing order protocol.
3. The patient is questioned about any previous large local or systemic reaction. The patient is also asked about potential contraindications, particularly poorly controlled asthma, recent start of a β-blocker and pregnancy.
4. The dose to be given is documented in the shot record. If more than one injection is to be administered, perform each step individually, as all vials may not be at the same dose level.
5. The proper vials for the patient are retrieved. Care should be taken to ensure that the correct vials are administered to the correct patient. Double-check labels to ensure patient safety.
6. Draw up the serum as documented in the chart. Take your time.
7. Call the patient by his/her complete name and re-verify his/her identity.
8. The injection is given subcutaneously at a 45- or 90-degree angle in the upper arm. Prior to injecting, ensure that you aspirate for blood. If blood appears, the needle is in a vein. Remove the needle immediately without giving the shot. Discard the needle and serum into a sharps container and begin the process of drawing up a new dose.
9. The patient should be observed in the waiting area for at least 30 minutes.

Post-injection Care. All patients are to wait for at least 30 minutes after their injection(s). In high-risk patients, the wait time can be extended at the physician's discretion. The patient may choose to place ice packs over the injection site(s) if susceptible to large local reactions. If the patient does not wait, document it in the patient's chart and follow your clinic's procedures. Most clinics elect to issue a warning for the first offence but discontinue immunotherapy after the second or third offence. Bear in mind that the physician is ultimately liable for any immunotherapy-related adverse reactions that may occur.

After the patient's designated waiting period, check the arms for any local reaction. Document the size of any induration or erythema. Large local reactions are not predictive of systemic reactions, and can usually be prevented by pretreatment with oral antihistamines and application of ice. Nonetheless, some physicians prefer to reduce the dose. In such case, the treating physician should formulate an easy-to-follow dose-adjustment protocol.

Treatment of Large Local Reactions. For local reactions that are 2.5–3 cm in size, apply ice and have the patient wait an additional 5 minutes. For a reaction > 3 cm, apply ice and administer an additional antihistamine. Oral corticosteroids are generally not necessary.

Treatment of Systemic Reactions. The diagnosis and treatment of anaphylaxis is beyond the scope of this chapter, and so will be discussed only briefly. For a more detailed discussion, please refer to the Practice Parameter on the diagnosis and management of anaphylaxis (Lieberman et al. 2015).

Systemic reaction protocol

1. Notify the physician immediately, and transfer the patient to an examination room if safe to do so.

2. In some clinics, the clinical staff may be authorized to administer epinephrine even before the patient is seen by the physician. In other clinics, the protocol calls for epinephrine to be drawn up but not administered. Note that antihistamines and corticosteroids are secondary medications that should never replace epinephrine in the treatment of anaphylaxis.
3. Assess airway, breathing, circulation and mental status. Record vital signs, including O_2 saturation on an emergency flow sheet.
4. Place the patient in a supine position and elevate the lower extremities, particularly when there is concern for hemodynamic compromise.
5. Administer oxygen. Titrate to keep O_2 saturation > 92%.
6. Administer an IV saline bolus in patients who remain hypotensive in spite of epinephrine.
7. For patients who develop bronchospasm, administer nebulized beta-$_2$ agonists.
8. If the patient's condition does not improve in spite of administration of an adequate dose of epinephrine, consider prompt transfer to the emergency department.
9. Once the patient has stabilized, antihistamines and corticosteroids can be administered as ancillary measures.
10. Inform the treating allergist of the systemic reaction, and note the dose adjustment in the shot chart.
11. Patients with systemic reactions should carry an epinephrine auto-injector. The auto-injector is also useful for delayed systemic reactions that have occurred after the patient has left the physician's office.

Technician Training. Staff who administer allergen immunotherapy must be thoroughly trained to recognize the symptoms of anaphylaxis, particularly in children, who may not be able to verbalize symptoms. Staff should regularly run mock drills simulating shot reactions, and should possess at least Basic Life Support certification.

Immunotherapy dosing schedule. Allergy injections are conventionally given once or twice a week during the build-up phase. Once a patient reaches a maintenance dose, the interval between injections can be progressively increased, as tolerated, up to an interval of 4 weeks for inhalant allergens and up to eight weeks for venom. Accelerated schedules such as cluster or rush immunotherapy, where several sets of injections are administered per visit, allow patients to achieve a maintenance dose much more rapidly. In the case of rush, the risk of both local and systemic reactions is greatly increased. Pre-medication is strongly recommended, and patients should remain in the office for a longer period after their injections (up to 3 hours).

Although there is no published evidence to support modification of immunotherapy doses due to treatment gaps during the build-up or maintenance phases, it is customary to reduce the dose when the interval between injections is prolonged. One suggestion is to reduce the previous dose by 25%, 14–21 days after the missed scheduled injection and by 50%, 21–28 days after the missed scheduled injection (Cox et al. 2011). A similar dose-reduction protocol may be used for gaps in maintenance immunotherapy.

As mentioned earlier, large local reactions are not predictive of subsequent systemic reactions. However, some allergists feel more comfortable decreasing the dose. Similarly, some allergists reduce the dose during high-pollen season, although several published studies have not found an association between pollen counts and systemic reactions. Finally, some authorities advocate reducing the dose when starting a patient on a new maintenance vial.

A pregnant patient may continue allergen immunotherapy, but her dose should not be increased until after delivery because of fetal risk in the event of a systemic reaction. If a pregnant patient's dose is decreased for any reason (e.g., new vial, large local reaction), her dose should be held at the decreased level until after delivery.

Contra-indications. The staff should be aware of certain situations that would dictate withholding immunotherapy. In particular, an asthmatic patient whose asthma is poorly controlled should not receive their allergy injection due to a high risk of a severe bronchoconstrictive reaction. For this reason, some allergists advocate measuring peak expiratory flow readings in all asthmatics and withholding injections if the reading is less than 70% of that predicted. Additional situations that dictate withholding immunotherapy include a patient who is experiencing fever or is acutely ill; is unable to wait for the entire waiting period; has skipped prior waiting periods; appears intoxicated or impaired; or has recently started beta-blocker therapy without the allergist's prior knowledge.

Equipment. The equipment necessary to perform immunotherapy includes syringes, cotton balls, alcohol prep pads, individualized allergen extracts, emergency equipment including epinephrine, oxygen, nebulizer machine, IV saline and an Automated External Defibrillator (AED). An easy-to-understand written anaphylaxis protocol that has been thoroughly reviewed and practiced with the staff is of critical importance.

Documentation. Prior to initiating allergen immunotherapy, patients should be informed of the clinic's immunotherapy procedures, including the mandatory 30-minute wait time. Asthmatic patients in particular should be reminded not to discontinue their maintenance asthma medications without their physician's permission and to defer immunotherapy if their asthma is not well controlled. Potential adverse reactions, including both local and systemic reactions, should be reviewed. All patients should sign an informed consent form prior to receiving their first injection. If the clinic's protocol requires carrying an epinephrine auto-injector, a prescription should be given to the patient with a reminder to carry it each time the patient comes in for an allergy injection.

Oral food challenge

An oral food challenge provides the most definitive means to diagnose a food allergy. It is used to identify, confirm or rule out a suspected food allergy, and may prevent unnecessary food restrictions (Boyce et al. 2010). An oral food challenge in the outpatient setting should only be performed if the benefit to the patient of a negative result is greater than the risk of the testing, and only if previous skin prick or *in vitro* tests have concluded a high probability of a negative result. The Food Allergy & Anaphylaxis Network has published *A Health Professional's Guide to Food Challenges*, which provides detailed information on conducting oral food challenges (Mofidi and Bock 2004).

Procedure. Testing can be an open, single-blind or double-blind challenge. Open challenges are the simplest to perform and the less time-consuming. They are ideal for situations where multiple foods are in question. However, as open challenges are prone to patient bias, positive results must be viewed with caution. Foods that result in symptoms should be further investigated in a blinded controlled challenge.

As opposed to an open challenge, the single-blind challenge helps eliminate patient bias. Single-blind challenges are technically easier to perform, because they do not involve an additional un-blinded participant to prepare the placebo and active doses. Single-blind challenges have more flexibility in design, such as the addition of multiple initial placebo doses. This can be particularly helpful in patients in whom reactions are not causally related to foods.

The double-blind placebo-controlled food challenge remains the gold standard for the diagnosis of food allergy. Although the single-blind challenge helps eliminate patient bias, the individual performing the food challenge has the potential to be biased in the interpretation of the results. Nevertheless, double-blind placebo-controlled food challenges are usually not necessary in most clinical situations.

Food challenges may be performed in the office, hospital or in rare circumstances, at home. The setting is dependent on the patient's history and likelihood of a positive challenge.

An oral food challenge may be considered after a negative skin prick test to the suspected food or low food-specific IgE antibodies. Foods that are identified by positive IgE tests with no clinical history of reactivity or those that are unlikely to provoke a reaction, may be screened with open food challenges.

A standardized food challenge procedure has been proposed (Perry et al. 2004). The challenge is performed over a 90-minute period. The total amount of food protein to be administered is 4 g for children ≤ 4 years of age and 8 g for those ≥ 5 years of age. Doses are administered at 15-minute intervals. The amount of food is increased with each dose, beginning with 5% of the total dose and increasing by

5% increments with each subsequent dose, with the final two doses being 25% of the total amount to administer (see Table 17.5).

Sicherer described a similar procedure for oral food challenge (Sicherer 1999). In his procedure, 8–10 g of dry food or 100 mL of wet food are administered on an incremental basis, with a doubling of the amount over 10–15 minutes for a total of 90 minutes. Details on how to prepare an oral food challenge, including challenge substances, placebos and vehicles, are given in the above-referenced article on oral food challenges.

Technician Training. Technicians who are assisting with the oral food challenge should be well versed in recognizing and treating anaphylaxis. At the first symptoms of an IgE-mediated reaction, the challenge should be immediately stopped and appropriate treatment should be given. Symptoms to watch for include hives, flushing, cough, difficulty in breathing and vomiting. A physician should be present during the entire procedure.

Emergency medications and supplies should be readily available prior to beginning the challenge. The following is a sample listing of medication and supplies to have on hand:

- Epinephrine solution 1:1000
- Normal saline
- Diphenhydramine
- Albuterol sulfate
- Nebulizer machine
- Methylprednisolone sodium succinate
- Prednisolone sodium phosphate
- Glucagon
- Dopamine
- Oxygen
- Large-bore catheter
- Peak flow meter
- Pulse oximeter
- Sphygmomanometer
- Automated External Defibrillator (AED)

Any patient considered at high risk for anaphylaxis should be challenged in the inpatient setting (hospital or even ICU) where highly-skilled personnel are available to promptly intervene in case of a life-threatening situation.

Table 17.5. Oral food challenge procedure.

Example: Total of 8 grams to administer	
5%	0.4 g
10%	0.8 g
15%	1.2 g
20%	1.6 g
25%	2.0 g
25%	2.0 g
Total	8.0 g

Source: Perry et al. 2004

Documentation. The oral food challenge should be documented in the patient's medical record, along with the reason for performing the challenge. The details of the challenge, including the time and amount of each dose and any reactions that are observed, should be fully documented. All patients should sign an informed consent form prior to the challenge.

Aspirin desensitization

Aspirin desensitization is indicated for patients who have Aspirin-Exacerbated Respiratory Disease (AERD) and whose asthma and/or rhinosinusitis is sub optimally controlled (Solensky et al. 2010). It is also indicated for cardiac patients who require aspirin for antiplatelet therapy. Additionally, aspirin desensitization may be offered to individuals without AERD but with a history of urticaria/ angioedema to aspirin or NSAIDs. However, it is generally not given to patients who have experienced systemic reactions. Similar to other drug desensitizations, tolerance is maintained only as long as aspirin is continuously taken. Loss of tolerance generally occurs in 2 to 4 days after discontinuation of therapy.

Reactions to aspirin and NSAIDs can be categorized as either pseudo allergic or allergic. Pseudo allergic reactions are related to COX-1 inhibition and are elicited by aspirin and multiple NSAIDs. These

Table 17.6. Aspirin induction of drug tolerance scripps protocol.

Assessment and premedication (1–7 days before procedure)	$FEV_1 > 60\%$ predicted (> 1.5 L) Start or continue treatment with montelukast, 10 mg daily Start or continue treatment with inhaled corticosteroid and long-acting β-agonist Systemic steroid burst if low FEV_1 or bronchial instability
Protocol	
Time	Aspirin Dose
Day 1:0	30 mg
Day 1:3 hours	60 mg
Day 1:6 hours	100 mg
Day 2:0	150 mg
Day 2:3 hours	325 mg
Day 2:6 hours	650 mg
\multicolumn{2}{l}{Start intravenous catheter with heparin lock (keep in for 2–3 days)}	

Start intravenous catheter with heparin lock (keep in for 2–3 days)
FEV_1 and clinical assessment every hour and with symptoms.
Reactions typically occur with a provoking dose of 20–101 mg. Treat with medications described below. Chance of reaction to repeated threshold dose is small, but if occurs, repeat dose until reactions cease and then proceed.
After patient completely stabilized, provoking dose can be repeated (assuming another 3 hours of observation time), otherwise start with provoking dose on day 2.
If nasal, gastrointestinal, or cutaneous reactions occur on day 1, pretreat with histamine$_1$ and histamine$_2$ receptor antagonists for remainder of procedure.

Medication for treatment of aspirin-induced reactions	
Ocular	Topical antihistamines
Nasal	Antihistamine, topical decongestant
Laryngeal	Racemic epinephrine nebulization
Bronchial	β-Agonists
Gastrointestinal	Histamine$_2$-receptor antagonists
Urticaria/angioedema	Antihistamine
Hypotension	Epinephrine

Abbreviation: FEV1, forced expiratory volume in 1 second.
Source: Stevenson and Simon 2006

typically occur in patients with AERD or chronic urticaria. Allergic reactions, on the other hand, are IgE-mediated reactions that are elicited by either aspirin or a single NSAID.

Desensitization protocol for AERD

In general, patients are treated with increasing incremental doses of aspirin over set time intervals. After a positive response to aspirin and subsequent recovery, the dose at which the response occurred is repeated until no reaction occurs and the dose is increased until a maximum dose is reached. The most commonly cited protocol involves incremental oral administration of aspirin during 2-day course starting at 30 mg and finishing at 650 mg (Table 17.6).

Alternatively, the Joint Task Force recently published a shorter protocol (Macy et al. 2007) with a starting dose of 20.25 mg and a final dose of 325 mg (Table 17.7). Note that both protocols recommend starting a leukotriene modifier prior to desensitization to diminish the likelihood of lower

Table 17.7. Aspirin induction of drug tolerance joint task force recommendations.

Assessment and premedication within 1 week before procedure	FEV_1 > 70% predicted Consider starting or continuing leukotriene modifier therapy Start or continue treatment with high-dose inhaled corticosteroid and long-acting β-agonist if poorly controlled asthma Systemic steroid burst if low FEV_1 or bronchial instability If receiving maintenance systemic steriod, consider doubling daily dose (if on alternate day steroids, change to daily dose)
Protocol	
Time	Aspirin Dose
0 min	20.25 mg
90 min	40.5 mg
180 min	81 mg
270 min	162.5 mg
360 min	325 mg

Document informed consent and advise patient it may take several days to complete (most will take 2 days).
Establish intravenous access.
FEV_1 and clinical assessment every 90 minutes and with symptoms.
Dosing interval may be extented to 3 hours based on individual patient characteristics.
Reactions will likely occur with early doses, usually 81 mg.
Treat reactions as indicated below.
After patient completely stabilized (but not less than 3 hours after the last dose), the provoking dose can be repeated. A persistent > 15 % decrease in FEV_1, with or without associated symptoms, lasting longer than 3 hours despite therapy, is an indication to discontinue the desensitization process for the day.
If nasal, gastrointestinal, or cutaneous reactions occur on day 1, pretreat with histamine$_1$ and histamine$_2$ receptor antagonists for remainder of procedure.

Medication for treatment of aspirin-induced reactions	
Ocular	Oral antihistamines
Nasal	Oral antihistamine, topical decongestant
Laryngeal	Racemic epinephrine nebulization and/or intramuscular epinephrine
Bronchial	β-Agonists
Urticaria/angioedema	Oral or intravenous antihistamine
Hypotension	Parenteral epinephrine

Abbreviation: FEV1, forced expiratory volume in 1 second.

* This recommended protocol is intended to be more practical, using doses based on commercially available 81 mg aspirin products and a shorter dosing interval. There are no data on safety and efficacy of this protocol.

Source: Macy et al. 2007

airway symptoms. Once patients are desensitized, continued daily administration of 325 to 650 mg of aspirin is recommended in order for patients to remain in a tolerant state. At that dose, universal cross-desensitization to all NSAIDs is also achieved.

Desensitization protocol for aspirin-induced urticaria/angioedema

Desensitization protocols for aspirin-induced urticaria/angioedema are typically shorter, but they start at a lower dose of aspirin. They are often used in patients in urgent need of aspirin in the context of an acute coronary syndrome or a coronary stent placement. An example of a protocol is highlighted in Table 17.8. Although their aggregate success rate exceeds 90%, no confirmatory challenge studies were ever performed to determine whether these patients were truly aspirin sensitive.

Nebulized aerosol treatments

Nebulized aerosol treatments are frequently given in the allergist's office to treat an acute asthma exacerbation. The choice of medication is up to the physician, and it is a good idea to keep a variety of nebulized medications in stock in your office.

Procedure. Begin by gathering the needed equipment. As with the administration of any medication, the staff should ensure that the right patient is being treated with the correct medication and dose. Nebulization is generally done with a compressor device, but if the patient is hypoxemic, nebulization can be performed with oxygen and a flowmeter.

To use the nebulizer with oxygen, connect the oxygen tubing to the nebulizer with a flowmeter in place. Place the ordered medication in the nebulizer cup, and set the oxygen rate to 4–6 L/min. If a portable compressor is used, attach the tubing to the cup and assemble as per the manufacturer's instructions. Continue nebulization for the prescribed time or until all of the medication has been given.

During nebulization, instruct the patient to sit upright and breathe deeply through the mouth at a normal rate. Care should be taken to prevent hyperventilation. The details of the treatment, along with any adverse reactions, should be recorded in the patient's chart.

Technician Training. The technician administering the treatment should be skilled at detecting adverse reactions to bronchodilators. The following adverse reactions may occur:

- **Increase in pulse rate.** Bronchodilators may cause a significant increase in pulse rate. In some clinics, pulse rates are checked regularly and treatment is discontinued if the pulse rate increases by

Table 17.8. Rapid aspirin desensitization protocol for patients with coronary artery disease requiring aspirin.

Time*	Aspirin dose, mg
0	0.1
15	0.3
30	1
45	3
60	10
75	20
90	40
105	81
120	162
135	325

* Dosing interval shown is 15 minutes but may dose every 20 minutes with premedication with oral antihistamine.
Source: Wong et al. 2000

50% from baseline. In such a case, note the reason for discontinuing aerosol therapy and notify the physician.
- **Chest pain.** If the patient complains of sudden chest pain during aerosol therapy, stop the treatment immediately, listen for bilateral breath sounds, monitor pulse for rate and regularity and report your findings to the physician.
- **Cardiac or respiratory arrest.** If the patient experiences cardiac or respiratory arrest during treatment, immediately call the physician, begin cardiopulmonary resuscitation and summon assistance to call 911.

Equipment. To perform nebulization in your office, you should have either oxygen with a flowmeter or a portable compressor. There are many choices of nebulizers, but if you plan to administer nebulized budesonide, ultrasonic nebulizers are not recommended. It is a good idea to have a variety of nebulized medications on hand so that you have a choice of what medication to use.

Documentation. Any nebulized treatment should be documented in the medical record. This includes the name of the medication, the route, the dose and the time given. In addition, any adverse reactions should be documented.

Rhinoscopy

Fiberoptic rhinopharyngolaryngoscopy (commonly known as rhinoscopy) is a procedure that is being increasingly performed in the allergist's office. The procedure is conducted with a rhinoscope, a device used to view anatomic structures in the nasal passages, sinuses, pharynx and larynx. The rhinoscope can be used in the diagnosis of diseases of the upper airway, including sinusitis, nasal polyps and vocal cord dysfunction. In the diagnosis of sinusitis, rhinoscopy has been shown to be more sensitive than sinus X-rays, but less so than a CT scan or MRI. On the other hand, in-office rhinoscopy is far less expensive compared to the latter. Moreover, it is useful in monitoring disease progression and response to therapy.

Procedure. Briefly explain to the patient the procedure and obtain written consent. Ensure that he or she is seated comfortably. The procedure will be performed most easily if the examination is done in a chair that has the capacity to adjust height and that has a headrest to stabilize the patient's head.

Administer a topical nasal decongestant (either 1% epinephrine or 1% ephedrine) via a nasal atomizer. Alternatively, an over-the-counter decongestant spray, such as oxymetazoline, can be administered using a nasal speculum to preserve sterility of the applicator. The patient should be warned that the decongestant solution may drip down the back of the throat and impart an unpleasant taste.

Administer topical anesthesia in the form of 4% lidocaine solution in a spray bottle or 4% viscous lidocaine on a sterile swab applied between the nasal septum and the middle and inferior nasal turbinates for 5 minutes. When using lidocaine, ensure that the administered dose is safe. The adult dosing for lidocaine is 0.3–1.5 mg/kg. Lidocaine solution is self-administered from a primed atomizer. Instruct the patient to sniff gently. Ideally, administer two sprays on each side and wait 1–2 minutes. Assess the patient for numbness, then repeat administration until the patient is sufficiently numb or the maximum dosage is reached. Viscous lidocaine can be added to the tip of the scope as an adjuvant to the anesthesia and to lubricate the insertion. If using lidocaine, instruct the patient not to have any food or drink for 1 hour afterward to reduce the risk of aspiration resulting from numbness.

The physician should stand in front of the patient and look directly into the eyepiece if a camera is not attached to the scope. If the scope has video capability, ensure that the monitor is in a position that allows for comfortable viewing by the physician. The chair should be positioned so that the patient is eye-to-eye.

When choosing a method for performing rhinoscopy, some find it helpful to always scope the most patent nare first, whereas others always start with their preference of the left or right nare. Ensure that the light source or battery attachment on the scope is in the 'on' position and adjusted to the appropriate brightness. Ensure that the optical focus is adjusted properly. If the angulation control has a locking mechanism, ensure that the lock is disengaged so that the scope moves freely. Use the minimum illumination necessary for adequate viewing to avoid mucosal burns to the patient, as the distal end of the endoscope may get hot.

Systematically insert the scope to view the anatomic features. While inserting the scope, instruct the patient to open his or her mouth and breathe. Warming the tip of the scope with warm water prior to insertion can help prevent fogging of the view. In patients with suspected sinusitis, care should be taken around the osteomeatal complex, as this area can be quite painful when touched with the distal end of the scope.

If assessing the patient for vocal cord dysfunction, the procedure above can be combined with the exercise challenge procedure to view the vocal cords after exercise. Patient preparation steps should be completed prior to exercise so that the scope can be inserted immediately following the challenge. When the true vocal cords are viewed, the patient should be instructed to perform high- and low-pitch phonation, normal respiration and forced expiration to induce paradoxical vocal fold motion. Davis, Brugman and Larsen performed a combination exercise and laryngoscopy procedure with video recording. The video clips can be seen by viewing their article online (Davis et al. 2007).

After the procedure, the scope should be cleaned with soap and water and sterilized with either ethylene oxide or 2–3% glutaraldehyde solution. Use care to follow the manufacturer's recommended cleaning and sterilization procedures, as a stronger solution may harm the scope.

Equipment. Several manufacturers produce high-quality rhinoscopes. Prior to purchasing a scope, be sure that the desired functionality is present. Consider whether you will want multiple light sources of varying intensity, video capability and comfort for the subject based on scope diameter. Light sources may be incorporated or provided in a separate unit. Both flexible and rigid scopes are available. Although a rigid scope allows visualization of airway areas that are not accessible with a flexible scope, the procedure is significantly less comfortable for the patient. The serviceability of the scope is another consideration prior to purchasing your equipment, as the scope may become damaged and need repair.

Documentation. Documentation in the medical record should include the indication for rhinoscopy, patient consent, pre-procedure and post-procedure diagnosis, list of medications used, significant findings on examination and the patient's tolerance of the procedure.

Acknowledgment

This chapter is adapted from Chapter 8 of the AAAAI Practice Management Resource Guide (2014). The author would like to acknowledge and thank the AAAAI for permission to use its content for this book chapter.

Conclusion

In summary, the accurate diagnosis and management of allergic disorders is largely dependent on a handful of office tests and procedures. It is therefore vital for both the allergist and clinical staff to continuously practice these skills in order to maintain proficiency.

References

Bernstein IL, Li JT, Bernstein DI, Hamilton R, Spector SL, Tan R, et al. Allergy diagnostic testing: An updated practice parameter. Ann Allergy Asthma Immunol 2008; 100: S1–S148.

Boyce JA, Assa'ad A, Burks AW, Jones SM, Sampson HA, Wood RA, et al. Guidelines for the diagnosis and management of food allergy in the United States: Report of the NIAID-sponsored expert panel. J Allergy Clin Immunol 2010; 126: S1–S58.

Cox L, Nelson H, Lockey R, Calabria C, Chacko T, Finegold I, et al. Allergen immunotherapy: A practice parameter third update. J Allergy Clin Immunol 2011; 127: S1–S55.

Crapo RO, Casaburi R, Coates AL, Enright PL, Hankinson JL, Irvin CG, et al. Guidelines for methacholine and exercise challenge testing-1999. Am J Respir Crit Care Med 2000; 161: 309–29.

Davis R, Brugman S, Larsen G. Use of videography in the diagnosis of exercise-induced vocal cord dysfunction: A case report with video clips. J Allergy Clin Immunol 2007; 119: 1329–1331.

Dweik RA, Boggs PB, Erzurum SC, Irvin CG, Leigh MW, Lundberg JO, et al. American Thoracic Society Committee on interpretation of exhaled nitric oxide levels (FENO) for clinical applications. Am J Respir Crit Care Med 2011; 184: 602–615.

Fox SJ, Park MA. Penicillin skin testing is a safe and effective tool for evaluating penicillin allergy in the pediatric population. J Allergy Clin Immunol Pract 2014; 4: 439–44.

Golden DB, Demain J, Freeman T, Graft D, Tankersley M, Tracy J, et al. Stinging insect hypersensitivity: A practice parameter update 2016. Ann Allergy Asthma Immunol 2017; 118: 28–54.

Lieberman P, Nicklas R, Randolph C, Oppenheimer J, Bernstein D, Bernstein J, et al. Anaphylaxis—a practice parameter update. Ann Allergy Asthma Immunol 2015; 115: 341–84.

Macy E, Bernstein JA, Castells MC, Gawchik SM, Lee TH, Settipane RA, et al. Aspirin challenge and desensitization for aspirin-exacerbated respiratory disease: a practice paper. Ann Allergy Asthma Immunol 2007; 98: 172–174.

Miller MR, Crapo R, Hankinson J, Brusasco V, Burgos F, Casaburi R, et al. General considerations for lung function testing. Eur Respir J 2005a; 26: 153–161.

Miller MR, Hankinson J, Brusasco V, Burgos F, Casaburi R, Coates A, et al. Mofidi, S. and Bock Standardisation of Spirometry. Eur Respir J 2005b; 26: 319–338.

Mofidi S, Bock SA. A Health Professional's Guide to Food Challenges. Fairfax, VA: The Food Allergy and Anaphylaxis Network 2004.

National Heart, Lung, and Blood Institute. 2007. National Asthma Education and Prevention Program, Third Expert Panel on the Diagnosis and Management of Asthma. Expert Panel Report 3: Guidelines for the Diagnosis and Management of Asthma. Available from https://www.ncbi.nlm.nih.gov/books/NBK7232.

Perry TT, Matsui EC, Conover-Walker MK, Wood RA. The relationship of allergen IgE levels and oral food challenge outcome. J Allergy Clin Immunol 2004; 114: 144–149.

Shah KM, Rank MA, Davé SA, Oslie CL, Butterfield JH. Predicting which medication classes interfere with allergy skin testing. Allergy Asthma Proc 2010; 31: 477–482.

Sicherer SH. Food allergy: When and how to perform oral food challenges. Pediatr Allergy Immunol 1999; 10: 226–234.

Solensky R, Khan DA, Bernstein IL, Bloomberg GR, Castells MC, Mendelson LM, et al. Drug allergy: an updated practice parameter. Ann Allergy Asthma Immunol 2010; 105: 259–273.

Stevenson DD, Simon RA. Selection of patients for aspirin desensitization treatment. J Allergy Clin Immunol 2006; 118: 801–804.

Trautmann A, Goebeler M, Stoevesandt J. Twenty years' experience with anaphylaxis-like reactions to local anesthetics: genuine allergy is rare. J Allergy Clin Immunol Pract 2018; 6: 2051–2058.

Wilkinson DS, Fregert S, Magnusson B, Bandmann HJ, Calnan CD, Cronin E, et al. 1970. Terminology of contact dermatitis. Acta Derm Venereol 2018; 50: 287–92.

Wong JT, Nagy CS, Krinzman SJ, Maclean JA, Bloch KJ. Rapid oral challenge-desensitization for patients with aspirin-related urticaria-angioedema. J Allergy Clin Immunol 2000; 105: 997–1001.

18

Environment and Lifestyle in Allergic Disease

Anubha Tripathi* and *Thomas AE Platts-Mills*

INTRODUCTION

Although case reports of allergic reactions go back to the Pharaohs, the rise of allergic disease to become one of the common diseases of mankind has occurred over the last 150 years. Here it can be argued that the rise is related not only to changes in exposure to allergens but equally to changes in the way that one chooses to live.

Three main phases of the increase can be recognized:

(1) Hay fever first became well known during the last 30 years of the 19th century and continued to increase through the first half of the 20th century.
(2) Asthma remained low in prevalence particularly among children up to 1950. After that, asthma prevalence and severity rose steadily for 50 years.
(3) Peanut allergy is not new but has dramatically increased both in severity and prevalence from 1990's and into the 21st century.

Each of these changes has been dependent upon exposure: (i) grass pollen, (ii) indoor allergens, and (iii) peanut butter; but the increases in exposure cannot logically explain either the timing or the scale of the increases in any of the diseases. Understanding the elements involved in the increase is essential in both combating the present disease and attempting to predict future changes. In addition, understanding what has happened in western countries is essential to understanding the ways in which allergic diseases will change or are currently changing in developing countries.

The changes in exposure to foreign antigens are complex and can only be described in outline. However, there were major changes in agriculture in the second half of the 19th century which increased pollen. In England, the rise of the dairy herds led to the introduction of meadow grasses which pollinate far more heavily than the traditional hill grass (Blackley 1873, Salter 1882, Wyman 1872). In the United States, major increases in farming led to a massive increase in ragweed, which flourishes in parallel with agriculture. By 1920, the island of Helgoland in the North Sea had been established as a refuge for hay fever sufferers, and in the United States it was already common practice for ragweed hay fever sufferers to escape the weed season by going to resorts in the mountains of New England. What is even more impressive is that New York City started a campaign to eradicate ragweed from the city in 1946 because

---

Division of Allergy & Immunology, University of Virginia Health System, Charlottesville, Virginia, USA.
 Email: tap2z@virginia.edu
* Corresponding author: anubha.tripathi@gmail.com

hay fever was such a problem for the citizens (Walzer and Siegel 1956). Although some epidemiological studies maintain that hay fever has continued to increase, those studies generally have a very low key definition of allergic rhinitis. More impressive has been the move indoors that started with the advent of television and that was reinforced in many areas by air conditioning. Today, many sufferers with hay fever simply withdraw from the outdoors. Indeed, the average amount of time that Americans spend outdoors is less than 30 minutes per day!

The progressive rise in asthma from 1960 onwards has been documented as the increase in the number of children wheezing, the number of cases on therapeutic treatment, and the number of admissions to hospital (Smith et al. 1969, Woolcock and Peat 1997, Crater et al. 2001, Eder et al. 2006). In the United States, there was also a major change in demographics of the disease. Between 1970 and 1990, both hospital admissions and mortality due to asthma became more common among children living in poverty, particularly among African American children (Grant et al. 2000, Weiss et al. 1993). This change has not been obvious in other countries and clearly raises questions about what is special about poverty in the United States? The possible explanations for the increase in asthma between 1960 and 2000 range from: increases in exposure to indoor allergens, progressive increases in public hygiene and progressive decreases in physical activity (with the associated rise in obesity in the USA) to increased use of antibiotics and even the shift from the use of aspirin to paracetamol in the treatment of childhood infections (Platts-Mills et al. 1997b, Matricardi et al. 1997, Perzanowski et al. 2010).

The most recent change is the rise in food allergy, particularly in peanut allergy from 1990 to the present. In this case, it is difficult to implicate traditional changes in hygiene such as enteric infections, helminths, parasites, etc. However, over this period, evidence has accumulated that sensitization to peanuts and perhaps other foods may occur primarily through exposure to the skin (Lack et al. 2003, Du Toit et al. 2008), a process that may be facilitated by the increased presence of peanut butter and foods containing peanut-derived products in households. This brings up the issue as to whether the skin has changed. While there is no firm evidence as yet, it is very clear that children's skin is being exposed to many chemicals including detergents (Smith and Lourie 2011). Though washing skin is not a new idea, the frequency and enthusiasm with which young children are bathed has increased dramatically (Figure 18.1).

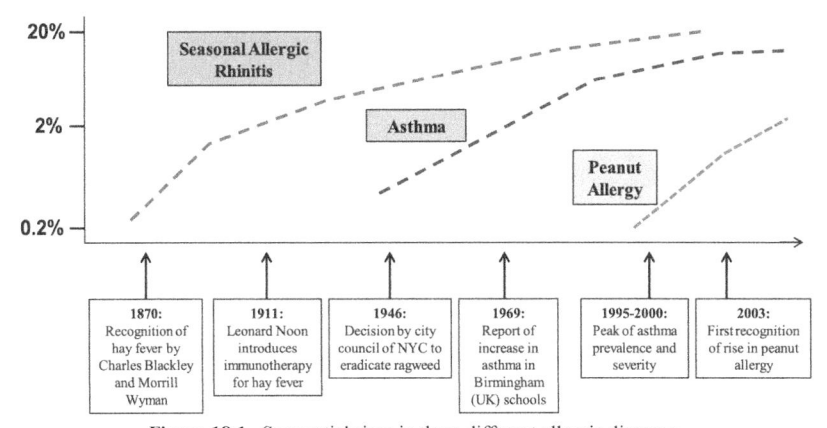

Figure 18.1. Sequential rises in three different allergic diseases.

Environmental exposure

Without some form of exposure, sensitization to common inhalant allergens does not occur. Thus, very few children raised in Los Alamos, New Mexico or the Norbotten region of Sweden are sensitized to mite or cockroach because these allergens are neither present in their homes nor in the homes of their neighbors (Perzanowski et al. 2002, Erwin et al. 2007, Spork et al. 1995). Furthermore, the symptoms of allergic diseases can be controlled by moving to a region where exposure does not occur. The clear implication is that allergen avoidance should be able to control both sensitization and the disease. Before considering the effects of avoidance, first the form in which exposure occurs and the ways in which allergens can enter the body should be considered.

The nature of exposure to antigens and allergens

Foreign antigens reach the body and, more importantly the immune system, in many different ways. However, only a limited number of these exposures induce IgE antibodies. With viral infections, bacterial infections and most immunization regimes, hypersensitivity (IgE production) to the relevant proteins is rare or has not been described. There are very effective controls in the immune system that prevent IgE production. The best understood of these is the apoptosis of IgE-switched B cells in germinal centers (Aalberse and Platts-Mills 2004). By contrast, IgE production is an important element of the immune response to: non-infective foreign antigens that are repeatedly inhaled, some food antigens, helminths that live in the gut, and foreign antigens, including endo- or ecto-parasites that enter through the skin.

Exposure to inhaled antigens

The first rule is that inhaled allergens only enter the system on particles. Thus, understanding exposure is as much about the nature of the particles as it is about the properties of the relevant proteins. The best defined inhaled particles are pollen grains, fungal spores, mite feces and the dander of cats and dogs (Table 18.1) (Tovey et al. 1981a, Tovey et al. 1981b, Luczynska et al. 1990). Pollen grains were first recognized as an allergen by Charles Blackley in 1873 (Blackley 1873). He also calculated the weight of pollen grains in the air and was astonished by how little pollen was necessary to cause these symptoms. Subsequent calculations were made in the 1970's by David Marsh at Johns Hopkins. He calculated annual exposure for specific ragweed allergens, and again the quantities inhaled were found to be very low (Marsh 1975). Those calculations suggested that even conditions of 'high' pollen exposure may not represent more than one microgram of pollen allergen inhaled per year. David Marsh also demonstrated that most pollen allergens elute from pollen grains within a few minutes of landing on a fluid surface (Marsh 1975).

After Der p 1 was first purified, mite fecal particles were identified as the form in which this allergen accumulates in a culture of mites and becomes airborne in houses (Tovey et al. 1981a, Tovey et al. 1981b). Further investigation of the fecal particles showed that the rate of elution of mite allergens and the quantities of allergen inhaled per day were similar to pollen allergens. However, there was a major difference in that the quantity of mite allergen airborne in homes was dependent to a large degree on the furnishings, which act as reservoirs of allergen, and on the behavior of the occupants. Mite growth in homes depends on temperature, humidity, the presence of human skin scales and 'nests' (Voorhorst et al. 1967). All of this is relevant to the approaches used for controlling exposure. The fecal particles of dust mites carry a striking collection of substances that could contribute to their ability to induce an IgE antibody response. These include: mite DNA and bacterial DNA (both of which are unmethylated, i.e., TLR-9 agonists), endotoxin (a TLR-4 agonist), chitin (which acts on TLR-2), as well as the potent proteinase Der p 1 and finally Der p 2 which can act as an MD-2 agonist (Fig. 18.2) (Trompette et al. 2009, Lee et al. 2011).

Cats and dogs are present in large numbers of homes and are an important cause of sensitization and allergic symptoms. However, there are major differences between cat exposure and mite exposure which may be relevant to the relationship of these allergens to disease (Platts-Mills et al. 2002). The aerodynamic sizes of particles carrying the cat allergen Fel d 1 are smaller (2–20 μm) than those of pollen grains (25–45 μm) or mite feces (20–40 μm). As a direct consequence of their smaller size, particles carrying cat allergen remain airborne in homes for a longer time, i.e., hours after disturbance and the overall quantities inhaled are much higher (Luczynska 1990). Indeed some estimates suggest that exposure in a home with a cat can be as high as one microgram per day. The particles carrying cat allergen carry Fel d 1 and endotoxin. Interestingly, while many cat proteins have major homology with the proteins of other mammals, this is not true of Fel d 1. This protein is present in all cats and has very little homology with other mammalian proteins. In addition, the DNA of cats is fully methylated and

Table 18.1. Allergen particles are derived from many sources and can multiple allergenic proteins.

Sources	Particles	Particle size†	Proteins*
Oak trees	Pollen	20–30 µm	Que a 1
Ryegrass	Pollen	20–30 µm	Lol p 1, Lol p 2
Ragweed	Pollen	20–30 µm	Amb a 1 Amba a 2
Dust mite	Fecal particles	15–40 µm	Der p 1, Der p 2, Der p 7
Cockroach	Debris	10–40 µm	Bla g 1, Bla g 2
Cat	Dander and epithelium	2–25 µm	Fel d 1, Fel d 2, Fel d 5
Aitemaria	Spores	10×14 µm	Alt a 1, Alt a 2
Aspergillus	Spores	2–3 µm	Asp f 1, Asp f 2

† Falling velocity of particles in still air is a function of their size. Particles greater than 20 µm in diameter fall within 10 minutes.
* Allergen protein molecules range in size from 13 kDa to 60 kDa (see www.allergen.org).

Component	Function
Der p 1 (0.2 ng)	Cysteine protease
Der p 2 (0.1 ng)	MD2 analog
Mite DNA	TLR9 agonist
Bacterial DNA	TLR9 agonist
Endotoxin	TLR4 agonist and MD2 analog
Chitin	TLR2 agonist and dectin 1

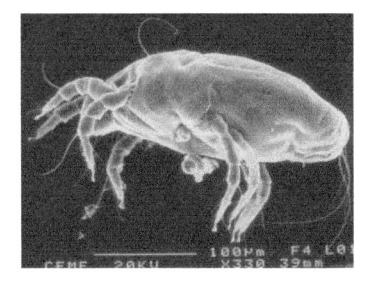

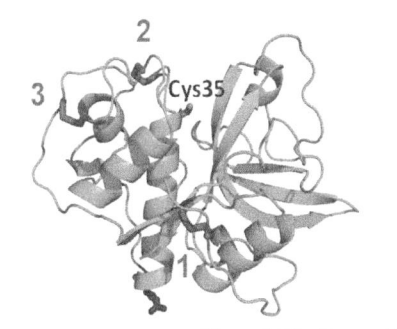

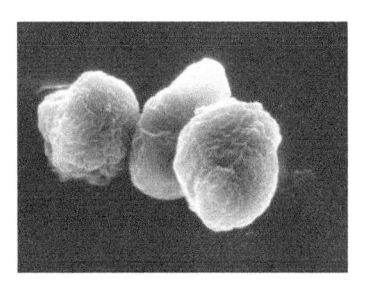

Figure 18.2. Composition of Mite Fecal particles.

does not act as a TLR-9 agonist. Finally, although the cat particles remain airborne and have a smaller aerodynamic size, many of the particles take the form of a flake, which decreases their falling velocity and apparent size (Luczynska 1990).

Fungal spores are routinely identified in 'pollen counts' and in many reports there are large or very large numbers. However, there are three elements of this exposure that are often not well understood. First, fungal 'spores' are seeds that have evolved to withstand long periods of dry conditions. Thus, they do not release proteins rapidly and, indeed, in some cases, the relevant allergens are not expressed until the spore germinates (Esch and Bush 2009, Arruda et al. 1992). Second, although fungal spores are the most easily identified part of these fungi, they may not be the most important form of exposure. Fungal hyphae also carry antigens and may release antigens more freely, but the hyphae of different species cannot be distinguished microscopically. Third, many of the fungal spores are much smaller than pollen grains. Penicillium and Aspergillus spores are approximately 2 µm in diameter, which is one thousandth of the volume of a pollen grain. At present, despite the availability of purified or recombinant fungal allergens from many fungal genera as well as classic crystal structures of the molecules, only limited data on exposure in homes either from airborne or dust samples is available.

The relevance of changes in lifestyle to understanding sequential changes in allergic disease

Introduction: There are many people who are active today who can recall the scale of changes in lifestyle that have occurred over the last 50 years. However, no one predicted the impact that these changes would have on general health or on specific diseases. Equally, there were major changes in lifestyle over the period of the 100 years before the last 50 which may have had greater impact. Concerning changes in lifestyle, it can be divided into those changes that could have: (i) directly altered the quantities of allergen to which patients were exposed, (ii) enhanced allergic immune responses, and (iii) had a physiological effect on allergic disease. The last of these is thought to be primarily relevant to asthma.

Hay Fever: The second half of the 19th century saw dramatic changes in our understanding of disease in general and in the widespread introduction of public hygiene. By 1900, clean water was common, helminth eradication was well underway, and shoes were almost universally used in cities in northern Europe and the United States. Looking at recent studies from many parts of the world, it is easy to argue in favor of these changes leading to production of high titer IgE antibody responses to inhalant allergens. In keeping with this, the first convincing studies of hay fever appeared in 1870, and the disease increased steadily until 1900. However, there were changes in agriculture occurring at the same time. Following the reform of the Corn Laws in 1847, wheat farming in England collapsed. This was followed by major increases in dairy herds and in the growth of meadow grasses, particularly heavily pollinating grasses such as Italian rye grass and timothy (Blackley 1873, Salter 1882, Wyman 1872). Thus, changes in hygiene and increased pollen exposure were occurring in parallel. Obviously, the changes that could have influenced hygiene were complex. However, some major changes match the changes in allergic disease, while others do not. The control of enteric disease mortality in the 19th century preceded the control of TB which only came under control in the 1940s. Indeed, Noon died of Phthisis in 1913 shortly after he introduced immunotherapy for hay fever, a disease which was already common (Noon 1911).

Allergic Asthma: Many authors have attempted to understand the changes in lifestyle that occurred over the period during which one observed the largest changes in allergic asthma. The problem, again, is that many changes were occurring during this period and that much of the epidemiology is contradictory. There is published evidence about the relevance of: (i) enteric infections, (ii) changes in vaccination, (iii) the introduction of broad-spectrum antibiotics, and (iv) the shift from use of aspirin to paracetamol in the treatment of fever in childhood (Shirakawa et al. 1997, Downs et al. 2001). In the UK, it was possible to state that not only was mite sensitization a risk factor for asthma, but also that increased exposure to mites could have had an important role in the increase in this disease (Platts-Mills et al. 1984). Between 1950 and 1980, there were extensive improvements in the insulation of homes, widespread use of fitted carpets, a rise in indoor temperatures, as well as the steady increase in time spent indoors. Each of these could have increased mite growth and, therefore augmented exposure. However, considering increased mite exposure as the primary cause for the growth in asthma was only convincing because, until 1985, the rise in asthma had only been documented in countries where dust mite sensitivity dominated asthma, such as New Zealand, Australia, Japan and the UK. After 1985, it became clear that asthma was also increasing in countries like Scandinavia, in the American inner city and in mountain towns such as Los Alamos, New Mexico, where dust mites were not an important part of the pathology (Sporik et al. 1995, Braback et al. 2004). Looking at the time course of the increase in asthma, the most persistent, and influential changes in lifestyle have been those related to the progressive increase in indoor entertainment (McWilliams et al. 2009, Gortmacher et al. 1996). Children first started watching television in earnest in the mid 1950's. Over the next 20 years, the portion of their time spent watching a screen rose steadily. However, the secondary results of this change have been very complicated:

(i) Increased time spent indoors sitting, often in a ' trance'.

(ii) Major loss of exercise or play outside.

(iii) Increased efforts to make homes draft-free and comfortable, i.e., warm.

(iv) Secondary changes in diet.

(v) Less time in the sun, i.e., less Vitamin D.

The growth in overall time spent indoors was relatively modest—from 21 hours per day to 23 hours per day. By contrast, the decrease in time spent playing outdoors has been dramatic, in many cases over 90% (Goran and Treuth 2001). This could pose the question of whether playing outdoors is protective or whether sitting still in a 'trance' is harmful. One of the consequences of sitting still is a decrease in the frequency of deep breaths or sigh rates (Hark et al. 2005). Interestingly, in 1873, Salter recognized that taking a deep breath could relieve wheezing (Salter 1882). More recently, both Fredberg and Togias provided clear evidence that full expansion of the lungs should be regarded as a primary prevention technique against bronchospasm (Fredberg 1998, Skloot et al. 1995). Thus, it is likely that both decreased outdoor activity and prolonged sedentary time watching a screen have contributed to the harmful effects on breathing over the period from 1960–2000. If, as seems likely, voluntary deep breathing can produce a significant relaxing effect on bronchial smooth muscle, it is perfectly possible that semi-cognitive processes such as using a computer or texting would be less harmful to lung function than TV! What matters over all is that we need to be aware that there are multiple ways in which lifestyle changes could influence a disease such as asthma.

Some investigators have tried to equate the changes in lifestyle with the rise in obesity. Indeed, there are multiple studies reporting an association between obesity and asthma (Mannino et al. 2006, Gilliland et al. 2003). However, most of those studies, particularly the ones with large cohorts, are deficient in mechanistic evaluation of lung function. Several have commented that asthma in obese children is less allergic in nature and has less evidence of bronchial inflammation (Chen et al. 2006). One study on 17,000 children used a parental report of a 'health care worker's diagnosis of asthma' as the definition (Cottrell et al. 2011). Recently the response of obese teenagers to full cardiopulmonary exercise testing (CPET) was compared with those without a 'physician diagnosis' of asthma. The result was clear, i.e., that the primary cause of breathlessness on exercise was cardiopulmonary deconditioning and that we could see no difference in lung function during exercise between the groups with or without a diagnosis of asthma (Shim et al. 2012). Thus, there is a real trap in giving a diagnosis of asthma to obese children, because a likely outcome is a decrease in exercise. This occurs because of the child's or the parent's fear that exercise could induce an attack of asthma. If fear of inducing wheezing is a reason for not doing exercise, then these children need pulmonary rehabilitation. An exercise prescription, however, should be part of the management of any obese child with asthma.

The importance of the skin as a route for sensitization

The first indication that the skin might be a route for sensitization came in 1931 when Taliafero demonstrated that patients with schistosomiasis had serum reagins to schistosomules (Taliafero 1931). The implications were clear: schistosomules going through the skin could induce sensitization and this sensitization might play a role in protection against further infestation. Normal skin has a layer of lipid and is generally considered to be impermeable to proteins but easily penetrated by small, fat-soluble molecules, such as Dinitrochlorobenzene (DNCB) or urushiol from poison ivy. However, detergents, including those used in shampoos, can dissolve fat and reduce the protective effects of the skin's lipid layer. Equally, mild abrasion of the skin will allow entry of proteins through the skin. In patients with atopic dermatitis, entry of proteins through the skin can induce a patch of eczema (Mitchell et al. 1982). In 2003, Gideon Lack took the whole argument about the skin one step further when he suggested that early sensitization to peanuts occurred through the skin (Lack et al. 2003, Du Toit et al. 2008). His data came from several different observations, but the central argument was that proteins taken by mouth normally induce tolerance, while the skin is a very effective route for inducing sensitization. The recent discovery that IgE responses to the mammalian oligosaccharide galactose alpha-1, 3-galactose are induced by tick bites provides further evidence that the skin is a good route for inducing IgE antibody responses

(Commins et al. 2011). However, equally the fact that IgE antibody responses induced by a tick bite are associated with delayed anaphylaxis after eating red meat, provides yet another example of sensitization occurring through a different route, the skin, rather than the conventional routes of allergen exposure (Commins et al. 2012). The question now is whether other environmental proteins can go through the skin and whether we have changed the skin by changes in lifestyle. Recent evidence has strongly argued that changes in the skin due to repeated washing or the use of chemicals on the skin such as Triclosan, may be decreasing the barrier function of the skin (Smith and Lourie 2011, Savage et al. 2012).

Environmental control measures for allergen exposure

Decreasing exposure to allergens is a central part of the treatment of allergic disease. For many types of allergens, the form of exposure, the measures necessary to control exposure and the results, are obvious. Thus, measures such as: removing a patient from an occupational exposure to rats or mice, eliminating shellfish from a patient's diet, removing a caged rabbit or hamster from a patient's home, recommending a patient stay inside the air-conditioned workplace or home during the pollen season, eliminating apples from the diet of a patient with oral allergy syndrome, and eliminating red meat from the diet of a patient with IgE to alpha-gal are all examples of tertiary prevention, which aims to control symptoms in a patient who is already allergic. Primary prevention, i.e., avoidance of sensitization, is complicated, especially in the case of the major indoor allergens, for which the sources and sites of exposure are much less obvious.

Indoor allergens

Dust Mite: There are two primary observations that have influenced the development of environmental control measures for dust mite allergen. Firstly, children raised in a region where the climate prevents mite growth are generally not sensitized to dust mites; in addition, mite sensitization that is present is not significantly associated with asthma. Secondly, mite-allergic patients with asthma who are moved to sanatoria or hospital rooms with 'no' mite exposure improve clinically and can exhibit significant decreases in non-specific Bronchial Hyper Reactivity (BHR) (Kerrebijn 1970, Platts-Mills et al. 1982, Peroni 2002). Thus, there is no doubt that decreased or absent exposure can: (i) prevent sensitization, and (ii) produce major benefit with regard to symptoms in allergic patients.

The results of studies on dust mite avoidance measures in patients' homes have been 'less consistent', both of studies designed to prevent primary sensitization and of studies on the treatment of allergic subjects (Platts-Mills 2008). The most common reason for inconsistency of results of these studies is insufficient or even insignificant reduction in exposure by the intervention. This raises the question of whether we know how much of a reduction is, in fact, sufficient? Should exposure be reduced by $\geq 80\%$, or should exposure be reduced to a level below a finite concentration, such as 1 µg Der p 1/g? An 80% reduction from exposure to 20 µg Der p 1/g would still be relatively high; by contrast, a 70% reduction from 2 µg/g would be well below the reported threshold (Platts-Mills et al. 1997a).

Another equally important reason is the presence of poly-sensitization to allergens present in the environment for which control measures are not being implemented (Morgan et al. 2004). The protocols recommended for dust mite control would have relatively little effect on the levels of cat or cockroach allergens in a house. Many or most controlled trials of mite avoidance do not adequately address sensitization to other allergens. Correct approaches would be to either identify patients who are only allergic to mites (Ehnert et al. 1992) or to apply avoidance measures relevant to each of a patient's sensitizations (Morgan et al. 2004). Both these approaches have yielded successful results in a limited number of studies. By contrast, the bulk of the studies included in the so-called 'meta-analysis' did not use either of these approaches (Platts-Mills 2008).

Different issues exist with studies on primary avoidance. In some studies, avoidance measures put in place early on in life have produced significant effects, but in others there has been very little effect on sensitization. In an important study in Manchester, England, Custovic and his colleague achieved highly reduced levels of mite allergen in children's homes but still failed to prevent sensitization in the children

(Simpson and Custovic 2004). They thought that the sensitization was due to exposure to endotoxin despite decreased levels in those homes where avoidance measures had been successfully carried out.

We believe that exposure in places other than their own homes is a more likely explanation. Thus, in Manchester, the homes of grandmothers, cousins or friends were likely to have significant mite allergens, and it was likely there that the children were exposed, however carefully avoidance was carried out in their own home. By contrast, children living in Los Alamos, New Mexico or the Norbotten region of Sweden, where none of the homes have significant mite allergen, did not develop significant sensitization.

Cat Dander: Avoiding cat exposure is more of a problem because cat allergen is carried on clothing and is, therefore, present in all homes. Children do not need to live in a home with a cat to become sensitized (Sporik et al. 1995, Almqvist et al. 2001). Indeed, in multiple studies, the presence of a cat in the home, particularly in the first year of life, has been associated with lower prevalence of sensitization (Perzanowski et al. 2002, Platts-Mills et al. 2001, Ownby et al. 2002). Thus, it is not clear how we should go about controlling exposure. Certainly, effective avoidance would have to include measures designed to decrease exposure to cat allergens in homes without a cat. Measures to control exposure with the cat in the house are not easy. De Blay showed that a combination of removal of carpeting, air filtration, vacuum cleaning and regular bathing of the cat could decrease exposure (De Blay et al. 1991). Use of single exposure control measures such as air filtration alone is unlikely to achieve much change if the cat remains in the home (Wood et al. 1989, Wood et al. 1998).

Dog Dander: Control measures for exposure to dog dander are similar to those for cat dander. Allergens from both of these domesticated animals are airborne. While keeping dogs from residing in the home is the most effective control measure, keeping dogs from being present inside rooms of the home in which a significant portion of time is spent (e.g., the bedroom), the use of High-Efficiency Particulate Arrestance (HEPA) Air filters in the home and the regular bathing of dogs have also been shown to significantly decrease airborne dog allergen levels (Hodson et al. 1999).

Cockroach and Indoor Fungi: Avoidance measures for cockroach allergens, the most common cause of inner-city asthma, have been shown to be effective when used in combination. Strategies include: use of poison bait applied in the form of traps or paste, enclosure of all sources of food in the home, regular cleaning of the home (especially the kitchen) to remove any accumulated allergen and sealing of as many access points to the home as possible (Morgan et al. 2004).

Avoidance measures for indoor fungi (e.g., Aspergillus and Alternaria) include control of humidity levels, removal of sites that provide favorable growth factors for fungi, cleaning of surfaces with fungicides, and avoidance of inhabitation of the basements of homes by allergic individuals (Platts-Mills, 2013).

Outdoor Allergens: Control of exposure to outdoor allergens is difficult to achieve since control involves limitation of exposure to the outdoor environment during the season(s) in which the allergens relevant to clinical allergy are prevalent. Avoidance of being present outdoors during peak exposure times may be a possible strategy since peak presence of the various seasonal allergens is dependent on certain environmental elements including outdoor temperature, humidity, wind, precipitation, time of day and proximity to pollen plants (Martorano and Erwin 2018). However, strategies limiting the spread of or the presence of particles carrying outdoor allergens to the indoor environment such as keeping windows and doors of the home closed and use of HEPA air filtration may be more effective in reducing outdoor allergen levels in the indoor environment.

Food Allergens: Studies on the effectiveness of primary prevention of food allergy in childhood have raised issues in our current management. Around the year 2000, in an effort to curtail the rise in prevalence of food allergy in children, the American Academy of Pediatrics along with the European Societies for Pediatric Allergology and Gastroenterology recommended maternal avoidance of ingestion of particular food allergens during pregnancy and lactation (namely peanuts), as well as delayed introduction of certain allergenic foods (Zeiger 2003). However, despite general adherence to this recommendation, the prevalence of food allergy continued to increase (Du Toit et al. 2008). Later studies, including the results of the LEAP study, were not able to provide sufficient evidence to support a major role for maternal dietary restriction or delayed introduction of foods in the development of atopic disease, including food allergy (Du Toit et al. 2015). The recommendations were therefore amended in 2008 to reflect these findings (Greer 2008).

Conclusions on Allergen Avoidance: In our view, reducing exposure should remain the focus of the treatment of allergic subjects. There are many situations where simply defining the patient's sensitivity is sufficient to convince them to avoid the relevant exposure. For perennial indoor exposures, the measures necessary to control exposure are more complex. It may prove difficult to persuade some patients about the importance of making relevant changes. However, other patients will quickly and effectively adopt the relevant measures and derive major clinical benefit. For mite and cockroach exposure, the bulk of the evidence suggests that there is a simple dose response relationship between exposure and both sensitization and disease.

By contrast, for cat allergens, the relationship between exposure and sensitization may plateau or can even be bell-shaped (Platts-Mills et al. 2002). Indeed, there may be many patients who have positive skin tests but will actually become more allergic if they have lower levels of exposure (i.e., higher levels of exposure can maintain tolerance). Thus, recommendations made about cat avoidance should take into account the probability of successfully persuading patients to find a new home for their pets.

In keeping with the evidence that avoidance of oral ingestion of food allergens in pregnancy, lactation and early childhood may not prevent sensitization, possibly because it can still occur through the skin, along with the statement that oral ingestion may actually induce tolerance (Du Toit et al. 2008), it seems that avoidance, in the case of food allergy, may actually not be the path to preventing or reducing the incidence of this disease.

Conclusions

The scale of changes in allergic disease over the last 60 years has been difficult to believe, and the implication is that these diseases will continue to change. Clearly, this reflects many different aspects of how we live, starting with primary hygiene, but continuing with diet, housing design and the ravages of electronic entertainment. Given the pace of these changes, it is unwise to try to predict the future. However, we do believe that understanding what has happened will help us react to changes as they occur and may make it possible to give better advice about lifestyle.

The first, and perhaps the biggest changes came from the initial introduction of 'hygiene', which was necessary to control typhoid, malaria, helminths, etc. The majority of these changes were made in New York, London, Munich and Berlin between 1850 and 1920; these changes can be temporally related to the development of hay fever as an allergic disease. There is excellent modern evidence that living on a farm can change the bacterial composition of dust in the home and can alter the microbiome and allergic sensitization of the children. However, the majority of western population do not live on farms and have not lived on farms anytime in the last 50 years. Recently, evidence has developed that dogs may have the same effect as farms on the microbiome (Wood et al. 1998). It is tempting to think that artificial manipulation of the microbiome early in life could produce the effects of a pre-hygiene society without the risk of an infectious disease. However, there are many hurdles that would have to be crossed, and simply eating worms will not do it!

The first phase of electronic entertainment was radio, but the effects of radio on children were modest because radio does not discourage movement within the house. By contrast, it is difficult to exaggerate the effect that television has had on children's lives. Over a period of 20 years (~ 1955–1975), children almost stopped going outside to play and were spending up to 3 hours per day sitting indoors. The secondary effects include: (i) warmer, unventilated houses providing better conditions for mite growth and for the accumulation of other indoor allergens; (ii) changes in diet combined with decreased exercise, leading to the truly horrific rise in childhood obesity in the United States; and (iii) breathing changes, including a decreased sigh rate or simply more shallow breathing, as a result of the trance-like state children often enter while sitting still. Most recently, there have been several changes that may have decreased the harmful effects of television. First, computers are much more interactive and children are generally not in a 'trance'. Second, innovations such as *Wii Fit* encourage activity indoors. Third, cell phones allow children and adults to talk while they are walking. Whether these recent changes have had a significant beneficial effect on asthma is difficult to evaluate because there have also been significant changes in treatment, including the combinations of inhaled steroids and long-acting bronchodilator drugs. However, the mortality rate for asthma in the United States has declined by almost 30% in the last 10 years.

In complete contrast to the decline or stabilization of asthma over the recent past is the major increase in food allergy. This is true both for peanut allergy and eosinophilic esophagitis (EoE). For peanut allergy, the pattern of disease is typical of most forms of anaphylactic food allergy, but the prevalence of *high* titer IgE antibodies to peanut allergens in the community compared to other foods is now remarkably high. As we have discussed, there is increasing evidence that sensitization to peanuts can occur through the skin rather than through oral exposure. This raises the question of whether composition of the skin and its function as a barrier has changed. The data on prevalence of high titer IgE to peanuts (during the period in which avoidance of ingestion was being recommended) clearly adds to a body of evidence that supports not only that sensitization can occur through the skin but also that high titers of IgE can be induced through this route. In contrast, EoE is associated with low titer of IgE antibodies to food allergens; at present, there is no evidence on the route of sensitization in this disease (Clayton et al. 2014, Schuyler et al. 2018).

In conclusion, the sequence of changes in allergic disease cannot be explained simply by hygiene or lifestyle, and one should be willing to recognize a role for many different changes over the last 100 years. There are ways in which one could identify changes in advance and predict or even avoid future changes in allergic disease. However, this involves some remarkable optimism about the ability for human society to plan and carry out a change in lifestyle as a conscious positive decision.

References

Aalberse RC, Platts-Mills TA. How do we avoid developing allergy: modifications of the TH2 response from a B-cell perspective. J Allergy Clin Immunol 2004; 113(5): 983–6.

Almqvist C, Wickman M, Perfetti L, Berglind N, Renstrom A, Hedren M, et al. Worsening of asthma in children allergic to cats, after indirect exposure to cat at school. Am J Respir Crit Care Med 2001; 163(3 Pt 1): 694–8.

Arruda LK, Mann BJ, Chapman MD. Selective expression of a major allergen and cytotoxin, Asp f I, in *Aspergillus fumigatus*. Implications for the immunopathogenesis of Aspergillus-related diseases. J Immunol, 1992; 149(10): 3354–9.

Blackley CH. Experimental Researches on the Causes and Nature of Catarrhusaestivus. Balliere, London, 1873.

Braback L, Hjern A, Rasmussen F. Trends in asthma, allergic rhinitis and eczema among Swedish conscripts from farming and non-farming environments. A nationwide study over three decades. Clin Exp Allergy 2004; 34(1): 38–43.

Chen Y, Dales R, Jiang Y. The association between obesity and asthma is stronger in nonallergic than allergic adults. Chest 2006; 130(3): 890–5.

Clayton F, Fang JC, Gleich GJ, Lucendo AJ, Olalla JM, Vinson LA, et al. Eosinophilic Esophagitis in Adults is associated with IgG4 and not mediated by IgE. Gastroenterology 2014 Sep; 147(3): 602–9.

Commins SP, Kelly LA, Ronmark E, James HR, Pochan SL, Peters EJ, et al. The relevance of tick bites to the production of IgE antibodies to the mammalian oligosaccharide galactose-α-1,3-galactose. JACI 2011; 127(5): 1286–1293.

Commins SP, et al. Galactose-alpha-1,3-galactose-specific IgE is associated with anaphylaxis but not asthma. Am J Respir Crit Care Med 2012; 185(7): 723–30.

Cottrell L, Neal WA, Ice C, Perez MK, Piedmonte G. Metabolic abnormalities in children with asthma. Am J Respir Crit Care Med 2011; 183(4): 441–8.

Crater DD, Heise S, Perzanowski M, Herbert R, Morse CG, Hulsey TC, et al. Asthma hospitalization trends in Charleston, South Carolina, 1956 to 1997: twenty-fold increase among black children during a 30-year period. Pediatrics 2001; 108(6): E97.

De Blay F, Chapman MD, Platts-Mills TA. Airborne cat allergen (Fel d I). Environmental control with the cat *in situ*. Am Rev Respir Dis 1991; 143(6): 1334–9.

Downs SH, Marks GB, Sporik R, Belosouva EG, Car NG, Peat JK. Continued increase in the prevalence of asthma and atopy. Arch Dis Child 2001; 84(1): 20–23.

Du Toit G, Katz Y, Sasieni P, Mesher D, Maleki SJ, Fisher HR, et al. Early consumption of peanuts in infancy is associated with a low prevalence of peanut allergy. J Allergy Clin Immunol 2008; 122(5): 984–91.

Du Toit G, Roberts G, Sayre PH, Bahnson HT, Radulovic S, Santos AF, et al. Randomized trial of peanut consumption in infants at risk for peanut allergy. N Engl J Med 2015 Feb 26; 372(9): 803–13.

Eder W, Ege MJ, von Mutius E. The asthma epidemic. N Engl J Med 2006; 355(21): 2226–35.

Ehnert B, Lau-Schadendorf S, Weber A, Buettner P, Schou C, Wahn U, et al. Reducing domestic exposure to dust mite allergen reduces bronchial hyperractivity in sensitive children with asthma. J All Clin Immunol 1992; 90(1): 135–8.

Erwin EA, et al. Cat and dust mite sensitivity and tolerance in relation to wheezing among children raised with high exposure to both allergens. J Allergy Clin Immunol 2005; 115(1): 74–9.

Erwin EA, Ronmark E, Wickens K, Perzanowski MS, Barry D, Lundback B, et al. Contribution of dust mite and cat specific IgE to total IgE: relevance to asthma prevalence. J Allergy Clin Immunol 2007; 119(2): 359–65.

Esch RE, Bush RK. Chapter 32: Aerobiology of Outdoor Allergens. Middleton's Allergy Principals and Practice, 2009. Seventh Edition: 509–538.

Fredberg JJ. Airway smooth muscle in asthma: flirting with disaster. Eur Respir J 1998; 12(6): 1252–6.

Gilliland FD, Berhand K, Islam T, McConnell R, Gauderman WJ, Gilliland SS, et al. Obesity and the risk of newly diagnosed asthma in school-age children. Am J Epidemiol 2003; 158(5): 406–15.

Goran MI, Treuth MS. Energy expenditure, physical activity, and obesity in children.Pediatr Clin North Am 2001; 48(4): 931–53.

Gortmaker SL, Must A, Sobol AM, Peterson K, Colditz GA, Dietz WH, et al. Television viewing as a causse of increasing obesity among children in the United States. Arch PediatrAdolesc Med 1996; 150: 356–362.

Grant EN, Lyttle CS, Weiss KB. The relation of socioeconomic factors and racial/ethnic differences in US asthma mortality. Am J Public Health 2000; 90(12): 1923–5.

Greer FR, Sicherer SH, Burks AW. Effects of early nutritional interventions on the development of atopic disease in infants and children: the role of maternal dietary restriction, breastfeeding, timing of introduction of complementary foods, and hydrolyzed formulas. Pediatrics 2008; 121(1): 183–191.

Hark WT, Thompson WM, McLaughlin TE, Wheatley LM, Platts-Mills TAE. Spontaneous sigh rates during sedentary activity: watching television vs reading. Ann Allergy Asthma Immunol 2005; 94(2): 247–50.

HodsonT, Custovic A, Simpson A, Chapman M, Woodcock A, Green R. Washing the dog reduces dog allergen levels, but the dog needs to be washed twice a week. J Allergy Clin Immunol 1999; 103: 581–5.

Kerrebijn KF. Endogenous factors in childhood CNSLD. Methodological aspects in populations studies. In "Bronchitis III". Royal Vangorcum, Assen, The Netherlands, 1970: p. 38–48.

Lack G, Fox D, Northstone K, Golding J. Factors associated with the development of peanut allergy in childhood. N Engl J Med 2003; 348(11): 977–85.

Lee CG, Da Silva CA, Dela Cruz CS, Ahangari F, Ma B, Kang M-J, et al. Role of chitin and chitinase/chitinase-like proteins in inflammation, tissue remodeling, and injury.AnnuRevPhysiol 2011; 73: 479–501.

Luczynska CM, Li Y, Chapman MD, Platts-Mills TA. Airborne concentrations and particle size distribution of allergen derived from domestic cats (Felis domesticus). Measurements using cascade impactor, liquid impinger, and a two-site monoclonal antibody assay for Fel d I. Am Rev Respir Dis 1990; 141(2): 361–7.

Mannino DM, Mott J, Ferdinands JM, Camargo CA, Friedman M, Groves HM. Boys with high body masses have an increased risk of developing asthma: findings from the National Longitudinal Survey of Youth (NLSY). Int J Obes (Lond) 2006; 30(1): 6–13.

Marsh DG. Allergens and the genetics of allergy. *In*: M. Sela (ed.). The Antigens, Academic Press, New York, 1975. III: p. 271.

Martorano L, Erwin EA. Aeroallergen exposure and spread in the modern era. J Allergy Clin Immunol Pract 2018; 6: 1835–42.

Matricardi PM, Rosmini F, Ferrigno L, Nisini R, Rapicetta M, Chionne P, et al. Cross sectional retrospective study of prevalence of atopy among Italian military students with antibodies against hepatitis A virus. BMJ 1997; 314(7086): 999–1003.

McWilliams C, Ball SC, Benjamin SE, Hales D, Vaughn A, Ward DS. Best-practice guidelines for physical activity at child care. Pediatrics 2009; 124(6): 1650–9.

Mitchel EB, Crow J, Chapman MD, Jouhal SS, Pope FM, Platts-Mills TA. Basophils in allergen-induced patch test sites in atopic dermatitis. Lancet 1982; 1(8264): 127–30.

Morgan WJ, Crain EF, Gruchalla RS, O'Connor GT, Kattan M, Evans, R 3rd, et al. Results of a home-based environmental intervention among urban children with asthma. N Engl J Med 2004; 351(11): 1068–80.

National Heart, Lung, and Blood Institute. 2007. Expert Panel Report 3: Guidelines for the Diagnosis and Management of Asthma.

Noon L. Prophylactic innoculation for hay fever. Lancet 1911; i: 1572.

Ownby DR, Johnson CC, Peterson EL. Exposure to dogs and cats in the first year of life and risk of allergic sensitization at 6 to 7 years of age. JAMA 2002; 288(8): 963–72.

Peroni DG, Piacentini GL, Costella S, Pietrobelli A, Bodini A, Loiacono A, et al. Mite avoidance can reduce air trapping and airway inflammation in allergic asthmatic children. Clin Exp Allergy 2002; 32(6): 850–5.

Perzanowski MS, Ronmark E, Platts-Mills TAE, Lundback B. Effect of cat and dog ownership on sensitization and development of asthma among preteenage children. Am J Respir Crit Care Med 2002; 166(5): 696–702.

Perzanowski MS, Miller RL, Tang D, Ali D, Garfinkel RS, Chew GL, et al. Prenatal acetaminophen exposure and risk of wheeze at age 5 years in an urban low-income cohort. Thorax 2010; 65(2): 118–23.

Platts-Mills TA, Tovey ER, Mitchell EB, Moszoro H, Nock P, Wilkins SR. Reduction of bronchial hyperreactivity during prolonged allergen avoidance. Lancet 1982; 2(8300): 675–8.

Platts-Mills T, Mitchell E, Tovey E, Chapman M, Wilkins S. Airborne allergen exposure, allergen avoidance and bronchial hyperreactivity. pp. 297–314. *In*: Kay AB, Austen KF, Lichtenstein LM (eds.). Asthma: Physiology, Immunopharmacology and Treatment. Third International Symposium. London: Academic Press, 1984.

Platts-Mills TA, Vervloet D, Thomas WR, Aslberse RC, Chapman MD. Indoor allergens and asthma: report of the Third International Workshop. J Allergy Clin Immunol 1997a; 100(6 Pt 1): S2–24.

Platts-Mills TA, Sporik RB, Chapman MD, Heymann PW. The role of domestic allergens. The rising trends in Asthma, 1997. Ciba Foundation Symp 1997b: pp. 173–189.

Platts-Mills T, Vaughan J, Squillace S, Woodfolk J, Sporik R. Sensitisation, asthma, and a modified Th2 response in children exposed to cat allergen: a population-based cross-sectional study. Lancet 2001; 357(9258): 752–6.

Platts-Mills TAE, Perzanowski M, Woodfolk JA, Lundback B. Relevance of early or current pet ownership to the prevalence of allergic disease. Clin Exp Allergy 2002; 32(3): 335–8.

Platts-Mills TA. Allergen avoidance in the treatment of asthma: problems with the meta-analyses. J Allergy Clin Immunol 2008; 122(4): 694–6.

Platts-Mills TAE. Indoor Allergens. pp. 453–469. *In*: Adkinson N, Bochner B, Burks A, Busse W, Holgate S, Lemanske R, O'Hehir R (eds.). Middleton's Allergy: Principles and Practice: 8th edition. Elsevier, 2013.

Salter HH. Asthma: Its Pathology and Treatment. William Wood, New York, 1882.

Savage JH, Matsui EC, Wood RA, Keet CA. Urinary levels of triclosan and parabens are associated with aeroallergen and food sensitization. J Allergy Clin Immunol 2012; 130(2): 453–60 e7.

Schuyler AJ, Wilson JM, Tripathi A, Commins SP, Ogbogu PU, Kruzsewski PG, et al. Specific IgG4 antibodies to cow's milk proteins in pediatric patients with eosinophilic esophagitis. J Allergy Clin. Immunol 2018 Jul; 142(1): 139–148.

Shim YM, Burnette A, Lucas S, Herring RC, Weltman J, Patrie JT, et al. Physical deconditioning as a cause of breathlessness among obese adolescents with a diagnosis of asthma. 2012 submitted.

Shirakawa T, Enomoto T, Shimazu S, Hopkin JM. The inverse association between tuberculin responses and atopic disorder. Science 1997; 3(275): 77–9.

Simpson A, Custovic A. Allergen avoidance in the primary prevention of asthma. CurrOpin Allergy Clin Immunol 2004; 4(1): 45–51.

Skloot G, Permutt S, Togias A. Airway hyperresponsiveness in asthma: a problem of limited smooth muscle relaxation with inspiration. J Clin Invest 1995; 96(5): 2393–403.

Smith J, Disney ME, Williams JD, Goels ZA. Clinical significance of skin reactions to mite extracts in children with asthma. Br Med J 1969; 2(5659): 723–6.

Smith R, Lourie B. Slow Death by Rubber Duck: The Secret Danger of Everyday Things. Counterpoint, Berkeley, CA, USA 2011.

Sporik R, Ingram JM, Price W, Sussman JH, Honsinger RW, Platts-Mils TA. Association of asthma with serum IgE and skin test reactivity to allergens among children living at high altitude. Tickling the dragon's breath. Am J Respir Crit Care Med 1995; 151(5): 1388–92.

Taliafero TA. Skin reactions in Schistosomiasis. Puerto Rico J Publ Health 1931; 7(23).

Tovey ER, Chapman MD, Platts-Mills TA. Mite faeces are a major source of house dust allergens. Nature 1981a; 289(5798): 592–3.

Tovey ER, Chapman MD, Wells CW, Platts-Mills TA. The distribution of dust mite allergen in the houses of patients with asthma. Am Rev Respir Dis 1981b; 124(5): 630–5.

Trompette A, Divanovic S, Visintin A, Blanchard C, Hegde, Madan R, et al. Allergenicity resulting from functional mimicry of a Toll-like receptor complex protein. Nature 2009; 457(7229): 585–8.

Voorhorst R, Spieksma FThM, Varekamp H, Leupen MJ, Lyklema AW. The house dust mite (Dermatophagoides pteronyssinus) and the allergens it produces. Identify with the house dust allergen. J Allergy 1967(39): 325.

Walzer M, Siegel BB. The effectiveness of the ragweed eradication campaigns in New York City; a 9-year study; 1946–1954. J Allergy 1956; 27(2): 113–26.

Weiss KB, Gergen PJ, Wagener DK. Breathing better or wheezing worse? The changing epidemiology of asthma morbidity and mortality. Annu Rev Public Health 1993; 14: 491–513.

Wood RA, Chapman MD, Adkinson NF, Jr, Eggleston PA. The effect of cat removal on allergen content in household-dust samples. J Allergy Clin Immunol 1989; 83(4): 730–4.

Wood RA, Johnson EF, Van Natta ML, Chen PH, Eggleston PA. A placebo-controlled trial of a HEPA air cleaner in the treatment of cat allergy. Am J Respir Crit Care Med 1998; 1998(158): 1.

Woolcock AJ, Peat JK. Evidence for the increase in asthma worldwide. Ciba Found Symp 1997; 206: 157–9.

Wyman M. Autumnal catarrh (Hay fever). Huro& Houghton, Cambridge, Mass, 1872.

Zeiger RS. Food allergen avoidance in the prevention of food allergy in infants and children. Pediatrics 2003; 111(6): 1662–1671.

19

Effects of Air Pollution on Allergy and Asthma

Sundeep Salvi[1,*] *and Sneha Limaye*[2]

INTRODUCTION

Human beings inhale a total of around 10,000 litres of air everyday into the lungs, which gets distributed via thousands of branching tubes to a large alveolar surface area of around 75 m^2 made up of thin epithelial and endothelial cell layers that are in contact directly with the blood circulation. It is therefore not surprising that the quality of air we breathe determines not only the health of our lungs but also the health of other body organs. With rapidly increasing industrialization and urbanization the quality of air we breathe has deteriorated markedly over the years, and it has been argued that this has been a major driving factor behind the growing problem of allergic diseases worldwide.

John Bostock first described allergic rhinitis in the UK in 1819 and it took him 9 years to collect a total of 27 cases. Today allergic rhinitis is one of the most common allergic diseases worldwide and affects around 20–30% of the global population. Such a rapid growth in allergic rhinitis over a relatively short period of time cannot be attributed purely to genetic factors or a growth in the number of allergens in the air, but seems to be due to a number of factors, including rapidly increasing ambient air pollution. In the same way, the prevalence of asthma which was as low as 1% during the 1950's, has grown rapidly over the last six decades to affect between 5–15% of the world's population. A significant proportion of asthma occurs because of allergen sensitization and is related to allergic rhinitis, such a rapid increase in allergic asthma over the last few decades cannot be due to increase in the number of allergens in the air or due to genetic factors, but seems most likely to be due to changes in lifestyle, including worsening of air quality. Unless one recognizes the fact that air pollution is a major cause of the growing allergic disease burden worldwide, one will not be able to take active measures to help reduce the burden of this important risk factor. This chapter describes evidence generated over the years which highlights the important role of air pollution as an important contributor to the growing prevalence of allergic diseases.

Exposure to air pollutants during foetal growth and the risk of allergic diseases during childhood

Exposure to air pollutants starts even before one is born. It was believed for a long time that the placenta offers an efficient barrier (called placental barrier) that prevents the passage of harmful substances from

---

[1] Pulmocare Research and Education (PURE), Pune, INDIA.
[2] Dataction Analytics Pvt. Ltd., Pune, Maharashtra, INDIA, Email: drsnehalimaye@gmail.com
* Corresponding author: sundeepsalvi@gmail.com

entering into the growing foetus. However, several studies have shown that the placenta not only allows the passage of aero-allergens (e.g., house dust mite allergens) that are circulating in the maternal blood (Peters et al 2009), but also allows passage of several air pollutants into the foetal circulation. A study from New York, USA, reported that blood collected from the umbilical cord of new born babies showed the presence of 287 different air pollutants, including industrial chemicals and pesticides which the mother had inhaled during pregnancy (Body Burden 2005) (Fig. 19.1). Chinese mothers exposed to high levels of ambient volatile organic compounds, such as benzo[a]anthracene, chrysene and benzo[a] pyrene during pregnancy were shown to pass on these pollutants into the foetal circulation, with significant adverse effects on neonatal growth (Guo et al. 2012). As will be described later in the chapter, volatile organic compounds such as the ones reported in this chapter have the ability to tamper the immune system in such a way that it amplifies the allergic responses to several allergens. Circulating levels of lead have been reported in the umbilical cord blood of babies born to mothers living near industrial areas (Privalova et al. 2007), and more recently, a study from China showed that children born to mothers exposed to high levels of ambient air pollutants had poor cognitive function at the age of 5 years (Perera et al. 2012), indicating that air pollutants that enter into the foetal circulation have significant systemic impacts. Home renovation and painting during pregnancy has been found to be an important predictor of atopic dermatitis amongst infants born to these mothers (Wen et al. 2009).

A recent study from the Netherlands showed that mothers exposed to even modest levels of air pollutants, especially particulate matter and nitrogen dioxide during pregnancy, not only have higher levels of Circulating C-Reactive Protein (CRP), a systemic inflammatory biomarker, but even babies born to them show higher levels of circulating CRP (Van den Hooven et al. 2012). Latzin et al. (2011) reported that particulate matter exposure during the last 3 days of pregnancy were significantly associated with reduced IL-10 levels and during the last 3 months of pregnancy with significantly increased IL-1β levels in the cord blood after adjustment for relevant confounders, indicating that foetal exposure to air pollutants has a significant impact on cytokine synthesis that are implicated in allergic responses.

Pregnant mothers from the USA living in relatively poor socio-economic conditions and exposed to high levels of indoor air pollutants were shown to give birth to babies who had high circulating IgE levels associated with increased prevalence of wheezing during early childhood (Sternthal et al. 2011). Similar observations were reported earlier from Poland (Perera et al. 1999). A Japanese birth cohort study that examined the association between proximity to main roads as a surrogate for exposure to motor vehicular air pollutants in pregnant women and the prevalence of asthma and atopic eczema born to these mothers up to the age of 2 years, reported that living within 50 metres from the main road was associated with a significantly increased risk of asthma (odds ratio 4.01; CI: 1.4-11.2) and eczema (odds ratio 2.26; CI: 1.08-4.6) as compared to babies born to mothers who lived more than 200 metres from the main road (Miyake et al. 2009). An earlier birth cohort study from California, USA also reported

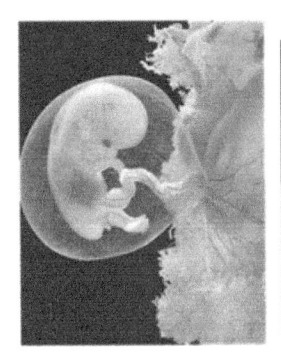

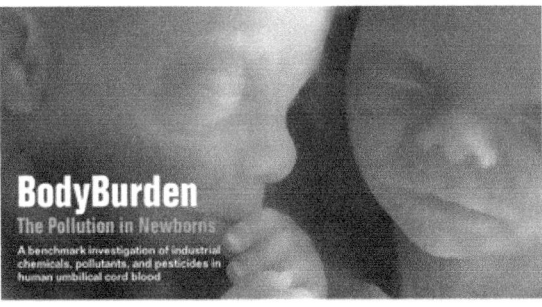

287 pollutants, chemicals, pesticides identified in the umbilical cord blood

Figure 19.1. Air pollutants that are inhaled by pregnant mother enters into the growing foetus through umbilical cord [Adapted from Report of Body Burden—The Pollution in Newborns].

that maternal exposure to high levels of vehicular air pollutants during pregnancy was associated with increased risk of allergen sensitization in the newborn children (Mortimer et al. 2008). These results support the hypothesis that intra-uterine exposures to traffic-related air pollutants significantly increase the risk of allergic diseases.

Although the biological mechanism that drives increased risk of asthma and allergic diseases in children following exposure to air pollutants during foetal growth is not yet known, several mechanisms have been postulated, including direct toxicity of particles due to particle translocation across tissue barriers or particle penetration across cellular membranes, induction of oxidative stress leading to systemic inflammation in the growing foetus and interference with the immune development in such a way that it deviates the immune responses towards the allergic phenotype (Proietti et al. 2011). More recently, Baiz et al. (2011) reported that exposure to particulate matter air pollution during foetal growth was associated with a significant decrease in activated T-helper lymphocytes (CD4+CD25+ T cells) in cord blood, while exposure to NO_2 was associated with significant increase in CD8+ T cells, indicating that maternal exposure to air pollutants during pregnancy can potentially alter the immune competence in the offspring and thereby increase the risk of the child developing allergic diseases and asthma.

Although our knowledge about prenatal exposures to air pollutants as a risk factor for the development of allergic diseases is still evolving, it underscores the importance of further defining the events occurring during the early life period, especially exposure to air pollutants, to determine causal pathways and better strategies for prevention.

Exposure to air pollutants during neonatal and the early childhood period and the risk of allergic diseases

Neonatal periods as well as early childhood are critical periods of development of not only the immune system, but also of the lungs. Exposure to air pollutants during early life may therefore have a significant impact on the risk of developing allergic airways disease. When newborn babies come home, they are usually welcomed with new clothes, new bedding, new upholstery, new carpet and sometimes even new painting of the walls of the home (Fig. 19.2). Little do people realize that these are all important sources of indoor volatile organic compounds that have the potential to increase the risk of allergic diseases. A birth cohort study from Paris has recently reported that carpeted flooring in the child's bedroom, use of cleaning sprays and renovation activities are associated with a significantly increased risk of wheezing among infants (Herr et al. 2012). It has been shown that synthetic pillows not only harbour 7–8 times more allergens than feather pillows, but also emit significantly higher levels of volatile organic compounds. Wooden beds made up of compact wood dust held together by strong adhesives (compressed wood) also emit significant amounts of VOCs (Jinno et al. 2011). Indoor air has therefore been shown to contain 3-times more VOCs than outdoor air (Siebers and Crane 2011). Outdoor air pollution also enters indoors and this has been shown to be significantly associated with the risk of developing asthma (Jung et al. 2012).

In developing countries, there are other sources of indoor air pollutants, such as biomass fuel (wood, animal dung, crop residues) smoke (Fig. 19.3), kerosene fuel smoke, both of which have been associated with increased risk of childhood asthma (Noonan and Ward 2007). Incense stick burning (Fig. 19.4) is common in India, China and many South East Asian countries. It is composed of aromatic plant materials often combined with essential oils, which release fragrant smoke when burned. It is used at homes as a part of religious rituals, for aromatherapy and to mask unpleasant odours. Incense smoke contains various gaseous air pollutants, including carbon monoxide, nitrogen oxides, sulphur oxides and volatile organic compounds. The smoke is made of particles between the sizes of 10 to 500 nm containing polyaromatic hydrocarbons and toxic metals. An earlier study from Taiwan showed that these pollutants were carcinogenic (Lin and Wang 1994). More recently, burning of incense has been shown to be associated with an increased risk of childhood asthma and asthma exacerbations in Taiwan (Wang et al. 2011) and in Oman, Muscat (Al-Rowas et al. 2009). Mosquito coils are mosquito-repelling incense materials, usually shaped into a spiral made from dried paste of pyrethrum powder and are widely used in Asia, Africa and South America (en-wikepedia 2012). Burning of mosquito coils produce smoke particles comprised of

222   Textbook of Allergy for the Clinician

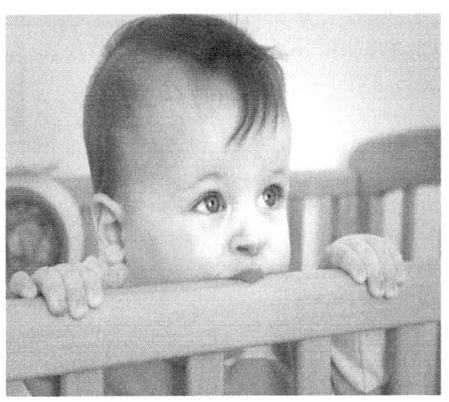

Figure 19.2. Beds made of compressed wood dust, new upholstery, carpets and new wall paints are important sources of volatile organic compounds to new born babies.

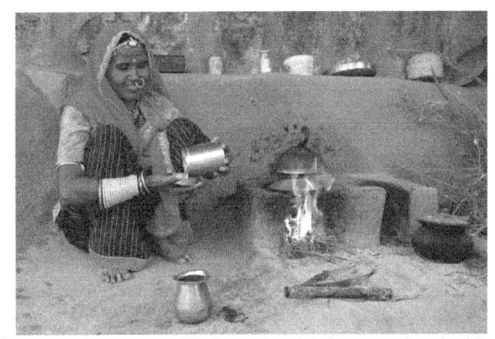

Figure 19.3. Biomass smoke—a major source of indoor air pollution associated with childhood and adult asthma.

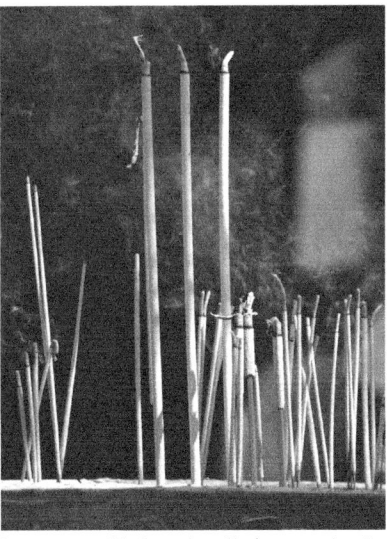

Figure 19.4. Incense stick burning: source of indoor air pollution associated with childhood and adult asthma.

volatile organic compounds and polyaromatic hydrocarbons that have the potential to cause significant respiratory health effects. Burning one mosquito coil produces the same amount of particulate mass of a diameter of 2.5 microns as 75–137 burning cigarettes would, and the emission of formaldehyde can be as high as that released from 51 burning cigarettes (Liu et al. 2003). While some studies have shown an association between burning mosquito coils at home and increased risk of asthma in children (Azizi et al. 1995, Fagbule et al. 1994, Yang et al. 1998), other studies have not confirmed this association (Quah et al. 2000).

Exposure to air pollutants during the childhood period and the risk of allergic diseases

The ISAAC Phase III study conducted in 238 centres across 98 countries in 513,087 school children reported that residential proximity to the main road (less than 50 metres) was associated with significantly higher prevalence of allergic diseases, including asthma, eczema and rhinoconjunctivitis (Brunekreef et al. 2009). This association was especially strong with the truck traffic density, indicating that diesel exhaust was a strong risk factor for allergic diseases. Interestingly, associations between traffic density (Fig. 19.5) and asthma in school children are also found in countries like Sweden, Nigeria and the USA where ambient levels of air pollutants are relatively lower as compared to other countries (Iskander et al. 2012, Mustafa Adetoun et al. 2011, Svendsen et al. 2012). Modest elevations in exposure to some traffic-related air pollutants in Canada, especially during the year of birth have been shown to be associated with new onset asthma at the age of 7 years (Carlsten et al. 2010). Residential proximity has also been shown to be inversely associated with levels of serum IgE (Patel et al. 2010). Perez et al studied the burden of asthma attributable to proximity to a main road in Los Angeles county of the US and estimated that 27,100 cases of childhood asthma (8% of total) were at least attributable to pollution associated with residential location within 75 metres from the major road (Perez et al. 2009). This study underscores the relatively unappreciated public health consequences of air pollution in areas with dense traffic corridors. Whilst ambient levels of air pollutants affecting mucosal airways diseases (e.g., asthma, allergic rhinitis) are not surprising, the fact that they can worsen allergic skin diseases also seems amazing (Song et al. 2011).

Hospital admissions for childhood asthma in Copenhagen have been reported to be positively associated in a dose-dependent manner with ambient levels of oxides of nitrogen (OR: 1.11; CI: 1.05-1.17), nitrogen dioxide (OR: 1.10; CI: 1.04-1.16), PM10 (OR: 1.07; CI: 1.03-1.12) and PM2.5 (OR: 1.09;

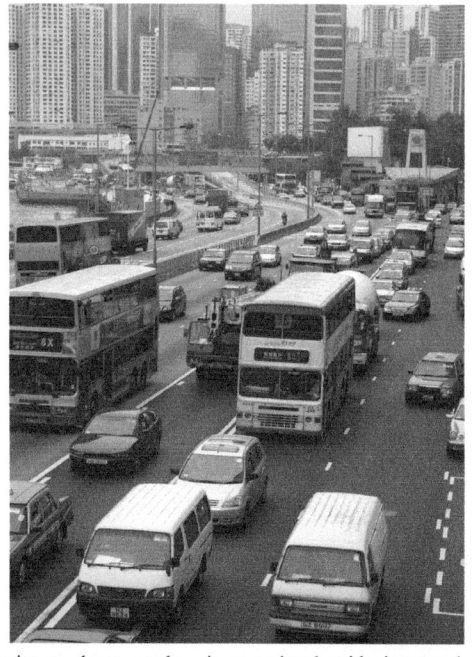

Figure 19.5. Residential proximity to busy roads is associated with increased prevalence of allergic asthma, rhinoconjunctivitis and eczema Picture: Wei Ming/Shutterstock.com.

CI: 1.04-1,13) (Iskander et al. 2012). Similar observations have also been reported from Perth, Australia (Cook et al. 2011), (Pereira et al. 2010) and Athens, Greece (Nastos et al. 2010).

We measured the levels of different gaseous air pollutants while travelling through three different modes of transport in the city of Pune in India, viz: motorcycle, autorickshaw and public transport bus. Figure 19.6 shows the minute-by-minute personal exposure levels to CO and SO_2, two common vehicular air pollutants while travelling by the three modes of transport. Travelling by autorickshaw and motorcycle were associated with the highest exposures to air pollutants, levels which were several times higher than the safety limits recommended by the World Health Organisation. Even travelling by bus, which was associated with the lowest exposures to CO, was higher than the recommended WHO safety standards. Children who travel to school by motorcycles and autorickshaws especially in developing countries are therefore exposed regularly to very high levels of ambient air pollutants, which may have significant adverse effects on their respiratory health.

The number of motor vehicles has increased exponentially over the last 2–3 decades worldwide. According to a report from Ward's Auto, the global number of cars exceeded 1 billion in 2010, which jumped from 980 million the year before (Sousanis 2011). This has led to growing and very high levels of vehicular air pollutants, both gaseous as well as particulate matter. Amongst all the motor vehicular air pollutants, diesel exhaust has been the most widely studied, especially because it is composed of tiny particles that are less than 100 nm in diameter and are made up of a carbon core adsorbed onto which are several thousand polyaromatic hydrocarbons, volatile organic compounds and toxic metals. Earlier it was reported by us that even 1-hour exposure to diesel exhaust at levels commonly encountered on roadsides of some of the most populated cities in the world, produces a systemic as well as bronchial cellular and mediator inflammatory response. Neutrophil, lymphocyte and mast cell numbers increase in the bronchial mucosa and this is accompanied by increased levels of histamine in the bronchial wash (Salvi et al. 1999) (Fig. 19.7). These effects are largely driven by oxidative stress (Laumbach and Kippen 2010), which also increases bronchial hyper responsiveness in asthmatic subjects (Ristovski et al. 2012). Administration of house dust mite allergens with diesel exhaust particles into dust mite sensitive human subjects, increases nasal histamine levels by 3-fold compared with those after house dust mite alone, and only 20% of the amount of intranasal dust mite normally required resulted in a symptomatic response (Diaz-Sanchez et al. 1999).

Diesel exhaust particles-induced oxidative stress and the resultant inflammation can be reduced by antioxidants such as N-acetyl cysteine (Li et al. 2010). It was earlier shown by us that bus drivers from India show high levels of lung oxidative stress and that administering N-acetyl cysteine (600 mg twice a

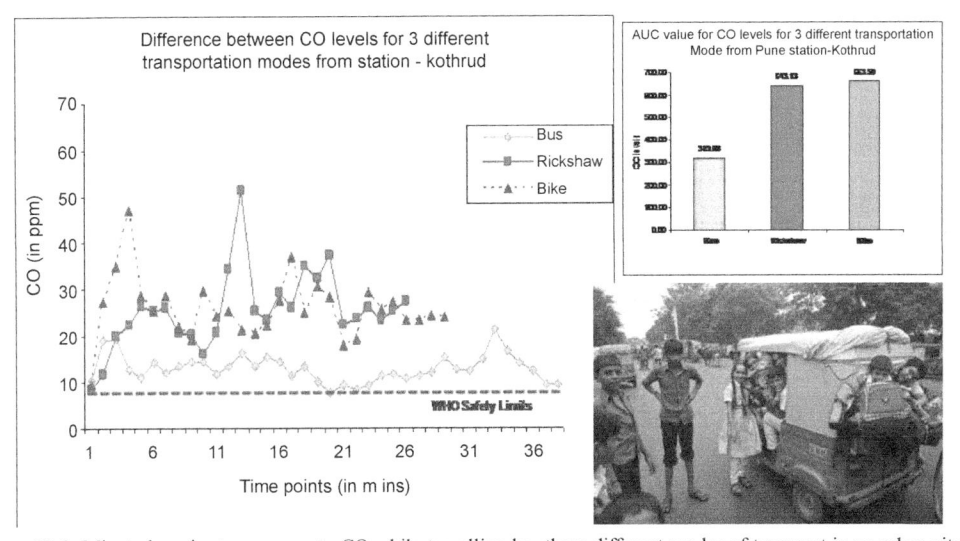

Figure 19.6. Minute by minute exposure to CO while travelling by there different modes of transport in an urban city in India. The dotted line is the WHO safety limit.

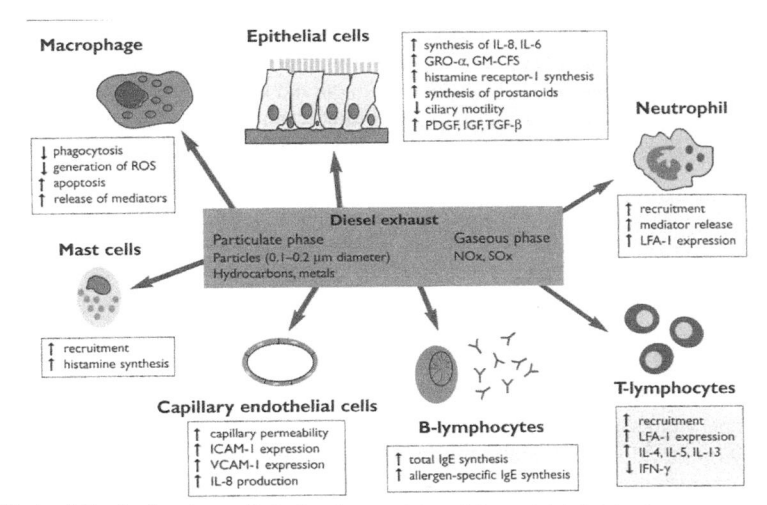

Figure 19.7. Effects of diesel exhaust on cells in the airways. Adapted from: Salvi S. Diesel Fumes and asthma: is there a link? The Asthma Journal; Mar 2002; 7(1): 15–21.

day), an anti oxidant for 4 weeks, reduces lung oxidative stress and also improves lung function (Brashier et al. 2009).

When exposed to Diesel Exhaust Particles (DEPs), alveolar macrophages as well as human bronchial epithelial cells actively phagocytose them, and this is followed by increased productions of the pro-inflammatory cytokines such as IL-6, IL-8 and GM-CSF (Salvi et al. 2000). Several lines of evidence suggest an important role for chemokines, such as IL-8 in the pathogenesis of chronic allergic airways disease. In addition to producing an acute cellular and mediator inflammatory response in the lungs, several studies have also demonstrated a role for diesel exhaust in enhancing the allergic inflammatory response (Fig. 19.6). Nasal and bronchial hyper responsiveness have been described as characteristic features of allergic rhinitis and bronchial asthma. DEPs have been shown to enhance airway hyper responsiveness via the up-regulation of the expression of histamine H1 receptor mRNA associated with enhanced effects of histamine on cytokine gene production (Salvi et al. 1999). Acting via H1 receptors, histamine increases epithelial and capillary endothelial permeability, mucus secretion, airway hyper responsiveness, smooth muscle contraction and also enhances mediator and cytokine release. Diesel exhaust particles have been shown to increase allergen-specific IgE levels by up to 50-times, but more importantly, also helps in development of new allergen-specific IgEs[1] (Takenaka et al. 1995), is therefore not surprising that pollen becomes more allergenic when they grow in an urban environment (Bryce et al. 2010).

Air pollution and allergies in the elderly

Air pollution is a health concern for everyone, but even more so for the elderly. Several factors contribute to this increased vulnerability, viz: longer life spent in the polluted air, weakening of the immune system with ageing and presence of underlying co-morbid conditions that are associated with increased age. Epidemiologic studies report associations between particulate matter air pollution and cardiopulmonary morbidity and mortality in the elderly. Although the underlying pathophysiologic mechanisms remain unclear, it has been hypothesized that altered autonomic function and pulmonary/systemic inflammation may play a role. Pope et al explored the effects of ambient air pollution on autonomic function measured by changes in Heart Rate Variability (HRV) and blood markers of inflammation in 88 elderly subjects and reported that exposure to PM2.5 may be one of multiple factors that influence heart rate variability and C-reactive proteins (Pope et al. 2004). Saldiva et al. have demonstrated that ambient PM10 levels are significantly and positively associated with daily mortality of the elderly. An increase in PM10 levels by 100 μg/m3 was associated with a 13% increase in overall mortality (Saldiva et al. 1995). A study done on 38,595 elderly subjects from India indicates that elderly men and women living in households using biomass fuels have a significantly higher prevalence of asthma than do those living in households using cleaner fuels [OR: 1.59 (1.30-1.94)] (Mishra 2003). The mechanisms of these harmful effects remain the same as discussed earlier. Exposures result in formation of reactive oxygen species, which in turn induce oxidative stress in the lungs that incites a powerful cellular and mediator inflammatory response, which spills into the systemic circulation and causes harmful effects in other body organs (Kelly 2003).

Air pollution and epigenetic changes

Epigenetics refers to changes in the genome that are not coded by the genomic sequence itself, but ultimately affect the expression of gene transcripts, and determine potentially heritable changes in gene expression. Changes that occur in the 'epigene' due to ageing, environmental factors, dietary factors or drugs can be transmitted for up to two subsequent generations without any alteration in the underlying genetic sequence. For example, transmission of asthma risk after maternal exposure to environmental tobacco smoke can continue across two generations (Li et al. 2005). The epigenome is an important target of environment-induced modification and can serve as an interface between the inherited genome and dynamic environment. The molecular mechanisms by which epigenetic changes are produced are: DNA methylation, posttranslational histone modification, histone variation, chromatin remodelling and non-coding RNA (Hong et al. 2012). These changes are usually implicated in cancer and increasingly associated with other common, chronic diseases affecting the heart and lungs (Madrigono et al. 2011). Epigenetic changes can occur prenatally, perinatally and later in life during developmental stages with unique susceptibility to the effects of environmental exposures. There is evolving evidence to suggest that exposure to air pollutants not only increases the risk of current allergic diseases, but that this risk can also be transmitted to subsequent generations. A six-month study of elderly men from Boston found that DNA methylation was reduced after exposures to higher levels of sulphates and black carbon (Madrigono et al. 2011). Human airway epithelial cells exposed to PM10 or diesel exhaust particles induce a global increase in histone H4 acetylation, which can increase the expression of the allergic pro-inflammatory gene IL-8. These epigenetic changes are mediated at least in part by oxidative stress because thiol anti-oxidant inhibition by N-acetyl cysteine ameliorated the effects of PM10 (Gilmour et al. 2003). Silveyra and Floros (2012) reviewed the recent findings on epigenetics and air pollution and discussed the epigenetic mechanisms affecting the expression of the two SP-A (surfactant proteins) genes and their variants by environmental challenges and proposed that surfactant proteins play a central role in pulmonary host defence by mediating pathogen clearance, modulating allergic responses and facilitating the resolution of lung inflammation.

Pollutants can affect the lung by altering its immune response and airway inflammation. Susceptibility to air pollutants differs among individuals, as exemplified by several diseases and conditions (e.g., asthma) in which both genetic and non-genetic factors seem to play a role in the individual response to ambient air pollution. In general, DNA methyltransferases are responsible for maintaining the methylation pattern from parental to daughter DNA strands upon cell division, and most cells have their epigenetic marks fixed when they differentiate or exit the cell cycle. However, in certain situations such as disease, or in normal development, these epigenetic marks are removed and re-established in a process called 'reprogramming'. Of all the epigenetic modifications mentioned above, DNA methylation holds a higher potential of being transmitted through generations, despite the reprogramming events mentioned.

Pollutants may differentially affect by epigenetic changes or other mechanisms, the function and/or regulation of different variants of innate immunity. In turn, due to these differences in their regulation and/or function, innate immune molecules may differentially 'set the ball rolling' as to who may be at disease risk and at what level of risk (Silveyra and Floros 2012). Identification of critical epigenetic marks associated with the development of allergic diseases and influenced by specific environmental factors at certain points, in utero or postnatally, would allow one to advise patients on limiting harmful exposures during the critical windows when these environmental factors have the strongest influence on the development of disease. Understanding the complex interactions between in utero exposures and epigenetic vulnerability will provide insight into future interventions for subjects at risk of allergic asthma and might lead to prevention of this disease altogether (Yang and Swartz 2012).

Prevention and treatment

Collectively, the knowledge available on the epidemiology and mechanisms of how air pollution impacts the burden of allergic diseases, leaves one with no specific antidote against air pollution and its harmful effects, but to manage this health problem at a broader level by reducing exposures, advocating policy changes and symptomatic management of the cases.

(I) Reduce Exposure

Despite the best intentions and efforts to reduce outdoor air pollution levels by most governments, outdoor air pollution levels are unlikely to reduce substantially in the near future. Likewise, occupational exposures and the use of biomass fuel and other indoor air pollutant sources are mostly not by choice but by lifestyle and financial compulsions. Therefore, advising patients to avoid the sources of exposures may not be the best option available to the healthcare providers. The only options at hand then are to reduce personal exposures and to decrease susceptibility. Patients with asthma and other allergic diseases need to be particularly educated to avoid high level exposures and to avoid outdoor activities during pollution advisories. They should be told to reduce outdoor activities when the air quality index is in the unhealthy range, increase peak flow checks during periods with poor air quality and exercise away from main roads. It is advisable to educate patients on good asthma control and the importance of compliance to maintenance therapy to avoid increased chances of suffering a pollution triggered exacerbation.

As children are most susceptible to the harmful effects of air pollutants as discussed earlier, attempts should be made to reduce maternal exposures during pregnancy and later during the growth phase of children. When new schools are being designed, they should be located further away from busy motorways. Encourage children to indulge in sports and physical activities involving running, exercise etc may be helpful in supporting good lung growth during initial years of life and lung development.

(II) Strengthen antioxidant defence

Antioxidant supplementation: The harmful effects of ambient air pollutants become pronounced when the antioxidant defence mechanism becomes weak. Supplementation with antioxidants may therefore strengthen defence mechanisms and reduce the harmful effects. More recently it was reported by us that supplementing bus drivers who are chronically exposed to high levels of vehicular air pollutants in India, with 1200 mg N-acetylcysteine per day significantly reduced lung oxidative stress and improved lung function parameters (Brashier et al. 2009). Preliminary evidence suggests that dietary supplementation with Sulforaphene, a potent inducer of antioxidant enzymes reduces inflammatory responses, especially for those exposed to diesel exhaust particles and therefore offers promise as an air pollution chemoprotective agent. Sulforaphene is naturally produced by cruciferous vegetables (vegetable that have cross-shaped petals), and include Brussels sprout, turnip, cabbage, broccoli and cauliflower among others.

Vitamin Supplementation: Lung lining fluid ascorbic acid (Vitamin C) and α-tocopherol (Vitamin E) concentrations are low in patients with mild asthma even though blood levels are normal or increased. There is evidence to support that Vitamin A (retinol) and its metabolite, retinoic acid, called natural retinoids, are major factors involved in differentiation and in maturation of the lungs in the perinatal period. Supplements with Vitamins C and A especially in high doses have shown some beneficial effects on small airways function in asthmatics exposed to the ozone, who inherently synthesize low levels of glutathione. Results of animal studies suggest that supplementations with Vitamins C and E modulates the pulmonary response to exposure to photo-oxidants, such as O3 or NO2 and that Vitamin C, uric acid and glutathione located in the respiratory tract lining fluid are consumed on exposure to O3 and NO2. However more evidence is required before recommending regular use of antioxidant supplements, but in the mean time it seems prudent to at least encourage vulnerable individuals to eat vegetables and fruits that are rich in antioxidants. Individuals who are most likely to benefit from regular antioxidant supplementation are those who have genetic defects in enzymes that are associated with reduced antioxidant production (e.g., GSTM1 null, GSTP1, NQO1). There is an urgent research need to develop

(III) Help reduce the burden of ambient air pollution

Advocate for policy change: A study in the United States has estimated that if ambient air pollution levels were reduced to match levels in the cleanest community, then annual asthma related emergency department visits and hospitalization rates would decrease from 22 to 6%, prevalence of bronchitis would decrease from 40 to 20%, asthma related school absenteeism would reduce by two thirds and new cases of asthma among the most active children living in polluted communities would decrease by 75%. With the realization that ambient levels of air pollutants in most cities and towns worldwide are associated with a significant impact on the health of the lungs, it is imperative to take appropriate steps to reduce the levels of key pollutants, such as particulate matter, oxides of nitrogen, sulphur dioxide and ozone in the ambient air.

Physicians and health care providers should advocate and educate governmental officials and policy makers and make them realize that the health of people should be at the top of the list of competing priorities for policy making. This can be achieved by good urban planning measures, innovative traffic management strategies, supporting technology advancements to use cleaner fuels and cleaner engines and enforcing strict legislative norms for industrial emissions.

Physicians should also advocate for the government to set air quality standards to protect the health of their citizens. The Government should routinely monitor important ambient air pollutants and the levels of these should be informed to the public when the levels are above the safety limits, so that necessary preventive measures could be advised to individuals who are susceptible to the harmful effects of air pollutants.

Conclusion and recommendation

Air pollution is one of the most important environmental factors associated with increased prevalence and worsening of allergic diseases. Exposure to air pollution starts from the womb and continues up to the tomb. Foetal, neonatal and post neonatal exposures to several air pollutants has been shown to be associated with increased risk of developing allergic diseases. This seems to be primarily mediated by oxidative stress-induced changes in the immune regulatory system as well as epigenetic changes. Further exposures to air pollutants both from indoor as well as outdoor sources during early and late childhood further drive the risk of development of allergic diseases. Exposures to motor vehicular pollutants and in particular, diesel exhaust have been shown to drive a whole host inflammatory changes that increase susceptibility to the development of allergic diseases. Supplementation with antioxidants has shown some protective role, although more research is required to substantiate this. Creating public awareness will be the most important intervention that will help not only in making people realize the harmful effects of air pollutants, but will also help develop preventative strategies at local, regional and national levels.

References

Al-Rawas OA, Al-Maniri AA, Al-Riyami BM. Home exposure to Arabian incense (bakhour) and asthma symptoms in children: a community survey in two regions in Oman. BMC Pulm Med 2009; 9: 23.

Azizi BH, Zulfkifli HI, Kasim S. Indoor air pollution and asthma in hospitalised children in a tropical environment. Journal of Asthma 1995; 32: 413–418.

Biaz N. Maternal exposure to air pollution before and during pregnancy related to changes in newborn's cord blood lymphocyte subpopulations. The EDEN study cohort. BMC Pregnancy and Childbirth 2011; doi: 10.1186/1471-2393-11-87.

Body Burden—The pollution in newborns. A benchmark investigation of industrial chemicals, pollutants and pesticides in umbilical cord blood. Environmental Working Group, July 14, 2005. Accessed from http://www.ewg.org/reports/bodyburden2/execsumm.php on 5th January 2010.

Brashier B, Ravindaran L, Kapoor S, Deshpande PK, Ghongane B, Madas S. Four weeks of treatment with n-acetyl cysteine (NAC) (1200 mg/day) reduces lung oxidative stress and improves lung function in moderate-to-severe COPD subjects. European Respiratory Society Congress 2009; Abstract 2016.

Brunekreef B, Stewart AW, Anderson HR, Lai CKW, Strachan DP, Pearce NE. The ISAAC phase three study group: self reported truck traffic in street of residence and symptoms of asthma and allergic disease: a global relationship in ISAAC phase three. Environ Health Perspect 2009; 117: 1791–1798.

Bryce M, Drews O, Schenk MF, Menzel A, Estrella N, Weichenmeier I, et al. Impact of urbanization on the proteome of birch pollen and its chemotactic activity on human granulocytes. Int Arch Allergy Immunol 2010; 151: 46–55.

Carlsten C, Dybuncio A, Becker A, Chan-Yeung M, Brauer M. Traffic-related air pollution and incident asthma in a high-risk birth cohort. Occup Environ Med 2010.

Cook AG, deVos AJ, Pereira G, Jardine A, Weinstein P. Use of a total traffic count metric to investigate the impact of roadways on asthma severity: a case-control study. Environ Health 2011 Jun 2; 10: 52.

Diaz-Sanchez D, Garcia MP, Wang M, Jyrala M, Saxon A. Nasal challenge with diesel exhaust particles can induce sensitization to a neoallergen in the human mucosa. J Allergy Clin Immunol 1999; 104: 1183–1188.

Fagbule D, Parakoyi DB, Spiegel R. Acute respiratory infections in Nigerian children: prospective cohort study of incidence and case management. Journal of Tropical Pediatrics 1994; 40: 279–84.

Guo Y, Huo X, Wu K, Liu J, Zhang Y, Xu X. Carcinogenic polycyclic aromatic hydrocarbons in umbilical cord blood of human neonates from Guiyu, China. Sci Total Environ 2012 Jun; 15(427-428): 35–40. Epub 2012 Apr 28.

Gilmour PS, Rahman I, Donaldson K, MacNee W. Histone acetylation regulates epithelial IL-8 release mediated by oxidative stress from environmental particles. Am J Physiol Lung Cell Mol Physiol 2003; 284: L533–L540.

Herr M, Just J, Nikasinovic L, Foucault C, Le Marec AM, Giordanella JP, et al. Influence of host and environmental factors on wheezing severity in infants: findings from the PARIS birth cohort. Clin Exp Allergy 2012 Feb; 42(2): 275–83. doi: 10.1111/j.1365-2222.2011.03933.x.

Hong Ji, Gurjit K. Khurana Hershey. Genetic and epigenetic influence on the response to environmental particulate matter. Journal of Allergy and Clinical Immunology 2012 Jan; 129(1): 33–41.

Iskandar A, Andersen ZJ, Bønnelykke K, Ellermann T, Andersen KK, Bisgaard H. Coarse and fine particles but not ultrafine particles in urban air trigger hospital admission for asthma in children. Thorax 2012 Mar; 67(3): 252–7.

Jinno H, Tanaka-Kagawa T, Furuta M, Shibatsuji M, Nishimura T. Volatile organic compounds (VOCs) emitted from wood furniture—estimation of emission rate by passive flux sampler. Kokuritsu Iyakuhin Shokuhin Eisei Kenkyusho Hokoku 2011; (129): 86–92.

Jung KH, Hsu SI, Yan B, Moors K, Chillrud SN, Ross J. Childhood exposure to fine particulate matter and black carbon and the development of new wheeze between ages 5 and 7 in an urban prospective cohort. Environ Int 2012 Sep 15; 45: 44–50.

Kelly FJ. Oxidative stress and its role in air pollution and adverse health effects. Occup Environ Med 2003; 60: 612–616.

Latzin P, Frey U, Armann J, Kieninger E, Fuchs O, Röösli M, et al. Exposure to moderate air pollution during late pregnancy and cord blood cytokine secretion in healthy neonates. PLoS One 2011 Aug 3; 6(8): e23130.

Laumbach RJ, Kipen HM. Acute effects of motor vehicle traffic-related air pollution exposures on measures of oxidative stress in human airways. Ann N Y Acad Sci 2010; 1203: 107–112.

Li YF, Langholz B, Salam MT, Gilliland FD. Maternal and grandmaternal smoking patterns are associated with early childhood asthma. Chest 2005; 127: 1232–1241.

Li YJ, Takizawa H, Kawada T. Role of oxidative stresses induced by diesel exhaust particles in airway inflammation, allergy and asthma: their potential as a target of chemoprevention. Inflammation and Allergy 2010; 9(4): 300–305.

Lin JM, Wang LH. Gaseous aliphatic aldehydes in Chinese incense smoke. Bulletin of Environmental Contamination and Toxicology 1994–09; 53(3): 374–381.

Liu Weili, Zhang Junfeng, Hashim Jamal H, Jalaludin Juliana, Hashim Zailina, Goldstein Bernard D. Mosquito coil emissions and health implications. Environmental Health Perspectives 2003 Sep; 111(12): 1454–1460.

Madrigano J, Baccarelli A, Mittleman MA, Wright RO, Sparrow D, Vokonas PS, et al. Epigenetic changes seen in elderly men after prolonged. Air Pollution Exposure Apr 25, 2011.

Madrigano J, Baccarelli A, Mittleman MA, Wright RO, Sparrow D, Vokonas PS, et al. Prolonged exposure to particulate pollution, genes associated with glutathione pathways, and DNA methylation in a cohort of older men. Environ Health Perspect 2011 Jul 1; 119(7): 977–82.

Mishra V. Indoor air pollution from biomass combustion and prevalence of asthma in the elderly. Environ Health Perspect 2003; 111: 71–77.

Miyake Y, Tanaka K, Fujiwara H, Mitani Y, Ikemi H, Sasaki S, et al. Residential proximity to main roads during pregnancy and the risk of allergic disorders in Japanese infants: the Osaka Maternal and Child Health Study. Pediatr Allergy Immunol 2010 Feb; 21(1 Pt 1): 22–8. Epub 2009 Sep 26.

Miyake Y, Tanaka K, Fujiwara H, Mitani Y, Ikemi H, Sasaki S, et al. Residential proximity to main roads during pregnancy and the risk of allergic disorders in Japanese infants: the Osaka Maternal and Child Health Study. Pediatric allergy and immunology. 2010 Feb; 21(1-Part-I): 22–8.

Mortimer K, Neugebauer R, Lurmann F, Alcorn S, Balmes J, Tager I. Early-lifetime exposure to air pollution and allergic sensitization in children with asthma. J Asthma 2008 Dec; 45(10): 874–81.

Mustapha BA, Blangiardo M, Briggs DJ, Hansell AL. Traffic air pollution and other risk factors for respiratory illness in schoolchildren in the niger-delta region of nigeria. Environ Health Perspect 2011 Oct; 119(10): 1478–82.

Nastos PT, Paliatsos AG, Anthracopoulos MB, Roma ES, Priftis KN. Outdoor particulate matter and childhood asthma admissions in Athens, Greece: a time-series study. Environ Health 2010; 9(45): http://dx.doi.org/10.1186/1476-069X-9-45.

Noonan CW, Ward TJ. Environmental tobacco smoke, woodstove heating and risk of asthma symptoms. J Asthma 2007; 44(9): 735–8.
Patel MM, Chillrud SN, Correa JC, Hazi Y, Feinberg M, KC D, et al. Traffic-related particulate matter and acute respiratory symptoms among New York City area adolescents. Environ Health Perspect 2010; 118: 1338–1343.
Pereira G, Cook A, De Vos AJ, Holman CD. A case-crossover analysis of traffic-related air pollution and emergency department presentations for asthma in Perth, Western Australia. Med J August 2010; 193: 511–514.
Perera F, Jedrychowski W, Rauh V, Whyatt RM. Molecular epidemiologic research on the effects of environmental pollutants on the fetus. Environ Health Perspect 1999; 107(suppl 3): 451–460.
Perera F, Li TY, Lin C, Tang D. Effects of prenatal polycyclic aromatic hydrocarbon exposure and environmental tobacco smoke on child IQ in a Chinese cohort. Environ Res 2012 Apr; 114: 40–6. Epub 2012 Mar 2.
Perez L, Künzli N, Avol E, Hricko AM, Lurmann F, Nicholas E, et al. Global goods movement and the local burden of childhood asthma in southern California. Am J Public Health 2009; 99(S3): S622–S628.
Peters JL, Suglia SF, Platts-Mills TAE, Hosen J, Gold DR, Wright RJ. Relationships among prenatal aeroallergen exposure and maternal and cord blood IgE: Project ACCESS J Allergy Clin Immunol 2009; 123: 1041–1046.
Pope 3rd CA, Hansen ML, Long RW, Nielsen KR, Eatough NL, Wilson WE, et al. Ambient particulate air pollution, heart rate variability, and blood markers of inflammation in a panel of elderly subjects. Environ Health Perspect 2004 Mar; 112(3): 339–45.
Privalova LI, Kosheleva AA, Brezgina SV. Analysis of time series to establish the relationship of respiratory symptomatology in children to ambient air pollution fluctuations. Gig Sanit 2007 May–Jun; (3): 64–7.
Proietti Elena, Martin Röösli, Urs Frey, Philipp Latzin. Air pollution during pregnancy and neonatal outcome: A review. Journal of Aerosol Medicine and Pulmonary Drug Delivery; ahead of print. doi:10.1089/jamp.2011.0932.
Quah BS, Mazidah AR, Simpson H. Risk factors for wheeze in the last 12 months in preschool children. Asia Pac J Allergy Immunol 2000; 18: 73–79.
Ristovski ZD, Miljevic B, Surawski NC, Morawska L, Fong KM, Goh F, et al. Respiratory health effects of diesel particulate matter. Respirology 2012 Feb; 17(2): 201–12.
Saldiva PH, Pope CA, 3rd, Schwartz J, Dockery DW, Lichtenfels AJ, Salge JM, et al. Air pollution and mortality in elderly people: a time-series study in Sao Paulo, Brazil. Arch Environ Health 1995 Mar–Apr; 50(2): 159–163.
Salvi S, Frew AJ, Holgate ST. Is diesel a cause for increasing allergies? Clin Exp Allergy 1999; 29: 4–8.
Salvi S, Blomberg A, Rudell B, Kelly F, Sandstrom T, Holgate ST, et al. Acute inflammatory responses in the airways and peripheral blood after short-term exposure to diesel exhaust in healthy human volunteers. Am J Respir Crit Care Med 1999 Mar 1; 159(3): 702–9.
Salvi SS, Nordenhall C, Blomberg A, Rudell B, Pourazar J, Kelly FJ, et al. Acute exposure to diesel exhaust increases IL-8 and GRO-α production in healthy human airways. Am J Respir Crit Care Med Feb 1; 161(2): 550–7.
Siebers RW, Crane J. Does bedding affect the airway and allergy? Int J Occup Environ Med 2011 Apr; 2(2): 65–75.
Silveyra P, Floros J. Air pollution and epigenetics: effects on SP-A and innate host defence in the lung Swiss Med. Wkly 2012; 142: w13579,b.
Song S, Lee K, Lee YM, Lee JH, Lee SI, Yu SD, et al. Acute health effects of urban fine and ultrafine particles on children with atopic dermatitis. Environ Res 2011; 111: 394–399 S.
Sousanis J. World Vehicle Population Tops 1 Billion Units. Aug. 15, 2011, WardsAuto, information from http://wardsauto.com/ar/world_vehicle_population_110815 accessed on 26.Nov.2012.
Sternthal MJ, Coull BA, Mathilda Chiu YH, Cohen S, Wright RJ. Associations among maternal childhood socioeconomic status, cord blood IgE levels, and repeated wheeze in urban children. J Allergy Clin Immunol 2011; 128: 337–345 e1.
Svendsen ER, Gonzales M, Mukerjee S, Smith L, Ross M, Walsh D, et al. GIS-modeled indicators of traffic-related air pollutants and adverse pulmonary health among children in El Paso, Texas. Am. J Epidemiol 2012 Oct 1; 176(suppl_7): S131–41.
Takenaka H, Zhang K, Diaz-Sanchez D, Tsien A, Saxon A. Enhanced human IgE production results from exposure to the aromatic hydrocarbons from diesel exhaust: direct effects on B-cell IgE production. J Allergy Clin Immunol 1995; 95: 103–115.
Van den Hooven EH, de Kluizenaar Y, Pierik FH, Hofman A, van Ratingen SW, Zandveld PY, et al. Chronic air pollution exposure during pregnancy and maternal and fetal C-reactive protein levels: the Generation R Study. Environ Health Perspect 2012; 120: 746–751.
Wang IJ, Tsai CH, Chen CH, Tung KY, Lee YL. Glutathione S-transferase, incense burning and asthma in children. Eur Respir J 2011 Jun 1; 37(6): 1371–7.
Wen HJ, Chen PC, Chiang TL, Lin SJ, Chuang YL, Guo YL. Predicting risk for early infantile atopic dermatitis by hereditary and environmental factors. Br J Dermatol 2009; 161: 1166–1172.
Wikipedia.org/wiki/Mosquito_coil accessed on 27/11/2012 at 13.15.
Yang CY, Lin MC, Hwang HC. Childhood asthma and the indoor environment in a subtropical area. Chest 1998; 114: 393–397.
Yang IV, Schwartz D. Epigenetic mechanisms and the development of asthma. JACI 2012; 130: 1243–1255.

20

Asthma and COPD
Similarities and Differences

Balamugesh Thangakunam and *Devasahayam J Christopher**

INTRODUCTION

COPD (Chronic Obstructive Pulmonary Disease) is a well know mimic of bronchial asthma, in adults and in practice, it is not uncommon to encounter misdiagnosis in both cases. There are of course similarities between asthma and COPD. Both are chronic diseases with varying degrees of airway inflammation and obstruction. They are associated with excess mucous production and bronchoconstriction, to different degrees. Treatment of both involves the use of bronchodilators. However, eosinophilic asthma is almost always steroid responsive, on the other hand, steroids are indicated only in a subset of severe COPD, and in any case, the benefits are very modest. From the point of view of treatment and prognostication, it is often necessary to differentiate between the two conditions. The frequent questions that are raised are: are they different ends of the spectrum of the same diseases? Is the diagnostic tag really important and will it radically change management or is it just a matter of semantics? These questions have resulted in several interesting pro/con debates, in scientific meetings and these discussions may continue in the future (Kraft 2006, Barnes 2006). One big drawback is that most of the studies in asthma and COPD have stringent entry criteria excluding patients with overlapping features and hence therapeutic interventions are not tested in this sub group.

Definitions

According to Global Initiative for Chronic Obstructive Lung Disease (GOLD) guidelines, COPD, a common preventable and treatable disease, is characterized by persistent airflow limitation that is due to airway and/or alveolar abnormalities usually caused by significant exposure to noxious particles or gases (COPDGold 2019). The course is punctuated by periods of acute symptomatic worsening termed as exacerbations. It is usually associated with significant concomitant chronic diseases which increase its morbidity and mortality (COPDGold 2019). Globally, mortality due to COPD is increasing and at present it has become the fourth leading cause of death (GINAsthma 2011).

Meanwhile, asthma is described by GINA (Global Initiatives for Asthma) as a heterogeneous disease usually characterized by chronic airway inflammation and associated with airway hyper responsiveness (GINAsthma 2019). It is defined by the history of respiratory symptoms such as wheezing, shortness of

---

Department of Pulmonary Medicine, Christian Medical College Hospital, Vellore, India. PIN- 632004.
  Email: drbalamugesh@yahoo.com
* Corresponding author: djchris@cmcvellore.ac.in

breath, tightness of the chest and coughing that vary over time and in intensity, together with variable expiratory air flow limitation (GINAsthma 2019).

Pathophysiology

Asthma is classically considered to be due to eosinophilic inflammation of the airways, which is driven by mast cells and activated T helper CD4 lymphocytes (Virchow et al. 1995). There is IgE mediated inflammation consequent to increased release of cytokines like IL-4, IL-5, IL-13, etc., which cause eosinophilic inflammation and bronchoconstrictor mediators, such as histamine, cysteinyl leukotrienes and prostaglandin D_2 (Uhm et al. 2012, Barnes et al. 1998). However up to 50% of asthma cannot be attributed to eosinophilic inflammation and in some patients neutrophils play a significant role (Gibson 2009). In COPD, the inflammation is characterized by increase in macrophages, neutrophils, dentritic cells and CD8+ lymphocytes (Jeffrey 1998). Neutrophils release elastases and proteases and cause permanent alveolar destruction (Tetley 2005). In a minority of stable COPD patients; eosinophilic inflammation also plays a role during exacerbations (Saha and Brightling 2006). The inflammatory mediator profile in COPD consists of neutrophil chemotactic mediators, such as leukotriene B_4 (LTB_4), CXCL8 (IL-8) and TNF-alpha (Barnes 2004).

The pathological changes in the airway wall are different between asthma and COPD. In asthma there is excess shedding of airway epithelial cells and subepithelial deposition of collagen resulting, in chronic cases, in subepithelial fibrosis. In COPD, the airway epithelium shows squamous metaplasia, hypertrophy of mucosal glands and globlet cell hyperplasia. In COPD, airway smooth muscle hypertrophy and bronchial hyper-vascularity is seen to a lesser degree as compared to asthma. In the emphysema phenotype of COPD, there is typically alveolar destruction which is not found in asthma. However, there is evidence that elastin degradation occurs in asthmatic alveoli; resulting in loss of elastic recoil and 'psuedo-emphysema' pattern (Gelb and Zamel 2000).

Genetic predisposition

The 'Dutch hypothesis' suggested that both asthma and COPD have common genetic origins with environmental factors playing a role in pathogenesis and clinical manifestation (Orie et al. 1961). In asthmatics many Single Nucleotide Polymophisms (SNPs) have been described in genes encoding Th2 cytokines like IL-4, IL-13 and their receptors (Barnes 2006). These are not associated with COPD. In COPD SNPs in genes are responsible for encoding various proteases, antiproteases and antioxidants. The classical genetic predisposition for COPD; alpa-1 antitrypsin deficiency is not associated with atopy or asthma. However, although most SNPs are different in asthma and COPD, there are some that are common to both like the polymorphisms in the promoter region of tumor necrosis factor-alpha (Sakao et al. 2001, Gao et al. 2006). Some novel asthma genes, like ADAM33 and DPP 10, have been associated with COPD as well as asthma (Holgate 2010, van Diemen et al. 2005, Arinir et al. 2004).

Contrary to the 'Dutch hypothesis', Airway Hyper-Responsiveness (AHR) and atopy, which are important determinants of asthma, are not linked to the development of COPD. The prevalence of atopy in COPD is not increased. The AHR, which is found in COPD, is a consequence of airway narrowing and not the cause of it.

Clinical features

Symptoms of asthma and COPD overlap since the airways have a limited range of responses to inflammation irrespective of the cause of the insult. The major differences in clinical features are given in Table 20.1. The onset of symptoms in the majority of asthmatics is during childhood, while in COPD patients; the symptoms usually start after 40 years of age. Patients with COPD usually have continuous symptoms which are progressive despite treatment. Whilst the majority of asthmatics have episodic symptoms, it is important to remember that severe asthma especially in smokers acts like COPD.

Corpulmonale and right heart failure are frequently found in advanced COPD patients and these are rare in asthmatics. Extra-pulmonary manifestations like weight loss, skeletal muscle wasting and

Table 20.1. Asthma and COPD—differences.

	Feature	Asthma	COPD
Clinical features	Age of onset	Childhood/Adolescence	> 40 years
	Smoking history	May be present	Present in majority
	Biomass fuel exposure	May be present	Present in female non-smokers
	Atopic/allergic manifestations	Common	May be present
	Family history	Common	May be present
	Course	Variable	Progressive
	Chronic productive cough	Uncommon	Common
	Breathlessness	Variable	Persistent and progressive
	Nocturnal worsening	Common	Rare
	Significant diurnal variability of symptoms	Common	Uncommon
	Cor-pulmonale & Systemic manifestations	Uncommon	Common
	Co-morbidities	Uncommon	Common
Pulmonary Function Test (PFT)	Spirometry reversibility	Frequently demonstrable	Absent
	Diurnal peak flow variability	Present	Absent
	Diffusing capacity	Normal/increased	Reduced
	TLC, RV/TLC	Normal in stable stage	Increased
	Exhaled NO	Increased	Normal
Pathology	Site of obstruction	Central airways	Peripheral airways
	Alveoli	Normal	Destroyed
	Airway microscopy	Excess airway epithelial cell shedding, basement membrane thickening, sub-epithelial fibrosis, smooth muscle hypertrophy, bronchial hypervascularity	Squamous metaplasia, glandular hypertrophy, globlet cell hyperplasia
	Inflammatory cells	Eosinophils, mast cells, , Activated CD4$^+$ T lymphocytes	Neutrophils, macrophages, Dendritic cells, CD8 lymphocytes
	Cytokines & mediators	IL-4,IL-5, IL-13, Histamine, cysteinyl leukotrienes, PG-D2	Elastses, proteases, LTB4, CXCL8, TNF-alpha

Treatment		Aim	Symptomatic & achieve normal lung function	Symptomatic
		Corticosteroids	Very responsive in the eosinophilic variant. At least a trial of inhaled steroids is indicated in all persistent asthmatics	Less responsive, Indicated only in severe cases/ repeated exacerbation
		Bronchodilators	Second line	First line
		Anticholinergic	Emerging role	Well established role
		Leukotriene antagonists	Well established role	Emerging role
Exacerbation		Role of bacteria	Less important	More important
		CO2 retention	Less common, indicates life threatening exacerbation	Common, particularly during exacerbation
		Role of MgSO4	Established	Not established
		Controlled oxygen therapy for SpO2 88–92%	Not important	Very important

osteoporosis are more common in COPD than asthmatics (Agusti and Faner 2012). This is because COPD is considered a systemic disease with release of pro-inflammatory cytokines and mediators into the systemic circulation. Co-morbidities like cardiovascular disease, depression and metabolic syndrome are more common in COPD patients and these are partly related to their advanced age and smoking status (Nussbaumer-Ochsner and Rabe 2011). Due to their effect on mortality, they should be actively looked for in COPD patients and treated, to the extent possible. COPD patients are at increased risk of lung cancer; which is related to smoking, genetic susceptibility, chronic inflammation and impaired clearance of carcinogens (De Torres et al 2011, Stavem et al. 2005).

Pulmonary function testing

Although both conditions are characterized by airflow obstruction there are important differences between the two. In both, there is airway narrowing due to mucosal inflammation and hyper-secretion. But unlike in asthma, in COPD, the peripheral airways play an important role in obstruction. This is due to the dynamic collapse of distal airways during expiration, due to destruction of surrounding alveoli and then loss of alveolar tethering (Kurosawa and Kohzuki 2004). In asthma, central airways are the site of predominant obstruction although in severe cases; peripheral airways are also involved.

Diurnal peak flow monitoring is an important tool in diagnosing and monitoring asthma. However its role in COPD is limited, since it is not a good tool for the assessment of small airway disorders.

Bronchodilator response: Asthma in early stages is associated with good response to bronchodilators and this property is often used to differentiate it from COPD. However in severe asthmatics, airway wall thickening due to airway remodeling leads to fixed airway obstruction. In COPD, the bronchodilator response is relatively reduced; but is a continuous variable that is normally distributed (Calverley et al. 2003). In COPD, there is no correlation of bronchodilator response to a smoking status, atopy, use of inhaled corticosteroids, rate of decline of FEV1 or exacerbation rate. Even if there is no bronchodilator reversibility as demonstrated by change in FEV1, a COPD patient may have improvement in symptoms and exercise capacity due to reduction in air trapping and dynamic hyperinflation (Berger and Smith 1988, Hay et al. 1992). Mannino and colleagues found that bronchodilator reversibility testing afforded only 44% sensitivity and 72% specificity in distinguishing asthma from COPD (Mannino et al. 2000). Typical spirometry and flow-volume loops of asthma and COPD subjects are given in Figs 20.1 and 20.2.

In stable COPD; Total Lung Capacity (TLC) is increased due to hyperinflation. There is increase in the Residual Volume (RV), and as a result of both these, there is an increase in RV/TLC ratio. This results in decrease in Inspiratory Capacity (IC), which is a good measure of air trapping and exercise capacity in COPD (O'Donnel et al. 2004). In asthmatics, normally RV and TLC may be increased only during exacerbations.

Diffusing capacity (DLCO) is usually normal in asthma, but it may increase due to augmented blood volume in the capillary bed; due to lung congestion (Mishima 2009). It is however reduced in COPD, due to alveolar destruction and co-existing pulmonary hypertension. DLCO, although thought to be the single best test to differentiate between asthma and COPD, is inadequate with a sensitivity of 77% and specificity of 71% in discriminating between them (Magnussen et al. 1998). Decreased elastic recoil or increased compliance is typical of COPD and is normal in asthma. Exhaled Nitric Oxide (NO), which

Figure 20.1a. Typical spirometry of an asthmatic patient showing significant bronchodilator reversibility.

	Predicted	Pre bronchodilator Lit. (% predicted)	Post bronchodilator	% improvement after bronchodilator
FVC (Lit)	3.57	2.12 (59.5%)	3.10	46.2
FEV 1(Lit)	2.84	1.05 (36.9%)	2.05	95.5
FEV1/FVC (%)		49.47		

The spirometry showed severe obstruction with FEV1/FVC ration of 49.47%. The pre-brochodilator (95.5% improvement) FEV1 was reduced to 1.05 litres (36.9% of predicted). This improved to 2.05 lit after bronchodilator (95.5%) improvement.

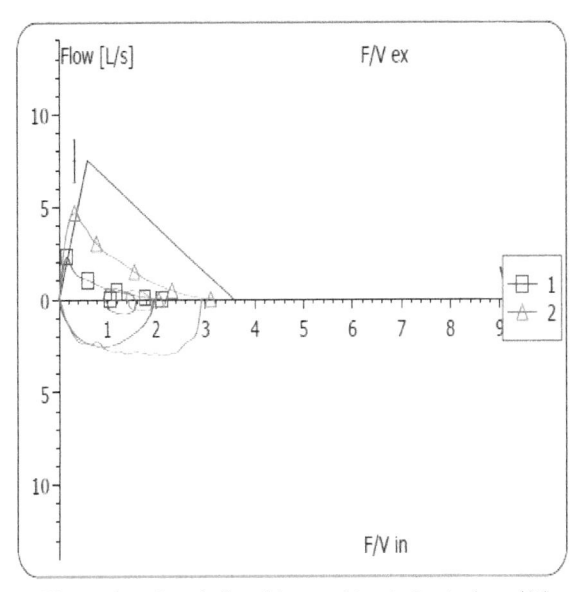

Figure 20.1b. Flow-volume loop before (blue graph) and after (red graph) bronchodilator.

Figure 20.2a: Typical spirometry of a patient with COPD.

	Predicted	Pre bronchodilator Lit. (% predicted)	Post bronchodilator	% improvement after bronchodilator
FVC (Lit)	1.90	1.40 (73.9%)	1.44	2.6
FEV 1(Lit)	1.51	0.48 (31.5%)	0.50	4.1
FEV1/FVC (%)		33.9		

The spirometry showed severe obstruction with FEV1/FVC ration of 33.9%. The pre-brochodilator (4.1% improvement) FEV1 was reduced to 0.48 litres (31.5% of predicted). This improved to 0.50 lit. after bronchodilator (4.1%) improvement. This shows no significant bronchodilator reversibility which is typical of COPD.

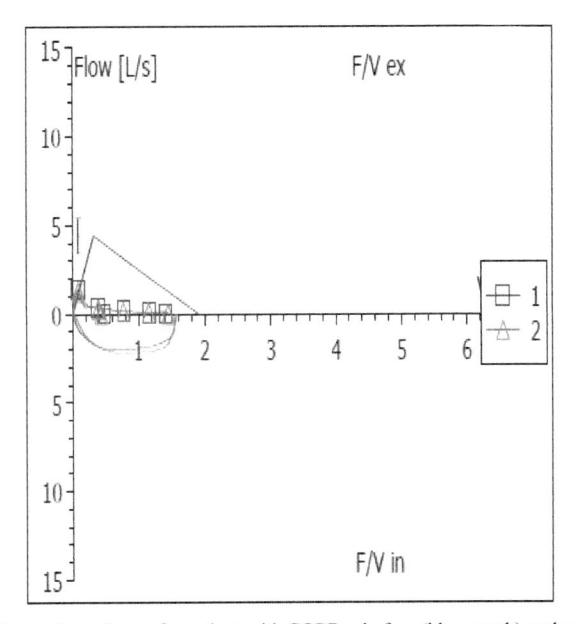

Figure 20.2. Flow volume loop of a patient with COPD—before (blue graph) and after (red graph).

is a marker of eosinophilic inflammation, is more often increased in asthmatics as compared to COPD patients.

Treatment

One of the goals of treatment in asthma is to minimize persistent airflow limitation (GINAsthma 2011). In COPD, normalization of pulmonary function is not possible and the goal is adequate symptom control (COPDGold 2019). Inflammation in asthma is usually steroid responsive; hence inhaled steroids are the cornerstone of treatment for all stages of persistent asthma-except mild intermittent asthma (Berger and Smith 1988). Regular bronchodilators are prescribed only when symptoms are not controlled with inhaled corticosteroids. In COPD, the inflammation is not so steroid responsive, hence the first line of treatment is usually an inhaled bronchodilator. However, there is evidence of usefulness of inhaled steroids in moderate to very severe COPD and in those with recurrent exacerbations (COPDGold 2019). Regular treatment with inhaled steroids in such patients; improves symptoms, lung function and quality of life and reduces the frequency of exacerbations (Jones 2003, Mahler et al. 2002, Szafranski et al. 2003). However, they may not prevent the long-term decline in lung function or improve mortality (Drummond et al. 2008).

Anticholinegics (Ipratropium and Tiotropium), by blocking the acetycholine effect on muscarinic receptors have an established role in the management COPD. Tiotropium improves symptoms, health status, reduces exacerbations and related hospitalizations (Barr et al. 2005). In stable asthma, the role of anticholinergics is less defined, because the cholinergic mechanism has a lesser role in bronchoconstriction. However, there is now an established role for Tiotropium as an add on therapy in severe asthma (Kerstjens et al. 2011, Peters et al. 2010).

Cysteinyl leukotriene antagonists have a well-established role in the management of asthma, which is uncontrolled on inhaled corticosteroids. Its role in management of COPD is less well defined, although there is some evidence to support its use (Rubinstein et al. 2004). Theophyllines are recommended in both conditions, when the symptoms are not controlled with inhaled medications. The Center for Disease Control and Prevention has recommended seasonal influenza vaccination and pneumococcal vaccination in both COPD and asthma (COPDGold 2019, Magnussen et al. 1998, CDC 2012).

Targeting the specific inflammatory pathway through various biological agents has a definitive role in the management of severe asthma, but such treatment is not available for COPD. Bronchial thermoplasty is a novel method of reducing the thickness of bronchial smooth muscle and has been found to be helpful in a subset of asthmatics. In severe COPD bronchoscopic treatments are available to reduce the volume of hyperinflated emphysematous lobes.

Exacerbations

Exacerbations of asthma and COPD are important adverse events in the natural history of the disease, which adversely affects the health status. Most of the interventional studies consider prevention of exacerbations as an important outcome (Pauwels 2004). In both conditions, exacerbations are considered as sustained worsening of the symptoms, mostly requiring treatment with systemic steroids. In both, there can be a preponderance of eosinophilic inflammation in the airways during the episode (Green et al. 2002, Saetta et al. 1994).

While there is some evidence that frequent exacerbations result in greater decline in the lung function in COPD patients, such a decline has not so far been described for asthma (Donaldson et al. 2002).

Viral infections, cigarette smoke and air pollution are well-established causes of exacerbation in both asthma and COPD. However, bacterial infections play a more important role in COPD exacerbation and so antibiotics are commonly prescribed (Sethi et al. 2002). In asthma exacerbations; antibiotics are recommended only if there is evidence of pneumonia or bacterial sinusitis. In a small percentage of asthmatics, Chlamydia and Mycoplasma have been found to have a role in worsening symptoms and treating with macrolides may be beneficial (Kraft et al. 2002, Specjalski 2010).

In asthma exacerbation, arterial blood gas analysis usually shows hypocapnia. A normal or elevated PaCO2 value suggests an impending respiratory arrest and requirement of intensive care. In contrast, hypercarbia and chronic type II respiratory failure are more common in COPD due to chronic fatigue of respiratory muscles, especially in severe cases (Virchow 2012).

Intravenous administration of magnesium sulfate has a role in the management of severe asthma exacerbation but not in COPD exacerbation (Rowe et al. 2000).

In COPD exacerbations, controlled oxygen therapy should be given to strictly maintain target saturation between 88 and 92% (Austin et al. 2010). Excess oxygen can cause hypercapnia and mortality. In contrast, during asthma exacerbation, oxygen administration can be more liberal to maintain saturation at 93–95% (Rodrigo et al. 2003, Perrin et al. 2011).

Non-Invasive Ventilation (NIV) has a well-established role in the management of COPD exacerbations with Type II respiratory failure. It has been proven to cause symptomatic and physiological improvement, reduce the need for intubation and in-hospital mortality rates and shorten hospital stay (Lightowler et al. 2003). The role of NIV in asthma exacerbations is less well established. It can be used in carefully selected and closely monitored patients with the intention to immediately go for intubation if there is no early improvement.

Asthma COPD overlap

In 2015 both GINA and GOLD recognized that distinguishing asthma from COPD can be problematic, particularly in smokers and older adults. In order to maintain awareness by clinicians, researchers and regulators a new terminology of Asthma COPD overlap (ACO) was coined. ACO does not describe a single disease entity (GINAsthma 2011). It includes patients with several different forms of airways disease phenotypes caused by a range of different underlying mechanisms. In epidemiological studies, the reported prevalence rates of ACO vary with the criteria used by different investigators. Between 15–20% of patients with concurrent asthma and COPD diagnosed by a doctor (GINAsthma 2011, McDonald et al. 2011, Krishnan et al. 2019). In a number of patients seen in our hospital 17.2% of the asthmatics and 2.8 % of the COPD patients qualified for a diagnosis of ACO (unpublished data CMC, Vellore).

There is high level of variability in lung function in ACO. Normal spirometry is not compatible with diagnosis of ACO and usually there is obstructive ventilatory defect. Significant bronchodilator reversibility is also common. In actual clinical practice when the patient has no pathognomonic features, the clinician has to weigh the evidence that is available and estimate the level of certainty and make a plan of treatment. If there is significant overlap in features and clear distinction is not possible, a diagnosis of ACO may be made. This is made easy by following the 'syndromic diagnosis of Airways disease', as stipulated by Global Initiative for Asthma (GINA) (Chronic Airflow Limitation 2015). The recommended default position is to treat these patients with ICS. This is because of the critical role of ICS in improving outcome in patients with uncontrolled asthma. Usually a LABA and/or LAMA are combined together with ICS.

Conclusion

In summary, although there are numerous similarities between asthma and COPD, yet there are significant differences which are important for patient care. A thorough knowledge of both the diseases as well as the ACO may facilitate the optimal management of patients.

References

Agusti A, Faner R. Systemic inflammation and comorbidities in chronic obstructive pulmonary disease. Proc Am Thorac Soc 2012; 9(2): 43–6.

Arinir U, Zhang Y, Holt R, Rohde G. Stemmler, Epplen JT, Schultze-Werninghaus G, et al. Polymorphisms in the PHF11and DPP10 genes and association with asthma and COPD. Am J Respir Crit Care Med 2004; 169: A273.

Austin MA, Wills KE, Blizzard L, Walters EH, Wood-Baker R. Effect of high flow oxygen on mortality in chronic obstructive pulmonary disease patients in prehospital setting: randomised controlled trial. BMJ 2010; 341: c5462.

Barnes PJ, Chung KF, Page CP. Inflammatory mediators of asthma: an update. Pharmacol Rev 1998; 50: 515–596.

Barnes PJ. Mediators of chronic obstructive pulmonary disease. Pharmacol Rev 2004; 56: 515–548.

Barnes PJ. Against the Dutch hypothesis: asthma and chronic obstructive pulmonary disease are distinct diseases. Am J Respir Crit Care Med 2006; 174: 240–243.

Barr RG, Bourbeau J, Camargo CA, Ram FS. Inhaled tiotropium for stable chronic obstructive pulmonary disease. Cochrane Database Syst Rev 2005; 18(2): CD002876.

Berger R, Smith D. Effect of inhaled metaproterenol on exercise performance in patients with stable "fixed" airway obstruction. Am Rev Respir Dis 1988; 138(3): 624–9.

Calverley PM, Burge PS, Spencer S, Anderson JA, Jones PW. Bronchodilator reversibility testing in chronic obstructive pulmonary disease. Thorax 2003; 58(8): 659–64.

CDC. Updated Recommendations for Prevention of Invasive Pneumococcal Disease Among Adults Using the 23-Valent Pneumococcal Polysaccharide Vaccine (PPSV23). Available from URL: http://www.cdc.gov/mmwr/preview/mmwrhtml/mm5934a3.htm#tab. 2012.

De Torres JP, Marín JM, Casanova C, Cote C, Carrizo S, Cordoba-Lanus E, et al. Lung cancer in patients with chronic obstructive pulmonary disease—incidence and predicting factors. Am J Respir Crit Care Med 2011; 184(8): 913–9.

Donaldson GC, Seemungal TA, Bhowmik A, Wedzicha JA. Relationship between exacerbation frequency and lung function decline in chronic obstructive pulmonary disease. Thorax 2002; 57(10): 847–52.

Drummond MB, Dasenbrook EC, Pitz MW, Murphy DJ, Fan E. Inhaled corticosteroids in patients with stable chronic obstructive pulmonary disease: a systematic review and meta-analysis. JAMA 2008; 300(20): 2407–16.

Gao J, Shan G, Sun B, Thompson PJ, Gao X. Association between polymorphism of tumour necrosis factor alpha-308 gene promoter and asthma: a meta-analysis. Thorax 2006; 61(6): 466–71.

Gelb AF, Zamel N. Unsuspected pseudophysiologic emphysema in chronic persistent asthma. Am J Respir Crit Care Med 2000; 162: 1778–1782.

Gibson PG. Inflammatory phenotypes in adult asthma: clinical applications. Clin Respir J. 2009 Oct; 3(4): 198–206.

GINA Report, Global Strategy for Asthma Management and Prevention. Updated Dec 2011. Available from URL: http://www.ginasthma.org.

Global Strategy. Diagnosis of Diseases of Chronic Airflow Limitation: Asthma, COPD, Asthma-COPD overlap syndrome. (ACOS). Based on the Global Strategy for Asthma management and prevention and the global strategy for the diagnosis, management and prevention of Chronic Obstructive Pulmonary Disease 2015.

Global Strategy for the Diagnosis, Management and Prevention of Chronic Obstructive Pulmonary Disease. Revised 2019. Available from URL: http://www.copdgold.org; 2019.

Global Strategy for Asthma Managment and Prevention guidelines. Global Initiative for Asthma. Revised 2019. Available from URL: www.ginasthma.org; Accessed on 3/7/2019.

Green RH, Brightling CE, McKenna S, Hargadon B, Parker D, Bradding P, et al. Asthma exacerbations and sputum eosinophil counts: a randomised controlled trial. Lancet 2002; 360: 1715–1721.

Hay JG, Stone P, Carter J, Church S, Eyre-Brook A, Pearson MG et al. Bronchodilator reversibility, exercise performance and breathlessness in stable chronic obstructive pulmonary disease. Eur Respir J 1992; 5(6): 659–64.

Holgate ST. ADAM metallopeptidase domain 33 (ADAM33): identification and role in airways disease. Drug News Perspect 2010; 23(6): 381–7.

Jeffery PK. Structural and inflammatory changes in COPD: a comparison with asthma. Thorax 1998; 53(2): 129–36.

Jones PW, Willits LR, Burge PS, Calverley PM. Inhaled Steroids in Obstructive Lung Disease in Europe study investigators. Disease severity and the effect of fluticasone propionate on chronic obstructive pulmonary disease exacerbations. Eur Respir J 2003; 21(1): 68–73.

Kerstjens HA, Disse B, Schröder-Babo W, Bantje TA, Gahlemann M, Sigmund R, et al. Tiotropium improves lung function in patients with severe uncontrolled asthma: a randomized controlled trial. J Allergy Clin Immunol 2011; 128(2): 308–14.

Kraft M, Cassell GH, Pak J, Martin RJ. Mycoplasma pneumoniae and Chlamydia pneumoniae in asthma: effect of clarithromycin. Chest 2002; 121: 1782–1788.

Kraft M. Asthma and chronic obstructive pulmonary disease exhibit common origins in any country. Am J Respir Crit Care Med 2006; 174: 238–240.

Krishnan JA, Nibber A, Chisholm A, Price D, Bateman ED, Bjermer L, et al. Prevalence and characteristics of asthma-COPD overlap in routine primary care practices. Ann Am Thorac Soc 2019; 16: 1143–1150.

Kurosawa H, Kohzuki M. Images in clinical medicine. Dynamic airway narrowing. N Engl J Med 2004; 350: 1036.

Lightowler JV, Wedzicha JA, Elliott MW, Ram FS. Non-invasive positive pressure ventilation to treat respiratory failure resulting from exacerbations of chronic obstructive pulmonary disease: Cochrane systematic review and meta-analysis. BMJ 2003; 326: 185.

Magnussen H, Richter K, Taube C. Are chronic obstructive pulmonary disease (COPD) and asthma different diseases? Clin Exp Allergy 1998; 28: 187–194.

Mahler DA, Wire P, Horstman D, Chang CN, Yates J, Fischer T, et al. Effectiveness of fluticasone propionate and salmeterol combination delivered via the Diskus device in the treatment of chronic obstructive pulmonary disease. Am J Respir Crit Care Med 2002; 166(8): 1084–91.

Mannino DM, Gagnon RC, Petty TL, Lydick E. Obstructive lung disease and low lung function in adults in the United States: data from the National Health and Nutrition Examination Survey, 1988–1994. Arch Intern Med 2000; 160: 1683–1689.

McDonald VM, Simpson JL, Higgins I, Gibson PG. Multidimensional assessment of older people with asthma and COPD: clinical management and health status. Age Ageing 2011 Jan; 40(1): 42–9.

Mishima M. Physiological Differences and Similarities in Asthma and COPD—Based on Respiratory Function Testing. Allergology International 2009; 58: 333–340.

Nussbaumer-Ochsner Y, Rabe KF. Systemic manifestations of COPD. Chest 2011; 139(1): 165–73.

O'Donnel DE, Fluge T, Gerken F, Hamilton A, Webb K, Aguilaniu B, et al. Effects of tiotropium on lung hyperinflation, dyspnoea and exercise tolerance in COPD. Eur Respir J 2004; 23: 832–40.

Orie NGM, Sluiter HJ, de Vries K, Tammeling GJ, Witkop J. The host factor in bronchitis. Orie, NGM Sluiter, HJ eds. Bronchitis Assen. Royal van Gorcum 1961; 43–59.

Pauwels RA. Similarities and differences in asthma and chronic obstructive pulmonary disease exacerbations. Proc Am Thorac Soc 2004; 1(2): 73–6.

Perrin K, Wijesinghe M, Healy B, Wadsworth K, Bowditch R, Bibby S, et al. Randomised controlled trial of high concentration versus titrated oxygen therapy in severe exacerbations of asthma. Thorax 2011 Nov; 66(11): 937–41.

Peters SP, Kunselman SJ, Icitovic N, Moore WC, Pascual R, Ameredes BT, et al. Tiotropium bromide step-up therapy for adults with uncontrolled asthma. N Engl J Med 2010; 363(18): 1715–26.

Rodrigo GJ, Rodriquez Verde M, Peregalli V, Rodrigo C. Effects of short-term 28% and 100% oxygen on PaCO2 and peak expiratory flow rate in acute asthma: a randomized trial. Chest 2003; 124(4): 1312–7.

Rowe BH, Bretzlaff JA, Bourdon C, Bota GW, Camargo CA Jr. Magnesium sulfate for treating exacerbations of acute asthma in the emergency department. Cochrane Database Syst Rev 2000; 2.

Rubinstein I, Kumar B, Schriever C. Long-term montelukast therapy in moderate to severe COPD—a preliminary observation. Respir Med 2004; 98(2): 134–8.

Saetta M, Di Stefano A, Maestrelli P, Turato G, Ruggieri MP, Roggeri A, et al. Airway eosinophilia in chronic bronchitis during exacerbations. Am J Respir Crit Care Med 1994; 150: 1646–1652.

Saha S, Brightling CE. Eosinophilic airway inflammation in COPD. Int J Chron Obstruct Pulmon Dis 2006; 1(1): 39–47.

Sakao S, Tatsumi K, Igari H, Shino Y, Shirasawa H, Kuriyama T. Association of tumor necrosis factor alpha gene promoter polymorphism with the presence of chronic obstructive pulmonary disease. Am J Respir Crit Care Med 2001; 163(2): 420–2.

Sethi S, Evans N, Grant BJ, Murphy TF. New strains of bacteria and exacerbations of chronic obstructive pulmonary disease. N Engl J Med 2002; 347(7): 465–71.

Specjalski K [Role of Chlamydia pneumoniae and Mycoplasma pneumoniae infections in the course of asthma]. Pneumonol Alergol Pol 2010; 78(4): 284–95.

Stavem K, Aaser E, Sandvik L, Bjørnholt JV, Erikssen G, Thaulow E, et al. Lung function, smoking and mortality in a 26-year follow-up of healthy middle-aged males. Eur Respir J 2005; 25(4): 618–25.

Szafranski W, Cukier A, Ramirez A, Menga G, Sansores R, Nahabedian S, et al. Efficacy and safety of budesonide/formoterol in the management of chronic obstructive pulmonary disease. Eur Respir J 2003; 21(1): 74–81.

Tetley TD. Inflammatory cells and chronic obstructive pulmonary disease. Curr Drug Targets Inflamm Allergy 2005; 4(6): 607–18.

Uhm TG, Kim BS, Chung IY. Eosinophil development, regulation of eosinophil-specific genes, and role of eosinophils in the pathogenesis of asthma. Allergy Asthma Immunol Res 2012 Mar; 4(2): 68–79.

Van Diemen CC, Postma DS, Vonk JM, ruinenberg M, Schouten JP, Boezen HM. A disintegrin and metalloprotease 33 polymorphisms and lung function decline in the general population. Am J Respir Crit Care Med 2005; 172: 329–333.

Virchow JC Jr, Walker C, Hafner D, ortsik C, Werner P, Matthys H, et al. T cells and cytokines in bronchoalveolar lavage fluid after segmental allergen provocation in atopic asthma. AmJ Respir Crit CareMed 1995; 151: 960–8.

Virchow JC. In: Similarities and differences in the pathophysiology of asthma and COPD. Advances in Combination Therapy for Asthma and COPD, First Edition. Edited by Jan L¨otvall. © 2012 John Wiley & Sons, Ltd. Published 2012 by John Wiley & Sons, Ltd.

21
Occupational Asthma

Bill Brashier[1,*] and *Amruta Wankhede*[2]

INTRODUCTION

Occupational asthma is one of the most prevalent lung diseases and is estimated to represent one in six cases of adult asthma (Ilgaz et al. 2019, Greiwe and Bernstein 2019, Walters et al. 2019, Dao and Bernstein 2018, Ellis and Walters 2017), forming a major public concern. Making an accurate diagnosis of Occupational Asthma (OA) is important not only because of the health consequences but also due to the socio-economic impact on workers, employers and the community (Greiwe and Bernstein 2019, Jacobsen et al. 2019).

Its annual incidence ranges between 22 and 40 cases per million of active workers and its prevalence is estimated around 16% of new onset adult asthma (Pralong and Cartier 2017). According to the Occupational Safety and Health Administration (OSHA), "an estimated 11 million workers in a wide range of industries and occupations are exposed to at least one of the numerous agents known to be associated with occupational asthma" (Greiwe and Bernstein 2019).

There are a number of medical conditions that can occur because of occupational exposures. There are a multitude of causative agents associated with this disease and numerous occupations at increased risk (Stevens and Grammer 2015). Occupational agents and industrial technologies are continuously being introduced to the work environment and require periodic health surveillance among exposed workers to detect early signs of disease (Quirce and Sastre 2019).

Occupational asthma is potentially preventable, by effective control of respiratory sensitizers in the workplace. Accordingly, identifying causal agents and associated risk factors is a key step towards optimal prevention of the disease (Vandenplas 2011). The basis for accurate diagnosis, management and prevention is the deeper knowledge of the allergic properties of the hazards and suitable diagnostic test methods as well as the identification of individual and occupational risk factors (Raulf et al. 2018). The disease conditions of occupational asthma do not differ from those of common forms of asthma. That is, obstruction of respiratory tract, high sensitivity of epithelial cells of respiratory tracts and inflammation of the tissue in the respiratory tract. The difference is that allergens that cause OA are usually found in the work place. If such allergens can be identified, it will help improve the diagnosis and treatment of occupational asthma (Maneechaeye et al. 2018). Thus, it is necessary to develop better standards and quality criteria for diagnosis, reliable biomarkers for severity assessment and prognosis, as well as new preventive and management strategies (Quirce and Sastre 2019).

---

[1] 802, B building, Dorabjee Paradise, Pune, Maharashtra, India.
[2] A-302, Ashtavinayak Darshan CHS, Mumbai-421201, Maharashtra, India, Email: amrutashaijesh@gmail.com
* Corresponding author: brashierbill@hotmail.com

Definition and classification

Occupational asthma is a "disease characterized by variable airway obstruction and/or airway hyperresponsiveness due to causes or conditions attributable to a particular occupational environment and not to stimuli encountered outside the workplace" (Greiwe and Bernstein 2019, Friedman-Jimenez et al. 2015, Balogun et al. 2018).

These are related to occupations (Table 21.1) and caused by antigens existing in the work place (Dobashi et al. 2017). Several hundred agents have been identified to cause occupational asthma (Beach et al. 2005). Pollutant and allergen exposures encountered at the work place can cause or exacerbate asthma, and these potential pollutants are numerous, varying and often under recognized (Kelly and Poole 2019). Chemicals which are known to be able to cause occupational asthma are usually identified on manufacturer's safety data sheets using the hazard statement H334—may cause allergy or asthma symptoms or breathing difficulties if inhaled or H335—may cause respiratory irritation (Beach et al. 2005).

Occupational asthma can be further divided into;

1. Hypersensitivity induced OA (immunologic OA) in which an immune response to a specific antigen is present, and
2. Irritant induced OA (non-immunologic OA) in which the airway inflammation is due to exposure to an irritant without specific sensitization (Greiwe and Bernstein 2019, Trivedi et al. 2017, Vandenplas et al. 2019, Dobashi et al. 2014, Quirce and Sastre 2019).

Hypersensitivity induced occupational asthma

Hypersensitivity-induced OA is the most common form of OA and is typically characterized by exposure to work place allergens or chemicals characterized by a latency period between first exposure to a substance at work and the onset of symptoms (Greiwe and Bernstein 2019). This type of OA is caused by physical contact with allergens in the workplace. The contact may occur in two ways (Table 21.2):

1. High-Molecular Weight (HMW) sensitizers: These are highly allergenic can cause hypersensitivity (allergy). A contact with high molecular weight allergens such as protein from animals which occurs in cattle farming, honey bee farming or seafood preparation process, high-molecular weights allergens from plants such as dyes, latex, starch or high-molecular weight allergens from fungi such as mushroom spore contacted by mushroom farmers or a scientist in a laboratory may lead to development of OA.
2. Low-Molecular Weight (LMW) sensitizers: These include reactive chemicals that readily take part in some chemical reaction. A contact with low-molecular weight allergens which are mostly chemicals or initial substances used in industrial manufacturing of other chemical substance such as organic solvents or organic compounds of metals may lead to OA occurrence (Maneechaeye et al. 2018, Perlman and Maier 2019, Beach et al. 2005, Dobashi et al. 2017, Kelly and Poole 2019).

Irritant induced occupational asthma

Irritant Induced Occupational Asthma (IIOA) consists of a spectrum of diseases from prolonged symptoms owing to a single large exposure, referred to a Reactive Airways Dysfunction Syndrome (RADS), to asthma induced by long-term, low-level exposure to irritant chemicals.

It is caused by physical contact with a substance irritant to the respiratory system at a high level within a short period of time which can directly damage the tissue within the respiratory tract of the patient. Examples of triggering events are swimming pool lifeguards inhaling chlorine gas at a high-level or a scientist in a laboratory inhaling intense vaporizing acidic or basic substance. A person may come into contact with the irritating substance by accident or being exposed to it in an unavoidable natural disaster incident. Naturally, human beings will not tolerate contact with intense irritants for a long period of time. From a study of patients who suffer irritant-induced occupational asthma caused by inhaling intense dust smog from the World Trade Center tragedy in the United States, it is found that many fire fighters and

Table 21.1. Aspirated substances and occupations assumed to induce occupational asthma

Aspirated substances inducing occupational asthma	Occupation or other
A. Plant-derived	
I. Powder dust	
1. Grain dust	
Buckwheat flour	Noodle makers & distributors
Wheat flour	Baking industry, rice millers
	Workers for milling factories
Barley flour	Animal feed business
	Families of rice millers
Animal feed dust	Rice millers
Rice	Rice farmers
Rice bran	
Rice straw	
2. Wood dust	
Red cedar	Red cedar wood industry
Clethra	Woodworkers
Magnolia	Wood industry
Rosewood	Furniture makers
Yellow pine	Carpenters
White ash	Furniture workers
3. Other powder dust	
Cotton dust	Curtain/flag makers
Coffee bean dust	Traders handling these beans
Powder dust of sunflower seeds	Confectioners handling them
Shoot of tea	Tea-picking workers
Tea packing business	Tea makers
Tomato stems	Planters in plastic greenhouses
Lettuce leaves	Food processors
Pepper	Food processors
Indian rice flour	Indian rice users
Smoke of tobacco	Resort hotel workers
II. Pollen and spores	
1. Occupational pollinosis	
Sugar beet pollen	Staff in research institutes, pollen researchers, growers
Rose pollen	
Hogweed pollen	
Cocksfoot pollen	
Strawberry pollen	Growers in plastic greenhouses
Peach pollen	Flowers picked at peach field
Pear pollen	Pear growers
Apple pollen	Hand pollinators
Grape pollen	Workers growing grapes
Green pepper pollen	Growers in plastic greenhouses
Corn pollen	Dairy farmers who raise corn
2. Spores	
Mushroom spore	Mushroom growers in plastic greenhouses
Club moss spore	Farmers growing wheat
Wheat smut fungus spore	
3. Fungus	
Trichophyton (fungus)	Contact with tinea patients

Table 21.1 contd. ...

...Table 21.1 contd.

Aspirated substances inducing occupational asthma	Occupation or other
B. Animal-derived	
1. Arthropod, insects	
Sericulture industry	Sericulturists
Mature silkworm urine	
Scary hair of moth of silkworm	
Carp food	Carp growers
Dried pupas	Silk handlers
Bee poison	Silk sericin
Tricopteran powder dust	Fishing gear business
House dust mite antigen	Researchers
Tetranychidae, mandarin orange spider mite	Workers cultivating yuzu
Pupas of arrowhead Coccoidea	Workers who clip mandarin trees
2. Fish	
Shrimp powder dust	Dried shrimp makers
Sardine powder dust	Dried sardine makers
3. Birds	
Chicken farming	
Chick feathers	Chicken hatching stations
Poultry manure and chicken feathers	Poultry dealers
4. Mammals	
Human dander	Person in charge of cosmetics
Pig stool powder dust	Pig industry
Dog skin	Managers of animal hospitals
Cat skin	Managers of animal hospitals
Cow hair/ furfur	Cattle farmers, horse-riders
Animal hair	Hair pencil makers
Sheep wool	Persons handling sheep wool
Furfur of guinea pig and rabbit, body components of frog	Personnel raising animals in university laboratories
5. Other	
Body components of ascidian	Oyster shuckers
Shell powder dust	Shell polishers
Pearl powder dust	Workers who form necklace holes
C. Drugs and food	
1. Drug powder dust	
Diastase, gentian, thyradin	Pharmacists
Pancreatin	Pharmacists
Matromycin, sigmamycin	Pharmaceutical company employees
Penicillin	Person in charge of experiments at pharmaceutical company
Kallikrein	Pharmacists
Gastropylore	Employees
Cetraxate hydrochloride pantothenic acid	
2. Foods	
Stevia powder	Traders adding stevia to sucrose
Galacto-oligosaccharide	Traders of oysters
Glycyrrhiza powder dust	Workers extracting pigment
Honey	Families of apiary workers
	Traders dividing royal jerry in sacks
Royal jerry	Sake brewers
Oxygen products containing amylase as a main component	Cheese plant employees
Milk curdling enzyme Rennin (for making cheese)	
Lysozyme, glycine, glucono delta lactone	Food preservative manufacturers
Food additive powder dust	Employees handling food additives

Table 21.1 contd. ...

...Table 21.1 contd.

Aspirated substances inducing occupational asthma	Occupation or other
D. Metals and Chemicals	
1. Chemicals	
Dyestuffs	
Dyestuff intermediates, Chicago Red, Pyrazolone derivatives	Employees of dye stuff factories
Reactive dyestuffs, Reactive Orange 7	
Arabian rubber powder dust	Printing by factory workers
Isocyanate	Polyurethane resin factory workers, house painters,
Toluene diisocyanate, methyl bisphenylisocynate	orthopedists fixing plaster casts
Cyanoacrylate adhesives, Cyanon	Plate makers
Anhydrous pyromellitic acid	Traders
Stimulation of anti-rust oil	Welders aspirating smoke
2. Metals	
Chrome	
Chrome in cement	Cement factory workers
Bichromate of soda	Metal factory workers
Chloroplatinic acid	Makers of platinum oxygen sensors
Tungsten	Workers at factory making cemented carbide tools
Cobalt	

Source: Greiwe and Bernstein 2019, Dobashi 2017, Daniels 2018, Dobashi 2014, Larco-Rojas et al. 2017, Le Moual et al. 2018, Lux et al. 2019

Table 21.2. Characteristics of high-molecular-weight and low-molecular-weight agents as causes of occupational asthma.

	High-molecular-weight agents	Low-molecular-weight agents
Structure	Proteins, polysaccharides	Chemicals, metals
Duration of latency period before getting 'sensitization'	Generally longer (ex: flour)	Generally shorter (ex: isocyanates)
Occulonasal symptoms	+++	+
Accompanying dermatitis	Rare	Possible
Immunologic mechanism	IgE-dependent	Generally not IgE-dependent IgG, MCP-1 (isocyanates)
Cellular component	Eosinophils	Eosinophils and neutrophils
Feasibility of skin testing to elicit immediate reactions	Yes	No
Type of asthmatic reaction after challenge	Immediate, dual	Isolated late or atypical
Frequency of referral	One third	Two third
Diagnostic means	Numerous	More limited

Source: Data from Malo and Chan-Yeung, 2009. Agents causing occupational asthma. J Allergy Clin Immunol. 545-550.

people situated within a close proximity of the World Trade Center suffered asthma-like symptoms. The condition of irritation-induced occupational asthma occurs in every patient who comes into contact with irritating substances at a high level. This is different from sensitizer-induced occupational asthma which occurs to only certain people who are allergic to the contacted substance (Maneechaeye et al. 2018).

Pathophysiological mechanism of occupational asthma

Hypersensitivity induced OA is characterized by a latency period between exposure and symptoms and involves IgE and non-IgE responses (Freidman-Jimenez et al. 2015). It involves development of IgE-specific antibodies produced by exposure to the antigen (Perlman and Maier 2019). Bonding of allergens to a specific IgE antibody on the surfaces of mast cells, basophils and possibly macrophages, dendritic cells, eosinophils and platelets subsequently gives rise to synthesis and/or release of inflammatory mediators that regulate the inflammatory process (Freidman-Jimenez et al. 2015).

Immunoglobulin E responses are mostly seen in HMW antigen exposure; it can also be seen in LMW exposure. High molecular weight agents act as complete antigens, whereas LMW chemicals must first react with autologous or heterologous proteins to produce a functioning allergen. In the cases of LMW that are IgE mediated (most notably platinum and other hard metal salts and acid anhydrides), the chemicals react with other proteins (endogenous or exogenous) to create an antigen capable of producing an allergic response. Most chemical sensitizers are organic molecules with reactive side chains, suggesting that the ability to cross-link proteins may be important in the immune mechanism of LMW OA; however, the mechanism of OA owing to LMW causes in many cases is unclear (Freidman-Jimenez et al. 2015, Perlman and Maier 2019, Maneechaeye et al. 2018).

Other mechanisms such as cell mediated immunity and T helper 2 type innate responses have been proposed. In the case of toluene diisocyanate, one of the most well-described LMW causes of OA, specific IgE antibodies are detected in some cases, although other data suggest an IgE-independent response. The phenotype of airway response is different in LMW versus HMW OA, and LMW-induced OA may have a tendency to be more severe compared with HMW agents. High molecular weight OA can often be associated with an immediate or dual phase reaction compared with LMW, which may result in greater difficulty in making a diagnosis of work relatedness (Perlman and Maier 2019).

Irritant Induced Occupational Asthma (IIOA) involves the breakdown of the epithelial barrier in the lung owing to an injury. The IIOA usually has a short latency period when compared with OA, particularly in cases of a high level of exposure. Conversely, long-term, low-level exposure has been shown to be associated with asthma, notably in cleaning products. In the latter cases, genetic susceptibility may play a role (Perlman and Maier 2019).

With RADS, the respiratory tract reacts to a massive irritant exposure producing a variety of respiratory symptoms for which the underlying histopathological mechanism is not clearly understood. Serial biopsies of two RADS cases during the acute and recovery phase helped elucidate the histopathologic process. Early changes show marked loss of epithelial cells and replacement of epithelium by fibrinohemorrhagic exudate. This was followed by subepithelial edema and signs of regeneration of the epithelial layer with proliferation of basal and parabasal cells. Inflammatory cells, mainly lymphocytes, are usually present. Airway remodeling leads to persistent structural changes, chronic airway inflammation and continual airway hyper responsiveness. One hypothesis is that injury to the airway epithelium stimulates the intrinsic repair pathway with healing by primary intention. Possibly, in RADS, there is an impaired airway repair response to injury that mimics the chronic wound scenario of healing by secondary intention. It is not known whether host susceptibility factors (e.g., cigarette smoking, genetic predisposition, pre-existing lung disease or atopy) are prerequisites for RADS development (Friedman-Jimenez et al. 2015, Maneechaeye et al. 2018).

Epidemiology and prevalence

The incidence of OA varies depending on the type of exposure and geographic location around the world. For example, OA has been reported in 8–12% of laboratory animal workers, 7–9% of bakers and 1.4% of healthcare workers exposed to natural rubber latex; however, these latter rates vary depending on the study cited. Overall, males have the higher attributable risk for OA (14%) compared to women (7%); however, women have a higher risk for OA in certain occupations such as drivers, cleaners, nurses and hairdressers. The use of spray products, especially chlorine bleach, ammonia and air freshening sprays, in occupations like spray-painters and janitorial cleaning seems to put these workers at greatest risk for developing OA and other respiratory disorders. Probably the best data on OA prevalence and occupational exposures comes from a public health surveillance program performed by the National Institute for Occupational Safety and Health (NIOSH) which identified > 4000 cases of work-related asthma from 1993 to 2002 in four states (California, Massachusetts, Michigan and New Jersey) with ~ 68% caused by occupational exposure and 20% represented pre-existing asthma aggravated by occupational exposure (Greiwe and Bernstein 2019). Occupational asthma can arise de novo, or in those with existing or reactivated childhood asthma, and its incidence is 74–300 cases per million workers per annum (Walters et al. 2019). Occupational asthma, according to existing national workplace health surveillance systems, has been the most commonly reported occupational respiratory disease in both the United States and Great Britain for more than two decades (Balogun et al. 2018).

Of all the work-related asthma cases from the states of California, Massachusetts, Michigan and New Jersey, ~ 20% were associated with miscellaneous chemicals, 13% with mineral and inorganic dust, 12% with cleaning materials, 11% with indoor air pollutants and 4% with exposures to polymers. Within agent categories, isocyanates and hydrocarbons, not otherwise specified, accounted for the greatest proportion of cases classified as occupational asthma, at 89 and 83%, respectively; pyrolysis products had the greatest proportion of cases classified as work-aggravated asthma, at 29% (Greiwe and Bernstein 2019).

In an analysis of US data from 2007, the total number of occupational injuries and illnesses reported was about nine million. Assuming a total number of employed people in the USA of 120 million, the prevalence is about 7.5%. As the number is likely an underestimation, the prevalence is probably higher (Stevens and Grammer 2015).

In an epidemiologic study of 13 European countries, 10 to 25% of new onset adult asthma was estimated to have been caused by work place exposures, including inhalation accidents and routine occupational exposures. A systematic review of international studies estimated 17.6% of adult asthma is caused by occupational exposures. From data from the Behavioral Risk Factor Surveillance System in the United States, the proportion of new onset adult asthma that was diagnosed as OA by a health professional was estimated as 4.7% plus an additional 13.5% that was self-reported by survey respondents to have been caused by work place exposures to chemicals, smoke, fumes or dust, although OA had not been diagnosed by a health professional. While there may be some variation by geographic location, occupation, definitions, methods and other factors, evidence is consistent that a substantial minority of cases of new onset adult asthma is caused by environmental exposures in the work place (Friedman-Jimenez et al. 2015).

An estimated 18 million people in the United States have asthma. OA prevalence is said to range between 2 and 6% of the asthmatic population. Consistent with this estimate, a recent large population-based study of OA estimated that between 5 and 10% of cases of asthma among adults in European and other industrialized countries were secondary to occupational exposures (Bardana 2003).

Very high incidence rates are reported by Scandinavian countries (7–18/100 000), with Finland reporting the highest incidence, western Europe and the USA having intermediate rates (2.4–4.3/100,000), while developing countries such as South Africa and Brazil (Sao Paulo) report a much lower incidence of 1.8/100 000 and 1.7/100,000, respectively. Despite this relatively low incidence in South Africa, regional differences exist, with a much higher incidence reported in the western Cape province, which is highly urbanized (2.5/100,000). The gender distribution of OA appears to be inconsistent, with some countries reporting a slightly higher incidence in men (Sweden, UK, France, Brazil), while others report higher rates for women (Finland, USA, Europe). Published data on OA incidence rates according to age are limited and demonstrate inconsistent trends, either increasing with age (UK) or with much higher rates in the 15–29 year age group (France) (Jeebhay and Quirce 2006).

Some common industries and occupations appear to be consistently associated with a higher incidence of OA. These include bakers and pastry makers (most European and Scandinavian countries, New Zealand), spray painters, especially in the car manufacturing industry (Norway, France, UK, Spain, New Zealand), and health care workers (France, Italy, Belgium). These patterns are also observed in developing countries such as South Africa. In certain countries, such as Norway, Germany and France, hairdressers appear to be at high risk. Interestingly, unlike other industrialized countries, in Finland the agricultural sector (farming, animal husbandry) has the second highest incidence rates among women workers. This pattern is very similar to developing countries such as Zambia. Countries such as New Zealand and South Africa have smelting aluminium and refining platinum operations that also report a high incidence of OA. Cleaners and janitors are commonly reported high-risk occupations in both industrialized (USA) and developing countries (Brazil, South Africa) (Jeebhay and Quirce 2006).

Diagnosis

The diagnosis of asthma follows a stepwise approach (Pralong and Cartier 2017) and is based on comprehensive and detailed history taking about work place exposures, temporal onset of asthma and atopic symptoms, physical examination and laboratory results such as peak expiratory flow rate and spirometry (Trivedi et al. 2017, Maneechaeye et al. 2018). Diagnosing OA early is associated with better clinical outcome for the worker (Fishwick and Forman 2018). The diagnosis of OA in terms of symptoms and signs does not differ from the diagnosis of general asthma. The difference is that the diagnosis of occupational asthma must be reassured to confirm that the exposure to allergens involves a contact to an irritating substance within the work place. This requires additional detailed information on the patient's work history, the nature of the work in the past, and his or her asthma history (in case the patient has an asthma history and the symptom has been aggravated during work, the symptom is called work-exacerbated asthma, not occupational asthma), asthma history in the patient's family and of the colleagues (Maneechaeye et al. 2018).

History and physical examination

The history taking steps that could lead to a conclusion that a patient has occupational asthma are as follows:

1. Medical evidence specifies asthma symptoms;
2. Major challenge posed is differential diagnosis of identical illness (such as previous asthma not related to work, COPD, etc.) which have to be carefully ruled out;
3. There is history or evidence showing patient's exposure to allergens at work and outside work;
4. The history of asthma symptoms to develop post exposures to work place sensitizers and there is a clear period of latency in which pathology develops;
5. Symptoms shown during certain periods have a correlation with the exposure to allergens in the area in question;
6. Symptoms during certain periods have improved as the patient is not exposed to the environment in the area in question;

Mere history taking is not sufficient to diagnose asthma. A further step may require a workplace survey by an occupational physician to collect additional information for the assessment of the surrounding environment at work to identify allergens in question (Maneechaeye et al. 2018). While the physical examination is generally unrevealing about specific causes of respiratory symptoms, it can be helpful in ruling out non-occupational causes of respiratory symptoms or diseases including cardiac or connective tissue disorders (Greiwe and Bernstein 2019).

Pulmonary function testing

Pulmonary function testing (normally spirometry) to assess the severity of airway obstruction and the presence of airway reversibility is the most important first objective assessment in an OA evaluation. If asthma is not confirmed with spirometry and there is high suspicion for OA, then additional provocation testing using direct approaches such as methacholine challenge or indirect methods (i.e., adenosine challenge) can help determine the presence of Airway Hyper Responsiveness (AHR) which is an essential characteristic for the diagnosis of asthma (Greiwe and Bernstein 2019). The allergen-Specific Inhalation Challenge (SIC) test is widely acknowledged as the gold standard for the diagnosis of OA (Suojalehto et al. 2019, Lux et al. 2019). It is important to recognize that a positive provocation test does not confirm a diagnosis of OA and neither does a negative test exclude AHR especially if performed when the patient is off work for a prolonged period of time and symptom free. Furthermore, a positive non-specific provocation test only indicates the presence of AHR suggestive for asthma but is not diagnostic of OA. However, if a challenge is performed when the patient is working and actively exposed to the suspected inciting agent(s) and is negative, then diagnosis of OA can in most circumstances be excluded. In some cases, a non-specific provocation test can be negative, whereas a specific provocation test can be positive, but this is uncommon and should only be pursued if the history is very compelling. If there is evidence of a restrictive pattern on screening spirometry, then additional testing should include full pulmonary function testing with lung volumes and a diffusion capacity (DLCO). In addition, radiographic imaging with a chest x-ray or if necessary a chest CT should be performed to rule out other conditions that can confound a diagnosis of OA (Greiwe and Bernstein 2019).

Once a diagnosis of asthma is confirmed, the next step is to establish a relationship between objective changes in lung function and symptoms in the work place. There are various approaches to help accomplish this goal; however, their sensitivity and validity are variable (Greiwe and Bernstein 2019). Serial measurements of Peak Expiratory Flow Rate (PEFR) are the most feasible and accurate tools in the diagnosis of occupational asthma. Studies indicate that in comparison to reference standard investigation (specific inhalation challenge) PEFR possesses sensitivity of 65% and specificity of 77%, while in comparison to expert diagnosis it is 75% sensitive and 94% specific (Tarlo and Vandenplas 2003, Mapp et al. 2005).

The sensitivity and specificity of serial PEFR can be further enhanced with increasing the frequency of PEFR measurements which can potentially project real time events of sensitizer exposures and asthma responses in airways. Ideally the PEFR readings should be recorded at intervals of 2 hours every day during working days and holidays. This entails considerable effort and consistent interest from the patient. However, studies have shown that recording of PEFR 4 times particularly before resumption of work in the morning, 2 hours after beginning work, at the end of the days work and before retiring to the bed, is also equivalently sensitive in diagnosing occupational asthma. Irrespective of PEFR measuring frequency, each time three readings have to be recorded and the best of three should be noted as the PEFR. To ensure that the best values are recorded, the reproducibility of the three readings has to be within 20 liter/minute. PEFR has to be measured over a period of 3 working weeks and 6–7 non-working days for a conclusive occupational asthma diagnosis. Newer technologies have provided a self-recording PEFR meter that automatically records time and PEFR values and comments on reproducibility (Tarlo and Vandenplas 2003, Mapp et al. 2005).

Patients with occupational asthma should exhibit a diurnal variation between the highest and lowest PEFR of more than 20% for at least 60–70% of the working days which remits during the weekends or days off from the work. In cases where a pre-existing asthmatic has also developed into an occupational asthma case, then PEFR evaluations have to be conducted after achieving stability in pre-existing asthma with stable dose of inhaled steroid treatment (Tarlo and Vandenplas 2003, Mapp et al. 2005).

Although, being a very sensitive and specific tool in diagnosis of occupational asthma the phenomenon of PEFR variation, during work exposure, is usually more prominent in earlier stages of the disease. This is the time when airway remodeling is minimal. Serial PEFR measurements have no diagnostic utility in RADS. Additional diagnostic tools to analyze lung function and airway inflammation at work are detailed in Table 21.3 (Greiwe and Bernstein 2019).

If possible, for workers with irritant-induced asthma measurement of an irritant exposure index which has previously been shown to be correlated with AHR may be a useful adjunctive tool but is not validated. This could potentially allow comparison of days when there is documented irritant exposure(s) with work-related symptoms and changes in lung function (Greiwe and Bernstein 2019). Confirmation of the diagnosis requires demonstration of bronchial hyper responsiveness by a positive methacholine test (Dao and Bernstein 2018).

Skin prick testing (SPT) or serologic testing for specific IgE (sIgE)

The first association between asthma and work-related exposures was documented by Hippocrates for occupations including metal workers, fishermen, farmhands, horsemen, and tailors. Over the ensuing centuries, greater than 400 agents have been described to cause OA, but only very few are characterized on the molecular level and available for routine diagnosis. A more thorough understanding of the relevant allergen components would significantly improve the diagnostic capability of testing. Both SPT and serum sIgE testing to aeroallergens to assess the worker's atopic status can sometimes be useful especially when

Table 21.3. Recommendations for diagnostic tools to help establish a relationship between objective changes in lung function and symptoms in the workplace

Peak expiratory flow rate (PEFR)
• PEFR measurements should be recorded every 2 hours in the workplace and every 3–4 hours at home while awake for at least 2 weeks • If feasible, PEFRs should be performed for 2 weeks while the worker is out of the workplace as well. • To improve worker adherence and the reliability of data, paper-free electronic devices that time and date stamp each reading in addition to quantifying effort are recommended PEFRs with 20% variability between workplace and home confirm workplace exposure airway hyper responsiveness
Cross-shift FEV_1
• Cross-shift FEV_1 measurements require the worker to undergo spirometry before and after the work-shift. • Reduction in FEV_1: 15–20% is suggestive of workplace exposure. • This method is currently not validated to confirm diagnosis of OA
Fractional concentration of exhaled nitric oxide (FeNO) and induced sputum eosinophil counts
• Noninvasive testing can identify increased inflammation within the airways. • Increased inflammation at the end of a period at work provides indirect evidence of OA • These methods are currently not validated to confirm diagnosis of OA

Source: Greiwe and Bernstein 2019, Fishwick and Forman 2018

Approaches to control occupational asthma in the worksite
Prevent the disease by reducing or eliminating environmental allergens and irritants
Detect the disease early, even before symptoms appear, by using surveillance measures
Avoid worsening symptoms by preventing exposure or using something less harmful

Source: Employers, Employees, and Worksites, NIH 2011

Primary prevention
Primary prevention includes worker education regarding occupational asthma, safe work practices, avoidance of known sensitizer agents, reducing/eliminating sensitizer exposure (where safe substitutes are not available) and continued monitoring of workplace exposures.

Secondary prevention
Secondary prevention (early detection) strategies include periodic monitoring that includes respiratory questionnaires, spirometry and continued education regarding occupational asthma symptoms and signs

Tertiary prevention
Reduction of exposure can lead to improvement or resolution of NSBHR and asthma symptoms, but this approach may be less useful than cessation of exposure. In cases when cessation of exposure is not possible, use of personal protective equipment maybe beneficial although few long-term data are available. One successful prevention strategy over the past decade has been the replacement of powdered allergen rich latex gloves in healthcare facilities. Use of immunotherapy has been described in small studies in sensitizer-mediated asthma but it is not currently recommended (Trivedi et al. 2017).

considering certain forms of OA where atopy is a risk factor. Skin prick testing is generally most useful for the diagnosis of OA caused by HMW agents, but there are circumstances where skin testing can also be useful for LMW agents such as acid anhydrides. If performed properly, these tests correlate very well with serologic testing for confirming sensitization. However, many workers may demonstrate sensitization to various HMW allergens by skin or serum testing but lack corresponding clinical symptoms, and therefore it is always important to correlate test results with exposure and symptoms (Jacobsen et al. 2019, Raulf et al. 2018).

Sensitization or allergenic cross-reactivity to allergens or epitopes from unrelated sources may interfere with specific IgE assays resulting in false-positive results. However, skin testing and/or serologic testing has been used very successfully as part of immunosurveillance programs. Enzymes and trimellitic anhydride (TMA) are two examples of HMW and LMW agents, respectively, where skin testing and serum-specific IgG and IgE assays have been effective at identifying sensitized workers who are at risk for subsequently developing OA.

Early removal of these workers from further work place exposure has been very effective at preventing development of OA (Walters et al. 2019, Griewe and Bernstein 2019). However, for most causes of OA, skin testing and specific serum assays are not available, and the approaches used for testing in these circumstances have not been well characterized or validated. Further knowledge of molecules relevant for some of the most prevalent causes of OA would allow for development of standardized *in vitro* IgE antibody assays that could aid in diagnosis. Component-resolved diagnosis is an attempt to address this unmet need by identifying relevant HMW molecules for OA like wheat flour components for baker's asthma, wood dust allergens and laboratory animal allergens (Greiwe and Bernstein 2019).

Treatment and management

Patients with occupational asthma due to a work place sensitizer should be completely removed from further exposure to the agent for the best medical outcome as supported by a Cochrane review and several other reviews and consensus statements (Bardana 2003, Greiwe and Bernstein 2019, Lau and Tarlo 2019). If simple avoidance fails to manage symptoms or is not feasible, workers may need medications to better control OA and prevent asthma attacks. Both the National Asthma Education and Prevention Program (NAEPP) and the Global Initiative for Asthma (GINA) provide guidelines that can be used to help guide therapy in a stepwise manner (Greiwe and Bernstein 2019).

Therapeutically, combination of anti-inflammatory and bronchodilator drugs are advocated (Bardana 2003). The two major categories of asthma medications are quick-relief and long term control medications. Quick-relief medications (a.k.a rescue medications) are used as needed for rapid, short-term symptom relief during an asthma attack. Short-acting beta agonists (albuterol, levalbuterol) act as smooth muscle bronchodilators within minutes to relieve symptoms. Ipratropium bromide is a long-acting M3 muscarinic receptor antagonist that is approved as a bronchodilator for acute COPD exacerbations. Long-term medications including inhaled corticosteroids (ICS), Long-Acting Beta-2-Agonists (LABA), leukotriene modifiers, combination ICS/LABA inhalers, Long-Acting Muscarinic Antagonists (LAMA) and biologics have all been approved for the treatment of asthma and should be used in a similar capacity in OA cases as appropriate. Oral and intravenous corticosteroids (prednisone, methylprednisolone) are reserved to treat more severe OA to aggressively relieve airway inflammation and as adjunctive therapy during an acute asthma exacerbation. Severe or poorly controlled cases of OA might require more frequent or prolonged use of oral corticosteroids to better control symptoms even after removal from the work place exposure (Greiwe and Bernstein 2019).

In cases where the diagnosis has been delayed for several years or the patient is close to retirement and does not wish to change work, there may be some benefit from reduction of exposure as able, by means of occupational hygiene measures such as improved local ventilation and use of respiratory protective equipment, but these measures have not been demonstrated to be as effective as complete removal of exposure. In addition, there have been a few deaths from occupational asthma associated with continued exposure at work. In the future, immune modulation might potentially allow safe ongoing exposure to the work place agent for those with sensitizer-induced occupational asthma. Although venom immunotherapy is effective for bee-keepers with anaphylaxis to bee venom, there have been relatively few studies to provide any support for specific immunotherapy for occupational allergens. Use of a biological agent such as omalizumab has been reported only in a small numbers of patients with occupational asthma, so further studies are needed to determine whether these will prevent responses to work place sensitizers in those with occupational asthma and whether cost/benefit estimates should be considered (Lau and Tarlo 2019).

For patients with occupational asthma and persistent symptoms or uncontrolled asthma despite optimal standard pharmacotherapy the use of new biologic agents (omalizumab, anti-interleukin-5 monoclonal antibodies) may be considered (Quirce and Sastre 2019).

Prognosis

Early recognition, early removal, well preserved lung function and less airway hyper reactivity are all characteristics associated with a better long-term prognosis (Greiwe and Bernstein 2019, Lau and Tarlo

2019). Older age and causation by high-molecular weight sensitizers are associated with worse outcome in a systematic review. Despite these recommendations, the mean time from the onset of symptoms to diagnosis is often 2 or more years (Lau and Tarlo 2019).

Although a majority of patients with occupational asthma from a sensitizer have improvement in asthma severity after removal from further exposure and improvement can continue over several years; nevertheless, the overall rate of symptomatic clearing of asthma at a mean of 31 months has previously been reported to be 32% from a pooled estimate. The advice to completely avoid the causative sensitizing agent at work can sometimes be achieved relatively simply by changing the material used at work (e.g., natural rubber latex gloves or a quaternary ammonium cleaning product), but often this is not feasible, so that the patient needs to be moved to a different work area or to a different company or job, leading potentially to significant socio-economic impact. The assistance of an effective workers' compensation system to provide economic support for lost or reduced earnings and for costs of asthma medications as well as for non-economic loss (disability) can be helpful in permitting patients to make such changes. Support from a workers' compensation system is usually dependent on having as much objective support for the diagnosis as possible, so that thorough and early investigations while the patient is still employed are important in this regard. For those who cannot stay in the same job, there may be support for retraining. Even with workers' compensation support, however, there can be significant income loss and socio-economic effects from the diagnosis (Lau and Tarlo 2019).

The principle determinants of patient outcome subsequent to removal from the offending agent include the total duration of exposure, asthma severity at diagnosis and the pathogenic mechanisms operative in the induction of OA. In addition, coexisting factors such as cigarette smoking, chronic sinusitis and gastroesophageal reflux may also play an important role as prognostic modifiers. Removal of the patient with OA from the offending immunogen or irritant should result in clinical improvement. In a study of 75 patients having western red cedar asthma, it was found that half of these patients recovered completely. A later follow-up study of 232 patients by the same group revealed that 60% had not completely recovered during a 4-year observation period. Most motivated patients achieve good control and are capable of resuming full employment in an alternative line of work (Bardana 2003).

In instances where the diagnosis of OA was delayed, or where the patient did not heed warnings about avoidance, chronic symptoms may remain indefinitely with concomitant pulmonary deterioration. On 48 patients with western red cedar asthma who had continuous exposure an average of 6.5 years after initial diagnosis, none of these patients had recovered and half demonstrated deterioration of lung function despite treatment. Specific BHR to an inciting agent may persist after removal from further exposure in subjects who no longer show evidence of asthma symptoms, use anti asthma medications or demonstrate nonspecific BHR (Bardana 2003).

Prevention

Since undiagnosed OA can cause considerable medical and economic consequences, aggressive prevention strategies are essential. Most preventive interventions focus on early recognition and removal of the worker from further exposure which can significantly improve overall outcomes by avoiding allergens (Greiwe and Bernstein 2019, Maneechaeye et al. 2018). While worker-focused interventions are crucial, additional efforts directed at improving the work place environment to reduce risk of exposure by other workers is also critical. Many public health-based and population-based interventions over the years have started with recognition of individual cases of occupational exposures causing health issues. These cases serve to increased clinical awareness that have led to the development of health surveillance programs which have been effective at defining the extent of these public health concerns. Several voluntary reporting programs have been established in the USA including the NIOSH Sentinel Event Notification System for Occupational Risk (SENSOR) program. The mission of the SENSOR program is to build and maintain occupational illness and injury surveillance registries within state health departments. Other countries have similar programs whose mission is to protect workers' safety and health. While NIOSH is not a regulatory agency, it may conduct thorough worksite evaluations, also referred to as Health Hazard

Evaluations (HHEs) in selected situations if requested by a worker or employer (Greiwe and Bernstein 2019).

The preventive measures may be constructed as follows:

1. **Primary prevention**

    It is the preferred method of prevention for both the types of occupational asthma.

    1.1. Primary prevention for hypersensitivity induced OA (immunologic OA): the primary prevention is focused on exposure prevention. Ideally, this consists of avoiding or terminating the use of agents that cause OA when possible and substituting safer substances for these agents, e.g., substituting orthophthalaldehyde for glutaraldehyde (ortho-phthalaldehyde has less commonly been reported to cause sensitization and asthma). For new chemicals, a quantitative structural analysis may potentially assist in predicting the likelihood that the agent will be a respiratory sensitizer, although there can be false negative predictive values. When complete avoidance of sensitizer use in a work place is not possible, reduced exposure to known respiratory sensitizers can be effective, such as using encapsulated enzymes, use of robots in place of workers, improved general and local ventilation and use of effective respiratory protective equipment for short potential exposure (Maneechaeye et al. 2018, Lau and Tarlo 2019).

    1.2. Primary prevention for irritant induced OA (non-immunologic OA): Enforced exposure limits for sensitizing chemicals would be expected to reduce rates of sensitization, since rates of sensitization are generally greater with higher exposure (Maneechaeye et al. 2018). Primary prevention for irritant-induced asthma would consist of preventing workers' exposure to high-level irritant vapor, gases, dusts and fumes. This is included in general occupational hygiene measures and most cases of irritant-induced asthma are accidental exposures that may be difficult to predict and prevent. When accidental exposure has occurred, it is appropriate for the work place to assess reasons for the exposure and measures that could be taken to prevent a further similar exposure at a later date (Lau and Tarlo 2019, Ilgaz et al. 2019).

2. **Secondary prevention**

    It comprises medical surveillance for early detection of affected workers so that early diagnosis and intervention can occur. Medical surveillance programs for occupational asthma usually include a pre-placement respiratory questionnaire, spirometry and if feasible specific immunologic test(s) and possibly other tests of airway inflammation such as exhaled nitric oxide, induced sputum variables or exhaled breath condensate (Lau and Tarlo 2019, Ilgaz et al. 2019, Maneechaeye et al. 2018).

3. **Tertiary prevention**

    To delay the progress of illness once the symptom has been seen and administer standard treatment forms the main focus of tertiary treatment. This might require switching the patient to a new department or assigning him or her to a new task. The physician should consider compensation for the patient's lost opportunity in relation to his or her medical welfare (Lau and Tarlo 2019, Maneechaeye et al. 2018).

Conclusion

In spite of having large data on sensitizing agents in the work place as well as improvements in work place safety and reporting, OA continues to affect the working population worldwide. The understanding of pathophysiology of OA is limited, especially regarding OA induced by LMW agents. Additional research is required to identify biological markers and more accurate ways of diagnosing OA as well as developing effective surveillance programs for use in high-risk workforces. To encourage industry-wide changes in health surveillance programs, occupational health professionals need to provide overwhelming evidence that early intervention leads to improved worker health in a cost-efficient manner. Fortification of larger collaboration between employers, employees and researchers can determine the most effective and economically feasible interventions for preventing OA in the work place.

References

Balogun RA, Siracusa A, Shusterman D. Occupational rhinitis and occupational asthma: association or progression? Am J Ind Med 2018; 1–15.

Bardana EJ. Occupational asthma and allergies. J Allergy Clin Immunol 2003; 111(2): S530–S539.

Beach J, Rowe BH, Blitz S, Crumley E, Hooton N, Russell K, et al. Diagnosis and Management of work-related asthma: summary, Evidence Report/Technology Assessment: Number 129. AHRQ Publication Number 06-E003-1, October 2005. Agency for Healthcare Research and Quality 2005, Rockville, MD. http://www.ahrq.gov/clinic/epcsums/asthworksum.htm.

Daniels RD. Occupational asthma risk from exposures to toluene diisocyanate: a review and risk assessment. Am J Ind Med 2018; 61(4): 282–292.

Dao A, Bernstein DI. Occupational exposure and asthma. Annals of Allergy, Asthma & Immunol 2018; 120(5): 468–475.

Dobashi K, Akiyama K, Usami A, Yokozeki H, Ikezawa Z, Tsurikisawa N, et al. Japanese guideline for occupational allergic diseases 2014. Allergol Int 2014; 63: 421–442.

Dobashi K, Akiyama K, Usami A, Yokozeki H, Ikezawa Z, Tsurikisawa N, et al. Japanese guidelines for occupational allergic diseases. Allergol Int 2017; 66: 265–280.

Ellis PR, Walters GI. Missed opportunities to identify occupational asthma in acute secondary care. Occup Med (Lond) 2017; 68: 56–59.

Employers, Employees, and Worksites, NIH 2011. Retrieved from:https://www.nhlbi.nih.gov/health-pro/resources/lung/naci/audiences/work.htm, last Updated February 2011.

Fishwick D, Forman S. Health surveillance for occupational asthma. CurrOpin Allergy Clin Immunol 2018; 18: 000–000.

Friedman-Jimenez G, Harrison D, Luo H. Occupational asthma and work-exacerbated asthma. SeminRespirCrit Care Med 2015; 36(03): 388–407.

Greiwe J, Bernstein JA. Occupational Asthma 2019; 10: 1–16.

Ilgaz A, Moore VC, Robertson AS, Walters GI, Burge PS. Occupational asthma; the limited role of air-fed respiratory protective equipment. Occup Med (Lond) 2019; 69(5): 329–335.

Jacobsen IB, Baelum J, Carstensen O, Skadhauge LR, Feary J, Cullinan P, et al. Delayed occupational asthma from epoxy exposure. Occup Med (Lond) 2019; Kqz088.

Jeebhay MF, Quirce S. Occupational asthma in the developing and industrialised world: a review. Int J Tuberc Lung Dis 2006; 11(2): 122–133.

Kelly KJ, Poole JA. Pollutants in the workplace: effect on occupational asthma. J Allergy Clin Immunol 2019; 143: 2014–5.

Larco-Rojas X, Gonzalez-Gutierrez ML, Vazquez-Cortes S, Úartolomé B, Pastor-Vargas C, Fernández-Rivas M, et al. Occupational asthma and urticaria in an fishmonger due to creatine kinase, a cross-reactive fish allergen. J InvestigAllergol Clin Immunol 2017; 27(6): 386–388.

Lau A, Tarlo SM. Update on management of occupational asthma and work-exacerbated asthma. Allergy Asthma Immunol Res 2019; 11(2): 188–200.

Le Moual N, Zock J, Dumas O, Lytras T, Andersson E, Lillienberg L, et al. Update of an occupational asthma-specific job exposure matrix to assess exposure to 30 specific agents. Occup Environ Med 2018; 0: 1–8.

Lux H, Lenz K, Budnik LT, Baur X. Performance of specific immunoglobulin E tests for diagnosing occupational asthma: as systemic review and meta-analysis. Occup Environ Med 2019; 0: 1–10.

Malo J, Chan-Yeung M. Agents causing occupational asthma. J Allergy Clin Immunol 2009; 545–550.

Maneechaeye W, Mitthamsiri W, Sangasapaviliya A, Pradubpongsa P. Asthma in workers: an overview. Am J Respir Crit Care Med 2018; 6(2): 121–124.

Mapp CE, Boschetto P, Maestrelli P, Fabbri LM. Occupational asthma. Am J Respir Crit Care Med 2005; 172: 280–305.

Perlman DM, Maier LA. Occupational lung disease. Med Clin N Am 2019; 103(3): 535–548.

Pralong JA, Cartier A. Review of diagnostic challenges in occupational asthma. Curr Allergy Asthma Rep 2017; 17: 1.

Quirce S, Sastre J. Occupational asthma: clinical phenotypes, biomarkers, and management. CurrOpinPulm Med 2019; 25: 59–63.

Raulf M, Quirce S, Vandenplas O. Addressing molecular diagnosis of occupational allergies. Curr Allergy Asthma Rep 2018; 18: 6.

Stevens WW, Grammer LC. Occupational Rhinitis: an update. Curr Allergy Asthma Rep 2015; 15: 487.

Suojalehto H, Suuronen K, Cullinan P. Specific challenge testing for occupational asthma: revised handbook. EurRespir J 2019; 54: 1901026.

Tarlo SM, Vandenplas O. Diagnosis and management of occupational Asthma. pp. 460–462. *In*: American Thoracic Society Workshop, Proceedings of the First Jack Pepys Occupational Asthma Symposium. This Statement of the American Thoracic Society (ATS) was Approved by the ATS Board of Directors, March 2002. 2003; 167: 450–471.

Trivedi V, Apala DR, Iyer VK. Occupational asthma: diagnostic challenges and management dilemmas. CurrOpinPulm Med 2017; 23: 177–183.

Vandenplas O. Occupational asthma: etiologies and risk factors. Allergy Asthma Immunol Res 2011; 3(3): 157–167.

Vandenplas O, Godet J, Hurdubaea L, Rifflart C, Suojalehto H, Walusiak-Skorupa J, et al. Severe occupational asthma: insights from a multicenter European cohort. J Allergy Clin Immunol Pract 2019; 7(7): 2309–2318.

Walters GI, Burge PS, Sahal A, Robertson AS, Moore VC. Hospital attendances and acute admissions preceding a diagnosis of occupational asthma. Lung 2019; 10.

22

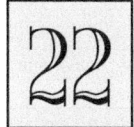

Anaphylaxis

*Amanda Cox** and *Julie Wang*

INTRODUCTION

Anaphylaxis is an acute systemic allergic reaction that varies in severity and may be rapidly progressive and can be life threatening. The term "*l'anaphylaxie*" was first proposed by Portier and Richet in a lecture given in 1902 at the Societé de Biologie in Paris (Portier and 1902). They presented their observations of a dog injected with sea anemone venom. While attempting to confer protective immunization against the toxin, they noted that the dog (called 'Neptune') initially tolerated a low dose of anemone venom, but some weeks later died within 25 minutes of an injection of a second same-sized dose of the venom. Immunization in this case resulted not in prophylaxis, but rather an opposite response, hence the Greek-derived term, 'ana-' (against) '-phylaxis' (protection). While they did not have a clear understanding of the pathophysiology, Portier and Richet did demonstrate that harmful effects could be induced by immunization, and their description and naming of the phenomenon 'anaphylaxis' marked the beginning of the field of allergology (Ring et al. 2014).

In this chapter, we will review the definition, clinical criteria, epidemiology, etiology, pathogenesis and the management of anaphylaxis.

Definition and diagnostic criteria

There is no universal definition or agreed-upon diagnostic criteria for anaphylaxis. However, a multi-disciplinary group of experts who met at the Second National Institute of Allergy and Infectious Disease/Food Allergy and Anaphylaxis Network (NIAID/FAAN) symposium in 2005/2006 published a definition and diagnostic criteria that are widely accepted (Sampson et al. 2005, Sampson et al. 2006). The expert panel defined anaphylaxis as "a severe allergic reaction that is rapid in onset and may cause death." With the goal of reducing confusion, expediting diagnosis and encouraging prompt and appropriate life-saving treatment of anaphylaxis, the symposium panel published three diagnostic criteria in order to aid clinicians (Table 22.1). Symposium participants felt that these diagnostic criteria should accurately identify anaphylactic reactions in more than 95% of cases (Sampson et al. 2005).

The clinical presentation of anaphylaxis varies, and there are many potential signs and symptoms that can occur in any combination, with the potential to involve the skin and mucosa, respiratory system, gastrointestinal tract and cardiovascular system (Simons 2010) (Table 22.2).

It is important to note that the signs, symptoms and organ involvement in anaphylaxis vary among individuals and even for different episodes that may occur in the same person. Cutaneous symptoms such

---

Icahn School of Medicine at Mount Sinai, New York, NY USA, Email: julie.wang@mssm.edu
* Corresponding author: amanda.cox@mssm.edu

Table 22.1. Clinical criteria for diagnosing anaphylaxis (1).

Anaphylaxis is highly likely when any ONE of the following 3 criteria is fulfilled:

1. Acute onset of an illness (minutes to several hours) involving the skin, mucosal tissue, or both (e.g., generalized hives, pruritus or flushing, swollen lips-tongue-uvula)
AND at least one of the following:
    a. Respiratory compromise (e.g., dyspnea, wheeze-bronchospasm, stridor, reduced PEF, hypoxemia)
    b. Reduced blood pressure (BP) or associated symptoms and signs of end-organ malperfusion (e.g., hypotonia [collapse], syncope, incontinence)

2. Two or more of the following that occur rapidly after exposure to a LIKELY allergen for that patient (minutes to several hours):
    a. Involvement of the skin-mucosal tissue (e.g., generalized hives, itch-flush, swollen lips-tongue-uvula)
    b. Respiratory compromise (e.g., dyspnea, wheeze-bronchospasm, stridor, reduced peak expiatory flow, hypoxemia)
    c. Reduced blood pressure or associated symptoms and signs of end-organ malperfusion (e.g., hypotonia [collapse], syncope, incontinence)
    d. Persistent gastrointestinal symptoms (e.g., crampy abdominal pain, vomiting)

3. Reduced BP after exposure to a KNOWN allergen for that patient (minutes to several hours):
    a. Infants and children: low systolic BP (age specific) or greater than 30% decrease in systolic BP*
    b. Adults: systolic BP of less than 90 mm Hg or greater than 30% decrease from that person's baseline systolic BP

PEF, Peak expiratory flow: *BP*, blood pressure. 'Low systolic blood pressure for children is defined as: • less than 70 mm Hg from 1 month to 1 year • less than (70 mm Hg + [2 × age]) from 1 to 10 year • less than 90 mm Hg from 11 to 17 years. Sampson HA, Munoz-Furlong A, Campbel RL, Ackinson NF, Jr., Bock SA, Branum A, et al. Second symposium on the definition and management of anaphylaxis: summary report-Second National Institute of Allergy and Infectious Disease/Food Allergy and Anaphylaxis Network symposium. J. Allergy Clin Immunol. 2006; 1177(2): 391–7.

Table 22.2. Symptoms and signs of anaphylaxis (2).

Cutaneous/subcutaneous/mucosal tissue
Flushing, pruritus, hives (urticaria), swelling, morbilliform rash, pilor erection Periorbital pruritus, erythema and swelling, conjunctival erythema, tearing Pruritus and swelling of lips, tongue, uvula/palate Pruritus in the external auditory canals Pruritus of genitalia, palms, soles
Respiratory
Nose: pruritus, congestion, rhinorrhea, sneezing Larynx: pruritus and tightness in the throat, dysphonia and hoarseness, dry staccato cough, stridor, dysphagia (difficulty swallowing) Lung: shortness of breath, chest tightness, deep cough, wheezing/bronchospasm (decreased peak expiratory flow) Cyanosis
Gastrointestinal
Nausea, cramping abdominal pain, vomiting (stringy mucus), diarrhea
Cardiovascular
Chest pain, palpitations, tachycardia, bradycardia, or other dysrhythmia Feeling faint, syncope, altered mental status, hypotension, urinary or fecal incontinence, shock, cardiac arrest
CNS
Aura of impending doom, uneasiness, throbbing headache, dizziness, confusion, tunnel vision; in infants and children, sudden behavioral changes, such as irritability, cessation of play, and clinging to parent
Other
Metallic taste in the mouth Dysphagia Uterine contractions in post-pubertal female patients
Sudden onset of symptoms and signs is characteristic of anaphylaxis.

Simon FE, Anaphalaxis. J Allergy clin Immunol. 2010; 125(2 Suppl 2): S 161–81.

as urticaria, pruritus, flushing and swelling, often help in making the diagnosis of anaphylaxis, but may be missed on examination or may not be present in up to 20% of anaphylaxis episodes (Simons 2006).

Anaphylaxis usually results after a specific exposure, and the time course for developing symptoms may be within seconds to minutes or up to hours later. The symptoms generally evolve rapidly, but overall Anaphylaxis symptoms are unpredictable. Anaphylaxis can be mild and can resolve spontaneously or may be severe and progress to a life-threatening clinical state. Fatal anaphylaxis may result from severe hypotensive shock, obstructive swelling of the upper airway, severe bronchoconstriction or cardiac arrhythmia (Greenberger 2015).

Making a diagnosis of anaphylaxis depends upon recognition of clinical signs and symptoms, identification of a known or likely trigger, and determination of the timing of likely exposure to a trigger. Other medical conditions of sudden multi-system onset should be ruled-out (differential diagnoses will be discussed later). There are no biomarkers or laboratory tests that immediately confirm the diagnosis of anaphylaxis, although laboratory tests taken during an anaphylaxis episode can be used to later confirm the diagnosis (Simons et al. 2013).

Several special anaphylaxis scenarios have been observed in practice and make for more challenging diagnosis and clinical management:

In biphasic anaphylaxis symptoms of anaphylaxis recur after initial anaphylaxis symptoms resolve or are treated, without further exposure to the precipitant for the initial reaction. An individual may be completely asymptomatic between the initial reaction and the recurrence of anaphylaxis symptoms. Biphasic reactions typically occur within 12 hours after the initial anaphylaxis, but have been reported to occur up to 72 hours later (Lieberman 2005). Biphasic reactions occur in 1 to 23% of anaphylactic reactions (Tole et al. 2007, Scranton et al. 2009).

Protracted anaphylaxis describes an anaphylactic reaction of more than 5 hours, up to days or even weeks in duration, and can be refractory to treatment (Stark and Sullivan 1986).

In delayed anaphylaxis, the initial onset of symptoms begins several hours after exposure to the triggering agent. This has primarily been observed in patients with galactose-alpha-1,3-galactose IgE in whom anaphylaxis is induced 3–6 hours after ingesting mammalian meats (such as beef, pork or lamb) (Commins et al. 2009).

In some cases of anaphylaxis, a detailed history and extensive diagnostic evaluation, including testing for foods, medications, latex, exercise and insect stings are non-contributory. Idiopathic anaphylaxis is diagnosed when there is no identifiable cause or trigger for anaphylaxis (Greenberger and Lieberman 2014). To make this diagnosis, especially if there are recurrent episodes, underlying mast cell disorders (including systemic mastocytosis and monoclonal mast cell activation syndrome) should be ruled-out (Theoharides et al. 2015).

Epidemiology of anaphylaxis

Determining accurate incidence and prevalence rates for anaphylaxisis is complicated by to a lack of universal terminology or diagnostic criteria, miscoding in medical record systems and lack of representative ICD codes, likely under-reporting, and the unfeasibility of prospective studies of anaphylaxis (Lieberman 2008). Most data on anaphylaxis comes from emergency departments, regional databases and from health information collected by health maintenance organizations (Tejedor-Alonso et al. 2015a).

Over the last two decades, there have been several studies seeking to determine incidence and prevalence rates for anaphylaxis. Evidence suggests that since the late 1990's and early 2000's, rates of anaphylaxis and anaphylaxis-related hospitalizations have been rising in the US, Australia, Europe and the UK (Lee et al. 2017, Turner et al. 2015, Lin et al. 2008, Sheikh et al. 2008, Mullins et al. 2015).

While prevalence estimates vary widely by study and by criteria, a 2004 expert working group review of population-based studies found that 0.05 to 2% of the population had at least one lifetime episode of anaphylaxis (Lieberman et al. 2006). Similarly, a nationwide cross-sectional survey of 1000 US adults performed in 2011 found a 1.6% prevalence rate of anaphylaxis in the general population (Wood et al. 2014). More recent publications estimate a prevalence of anaphylaxis between 0.3–5.1%

with rates almost three times higher in children 0–4 years when compared to other age groups (Tejedor-Alonso et al. 2015a, Tejedor-Alonso et al. 2015b).

Food-allergy in children seems to account for marked increases in anaphylaxis and anaphylaxis related hospitalizations, and this may explain the rise in anaphylaxis rates in children. A UK study found an increase between 1998 and 2012 of 137% for the incidence of food-induced anaphylaxis in 0–14 year olds (Turner et al. 2015). In a meta-analysis of studies of food anaphylaxis cases, an incidence rate of anaphylaxis for food-allergic 0–19 year olds was 0.2 per 100 person years, whereas the incidence rate for 0–4 year olds was 7.0 per 100 person years (Umasunthur et al. 2015). Another US report found that the rate of food-induced anaphylaxis related hospitalizations more than doubled (from 0.60 per 1000 to 1.26 per 1000) between 2000 and 2009 (Rudders et al. 2014).

Fatal anaphylaxis

Death due to anaphylaxis is usually secondary to upper or lower airway obstruction or cardiovascular collapse. Despite an apparent increase in anaphylaxis rates, anaphylaxis fatalities have not increased and death due to anaphylaxis remains rare. Across several studies, the rates of fatal anaphylaxis range from 0.12 to 1.06 deaths per million person-years, and the probability of death in patients with severe anaphylaxis ranges from 0.3 to 2% (Tejedor-Alonso et al. 2015a, Monerer-Vautrin et al. 2005, Ben-Shoshan et al. 2011, Liew et al. 2009, Pumphrey et al. 2004, Ma et al. 2014). Deaths due to anaphylaxis are caused most often by medications, insect stings and food (Tejedor-Alonso et al. 2015b). Insect and drug-induced anaphylaxis are more often fatal in adults older than 35–40 years, while food-induced anaphylaxis is more frequently fatal among children and younger adults (ages 5–35 years) (Liew et al. 2009, Jerschow et al. 2014, Turner et al. 2015) and within the pediatric age group, fatal anaphylaxis is more common in teenagers than in younger children (Gupta 2014). Death from anaphylaxis is often preceded by a prior non-fatal anaphylactic episode.

Causes (triggers) of anaphylaxis

There are multitudes of potential triggers for anaphylaxis (Table 22.3), and the predominant causes vary among different age groups. The most common substances to cause IgE-mediated anaphylaxis include medications, foods, insect bites/stings, latex and allergen immunotherapy injections. Anaphylaxis is possible to any medication, however antibiotics, NSAIDs, neuromuscular blocking agents, chemotherapeutic agents and monoclonal antibodies are most common (Simons et al. 2013) and parenteral administration of medication carries the highest risk. The most frequent foods triggering anaphylaxis are cow's milk, eggs, peanuts, tree nuts, fish, shellfish, soy and wheat. The most common stinging insects that trigger anaphylaxis are hymenoptera, which include bees, wasps, polistes, hornets and fire ants. Exercise can also be a trigger for anaphylaxis, sometimes in association with prior ingestion of a specific food (Feldweg 2017).

Risk factors and co-factors (Table 22.4)

Atopy is a risk factor for anaphylaxis in general and specifically for anaphylaxis related to latex, ingested antigens, exercise, radiographic contrast media, as well as idiopathic events (Lieberman 2008). Adolescence and advanced age are associated with increased risk for severe anaphylaxis, as are pre-existing medical conditions including asthma, cardiovascular disease, respiratory disease, mastocytosis and mast cell activation syndromes (Simon et al. 2015). Upper respiratory infections, fever, emotional stress and premenstrual status are also recognized cofactors for anaphylaxis. External factors, such as rigorous exercise, alcohol, concomitant use of certain medications, infection and stress can also augment the severity of an allergic reaction or make an individual more susceptible to anaphylaxis (Dhami and Sheikh 2017). Beta-adrenergic blockers, ACE inhibitors and alpha-adrenergic blocking medications interfere with treatment of anaphylaxis as well as prevent physiologic compensatory mechanisms for cardiovascular compromise.

Table 22.3. Causes of anaphylaxis.

Allergens (IgE-dependent immunologic mechanism)
Food • especially milk, egg, soy, wheat, peanut, tree nuts, fish, shellfish, sesame • delayed anaphylaxis to mammalian meats (alpha-gal syndrome) • food additives (e.g., spices, colorants including carmine, vegetable gums, gelatin)
Venoms as from stinging insects (hymenoptera) and insect bites (e.g., kissing bugs) Medications (B-lactam antibiotics, NSAIDs, monoclonal antibodies, chemotherapeutic agents, neuromuscular blocking agents) Vaccines (reaction is typically to an excipient in vaccine rather than microbial content) Subcutaneous allergen immunotherapy Natural rubber latex Inhalants (horse dander, cat dander, grass pollen) - rare Human seminal fluid (prostate-specific antigen) - rare Occupational allergens
Immunologic triggers (IgE-independent machanism)
IgG-dependent Ito high-molecular weight dextran, infliximab) - rare Coagulation system activation (e.g., heparin contaminated with oversulfated chondroitin sulfate)
Non-immunologic triggers (direct activation of mast cells and basophils)
Physical factors (e.g., cold, heat, UV radiation, exercise with or without a cofactor) Medications (opioids, NSAIDS) Radiocontrast media Alcohol (ethanol)
Idiopathic anaphylaxis
Consider the possibility of a hidden or previously unrecognized trigger
Consider the possibility of a mast cell activation syndrome, or monoclonal mast cell disorder

Adapted from UpToDate (www.uptodate.com/contents/anaphylaxis-acute-diagnosis)

Pathophysiology of anaphylaxis

Anaphylaxis can be immunologic or non-immunologic. Immunologic anaphylactic reactions in humans include IgE-mediated and immune-complex or complement-mediated reactions. In non-immunologic anaphylaxis, mast cells or basophils are stimulated to degranulate without IgE (or other antibodies) or immune complex involvement (Johansson et al. 2004).

IgE is bound to high-affinity receptor FcϵRI on the surfaces of blood basophils and tissue mast cells. In the classic IgE-mediated allergic reaction, a circulating allergen interacts with surface-bound FcϵRIIgE, cross-links two IgE molecules on the mast cell or basophil. This in turn initiates intracellular signaling for the cell to degranulate and release preformed mediators, enzymes, and cytokines as well as induces *de novo* synthesis of inflammatory mediators (Reber et al. 2017). These chemical mediators act directly on tissues and result in the previously described allergic symptoms. Figures 22.1 and 22.2 demonstrate mediators of anapyhylaxis and their tissue targets, resulting in anaphylaxis symptoms (Reber et al. 2017, Castells 2017). Additional inflammatory cells, in particular eosinophils, are recruited and stimulated to release additional chemical mediators. This results in full-blown allergic inflammation and the clinical signs of anaphylaxis.

IgG-mediated anaphylaxis has been demonstrated in mouse models and is postulated to be involved in anaphylaxis in humans to omalizumab or other monoclonal antibodies (Cox et al. 2007, Cheifetz et al. 2003). Immune complex/complement-mediated mechanisms may be involved in reactions to protamine and some other drugs. In reactions to Radio Contrast Media (RCM), RCM molecules may interact with the Fc portion of IgE or IgG already bound to mast cells or basophils, directly causing cross-linking and cell activation (Brockow and Ring 2011). Cytokine storm-like reactions, characterized by chills and fever, followed by hypotension, desaturation and cardiovascular collapse can occur with chimeric, humanized and human monoclonal antibodies and chemotherapy. Cytokine storm reactions are systemic

Table 22.4. Risk factors for severe anaphylaxis and fatal anaphylaxis.

Age
Infants
Adolescents and young adults
Elderly
Comorbidities
Asthma and other pulmonary disease (COPD, interstitial lung disease) especially if poorly-controlled cardiovascular disease (ischemic heart disease, hypertensive vascular disease, cardiomyopathy)
Mast cell disorder (systemic mastocytosis or mast cell activation syndrome)
Atopy (risk factor for anaphylaxis to food, exercise, and latex)
Depression and other psychiatric disorder
Medications
Affect recognition of anaphylaxis
• Sedatives, hypnotics, antidepressants, ethanol, recreational drugs
Increase anaphylaxis severity or interfere with epinephrine treatment
• Beta-adrenergic blockers
• Alpha-adrenergic blockers
• Angiotensin II receptor blockers
• Tricyclic antidepressants
• Monoamine oxidase inhibitors
• ADHD medications
Other factors
• Exercise
• Acute infection, fever
• Menses
• Emotional stress
• Parenteral route of medication or immunotherapy administration
• Previous history of anaphylaxis

Adapted from Simons FE. Anaphylaxis. J Allergy Clin Immunol. 2010; 125(2 Suppl 2): S161–81.

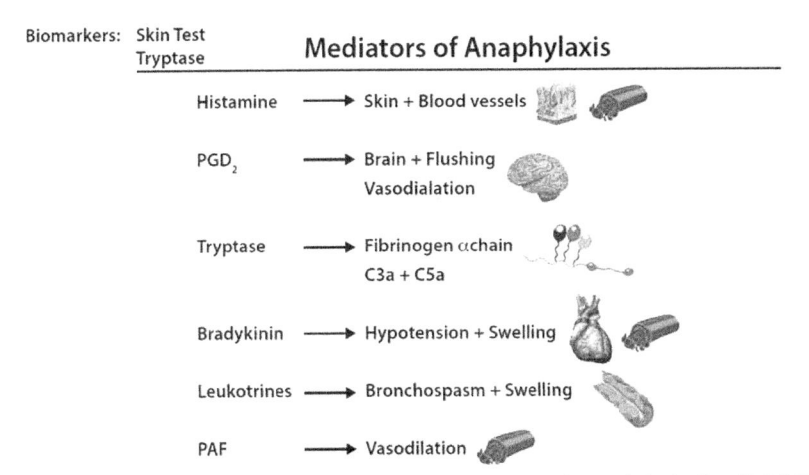

Figure 22.1. Mediators of anaphylaxis released from mast cells and basophils in anaphylaxis. Castells M. Diagnosis and management of anaphylaxis in precision medicine. J Allergy Clin Immunol. 2017; 140(2): 321–33.

inflammatory responses instigated by leukocyte release of pro-inflammatory cytokines (TNF-α, IL-1B, and IL-6) (Castells 2017).

In non-immune anaphylaxis, the mechanism of activating mast cells and basophils bypasses IgE. Examples include reactions to vancomycin and opiates, which can cause direct activation of mast cells

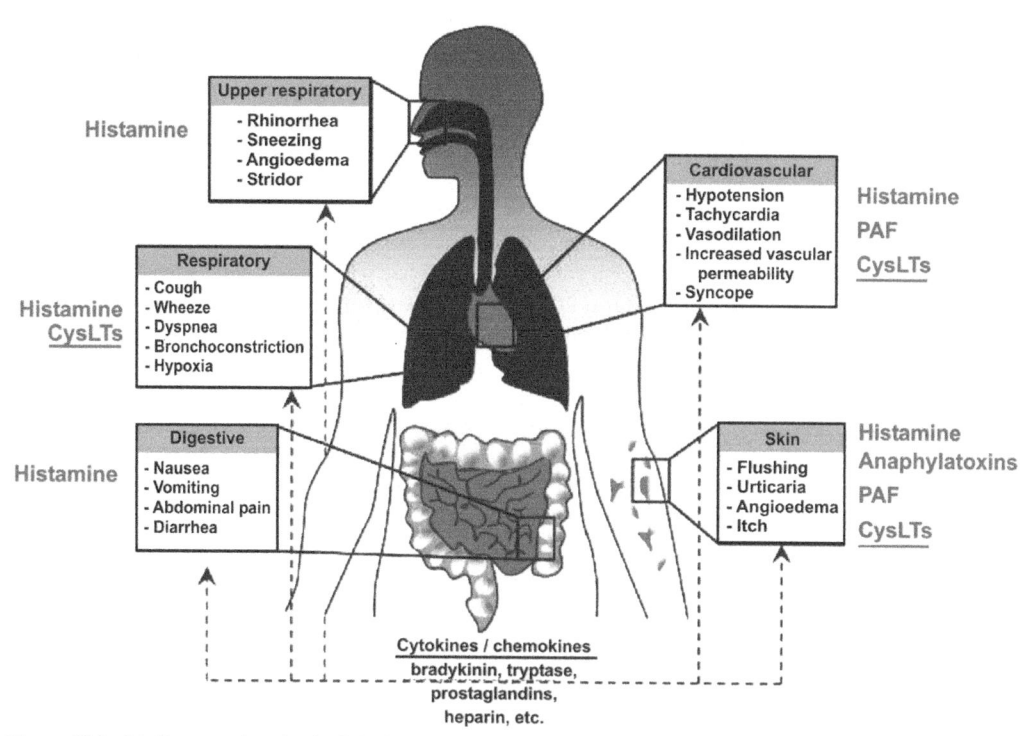

Figure 22.2. Mediators and pathophysiologic changes in anaphylaxis. From Reber LL, Hernandez JD, Galli SJ. The pathophysiology of anaphylaxis. J Allergy Clin Immunol. 2017;140(2):335-48.

and/or basophils to release histamine, and can result in symptoms of anaphylaxis, including hypotension flushing and urticaria.

Effector cells and chemical mediators of anaphylaxis

Mast cells are the dominant effector cells in anaphylaxis, while there is evidence that basophils also participate in the pathophysiology of anaphylaxis. Laboratory assays of mediators from neutrophils, monocytes/macrophages and platelets, all of which express activating FcγR suggest that these cell types may also be involved in anaphylaxis pathophysiology. The mediators released from degranulating mast cells during anaphylaxis bind to specific tissue receptors on target organs to induce the clinical symptoms of anaphylaxis and cause downstream effects on other immunologically active cells (Castells 2017). The primary chemical mediators of anaphylaxis include preformed intracellular granule substances (histamine, tryptase, chymase and heparin) and newly-generated lipid-derived mediators, including prostaglandin D2 (PGD_2), leukotriene B_4 (LTB_4), platelet-activating factor (PAF) and the cysteinyl leukotrienes (LTC_4, LTD_4, and LTE_4) (Reber et al. 2017).

Histamine is an important chemical mediator of allergic responses and the major clinical manifestations of anaphylaxis. Histamine is released by activated mast cells and basophils. Cutaneous histamine release causes urticaria and pruritus, while systemic release of histamine results in flushing, headache, bronchoconstriction, hypotension, tachycardia, as well as direct effects on coronary arteries and atrial and ventricular contractility (Reber et al. 2017). Histamine effects are mediated through four histamine receptors; H1, H2, H3 and H4, which are present on target cells in different organs (MacGlashan 2003). H1 and H2 receptors both mediate flushing, hypotension and headaches, whereas airway obstruction and tachycardia are primarily mediated via the H1 receptor (Kaliner et al. 1981, Vigorito et al. 1983). In animal models, H3 appears to influence cardiovascular response to norepinephrine, and H4 may be involved in chemotaxis, mast cell cytokine release and pruritus (Godot et al. 2007, Dunford et al. 2007).

Tryptase is primarily a mast cell derived protease but is produced by basophils in smaller amounts. Mature, enzymatically active β-tryptase is stored in mast cell granules and is released to the circulation when the cell is activated, such that increased levels can be detected during acute anaphylaxis (Schwartz 2006). Mast cells constitutively secrete α- and β-protryptases, and baseline high serum levels of these enzymes may indicate an underlying increased mast cell and basophil burden (Theoharides et al. 2015). Mast cell activation disorders and mastocytosis can be risk factors for anaphylaxis and for more severe anaphylaxis. While its functional role in anaphylaxis has not been fully determined, it is known that tryptase activates the complement (C3a and C5a) pathways, coagulation pathway, as well as the kallikrein-kinin contact system and that high tryptase levels largely correlate with more severe anaphylaxis, except in cases of food-triggered anaphylaxis (Reber 2017, Adkinson and Middleton 2009).

Arachidonic acid metabolites derived from membrane phospholipids generate pro-inflammatory mediators such as cysleukotrienes (CysLTs), prostaglandins and PAF that can be released during anaphylaxis. Studies have shown that circulating levels of leukotrienes (LTB_4, LTC_4, and LTD_4) increase during anaphylaxis, and are involved in enhanced vascular permeability and bronchoconstriction (Reber et al. 2017). Prostaglandin D2 (PGD_2), also released from activated mast cells, promotes vasodilation, vasopermeability and airway smooth muscle bronchoconstriction (Hardy et al. 1984). The role of PAF in anaphylaxis in humans is still not well defined, however studies suggest that PAF and platelet-activating factor acetylhydrolase (PAF-AH) activity are increased in anaphylaxis, and that PAF-AH is inversely correlated with anaphylaxis severity (Vadas et al. 2013).

Pathways activated during anaphylaxis

In severe anaphylaxis, complement and coagulation pathways and the kallikrein-kinin contact system may be activated when mast cells and basophils release various cytokines and inflammatory mediators. Activation of the complement cascade leads to the generation of inflammatory anaphylatoxins (C3a, C4a, and C5a), levels of which correlate with the severity of anaphylaxis (Brown et al. 2013). Clotting factors, including Factors V and VIII, can be depleted and, in extreme cases, result in disseminated intravascular coagulation (DIC), a coagulopathy characterized by microthrombi, tissue hypoxia and infarction and hemorrhages (Smith et al. 1980). Late, prolonged or recurrent (biphasic) symptoms may be the result of release of certain mediators, such as CysLTs, cytokines and chemokines (Reber et al. 2017, Lieberman 2005).

Differential diagnosis of anaphylaxis

Rapid recognition of anaphylaxis is necessary as this has implications for optimal and prompt medical management. Evaluation of a patient's clinical history (with emphasis on the history of exposures and chronology), presenting symptoms and physical examinations, as well as ruling-out of other sudden multi-system diseases, is critical. The signs and symptoms of anaphylaxis overlap with many other disorders and acute illnesses, so that, making a correct diagnosis of anaphylaxis can be challenging. The most common disorders that mimic anaphylaxis are acute generalized urticaria or angioedema, acute asthma, vasovagal syncope and panic attacks or acute anxiety (Simons 2010). These can be symptoms of anaphylaxis but may also occur as isolated problems. The differential diagnosis of anaphylaxis includes other respiratory and cardiac events, other causes of shock, flushing syndromes, postprandial syndromes, hematologic disorders and neurologic events, as listed in Table 22.5. In addition to the diagnostic criterion (Table 22.1), the algorithm in Fig. 22.3 is a tool that may aid in confirming the diagnosis of anaphylaxis (Castells 2017).

Suggested laboratory tests for the diagnosis of anaphylaxis

The diagnosis of anaphylaxis should be made clinically, and should be based on the presenting signs, symptoms and temporal history. Medical management should not be delayed for laboratory confirmation, and appropriate treatment should be initiated promptly when a diagnosis of anaphylaxis is suspected. While most laboratory testing for anaphylaxis is not sensitive or specific enough, laboratory samples

Table 22.5. Different diagnosis of anaphylaxis (2).

Common entities
• Acute generalized hives • Acute asthma • Syncope (fainting, vasovagal episode) • Panic attack • Aspiration of a foreign body • Cardiovascular event (myocardial infarction, pulmonary embolus) • Neurologic event (seizure, stroke)
Postprandial syndromes
• Pollen-food syndrome • Scombroidosis • Monosodium glutamate • Sulfites
Excess endogenous histamine production
• Mastocytosis/clonal mast cell disorders • Basophilic leukemia
Flush syndromes
• Perimenopause • Carcinoid • Autonomic epilepsy • Medullary carcinoma • Vancomycin flushing syndrome • Alcohol
Shock
• Hypovolemic • Cardiogenic • Distributive • Septic
Nonorganic disease
• Vocal cord dysfunction
Other
• Nonallergic angioedema, hereditary angioedema • Urticarial vasculitis • Hyper-IgE urticarial syndrome • Progesterone anaphylaxis • Pheochromocytoma • Idiopathic systemic capillary leak syndrome

Adopted from Simons FE. Anaphylaxis. J Allergy Clin Immunol. 2010: 125 (2 Suppl 2)S161–81.

obtained at the time of anaphylaxis, can however be used to confirm the diagnosis when there is doubt and to rule-out other underlying disorders or conditions with similar acute clinical presentations.

For instance, serum tryptase may be measured within 15 minutes to 3 hours of the onset of anaphylaxis. If the tryptase level during the event is greater than 11.4 ng/mL (or elevated $\geq 20\%$ above baseline plus 2 ng/mL), and returns to normal after the event, a diagnosis of anaphylaxis can be confirmed. An event-related normal tryptase, however, does not rule-out anaphylaxis, especially in cases of food-induced anaphylaxis in which tryptase does not typically rise. Elevated serum tryptase may also be present at baseline in the setting of elevated mast cell burden and in some other disease states (Simons 2010).

Plasma histamine levels begin to rise within 5–10 minutes of the onset of anaphylaxis, and remain elevated only for 30–60 minutes, thus this is a less than ideal test in the setting of anaphylaxis, in which acute management should supersede laboratory diagnostic testing. Urinary histamine, methylhistamine, PGD_2, 9-α-11-β PGF_2, LTE_4 and LTC_4 are elevated for a more prolonged period after anaphylaxis, and

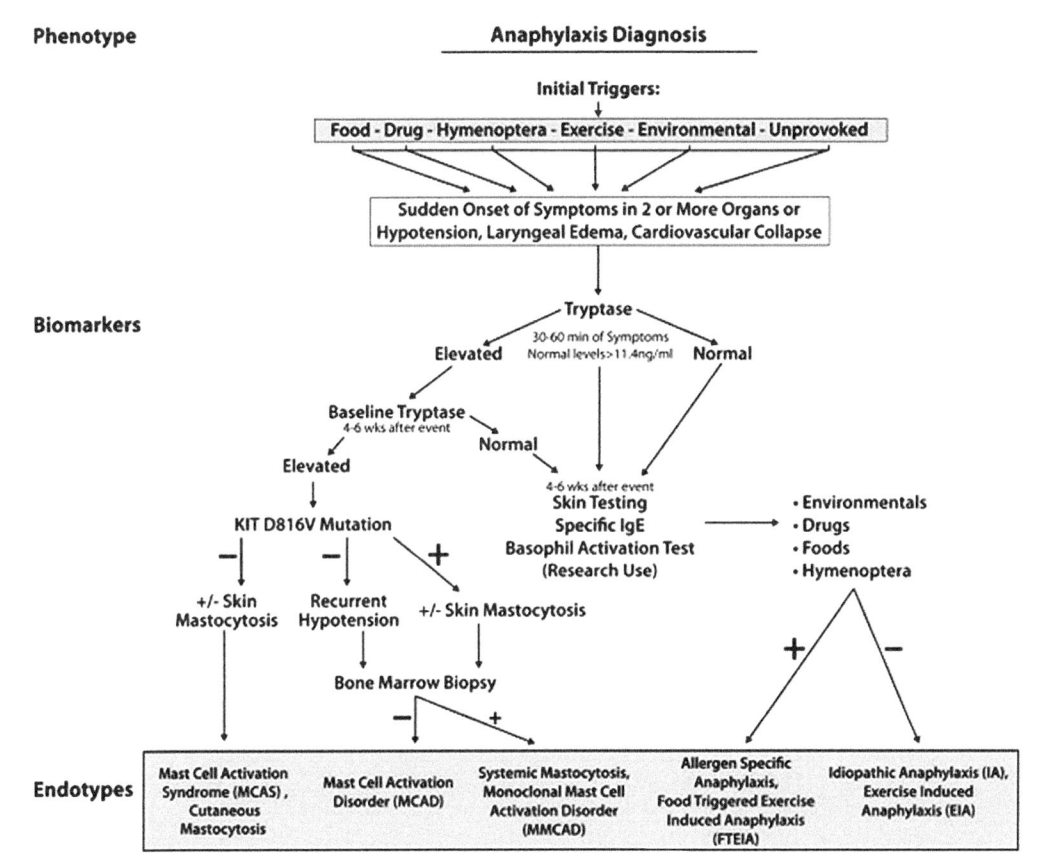

Figure 22.3. Proposed algorithm for the diagnosis of anaphylaxis. Castells M. Diagnosis and management of anaphylaxis in precision medicine. J Allergy Clin Immunol. 2017; 140(2): 321–33.

can be measured by 24-hour urine collection, however the timing and logistics of this testing may also not be feasible (Castells 2017).

Plasma free metanephrine and urinary vanillylmandelic acid level measurements may be considered to rule-out pheochromocytoma, serum serotonin and urinary 5-hydroxyindoleacetic acid may be evaluated to rule-out carcinoid syndrome and vasointestinal hormonal polypeptide (VIP) panel may be measured to rule-out VIP secreting tumors (Lieberman and Blaiss 2002).

Evaluating for potential cause of anaphylaxis

Identifying the cause of anaphylaxis is imperative so that the individual can avoid future exposures and prevent recurrence of anaphylaxis. The clinical history will often indicate the likely trigger, and careful evaluation of the patient's exposures (i.e., medications, foods, insect stings, activities) prior to the onset of symptoms will often reveal the cause. For IgE-mediated allergic reactions, allergen skin testing or *in vitro* measurement of allergen specific serum IgE levels can establish whether a patient is sensitized to an allergen, and if considered in the context of the clinical history, may lead to determination of the likely trigger. It may also be prudent to test for related allergens or similar substances, in cases of anaphylaxis to foods, medications and insect venoms.

While not yet commercially available, the Basophil Activation Test (BAT) is an emerging laboratory tool, in which basophils are stimulated *in vitro* with allergens, after which surface activation markers or mediators can be measured. This is thought to reflect the presence of sensitized mast cells that would mediate an allergic response, and may eventually aid in the diagnosis of an individual's anaphylaxis potential to food, hymenoptera venom and drug allergens (Castells 2017). Clinical utility still requires additional study.

In cases of anaphylaxis where the history and subsequent evaluation does not reveal a trigger, the clinician should address the list of differential diagnosis (Table 22.5), as well as consider unusual or hidden triggers, such as exercise-related phenomenon, delayed anaphylaxis to mammalian meats or reactions to physical triggers such as cold air, cold water or heat. In patients with recurrent anaphylaxis or anaphylaxis-like symptoms, systemic mastocytosis and mast cell activation disorders must be excluded (Mast cell disorders are reviewed elsewhere in this volume). An individual is diagnosed with idiopathic anaphylaxis when no trigger can be identified and when mast cell disorders have been ruled-out (Greenberger 2007).

Overview of anaphylaxis treatment

As respiratory or cardiac arrest and death can occur within minutes of onset of anaphylaxis, rapid assessment and treatment are crucial (Pumphrey 2000, Bock et al. 2001, Pumphrey et al. 2007). Epinephrine (adrenaline) remains the first line medication in the treatment of anaphylaxis (Simons et al. 2015). Fatal anaphylaxis has been associated with delayed injection of epinephrine (Shiekh et al. 2009, Simons 2008, McLean-Tooke et al. 2003). Thus, the early phases of anaphylaxis appear to be most responsive to treatment, and prompt treatment of suspected or impending anaphylaxis may prevent progression to shock and life-threatening symptoms.

In particular, for anaphylaxis, it is essential to identify, remove or discontinue the anaphylaxis trigger if exposure is ongoing (i.e., medication, latex, food ingestion, stinging vespid, exercise). Secondly, anyone responding to anaphylaxis should call for immediate help (such as 911 or an emergency medical service or resuscitation team).

As with any critically ill individual, airway, breathing and circulation should be assessed immediately. Furthermore, until the patient is completely stabilized, blood pressure, heart rate, respiratory rate and oxygen saturation should be continuously monitored during anaphylaxis.

Major components of medical management of anaphylaxis

Epinephrine: Administer intramuscular (IM) epinephrine as early as possible. The dose of IM epinephrine should be 0.01 mg/kg (maximum dose of 0.5 mg) and injection can be repeated every 5–15 minutes if needed. Intravenous epinephrine is associated with more dosing errors and cardiac complications but may be an option for a patient with severe hypotension or circulatory symptoms that are not responsive to IM epinephrine (Sampson et al. 2006).

Respiratory management: Supplemental high-flow oxygen (via non-rebreather mask, high flow oxygen mask or endotracheal tube) can be administered for hypoxemia, and inhaled β-2 agonists (such as albuterol) can be given for bronchospasm (bronchodilators are considered an adjunctive agent, and should never be used instead of epinephrine). If the airway is compromised by angioedema, intubation should be performed immediately.

Patient positioning: Placement of the patient in a recumbent or supine position, with legs elevated, may improve cardiac stroke volume and maximize vital organ perfusion. Studies of anaphylaxis-related deaths have suggested that postural changes to an upright position or failure of a patient to remain supine, have contributed to some fatal outcomes (Pumphrey 2003). Supine repositioning should not however be attempted in patients who are actively vomiting or who have respiratory distress.

Fluid resuscitation: The increased vascular permeability associated with severe anaphylaxis can lead to rapid redistribution of intravascular blood volume and can lead to distributive shock (Brown et al. 2004). If hypotension or orthostasis are present and not responsive to IM epinephrine, large bolus IV fluids should be administered immediately (Simons et al. 2011).

Rapid overview: Emergency management of anaphylaxis in adults

Diagnosis is made clinically:

The most common signs and symptoms are cutaneous (eg, sudden onset of generalized urticaria, angioedema, flushing, pruritus). However, 10 to 20% of patients have no skin findings.

Danger signs: Rapid progression of symptoms, respiratory distress (eg, stridor, wheezing, dyspnea, increased work of breathing, persistent cough, cyanosis), vomiting, abdominal pain, hypotension, dysrhythmia, chest pain, collapse.

Acute management:

The first and most important treatment in anaphylaxis is epinephrine. There are **NO absolute contraindications to epinephrine** in the setting of anaphylaxis.

Airway: Immediate intubation if evidence of impending airway obstruction from angioedema. Delay may lead to complete obstruction. Intubation can be difficult and should be performed by the most experienced clinician available. Cricothyrotomy may be necessary.

Promptly and simultaneously, give:

IM epinephrine (1 mg/mL preparation): Give epinephrine 0.3 to 0.5 mg intramuscularly, preferably in the mid-outer thigh. Can repeat every 5 to 15 minutes (or more frequently), as needed. If epinephrine is injected promptly IM, most patients respond to one, two, or at most, three doses. If symptoms are not responding to epinephrine injections, prepare IV epinephrine for infusion.

Place patient in recumbent position, if tolerated, and elevate lower extremities.

Oxygen: Give 8 to 10 L/minute via facemask or up to 100% oxygen, as needed.

Normal saline rapid bolus: Treat hypotension with rapid infusion of 1 to 2 liters IV. Repeat, as needed. Massive fluid shifts with severe loss of intravascular volume can occur.

Albuterol (salbutamol): For bronchospasm resistant to IM epinephrine, give 2.5 to 5 mg in 3 mL saline via nebulizer. Repeat, as needed.

Adjunctive therapies:

H1 antihistamine*: Consider giving diphenhydramine 25 to 50 mg IV (for relief of urticaria and itching only).

H2 antihistamine*: Consider giving ranitidine 50 mg IV.

Glucocorticoid*: Consider giving methylprednisolone 125 mg IV.

Monitoring: Continuous noninvasive hemodynamic monitoring and pulse oximetry monitoring should be performed. Urine output should be monitored in patients receiving IV fluid resuscitation for severe hypotension or shock.

Treatment of refractory symptoms:

Epinephrine infusion¶: For patients with inadequate response to IM epinephrine and IV saline, give epinephrine continuous infusion, beginning at **0.1 mcg/kg/minute** by infusion pumpΔ. Titrate the dose continuously according to blood pressure, cardiac rate and function, and oxygenation.

Vasopressors¶: Some patients may require a second vasopressor (in addition to epinephrine). All vasopressors should be given by infusion pump, with the doses titrated continuously according to blood pressure and cardiac rate/function and oxygenation monitored by pulse oximetry.

Glucagon: Patients on beta-blockers may not respond to epinephrine and can be given glucagon 1 to 5 mg IV over 5 minutes, followed by infusion of 5 to 15 mcg/minute. Rapid administration of glucagon can cause vomiting.

Instructions on how to prepare and administer epinephrine for IV continuous infusions are available as separate tables in UpToDate.

IM: intramuscular; IV: intravenous.
* These medications should not be used as initial or sole treatment.
¶ All patients receiving an infusion of epinephrine and another vasopressor require continuous noninvasive monitoring of blood pressure, heart rate and function, and oxygen saturation.
Δ For example, the initial infusion rate for a 70 kg patient would be 7 mcg/minute. This is consistent with the recommended range for non-weight-based dosing for adults, which is 2 to 10 mcg/minute. Non-weight-based dosing can be used if the patient's weight is not known and cannot be estimated.

Adapted from: Simons FER. Anaphylaxis. J Allergy Clin Immunol 2010; 125:S161.

Figure 22.4. Rapid overview of emergency management of anaphylaxis in adults.

Rapid overview: Emergency management of anaphylaxis in infants and children*

Diagnosis is made clinically:

The most common signs and symptoms are cutaneous (eg, sudden onset of generalized urticaria, angioedema, flushing, pruritus). However, 10 to 20% of patients have no skin findings.

Danger signs: Rapid progression of symptoms, evidence of respiratory distress (eg, stridor, wheezing, dyspnea, increased work of breathing, retractions, persistent cough, cyanosis), signs of poor perfusion, abdominal pain, vomiting, dysrhythmia, hypotension, collapse.

Acute management:

The first and most important therapy in anaphylaxis is epinephrine. There are **NO absolute contraindications to epinephrine** in the setting of anaphylaxis.

Airway: Immediate intubation if evidence of impending airway obstruction from angioedema. Delay may lead to complete obstruction. Intubation can be difficult and should be performed by the most experienced clinician available. Cricothyrotomy may be necessary.

IM epinephrine (1 mg/mL preparation): Epinephrine 0.01 mg/kg should be injected intramuscularly in the mid-outer thigh. For large children (>50 kg), the maximum is 0.5 mg per dose. If there is no response or the response is inadequate, the injection can be repeated in 5 to 15 minutes (or more frequently). If epinephrine is injected promptly IM, patients respond to one, two, or at most, three injections. If signs of poor perfusion are present or symptoms are not responding to epinephrine injections, prepare IV epinephrine for infusion (see below).

Place patient in recumbent position, if tolerated, and elevate lower extremities.

Oxygen: Give 8 to 10 L/minute via facemask or up to 100% oxygen, as needed.

Normal saline rapid bolus: Treat poor perfusion with rapid infusion of 20 mL/kg. Re-evaluate and repeat fluid boluses (20 mL/kg), as needed. Massive fluid shifts with severe loss of intravascular volume can occur. Monitor urine output.

Albuterol: For bronchospasm resistant to IM epinephrine, give albuterol 0.15 mg/kg (minimum dose: 2.5 mg) in 3 mL saline inhaled via nebulizer. Repeat, as needed.

H1 antihistamine: Consider giving diphenhydramine 1 mg/kg (max 40 mg) IV.

H2 antihistamine: Consider giving ranitidine 1 mg/kg (max 50 mg) IV.

Glucocorticoid: Consider giving methylprednisolone 1 mg/kg (max 125 mg) IV.

Monitoring: Continuous noninvasive hemodynamic monitoring and pulse oximetry monitoring should be performed. Urine output should be monitored in patients receiving IV fluid resuscitation for severe hypotension or shock.

Treatment of refractory symptoms:

Epinephrine infusion¶: In patients with inadequate response to IM epinephrine and IV saline, give epinephrine continuous infusion at 0.1 to 1 mcg/kg/minute, titrated to effect.

Vasopressors¶: Patients may require large amounts of IV crystalloid to maintain blood pressure. Some patients may require a second vasopressor (in addition to epinephrine). All vasopressors should be given by infusion pump, with the doses titrated continuously according to blood pressure and cardiac rate/function monitored continuously and oxygenation monitored by pulse oximetry.

IM: intramuscular; IV: intravenous.
* A child is defined as a prepubertal patient weighing less than 40 kg.
¶ All patients receiving an infusion of epinephrine and/or another vasopressor require continuous noninvasive monitoring of blood pressure, heart rate and function, and oxygen saturation. We suggest that pediatric centers provide instructions for preparation of standard concentrations and also provide charts for established infusion rate for epinephrine and other vasopressors in infants and children.

Figure 22.5. Rapid overview of emergency management of anaphylaxis in infants and children.

Vasopressors may be needed for refractory anaphylaxis, in which epinephrine and fluid hydration fail to correct hypotension and vasodilation (Brown 2005). For patients who are on β-blockers, anaphylaxis may be more severe, as hypotension and bronchospasm may be refractory to epinephrine. In these cases, IV glucagon can be administered. The airway should be protected, as rapid administration of glucagon can induce vomiting.

Second-line agents

H1 and H2 antihistamines are usually administered for anaphylaxis. However, these medications should never be used as the initial or sole treatment, as they do not reverse life threatening respiratory or cardiovascular manifestations of anaphylaxis. H1 antihistamines (both first- and second-generation) relieve cutaneous symptoms of pruritus and urticaria that may be present in anaphylaxis. A first generation H1 antihistamine (diphenhydramine, chlorpheniramine, hydroxyzine) or a second generation H1 antihistamine (e.g., cetirizine) may be given. A combination of an H1 and H2 antihistamine (ranitidine or cimetidine) may provide superior relief from urticaria as compared to H1 antihistamine alone (Lin et al. 2000).

Despite lack of clear evidence for effectiveness in reversing the major clinical manifestations of anaphylaxis, glucocorticoids are also given very frequently. The onset of action for glucocorticoids is slow (several hours), so they should not be considered in the initial management of anaphylaxis. There is no evidence that glucocorticoids are harmful in the treatment of anaphylaxis, and there is some suggestion that glucocorticoids may prevent biphasic reactions and may attenuate protracted symptoms in patients who require hospitalization (Sampson et al. 2006).

There is no consensus suggesting the optimal observation period for a patient with anaphylaxis who responds successfully to treatment. The NIAAD/FAAN symposium suggested that the length of observation may be individualized for the patient, the severity of reaction and healthcare setting, but agreed that a post-anaphylaxis observation period of 4 to 6 hours is reasonable (Sampson et al. 2006). Patients with severe anaphylaxis, and those whose symptoms do not reverse promptly with epinephrine should be hospitalized for continued management and prolonged observation.

Any patient who experiences anaphylaxis should be discharged with (1) clear instructions for identifying and avoiding further exposure to the anaphylaxis trigger, (2) a prescription for an epinephrine auto-injector and instructions for its use, (3) an anaphylaxis emergency action plan, and (4) a plan or referral to follow-up with an allergist.

Figures 22.4 and 22.5 provide overviews for the emergency management of anaphylaxis in adults and children, respectively.

Conclusion

Anaphylaxis is a life-threatening condition and one of the most severe acute manifestations of allergy, and can present in patients of all ages. Prompt recognition of anaphylaxis is essential as symptoms may progress quickly, and treatment requires rapid treatment. Clinicians should be familiar with the pathophysiology, recognize symptoms, and possess knowledge of the diagnostic criteria for anaphylaxis. In addition, familiarity with common and rare triggers of anaphylaxis will aid in diagnosis and patient care. Most importantly, appropriate emergency treatment for acute anaphylaxis must be administered promptly in order to prevent progression to or reverse severe respiratory and circulatory compromise.

References

Adkinson NF, Middleton E. Middleton's allergy : principles & practice. 7th ed. Philadelphia, PA: Mosby/Elsevier; 2009.
Ben-Shoshan M, Clarke AE. Anaphylaxis: past, present and future. Allergy 2011; 66(1): 1–14.
Bock SA, Munoz-Furlong A, Sampson HA. Fatalities due to anaphylactic reactions to foods. J Allergy Clin Immunol 2001; 107(1): 191–3.
Brockow K, Ring J. Anaphylaxis to radiographic contrast media. Curr Opinion Allergy Clin Immunol 2011; 11(4): 326–31.
Brown SG, Blackman KE, Stenlake V, Heddle RJ. Insect sting anaphylaxis; prospective evaluation of treatment with intravenous adrenaline and volume resuscitation. Emerg Med J. 2004; 21(2): 149–54.

Brown SG. Cardiovascular aspects of anaphylaxis: implications for treatment and diagnosis. Curr Opin Allergy Clin Immunol 2005; 5(4): 359–64.
Brown SG, Stone SF, Fatovich DM, Burrows SA, Holdgate A, Celenza A, et al. Anaphylaxis: clinical patterns, mediator release, and severity. J Allergy Clin Immunol 2013; 132(5): 1141–9 e5.
Castells M. Diagnosis and management of anaphylaxis in precision medicine. J Allergy Clin Immunol 2017; 140(2): 321–33.
Cheifetz A, Smedley M, Martin S, Reiter M, Leone G, Mayer L, et al. The incidence and management of infusion reactions to infliximab: a large center experience. Am J Gastroenterol 2003; 98(6): 1315–24.
Commins SP, Satinover SM, Hosen J, Mozena J, Borish L, Lewis BD, et al. Delayed anaphylaxis, angioedema, or urticaria after consumption of red meat in patients with IgE antibodies specific for galactose-alpha-1,3-galactose. J Allergy Clin Immunol 2009; 123(2): 426–33.
Cox L, Platts-Mills TA, Finegold I, Schwartz LB, Simons FE, Wallace DV, et al. American academy of allergy, asthma & immunology/american college of allergy, asthma and immunology joint task force report on omalizumab-associated anaphylaxis. J Allergy Clin Immunol 2007; 120(6): 1373–7.
Dhami S, Sheikh A. Anaphylaxis: epidemiology, aetiology and relevance for the clinic. Expert Rev Clin Immunol 2017; 13(9): 889–95.
Dunford PJ, Williams KN, Desai PJ, Karlsson L, McQueen D, Thurmond RL. Histamine H4 receptor antagonists are superior to traditional antihistamines in the attenuation of experimental pruritus. J Allergy Clin Immunol 2007; 119(1): 176–83.
Feldweg AM. Food-Dependent, exercise-induced anaphylaxis: diagnosis and management in the outpatient setting. J Allergy Clin Immunol Pract 2017; 5(2): 283–8.
Godot V, Arock M, Garcia G, Capel F, Flys C, Dy M, et al. H4 histamine receptor mediates optimal migration of mast cell precursors to CXCL12. J Allergy Clin Immunol 2007; 120(4): 827–34.
Greenberger PA. Idiopathic anaphylaxis. Immunol Allergy Clin North Am 2007; 27(2): 273–93, vii–viii.
Greenberger PA, Lieberman P. Idiopathic anaphylaxis. J Allergy Clin Immunol Pract 2014; 2(3): 243–50; quiz 51.
Greenberger PA. Fatal and near-fatal anaphylaxis: factors that can worsen or contribute to fatal outcomes. Immunol Allergy Clin North Am 2015; 35(2): 375–86.
Gupta RS. Anaphylaxis in the young adult population. Am J Med 2014; 127(1 Suppl): S17–24.
Hardy CC, Robinson C, Tattersfield AE, Holgate ST. The bronchoconstrictor effect of inhaled prostaglandin D2 in normal and asthmatic men. N Engl J Med 1984; 311(4): 209–13.
Jerschow E, Lin RY, Scaperotti MM, McGinn AP. Fatal anaphylaxis in the United States, 1999–2010: temporal patterns and demographic associations. J Allergy Clin Immunol 2014; 134(6): 1318–28 e7.
Johansson SG, Bieber T, Dahl R, Friedmann PS, Lanier BQ, Lockey RF, et al. Revised nomenclature for allergy for global use: report of the nomenclature review committee of the world allergy organization, October 2003. J Allergy Clin Immunol 2004; 113(5): 832–6.
Kaliner M, Sigler R, Summers R, Shelhamer JH. Effects of infused histamine: analysis of the effects of H-1 and H-2 histamine receptor antagonists on cardiovascular and pulmonary responses. J Allergy Clin Immunol 1981; 68(5): 365–71.
Lee S, Hess EP, Lohse C, Gilani W, Chamberlain AM, Campbell RL. Trends, characteristics, and incidence of anaphylaxis in 2001-2010: A population-based study. J Allergy Clin Immunol 2017; 139(1): 182–8 e2.
Lieberman PL, Blaiss MS. Atlas of allergic diseases. Philadelphia: Developed by Current Medicine 2002; xii, 274 p.
Lieberman P. Biphasic anaphylactic reactions. Ann Allergy Asthma Immunol 2005; 95(3): 217–26; quiz 26, 58.
Lieberman P, Camargo CA, Jr, Bohlke K, Jick H, Miller RL, Sheikh A, et al. Epidemiology of anaphylaxis: findings of the american college of allergy, asthma and immunology epidemiology of anaphylaxis working group. Ann Allergy Asthma Immunol 2006; 97(5): 596–602.
Lieberman P. Epidemiology of anaphylaxis. Curr Opin Allergy Clin Immunol 2008; 8(4): 316–20.
Liew WK, Williamson E, Tang ML. Anaphylaxis fatalities and admissions in Australia. J Allergy Clin Immunol 2009; 123(2): 434–42.
Lin RY, Curry A, Pesola GR, Knight RJ, Lee HS, Bakalchuk L, et al. Improved outcomes in patients with acute allergic syndromes who are treated with combined H1 and H2 antagonists. Ann Emerg Med 2000; 36(5): 462–8.
Lin RY, Anderson AS, Shah SN, Nurruzzaman F. Increasing anaphylaxis hospitalizations in the first 2 decades of life: New York State, 1990–2006. Ann Allergy Asthma Immunol 2008; 101(4): 387–93.
Ma L, Danoff TM, Borish L. Case fatality and population mortality associated with anaphylaxis in the United States. J Allergy Clin Immunol 2014; 133(4): 1075–83.
MacGlashan D, Jr. Histamine: A mediator of inflammation. J Allergy Clin Immunol 2003; 112(4 Suppl): S53–9.
McLean-Tooke AP, Bethune CA, Fay AC, Spickett GP. Adrenaline in the treatment of anaphylaxis: what is the evidence? BMJ 2003; 327(7427): 1332–5.
Moneret-Vautrin DA, Morisset M, Flabbee J, Beaudouin E, Kanny G. Epidemiology of life-threatening and lethal anaphylaxis: a review. Allergy 2005; 60(4): 443–51.
Mullins RJ, Dear KB, Tang ML. Time trends in Australian hospital anaphylaxis admissions in 1998–1999 to 2011–2012. J Allergy Clin Immunol 2015; 136(2): 367–75.
Portier P, Richet CR (eds.). De l' action anaphylactique de certains venins. C Royal Societe de Biologie; 1902; Paris.
Pumphrey RS. Lessons for management of anaphylaxis from a study of fatal reactions. Clin Exp Allergy 2000; 30(8): 1144–50.
Pumphrey RS. Fatal posture in anaphylactic shock. J Allergy Clin Immunol 2003; 112(2): 451–2.

Pumphrey RS. Fatal anaphylaxis in the UK, 1992–2001. Novartis Found Symp 2004; 257: 116–28; discussion 28–32, 57–60, 276–85.

Pumphrey RS, Gowland MH. Further fatal allergic reactions to food in the United Kingdom, 1999–2006. J Allergy Clin Immunol 2007; 119(4): 1018–9.

Reber LL, Hernandez JD, Galli SJ. The pathophysiology of anaphylaxis. J Allergy Clin Immunol 2017; 140(2): 335–48.

Ring J, Grosber M, Brockow K, Bergmann K. Anaphylaxis. History of Allergy. Basel: Karger 2014; 54–61.

Rudders SA, Arias SA, Camargo CA, Jr. Trends in hospitalizations for food-induced anaphylaxis in US children, 2000–2009. J Allergy Clin Immunol 2014; 134(4): 960–2 e3.

Sampson HA, Munoz-Furlong A, Bock SA, Schmitt C, Bass R, Chowdhury BA, et al. Symposium on the definition and management of anaphylaxis: summary report. J Allergy Clin Immunol 2005; 115(3): 584–91.

Sampson HA, Munoz-Furlong A, Campbell RL, Adkinson NF, Jr, Bock SA, Branum A, et al. Second symposium on the definition and management of anaphylaxis: summary report—Second national institute of allergy and infectious disease/food allergy and anaphylaxis network symposium. J Allergy Clin Immunol 2006; 117(2): 391–7.

Schwartz LB. Diagnostic value of tryptase in anaphylaxis and mastocytosis. Immunol Allergy Clin North Am 2006; 26(3): 451–63.

Scranton SE, Gonzalez EG, Waibel KH. Incidence and characteristics of biphasic reactions after allergen immunotherapy. J Allergy Clin Immunol 2009; 123(2): 493–8.

Sheikh A, Hippisley-Cox J, Newton J, Fenty J. Trends in national incidence, lifetime prevalence and adrenaline prescribing for anaphylaxis in England. J R Soc Med 2008; 101(3): 139–43.

Sheikh A, Shehata YA, Brown SG, Simons FE. Adrenaline for the treatment of anaphylaxis: cochrane systematic review. Allergy 2009; 64(2): 204–12.

Simons FE. Anaphylaxis, killer allergy: long-term management in the community. J Allergy Clin Immunol 2006; 117(2): 367–77.

Simons FE. Emergency treatment of anaphylaxis. BMJ 2008; 336(7654): 1141–2.

Simons FE. Anaphylaxis. J Allergy Clin Immunol 2010; 125(2 Suppl 2): S161–81.

Simons FE, Ardusso LR, Bilo MB, El-Gamal YM, Ledford DK, Ring J, et al. World allergy organization guidelines for the assessment and management of anaphylaxis. World Allergy Organ J 2011; 4(2): 13–37.

Simons FE, Ardusso LR, Dimov V, Ebisawa M, El-Gamal YM, Lockey RF, et al. World allergy organization anaphylaxis guidelines: 2013 update of the evidence base. Int Arch Allergy Immunol 2013; 162(3): 193–204.

Simons FE, Ebisawa M, Sanchez-Borges M, Thong BY, Worm M, Tanno LK, et al. 2015 update of the evidence base: World Allergy Organization anaphylaxis guidelines. World Allergy Organ J 2015; 8(1): 32.

Smith PL, Kagey-Sobotka A, Bleecker ER, Traystman R, Kaplan AP, Gralnick H, et al. Physiologic manifestations of human anaphylaxis. J Clin Invest 1980; 66(5): 1072–80.

Stark BJ, Sullivan TJ. Biphasic and protracted anaphylaxis. J Allergy Clin Immunol 1986; 78(1 Pt 1): 76–83.

Tejedor-Alonso MA, Moro Moro M, Mugica Garcia MV. Epidemiology of anaphylaxis. Clin Exp Allergy 2015a; 45(6): 1027–39.

Tejedor-Alonso MA, Moro-Moro M, Mugica-Garcia MV. Epidemiology of anaphylaxis: contributions from the last 10 years. J Investig Allergol Clin Immunol 2015b; 25(3): 163–75; quiz follow 74–5.

Theoharides TC, Valent P, Akin C. Mast cells, mastocytosis, and related disorders. N Engl J Med 2015; 373(2): 163–72.

Tole JW, Lieberman P. Biphasic anaphylaxis: review of incidence, clinical predictors, and observation recommendations. Immunol Allergy Clin North Am 2007; 27(2): 309–26, viii.

Turner PJ, Gowland MH, Sharma V, Ierodiakonou D, Harper N, Garcez T, et al. Increase in anaphylaxis-related hospitalizations but no increase in fatalities: an analysis of United Kingdom national anaphylaxis data, 1992–2012. J Allergy Clin Immunol 2015;135(4): 956–63 e1.

Umasunthar T, Leonardi-Bee J, Turner PJ, Hodes M, Gore C, Warner JO, et al. Incidence of food anaphylaxis in people with food allergy: a systematic review and meta-analysis. Clin Exp Allergy 2015; 45(11): 1621–36.

Vadas P, Perelman B, Liss G. Platelet-activating factor, histamine, and tryptase levels in human anaphylaxis. J Allergy Clin Immunol 2013; 131(1): 144–9.

Vigorito C, Russo P, Picotti GB, Chiariello M, Poto S, Marone G. Cardiovascular effects of histamine infusion in man. J Cardiovasc Pharmacol 1983; 5(4): 531–7.

Wood RA, Camargo CA, Jr, Lieberman P, Sampson HA, Schwartz LB, Zitt M, et al. Anaphylaxis in America: the prevalence and characteristics of anaphylaxis in the United States. J Allergy Clin Immunol 2014; 133(2): 461–7.

23

Insect Venom Allergy

William H Bermingham,[1,]* Alex G Richter[2] and Mamidipudi T Krishna[2]

INTRODUCTION

The order of Hymenoptera includes a broad range of insects. Within this, three families account for the majority of insect venom allergy in humans:

- *Apidae* (including honey bees and bumblebees)
- *Vespidae* (including yellow jackets, hornets, paper wasps)
- *Formicidae* (including fire ants).

The risk of being stung depends on the distribution, the likelihood of coming into contact and aggressiveness of the insect. Venoms contain a complex mix of potentially allergenic molecules which are variably understood between species. Following an initial sting, sensitization may or may not occur and interestingly only a small proportion of sensitized individuals develop systemic reactions upon re-exposure.

This chapter will focus on *Apidae* and *Vespidae* venom-induced type I hypersensitivity (HSR).

Insect identification

It is not uncommon for a patient to be uncertain regarding the nature of the stinging insect and history alone is insufficient to confirm clinical reactivity. Knowledge of the classification, distribution, habitat, time of the year and whether a barbed stinger was left *in situ* (honeybees usually do) following a sting can guide specialist physicians in further investigations and management. Descriptions to aid identification of insects are summarized in Table 23.1.

Types of sting reactions

Clinical symptoms following a sting are highly variable and difficult to predict. Symptoms presenting as part of a sting reaction are detailed in Table 23.2. Classification of reactions is not standardized. Examples of grading systems include those postulated by Mueller (1996), Cox et al (2010), Ring and Messmer (1977) and Muraro et al (2018). For the purposes of this chapter, we will refer to reactions as

---

[1] Department of Allergy and Immunology, University Hospitals Birmingham NHS Trust, Birmingham, UK.
[2] Department of Allergy and Immunology, University Hospitals Birmingham NHS Trust; Institute of Immunology & Immunotherapy, University of Birmingham, Birmingham, UK, Emails: A.G.Richter@bham.ac.uk; mtkrishna@yahoo.com
* Corresponding author: william.bermingham@nhs.net

Table 23.1. Identifying the culprit insect.

Common name(s)	Scientific name	Distribution	Habitat	Appearance	Size of insect	Sting features
Honey bee	Apis Mellifera	Worldwide	Trees are natural nesting sites. Often farmed in hives	Short dense golden brown and black hair with a striped abdomen	13-25mm long	Barbed stinger often left behind and may continue to inject venom until removed.
Bumble bee	Bombus Apidae	Northern Hemisphere, New Zealand, Tasmania	Nest in underground holes or directly on the ground. Small colonies of up to 50 bees	Black and yellow soft body hair appears fuzzy and often in bands. Either orange/red in their bodies or entirely black	19-38mm long	Sting lacks barbs so can sting repeatedly. Not aggressive unless hive threatened
European Hornet	Vespa Crabro	Europe, Russia, North East Asia, Eastern North America	Nests typically in hollow trees or other cavities. Also active at night.	Reddish brown head, black and brown shaded thorax, yellow and black abdomen	Largest of wasp family. Queens reach 35mm	Larger venom sack than YJ – thought to be more a painful sting
Wasp / Yellow Jacket (YJ)	Vespula	Northern Hemisphere, Australia and New Zealand	Nests in cavities or subterranean.	Bright yellow. Abdomen is broad at both ends	12mm long	Aggressive, more likely to sting than other wasps. Lance-like stinger with small barbs, occasionally leave behind. Can sting repeatedly
Paper Wasps	Polistes	Mainland Europe, the Americas, parts of Asia and Australasia	Paper wasp nests are open and cells are not covered with a cap	P.dominula marking may be confused with YJs. Others vary in colour with brown, yellow or red markings. Abdomen is spindle-shaped and tapers	15-25 mm long	Rarely sting, mainly if nest is threatened
Imported fire ants	Formicidae	South Eastern states of USA. Other stinging ants occur in Asia and Australia (Jumper ants)	Large colonies in the ground, typically build mounds	Copper brown head and body with a darker abdomen	2-6mm	Multiple stings from multiple ants. Inject formic acid

(Source: Briesch and Greene; Buck, Marshall and Cheung, 2008)

Table 23.2. Symptoms of IgE mediated venom allergy.

System	Systemic symptoms of venom allergy
Cutaneous	Pruritus, urticaria and/or angioedema distal to sting site.
Gastrointestinal	Vomiting, diarrhoea, abdominal pain and incontinence
Cardiovascular	Tachycardia, hypotension. Isolated cardiovascular collapse can occur in some patients. Severe cases may culminate into myocardial ischaemia ± associated complications.
Neurological	light headedness, dizziness, altered vision, seizures, collapse, loss of consciousness, feeling of impending doom due to hypotension (Lockey et al., 1988)
Respiratory	Rhinitis, shortness of breath, tight chest, wheeze, stridor, laryngeal oedema

(Sources: Moffitt et al 2004; Krishna et al., 2011)

per the description detailed within the 2018 the European Academy of Allergy and Clinical Immunology (EAACI) guidelines on venom immunotherapy (VIT) (Sturm et al. 2018).

IgE mediated reactions

- **Large Local Reactions (LLR):** A LLR is a swelling of > 10 cm that lasts for longer than 24 hours. Such reactions can cause significant morbidity, but are not dangerous unless it affects the upper airway.
- **Systemic reactions (SR)**
  o Mild: Typically involve generalized skin symptoms, e.g., flushing, urticaria, angioedema
  o Moderate: Include symptoms such as dizziness, nausea and dyspnoea
  o Severe: May include shock, loss of consciousness and cardiac or respiratory arrest (Sturm et al. 2018).

Non-IgE mediated reactions

- These are extremely rare, but may be severe/serious. Examples are summarized in Table 23.3 and the underlying mechanism/s are not known. It is important to note that allergy tests and VIT are not indicated in such patients.

Epidemiology of insect sting reactions

- A sting resulting from an insect in the Hymenoptera order is common. It is estimated that 56.6–94.5% of the general population will receive a hymenoptera sting in their lifetime (Bilo and Bonifazi 2009).
- Large local reactions are estimated to occur after 2.4–26.4% of hymenoptera stings (Sturm et al. 2018).
- Systemic Reactions (SRs), ranging from mild to life threatening anaphylaxis, have been estimated to occur in 0.3–7.5% of adults in European studies (Bilo and Bonifazi 2008). SRs are less common in children, estimated at 3.4%. Specifically, SRs in children seldom lead to cardio-respiratory compromise stings (Sturm et al. 2018).
- *Hymenoptera* venom are one of the main causes of fatal anaphylaxis in the USA and UK (Pumphrey 2000, DB 2007), the second most frequent cause of anaphylaxis outside of medical settings (Pumphrey 1996). A review of animal-related deaths in 2005 determined that *Hymenoptera* stings accounted for 533 deaths in the United States from 1991–2001 (Langley 2005). Other studies estimate wasps and bees cause 30–120 deaths annually in the United States and 2–9 in the United Kingdom (Pumphrey 1996). In 1989, 32 deaths were reported from fire ant stings in Texas, Florida, Louisiana and Georgia (Rhoades et al. 1989). Studies investigating fatality rates have demonstrated

Table 23.3. Manifestations of non IgE mediated reactions to bee and wasp venom.

System	Non allergic symptoms
Cutaneous	Necrosis
Renal	Interstitial nephritis, rhabdomyolysis
Haematological	Haemolysis, cytopaenia's, Disseminated intravascular coagulopathy, vasculitis
Neurological	Guillain Barre syndrome, Myasthenia gravis, Neuropathies, Encephalitis
Respiratory	Alveolar haemorrhage

(Sources: Moffitt et al 2004; Krishna et al., 2011)

- similar results in Australia (0.09 per million), Canada (0.1 per million) and the USA (0.09–0.17 per million) (Stoevesandt et al. 2019).
- Whilst hospitalization due to stings are increasing, the number of fatality rates remained stable. In a large study of UK study between 1992 and 2012, the mean age for fatal anaphylaxis caused by insect stings was 59 years (Turner et al. 2015).

Who is at risk of a systemic/more severe reactions?

Predicting a patient's risk of future systemic reactions to insect stings represents a significant clinical challenge. Evidence for known risk factors has been generated both through epidemiological studies of all-cause anaphylaxis as well as typically smaller scale observational studies specifically in the context of venom allergy.

Risk factors for severe or systemic allergic reactions to insect venom

- Preceding reaction: A patient must be sensitized, due to a prior sting or venom exposure to suffer a subsequent IgE mediated reaction. However, the severity of subsequent reactions is hard to predict.
    o Following a severe anaphylactic reaction, the risk of having a recurrent episode to a further sting has been estimated to be between 60 and 79% (Biló et al. 2005).
    o Studies looking at whether LLRs can predict future SRs are not conclusive and range from a 4–24% risk of SR on re-sting (Moffitt et al. 2004, Bilò et al. 2019).
- Exposure: Beekeepers and their families are an interesting group that show high rates of sensitization and develop SRs and this is considered to be due to their high exposure. Systemic reactions are more common in those who are in the early years of beekeeping or who those who receive < 15–25 stings per year (Eich-Wanger and Müller 1998, Richter et al. 2011). Examples of groups that are at a high risk of wasps stings are pest controllers, gardeners, farmers and refuse collectors.
- Diagnosis of mastocytosis or evidence of a raised baseline tryptase level: Patients with an elevated baseline serum total tryptase ($\geq$ 11.4 mcg/l), with or without systemic or cutaneous mastocytosis, are predisposed to severe anaphylaxis (Ludolph-Hauser et al. 2001, Haeberli et al. 2003).
- Older age: Severe reactions have been found to be significantly more likely in older adults (median age > 38 years) (Ruëff et al. 2009a,b). It is important to note that children usually suffer from cutaneous SRs, whereas cardio-respiratory compromise is more common in adults. Near fatal or fatal anaphylaxis in children is exceptionally rare.
- Cardiovascular comorbidities: This has been connected with poor outcomes in all-cause anaphylaxis in numerous studies (Stoevesandt et al. 2019). Data are sparse for the specific context of venom allergy and results are variable. Kounis syndrome (cardiac ischaemia or infarction in the context of anaphylaxis) has been reported in case studies of venom allergy.
- Antihypertensive medications: Studies assessing the impact of beta-blocker and Angiotensin Converting Enzyme (ACE) inhibitors are challenging due to the confounder of co-existing cardiovascular comorbidities. A large European study reported ACE inhibitors as one of the risk

factors contributing to severity of anaphylaxis to bee and wasp stings (Ruëff et al. 2009b). Both have a rationale for an adverse impact, through inhibition of effect of endogenous/exogenous epinephrine or impaired bradykinin breakdown respectively. This is supported by evidence of adverse outcomes in anaphylaxis studies of all-cause anaphylaxis, but data for venom allergy is variable.

- Male sex: This has previously been associated with systemic venom reactions (Ruëff et al. 2009b). It is unclear if this represents a greater environmental sting exposure risk for males.
- Pulmonary disease, specifically asthma: This has been associated with adverse outcomes in all cases of anaphylaxis studies (Brown et al. 2013).

Risk factors for poor outcomes of systemic sting reactions

- Delayed administration of epinephrine: This has been strongly associated with adverse outcomes in both all cause and venom-specific anaphylaxis (Pumphrey 2003, 2008).
- Upright posture during hypotension in anaphylaxis: Associated in both all-cause and venom specific studies with sudden death in the context of anaphylaxis. This has been attributed to 'empty ventricle syndrome (Pumphrey 2003, 2008).'
- Other associations from studies of all-cause or other anaphylaxis setting include recent vigorous exercise and concomitant alcohol/recreational drug use (Worm et al. 2018).
- Data regarding the impact of location of sting or number of stings is not available. Mortality relating to patients who received a high number of stings may relate directly to venom toxicity rather than IgE mediated allergic mechanism.

Investigation of venom allergy

A systematic clinical approach to patients with a history/suspected history of an allergic reaction to hymenoptera sting is described as follows:

Key points of clinical history

- Severity of the reaction:
  o Are symptoms consistent with an IgE mediated response? (Table 23.2)
  o Did the patient seek medical attention?
  o What treatment did the patient receive, specifically was epinephrine (including number of doses) administered?
  o Are details of the contemporaneous assessment from emergency room and ambulance records available?
- Culprit insect: (Table 23.1)
  o Size and appearance of insect and/or hive.
  o Was a barbed stinger left *in situ* following sting?
- Risk of future sting reactions:
  o Patient's occupation or hobbies (these may have major implications on future management).
  o Atopy: Any history of asthma, hay fever, eczema or food allergy? Does the patient carry antihistamines or an epinephrine auto-injector?
  o Comorbid conditions: Any history of chronic respiratory or cardiovascular disease?
  o Concomitant medication: Beta Blockers or ACE inhibitors
- Other relevant points:
  o Access to emergency care.
  o Anxiety regarding future stings.
  o For beekeepers: presence of a 'buddy', intention to continue with beekeeping following a SR, preference for VIT (described later).
  o Ability/confidence to self-administer epinephrine.

Skin testing for venom allergy

- In many countries, the 'gold standard' investigation for hymenoptera venom allergy is skin testing. This is simple to perform, provides an immediate answer and has greater sensitivity and specificity than serum specific IgE (SsIgE) (Krishna et al. 2011).
- There are two principal steps to skin testing relevant in this context: First, Skin Prick Testing (SPT: using 10–100 mcg/ml of extract) and second intradermal testing (IDT: 0.0001–1.0 mcg/ml of extract). Appropriate positive and negative controls must be employed (Krishna et al. 2011).

Serum specific IgE testing

- Serum specific IgE (SsIgE) is reported to have a sensitivity of 76–91% and specificity of 85–100% in known venom allergic patients (Krishna et al. 2011, Sturm et al. 2018).
- Component Resolved Diagnostic (CRD) testing is being increasingly used in clinical practice. Commonly available CRD antigens include Api m1 (bee), Api m10 (bee), Ves v1 and Ves v5 (wasp) and MUXF (cross reactive carbohydrate determinant [CCD])[14]. This approach is particularly helpful in delineating 'true sensitization' in patients showing dual sensitization to bee and wasp venom (whole extracts). Also, sensitization to Api m10, has been associated with failure of bee venom VIT, as this antigen is not adequately represented in VIT extracts (Frick et al. 2016).
- The major allergens in bee and wasp venom are summarized in Table 23.5 (Krishna et al. 2011).

Basophil Activation Test (BAT)

- This is an '*ex vivo*' method of measuring basophil response to an allergen crosslinking specific IgE. It utilizes basophil activation markers (e.g., CD63, CD203C) which are detectable by flow cytometry (Hoffmann et al. 2015).
- In the context of a relevant clinical history, sensitivity and specificity have been estimated at 85–100% and 83–100%.
- BAT may be of particular use in patients where other tests have not provided clear evidence of causative sensitization in the context of a clinical history suggestive of hymenoptera venom allergy.
- Challenges relating to BAT remain including the stability of samples, a lack of standardization of platforms, requirement of skilled personnel in a specialist laboratory for analysis and a paucity of large multicentre studies to characterize diagnostic utility.

Other relevant investigations

- Serum total tryptase:
  - In the context of an acute assessment of an insect sting reaction, a raised acute serum total tryptase measurement [(baseline tryptase x 1.2) + 2 ug/L] is considered clinically significant for a diagnosis of anaphylaxis (Baretto et al. 2017).
  - A raised baseline serum total tryptase (bT) of $\geq$ 11.4 mcg/l, is an independent risk factor for systemic allergic reactions to venom (Blum et al. 2011).
- Assessment for evidence of clonal mast cell disease includes bone marrow studies and analysis for c-KIT mutations. A clonal mast cell disorder must be considered in patients presenting with severe cardiovascular anaphylaxis (with paucity of cutaneous signs and symptoms) and an unusually severe anaphylactic episode (e.g., cardio-pulmonary arrest, culminating into seizure and/or Kounis syndrome).

A summary of commonly available tests for venom allergy are summarised in Table 23.4.

Table 23.4. Summary of allergy tests used in the context of venom allergy.

Test	Details	Positive result
Skin prick test	SPT is performed with standardized venom (1–100 µg/ml). Graded testing starting at a lower concentration may be considered in patients with severe anaphylaxis.	≥ 3 mm wheal larger than negative control at 15 minutes
Intradermal test	IDT is undertaken with increasing concentrations of venom extract (0.001–1.0 µg/ml). 0.03 ml of extract is injected to raise a 3–5 mm bleb.	≥ 3 mm wheal larger than negative control at 20 minutes
Serum-specific IgE	An adjunct to skin testing as less sensitive and specific.	≥ 0.35 kU/L
Component testing	May offer superior discrimination between venoms when there is dual positivity on skin/serum testing with 'whole extracts'	≥ 0.35 kU/L
Total serum IgE	A non-specific marker. SSIgE data must be cautiously interpreted when total IgE is > 5,000 kU/	reference range varies with local laboratories
Baseline serum total tryptase (bT)	An elevated bT is an independent risk factor in hymenoptera venom anaphylaxis	≥ 11.4 µg/ml

(Source: Moffitt et al. 2004, Krishna et al. 2011, Sturm et al. 2018)

Table 23.5. Major allergens in Wasp and Bee venom.

Venom	Component	Protein
Wasp (Yellow jacket)	Ves v 1	Phospholipase A1
	Ves v 2	Hyaluronidase (glycoprotein with cross reactivity with honeybee)
	Ves v 5	Antigen 5, the major allergen
Honeybee	Api m 1	Phospholipase A2
	Api m 2	Hyaluronidase
	Apim 3	Acid phosphatase
	Apim 4	Melittin
	Apim 10	Icarapin

(Source: Biló et al. 2005)

Challenges in venom allergy diagnosis

- Challenges can arise at each step in the assessment of hymenoptera venom anaphylaxis. Prior to testing, common challenges include: lack of recognition of causative insect; lack of detail from the acute assessment/management of index reaction; a long lag time from index reaction to specialist review.
- Double sensitization to bee and wasp venoms.
    - This is frequently observed but 'true' dual clinical reactivity is rare. The frequency of double sensitization varies according to the test method used. SsIgE testing to whole venom is associated with rates as high as 50% but such a pattern is relatively lower with IDT and CRD (Sturm et al. 2011).
    - Cross reactive Carbohydrate Determinants (CCDs) on hymenoptera venom hyaluronidases have been identified as a frequent cause of double sensitization (Hemmer et al. 2001).
    - Basophil activation tests may be helpful in making this discrimination in some cases but a robust diagnostic test with 100% specificity for predicting clinical reactivity in sensitized individuals is not yet available (Jakob et al. 2017b).
    - Skin tests may be negative in the immediate aftermath of anaphylaxis to insect-sting/s, so tests should be repeated after few weeks to reduce false negative results.
- Cross-reactivity between hymenoptera venoms:
    - There is no clinically significant cross reactivity between bee and wasp venoms.

o There is significant cross-reactivity between wasp and hornet venoms.
o There is some limited clinically relevant cross reactivity between wasp/hornet and paper wasp venoms.
- Practise may vary depending on national and local guidelines. Algorithms guiding the selection of patients for VIT have been postulated, but data from large, multicentre randomized control studies are not available (Jakob et al. 2017a, Jakob et al. 2017b).

Management of hymenoptera venom allergy

The management largely depends on the severity of the reaction (Fig. 23.1), although avoidance advice is universal (Table 23.6).

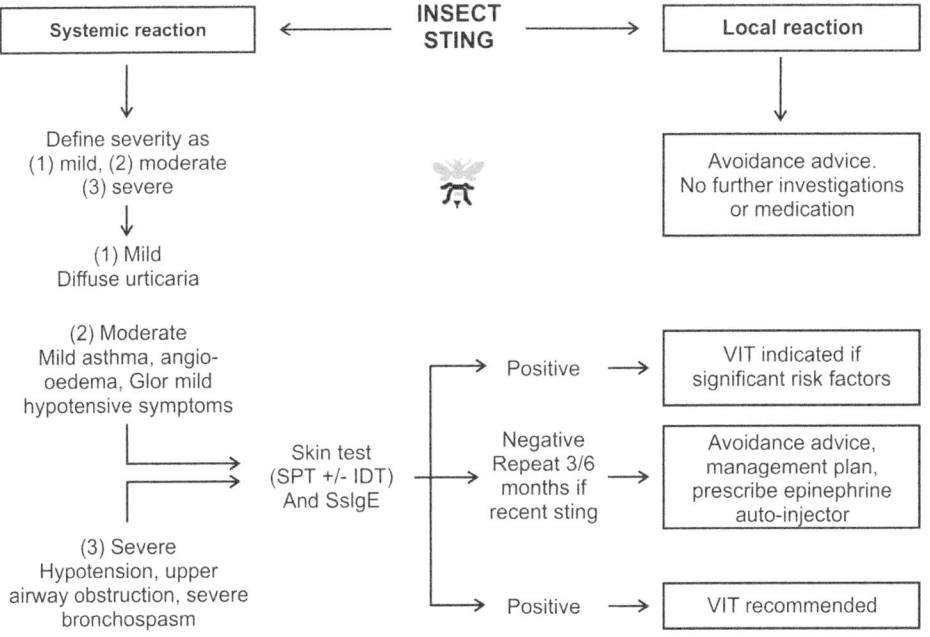

Figure 23.1. A flow diagram for the management of venom allergy.

Table 23.6. General advice in venom allergy.

	Advice
Avoidance	Eradicate infestations Insect repellents Wear long sleeves/shoes when outside Recognize careers/hobbies with increased exposure to insects
Non-medical	Remove stinger (for honeybees) Medical alert bracelet or like Management plan in case of reaction
Medical	Early antihistamines for pruritis and urticaria Prescribe and train patient for epinephrine auto injector Consider β_2 agonist inhaler, especially in asthmatics Ensure chronic asthma is well controlled

(Source: Moffitt et al. 2004, Krishna et al. 2011, Sturm et al. 2018)

Example avoidance advice for all patients (adapted from www.allergyuk.org):

- Patients should instruct professional exterminators if infestations may put the patient at risk.
- When working outside, wear protective covering and closed toed shoes.
- Avoid wearing bright colours or scented sprays.
- Stay indoors whilst eating and drinking during seasons when bees and wasps are prevalent. Avoid drinking from cans which insects may have crawled inside.
- Drive with windows closed.
- Careers/hobbies where the risk of sting is high (e.g., bee keeping and gardening) should be avoided.
- If a stinger remains in the skin (typical of a honeybee sting), it should be extracted carefully and quickly.

Acute treatment depends on the severity of the reaction

- Large local reactions may benefit from early antihistamines and for severe cases a short course of oral corticosteroids may be considered. Occasionally these become infected and antibiotics may be considered. Ice or cold-compresses at the sting site may reduce local swelling.
- Mild systemic reactions are usually treated with oral antihistamines when limited to non-life threatening muco-cutaneous symptoms (e.g., pruritis/urticaria).
- Moderate to severe systemic reactors: Anaphylaxis and moderate systemic reactions should be managed as per standard resuscitation guidelines. Prompt administration of epinephrine via intramuscular route and correct posture during treatment are the key to good clinical outcomes. At discharge, patients should be prescribed and trained in the use of self-injectable epinephrine. Medical alert bracelets or the like are recommended (Simons et al. 2011).

Paediatric hymenoptera sting reactions

- Sixty percent of sensitized children that are stung suffer mucocutaneous symptoms only. Respiratory involvement may occur, however, in contrast to adults symptomatic hypotension and loss of consciousness are uncommon in children.
- VIT is rarely indicated in children and should only be considered in those that experience moderate-severe SRs. Long-term efficacy of VIT has been reported in children and adults with venom allergy (Valentine et al. 1990, Golden et al. 2004).

Venom immunotherapy

Venom immunotherapy is the only specific treatment currently available for reducing/preventing systemic reactions/anaphylaxis to future stings. It must be used only in patients with demonstrable sensitization to the respective venom and with a history of systemic reaction/s or anaphylaxis (Moffitt et al. 2004, Krishna et al. 2011, Sturm et al. 2018). Guidelines, protocols and availability of VIT products may vary regionally and nationally (Mahler et al. 2019). It is important that clinicians familiarize themselves with local and regional guidelines where available, to guide their practise. A summary of key features of European, USA and UK guidelines can be found in Table 23.7.

Venom immunotherapy is delivered by subcutaneous injections. Centres typically use a combination of conventional (over 12 weeks) or clustered up-dosing (over ~ 7 weeks). Accelerated regimens including rush (over few days) and ultra-rush (over 24 hours) may be used when induction of clinical tolerance is urgently required (e.g., beekeepers), but these are associated with higher rates of VIT-induced systemic reactions (Mosbech and Muller 2000, Sturm et al. 2002). See Table 23.8.

Sublingual VIT has been attempted but does not have proven efficacy (Ruëff et al. 2009).

Table 23.7. Comparison of key domains of American, UK and European guidelines on VIT.

Domain	AAAAI	BSACI	EAACI
When to offer VIT (adults)	• Recommended for those with sting anaphylaxis PLUS a specific IgE to venom allergens • Consider for sting large local reactions where frequent ongoing exposure is likely • Consider in special circumstances for cutaneous reactions with consideration of other risk factors • VIT is not indicated in those with positive tests without a relevant clinical history	• Recommended for those with a severe sting SR and many with a moderate SR • Usually not indicated for cutaneous SR, but considered in context of other risk factors • Not indicated for local sting reactions	• Recommended for those with a systemic sting reaction (other than cutaneous only) with evidence of sensitization • Recommended in cutaneous systemic sting reactions if quality of life is impaired • Consider in those with LLRs if recurrent and troublesome, with the intention of reducing LLR duration/size • VIT is not indicated in those with positive tests without a relevant clinical history • VIT is not recommended in non-IgE mediated reactions
When to stop VIT	• Standard course: 5 years • Consider extending duration in those with other risk factors	• Standard course: 3 years	• Standard course: > 3 years, but > 5 years for those with severe SRs • Consider lifelong VIT in those with a very severe SR, ongoing reactions whilst receiving VIT and those with a very high bee sting exposure risk
Epinephrine auto-injectors during and after VIT	• Consider during/after VIT based on physician/patient discussion. Particularly in settings where VIT is known to be less efficacious, e.g., bee	• Should carry during up-dosing • Should be carried after successful VIT in specific circumstances: Those at high ongoing risk of stings; those with a raised bT or mastocytosis; those with ongoing reactions during VIT	• During and after VIT, consider in those with an ongoing risk of multiple stings or risk factors for further SRs • During and after VIT, not recommended for those with a history of only mild or moderate sting reactions with no other risk factors

(Source Moffitt et al. 2004, Krishna et al. 2011, Sturm et al. 2018)

Table 23.8. VIT up-dosing protocols.

	Conventional	Cluster	Rush	Ultra-rush
Up-dosing phase	10–19 weeks	5–7 weeks	3–10 days	Hours-2 days
Location	Outpatient	Outpatient	Inpatient/outpatient	Inpatient
SR rate	12%	22%	24%	

In our experience, anaphylaxis is a rare event with conventional protocols. Severity of SRs have been variable in previous studies, some reporting low rates and others high. In part this may be explained by patient selection criteria and heterogeneity in dosage regimens. Importantly, baseline serum tryptase and clonal mast cell disorders were not factored into the analysis in most studies.
(Source: Mosbech and Muller 2000, Sturm et al. 2002, 2018, Moffitt et al. 2004, Krishna et al. 2011)

Indications

Venom immunotherapy is recommended for patients who have had anaphylaxis or severe systemic reaction/s unless there are contraindications to treatment. It may also be considered in patients who have had mild/moderate reactions with risk factors such as raised bT, increased likelihood of future stings, remoteness from emergency medical help, effect on Health-Rrelated Quality of Life (HRQoL), patient anxiety and co-morbid conditions (e.g., chronic asthma). Venom immunotherapy is not recommended for local reactions per se regardless of the severity. The clinician should familiarize themselves with specific guidance applicable to their area.

Protocols and safety

- Venom Immunotherapy involves a series of subcutaneous injections commencing at a low dose with gradual escalation until the maintenance dose (100 mcg) is achieved. A higher maintenance dose of 150–200 mcg may be considered in patients that develop SR/s to field sting/s despite being on a maintenance dose of 100 mcg (Krishna et al. 2011).
- Maintenance treatment is typically for 3–5 years, depending on the patient, and may be considered indefinitely for patients with clonal mast cell disorders. The optimum duration, safety and efficacy in patients with an elevated bT and/or mastocytosis has not yet been established.
- Systemic reactions are relatively more common during the up-dosing than during maintenance phase (Mosbech and Muller 2000).
- Although accelerated protocols (rush and ultra-rush) have been shown to be safe with respect to comparable rates of SRs with slower regimens (conventional and cluster), overall reaction rates are relatively higher with the former (Mosbech and Muller 2000, Sturm et al. 2002).
- The choice of protocol (Table 23.7 and Fig. 23.2) would depend on the expertise of the specialist and available facilities, patient availability and distance from centre, occupation and likelihood of future stings, co-morbidities including bT/clonal mast cell disorder and the ability to tolerate cardio-respiratory compromise.
- The consensus is that the different up-dosing protocols as stated above are clinically acceptable depending on the setting and are efficacious.
- Systemic reactions more frequent with honeybee (~ 25%) compared to wasp/hornet VIT (~ 5%) (Birnbaum et al. 1993, Wyss et al. 1993, Mosbech and Muller 2000, Sturm et al. 2002, Adamic et al. 2009).
- Omalizumab (anti-IgE monoclonal antibody) has been used in a number of small, 'off-label' allergen-specific immunotherapy studies, including VIT. Promising results have been demonstrated for reducing adverse events, but large scale, randomized control trials are needed (Dantzer and Wood 2018).
A summary of advice for providing a safe VIT service are summarized in Table 23.9.

282 Textbook of Allergy for the Clinician

- Occupation risk
- Lives too far away for conventional up-dosing

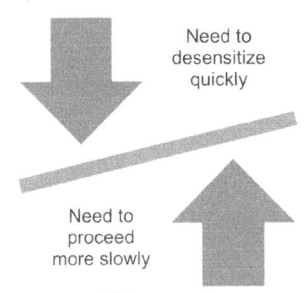

Need to desensitize quickly

Need to proceed more slowly

- Cardio-respiratory comorbidities
- Mastocytosis
- No in patient facilities

Figure 23.2. Weighing up the risk of up-dosing schedules.

Advise for providing a safe immunotherapy service.

Box 23.1. Routine measures recommended to be followed in an immunotherapy clinic.

- Ensure there is access to a medical emergency trolley
- Rapid access available to emergency medications for the treatment of anaphylaxis. This should include: intramuscular adrenaline; oral and intravenous antihistamine preparations; nebulised and inhaled beta 2 agonist preparations (e.g. salbutamol); intravenous and oral corticosteroid preparations.
- Identify patients by a minimum of name, date of birth and relevant venom used for VIT.
- Check dosage and shelf life of the vaccine with an experienced colleague prior to injection.
- Check baseline observations (these could include, peak expiratory flow, blood pressure and pulse rate) pre injection and after a 60 minute observation period and document this in the patient note's. Any local or systemic reactions should be clearly recorded in the patient's notes and reported through local medicines surveillance infrastructure as appropriate.
- Dose adjustments may be required in patients missing an injection or if significant systemic or local reactions are experienced.
- The minimum recommended observation time in clinic after receiving VIT is 60 minutes.

(Source: Moffitt et al. 2004, Krishna et al. 2011, Sturm et al. 2018)

Contraindications to VIT

Contra-indications to VIT has been described in national guidelines from the UK, Europe and N. America but patients need to be considered on an individual basis following a careful risk-benefit analysis. Commonly stated contraindications include (Moffitt et al. 2004, Krishna et al. 2011, Pitsios et al. 2015, Sturm et al. 2018):

- Uncontrolled asthma, severe asthma and/or brittle asthma.
- Severe chronic heart/lung diseases with poor cardio/respiratory reserve (unable to tolerate hypotension or bronchospasm)
- Pregnancy—As far as possible discontinue VIT in pregnancy. However, if there is an increased risk for future stings, VIT may be continued in a patient who has been established in the maintenance phase and treatment has been well tolerated. This must be clearly discussed and documented in patient's medical records. VIT should not be initiated during pregnancy.
- Treatment with β-blockers or ACE-inhibitors, particularly the former must be avoided. However, in exceptional circumstances, β-blockers may be temporarily withheld prior to injections but after liaison with the patient's cardiologist. ACE inhibitors are not an absolute contraindication to VIT.
- Active cancer or previous history* of cancer.

- Active systemic autoimmune disorders* (e.g., immune complex diseases, immune deficiency, active rheumatoid arthritis, etc.).
- Patients on immunosuppressive* or cytotoxic drugs or immunodeficiency*.

relative contraindications, so decision should be individualized based on risk-benefit analysis

Efficacy and deciding when to stop VIT

- Long term follow up studies have shown that the cumulative risk of SR following 3–5 years of VIT is 10–15% for adults (Reisman 1993, Graft and Schoenwetter 1994, Lerch and Müller 1998, Golden 2010). In those where a SR is experienced after VIT, a thorough assessment for evidence of an underlying clonal mast cell disorder should be undertaken. Treatment beyond 5 years may be considered in patients with evidence for a clonal mast cell disorder.
- There are no biomarkers to predict reactions to future stings.
- Majority of patients have detectable SsIgE at the end of 3–5 years of VIT despite being protected or developing immunological tolerance. Whilst demonstration of specific IgE is useful in the diagnosis of venom allergy, it has no place as a biomarker for assessment of treatment response.
- Due to small, but reduced risk of further SRs following completion of VIT, a 'selected group' of patients (e.g., beekeepers, 'index reaction' was severe anaphylaxis, clonal mast cell disorder, elevated bT) may be advised to carry an epinephrine auto-injector (Krishna et al. 2011).
- Decisions around 'when to stop VIT' may be difficult in some patients and there are no conclusive studies. Factors that are taken into account are summarized in Fig. 23.3 and include (Moffitt et al. 2004, Golden 2010, Krishna et al. 2011, Sturm et al. 2018):
  o Severity of 'index reaction'
  o Cardio-respiratory comorbidity
  o Any VIT-induced SRs
  o Field-sting reactions during VIT
  o Occupational factors and/or hobbies
  o Patients with elevated bT or clonal mast cell disorders.

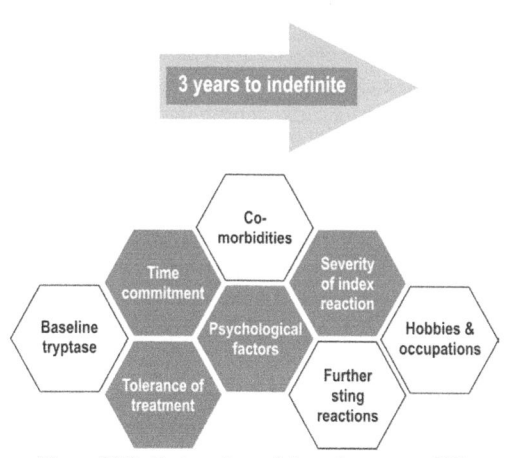

Figure 23.3. Factors determining when to stop VIT.

Clonal mast cell disorders and hymenoptera venom allergy

Mastocytosis refers to a continuum or a spectrum of disorders characterized by an abnormal, clonal proliferation of mast cells. Diagnostic criteria for distinct forms of these conditions has been produced by the World Health Organisation (WHO) (Valent et al. 2017).

An awareness of mastocytosis is important for specialists providing VIT. Recent evidence has indicated that as many as 4% of venom allergy patients may have an underlying mast cell disorder, and insect-sting anaphylaxis may be the first clinical presentation. Particular features that should flag patients for further investigation include: severe cardiovascular anaphylaxis with a paucity of cutaneous features; systemic reactions occurring during or after VIT; baseline tryptase > 11.4 mg/l. However, it is important to keep an open mind in the clinical assessment of patients, as some patients with systemic mastocytosis may not have an elevated bT (< 11.4 mg/l) (Bonadonna et al. 2009).

Investigation for mastocytosis will typically involve a detailed history, clinical examination for any hallmark features (e.g., urticaria pigmentosa), bT and bone marrow examination (including analysis for gain of function c-KIT mutations, e.g., D816V). There is some evidence of clinical utility of peripheral blood D816V screening, but this warrants further validation prior to widespread adoption (Jara-Acevedo et al. 2015). Patients with confirmed mastocytosis require specific management, including;

- Clear guidance on emergency management of allergic reaction, with a written management plan guiding the use of epinephrine auto-injectors.
- Information regarding avoidance of mast-cell stimulating medications, e.g., opiates, radio-contrast media, NSAIDs, etc.
- Information regarding advice for induction anaesthesia (i.e., use of neuromuscular blockers) if required in the future.
- Monitoring/treatment for osteopenia/osteoporosis.

Patients with suspected or confirmed mastocytosis and a history of SR to hymenoptera venom are at a high risk for severe future reactions. The evidence base for this cohort is sparse. VIT should be offered, but patients require counselling regarding the increased risk of reactions to VIT and the potential to require long term therapy. As stated earlier, efficacy of VIT in clonal mast cell disorders has not been established. The type of induction regime for VIT requires careful consideration, with conventional up-dosing protocols being preferable. This may also be a population who benefit from VIT in conjunction with anti-IgE therapy (Omalizumab) (Kontou-Fili and Filis 2009, Verburg et al. 2015) but this needs further research.

Conclusion

Hymenoptera stings are an important cause of systemic type 1 hypersensitivity reactions in adults. They represent a significant proportion of cases of fatal anaphylaxis, albeit rare. In this chapter, we have highlighted the importance of clinical history and appropriate use of available investigations, including component resolved diagnosis, in making an accurate diagnosis of insect venom allergy. Common diagnostic challenges, such as dual bee/wasp venom sensitisation have been discussed, with an aim to providing support to the practising Allergist.

We have presented key considerations for the management of patients with insect venom allergy, including detailed guidance on sting avoidance, the emergency management planfor acute allergic reactions and a summary of current guidance for the appropriate use of hymenoptera VIT. Special consideration has also been given to the importance of recognising a co-existing clonal mast cell disorder in the setting of hymenoptera venom allergy.

References

Adamic K, Zidarn M, Bajrovic N, Erzen R, Kopac P, Music E. The local and systemic side-effects of venom and inhaled-allergen subcutaneous immunotherapy. Wien Klin Wochenschr 2009; 121(9-10): 357–360.

Baretto RL, Heslegrave J, Melchlor C, Mohamed O, Ekbote A, et al. Validation of international consensus equation for acute serum total tryptase in mast cell activation: a perioperative perspective, Allergy. Wiley Online Library 2017; 72(12): 2031–2034.

Biló BM, Rueff F, Mosbech H, Bonifazi F, Oude-Elberink JNG, Birnbaum J, et al. Diagnosis of Hymenoptera venom allergy, Allergy Eur J Allergy Clin Immunol 2005; 60(11): 1339–1349. doi: 10.1111/j.1398-9995.2005.00963.x.

Bilo BM, Bonifazi F. Epidemiology of insect-venom anaphylaxis. Curr Opin Allergy Clin Immunol 2008; United States 8(4): 330–337. doi: 10.1097/ACI.0b013e32830638c5.

Bilo MB, Bonifazi F. The natural history and epidemiology of insect venom allergy: clinical implications. Clinical & Experimental Allergy. Wiley Online Library 2009; 39(10): 1467–1476.

Bilo MB, Martini M, Pravettoni D, Bonadonna P, Cortilleni G, et al. Large local reactions to Hymenoptera stings: Outcome of re-stings in real life. Allergy 2019 (April); pp. 1969–1976. doi: 10.1111/all.13863.

Birnbaum J, Charpin D, Vervloet D. Rapid Hymenoptera venom immunotherapy: comparative safety of three protocols', Clinical & Experimental Allergy. Wiley Online Library 1993; 23(3): 226–230.

Blum S, Gunzinger A, Müller UR, Helbling A. Influence of total and specific IgE, serum tryptase, and age on severity of allergic reactions to Hymenoptera stings. Allergy Eur J Allergy Clin Immunol 2011; 66(2): 222–228. doi: 10.1111/j.1398-9995.2010.02470.x.

Bonadonna P, Perbellini O, Passalacqua G, Caruso B, Colarossi S, Dal Fior D, et al. Clonal mast cell disorders in patients with systemic reactions to Hymenoptera stings and increased serum tryptase levels. J Allergy Clin Immunol 2009; United States, 123(3): 680–686. doi: 10.1016/j.jaci.2008.11.018.

Briesch N, Greene A (no date). Stinging insects: Biology and identification. UpToDate. Waltham, MA: UpToDate Inc. https://www.uptodate.com.

Brown SGA, Stone SF, Fatovich DM, Burrows SA, Holdgate A, Celenza A, et al. Anaphylaxis: clinical patterns, mediator release, and severity. J Allergy Clin Immunol. Elsevier 2013; 132(5): 1141–1149.

Buck M, Marshall SA, Cheung DKB. Identification Atlas of the Vespidae (Hymenoptera, Aculeata) of the northeastern Nearctic region. Canadian Journal of Arthropod Identification 2008; 5(1): 1–492.

Cox L, Larenas-Linnemann D, Lockey RF, Passalacqua G. Speaking the same language: the world allergy organization subcutaneous immunotherapy systemic reaction grading system. J Allergy Clin Immunol. Elsevier Ltd 2010; 125(3): 569–574.e7. doi: 10.1016/j.jaci.2009.10.060.

Dantzer JA, Wood RA. The use of omalizumab in allergen immunotherapy. Clinical & Experimental Allergy. Wiley Online Library 2018; 48(3): 232–240.

DB G. Insect sting anaphylaxis. Immunol Allergy Clin North Am 2007; 27(2): 261–272.

Eich-Wanger C, Müller UR. Bee sting allergy in beekeepers. Clinical and Experimental Allergy 1998; 28(10): 1292–1298. doi: 10.1046/j.1365-2222.1998.00411.x.

Frick M, Fischer J, Helbling A, Rueff F, Wieczorek D, Ollert M, et al. Predominant Api m 10 sensitization as risk factor for treatment failure in honey bee venom immunotherapy. J Allergy Clin Immunol. Elsevier 2016; 138(6): 1663–1671.

Golden DBK, Kagey-Sobotka A, Norman PS, Hamilton RG, Lichtenstein LM. Outcomes of Allergy to Insect Stings in Children, with and without Venom Immunotherapy. N Engl J Med. 2004; 351(7): 668–674. doi: 10.1056/NEJMoa022952.

Golden DBK. Long-term outcome after venom immunotherapy. Current Opinion in Allergy and Clinical Immunology. LWW 2010; 10(4): 337–341.

Graft DF, Schoenwetter WF. Insect sting allergy: analysis of a cohort of patients who initiated venom immunotherapy from 1978 to 1986. Annals of Allergy 1994; 73(6): 481–485.

Haeberli G, Bronnimannw M, Hunziker T, Muller U. Elevated basal serum tryptase and hymenoptera venom allergy: relation to severity of sting reactions and to safety and efficacy of venom immunotherapy. Clin Exp Allergy 2003; 33: 1216–1220.

Hemmer W, Focke M, Kolarich D, Wilson IBH, Altmann F, Wöhrl S, et al. Antibody binding to venom carbohydrates is a frequent cause for double positivity to honeybee and yellow jacket venom in patients with stinging-insect allergy. J Allergy Clin Immunol 2001; 108(6): 1045–1052. doi: 10.1067/mai.2001.120013.

Hoffmann, HJ, Santos AF, Mayorga C, Nopp A, Eberlein B, Ferrer M, et al. The clinical utility of basophil activation testing in diagnosis and monitoring of allergic disease. Allergy Eur J Allergy Clin Immunol 2015; 70(11): 1393–1405. doi: 10.1111/all.12698.

Jakob T, Müller U, Helbling A, Spillner E. Component resolved diagnostics for hymenoptera venom allergy. Curr Opin Allergy Clin Immunol 2017a; 17(5): 363–372. doi: 10.1097/ACI.0000000000000390.

Jakob T, Rafei-Shamsabadi D, Spillner E, Müller S. Diagnostics in Hymenoptera venom allergy: current concepts and developments with special focus on molecular allergy diagnostics. Allergo J Int 2017/04/11. Springer Medizin 2017b; 26(3): 93–105. doi: 10.1007/s40629-017-0014-2.

Jara-Acevedo M, Teodosio C, Sanchez-Muñoz L, Álvarez-Twose I, Mayado A, Caldas C, et al. Detection of the KIT D816V mutation in peripheral blood of systemic mastocytosis: Diagnostic implications. Mod Pathol 2015; 28(8): 1138–1149. doi: 10.1038/modpathol.2015.72.

Kontou-Fili K, Filis, CI. Prolonged high-dose omalizumab is required to control reactions to venom immunotherapy in mastocytosis, Allergy. Wiley Online Library 2009; 64(9): 1384–1385.

Krishna MT, et al. Diagnosis and management of hymenoptera venom allergy: British Society for Allergy and Clinical Immunology (BSACI) guidelines. Clinical & Experimental Allergy. Wiley Online Library 2011; 41(9): 1201–1220.

Langley RL. Animal-related fatalities in the United States-an update. Wilderness Environ Med 2005; 16(2): 67–74.

Lerch E, Müller UR. Long-term protection after stopping venom immunotherapy: results of re-stings in 200 patients. Journal of Allergy and Clinical Immunology. Elsevier 1998; 101(5): 606–612.

Lockey RF, Turkeltaub PC, Baird-Warren IA, Olive CA, Olive ES, Peppe BC, et al. The Hymenoptera venom study I, 1979–1982. Demographics and history-sting data. J Allergy Clin Immunol 1988; 82(3 PART 1), pp. 370–381. doi: 10.1016/0091-6749(88)90008-5.

Ludolph-Hauser D, Ruëff F, Fries C, Schöpf P, Przybilla B. Constitutively raised serum concentrations of mast-cell tryptase and severe anaphylactic reactions to Hymenoptera stings. Lancet 2001; 357(9253): 361–362. doi: 10.1016/S0140-6736(00)03647-3.

Mahler V, Esch RE, Kleine-Tebbe J, Lavery WJ, Plunkett G, Vieths S, et al. Understanding differences in allergen immunotherapy products and practices in North America and Europe. J Allergy Clin Immunol 2019; 143(3): 813–828.

Moffitt JE, Golden DBK, Reisman RE, Lee R, Ni R. Stinging insect hypersensitivity: A practice parameter update. Journal Allergy Clinical Immunology. Elsevier Inc 2004; 114(4): 869–886. doi: 10.1016/j.anai.2016.10.031.

Mosbech H, Muller U. Side-effects of insect venom immunotherapy: results from an EAACI multicenter study. European Academy of Allergology and Clinical Immunology. Allergy. Denmark 2000; 55(11): 1005–1010. doi: 10.1034/j.1398-9995.2000.00587.x.

Mueller HL. Diagnosis and treatment of insect sensitivity. Journal of Asthma Research. Taylor & Francis 1966; 3(4): 331–333.

Muraro A, Fernandez-Rivas M, Beyer K, Cardona V, Clark A, Eller E, et al. The urgent need for a harmonized severity scoring system for acute allergic reactions. Allergy 2018; 73(9): 1792–1800.

Pitsios C, Demoly P, Bilò MB, Gerth van Wijk R, Pfaar O, Sturm GJ, et al. Clinical contraindications to allergen immunotherapy: an EAACI position paper. Allergy 2015; 70(8): 897–909.

Pumphrey R. The clinical spectrum of anaphylaxis in north-west England. Clin Exp Allergy 1996; 26(12): 1364–70.

Pumphrey R. Lessons for management of anaphylaxis from a study of fatal reactions. Clin Exp Allergy 2000; 30(8): 1144–50.

Pumphrey RSH. Fatal posture in anaphylactic shock. Journal of Allergy and Clinical Immunology. Elsevier 2003; 112(2): 451–452.

Pumphrey RSH. When should self-injectible epinephrine be prescribed for food allergy and when should it be used? Current Opinion in Allergy and Clinical Immunology. LWW 2008; 8(3): 254–260.

Reisman RE. Duration of venom immunotherapy: relationship to the severity of symptoms of initial insect sting anaphylaxis. Journal of Allergy and Clinical Immunology. Elsevier 1993; 92(6): 831–836.

Rhoades RB, Stafford CT, James FK. Survey of fatal anaphylactic reactions to imported fire ant stings. The Journal of Allergy and Clinical Immunology 1989; 84(2): 159–162. doi: 10.1016/0091-6749(89)90319-9.

Richter AG, Nightingale P, Huissoon AP, Krishna MT. Risk factors for systemic reactions to bee venom in British beekeepers. Ann. Allergy, Asthma Immunol 2011; 106(2): 159–163. doi: 10.1016/j.anai.2010.11.005.

Ring J, Messmer K. Incidence and severity of anaphylactoid reactions to colloid volume substitutes. The Lancet. Elsevier 1977; 309(8009): 466–469.

Ruëff F, Bilò MB, Jutel M, Mosbech H, Müller U, Przybilla B. 'Sublingual immunotherapy with venom is not recommended for patients with Hymenoptera venom allergy. J Allergy Clin Immunol 2009a; 123(1): 272.

Ruëff F, Przybilla B, Biló MB, Müller U, Scheipl F, Aberer W, et al. Predictors of severe systemic anaphylactic reactions in patients with Hymenoptera venom allergy: importance of baseline serum tryptase—a study of the European Academy of Allergology and Clinical Immunology Interest Group on Insect Venom Hypersensitivity. J Allergy Clin Immunol 2009b; 124(5): 1047–1054.

Simons FER, Ardusso LRF, Bilo MB, El-Gamal YM, Ledford DK, Ring J, et al. World Allergy Organization anaphylaxis guidelines: summary. J Allergy Clin Immunol 2011; 127(3): 522–587. doi: 10.1016/j.jaci.2011.01.038.

Stoevesandt J, Sturm GJ, Bonadonna P, Oude Elberink JNG, Trautmann A. Risk factors and indicators of severe systemic insect sting reactions. Allergy 2019 (June); pp. 1–11. doi: 10.1111/all.13945.

Sturm G, Kränke B, Rudolph C, Aberer W. Rush Hymenoptera venom immunotherapy: a safe and practical protocol for high-risk patients. J Allergy Clin Immunol 2002; 110(6): 928–933.

Sturm GJ, Jin C, Kranzelbinder B, Hemmer W, Sturm EM, Griesbacher A, et al. Inconsistent results of diagnostic tools hamper the differentiation between bee and vespid venom allergy. PLoS One 2011; 6(6): 1–8. doi: 10.1371/journal.pone.0020842.

Sturm GJ, Varga EM, Roberts G, Mosbech H, Bilò MB, Akdis CA, et al. EAACI guidelines on allergen immunotherapy: Hymenoptera venom allergy. Allergy Eur J Allergy Clin Immunol 2018; 73(4): 744–764. doi: 10.1111/all.13262.

Turner PJ, Gowland BH, Sharma V, Lerodiakonou D, Harper N, Garcez T, et al.. Increase in anaphylaxis-related hospitalizations but no increase in fatalities: An analysis of United Kingdom national anaphylaxis data, 1992–2012. Journal of Allergy and Clinical Immunology. Elsevier Inc 2015; 135(4): 956–963.e1. doi: 10.1016/j.jaci.2014.10.021.

Valent P, Akin C, Metcalfe DD. Mastocytosis : 2016 updated WHO classification and novel emerging treatment concepts. Blood 2017; 129(11): 1420–1428. doi: 10.1182/blood-2016-09-731893.effective.

Valentine MD, Schuberth K, Kagey-Sobotka A, Graft D, Kwiterovich K, Szklo M. The Value of Immunotherapy with Venom in Children with Allergy to Insect Stings. New Eng J Med 1990; 323(23): 1601–3.

Verburg M, Oldhoff JM, Klemans RJ, Lahey-de AB, Röckmann H, Sanders C, et al. Rush immunotherapy for wasp venom allergy seems safe and effective in patients with mastocytosis. Eur Ann Allergy Clin Immunol 2015; 47(6): 192–196.

Worm M, Francuzik W, Renaudin J, Bilo MB, Cardona V, Scherer Hofmeier K et al. Factors increasing the risk for a severe reaction in anaphylaxis: an analysis of data from The European Anaphylaxis Registry. Allergy 2018; 73(6): 1322–1330.

Wyss M, Scheitlin T, Stadler BM, Wüthrich B. Immunotherapy with aluminum hydroxide adsorbed insect venom extracts (Alutard SQ): immunologic and clinical results of a prospective study over 3 years. Allergy 1993; 48(2): 81–86.

24

Urticaria and Angioedema

Jenny M Stitt[1,*] and *Stephen C Dreskin*[2]

INTRODUCTION

Urticaria (hives) are lesions that are edematous with raised round or oval centers (wheals), of varying size and may occur anywhere on the body (Fig. 24.1). The area surrounding the wheal is erythematous, well circumscribed and blanches with pressure. Urticaria may coalesce and create an appearance of irregular margins, but lesions remain well defined. Urticaria is transient skin lesions that last for minutes to hours and resolve completely within about 24 hours. This is sometimes described as 'evanescence'. Typical lesions are pruritic and are not associated with pain or burning sensations (Dreskin 2012, Kaplan 2009, Powell et al. 2007, Zuberbier et al. 2006). Atypical urticaria lesions can be non-blanching, burning in character, last more than 24 hours, cause residual skin hyperpigmentation, bruising or scarring. These may represent vasculitic disease and warrant further evaluation (Davis and Brewer 2004).

The majority of urticaria cases are acute, lasting less than 6 weeks. Hives may occur in one isolated outbreak or hives may occur daily or almost daily for several weeks and then resolve. In as many as 30% of patients, hives continue to occur on most days of the week for longer than 6 weeks and are referred to as chronic urticaria (Powell et al. 2007, Grigoriadou and Longhurst 2009, Kulthanan et al. 2007, Pickering et al. 1969).

Angioedema is non-pitting edema that affects deeper tissue layers and is associated with approximately 40% of urticaria cases. The edema occurs in the deep dermis and subcutaneous tissues.

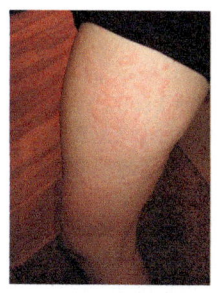

Figure 24.1. Well demarcated urticarial lesions of varying sizes with some coalescence and irregular margins.

---

[1] University of Colorado Hospital Allergy, Asthma, and Immunology Practice, Division of Allergy and Clinical Immunology, University of Colorado, Anschutz Medical Campus, Aurora, Colorado USA.
[2] Division of Allergy and Clinical Immunology, University of Colorado, Anschutz Medical Campus, Aurora, Colorado USA.
  Email: stephen.dreskin@cuanschutz.edu
* Corresponding author: jenny.stitt@cuanschutz.edu

Areas of angioedema may be of normal skin coloration or erythematous. Angioedema is not typically accompanied with pruritus, but can be associated with sensations of pressure, aching or burning. The distribution of angioedema may vary, although it often affects the lips, face or hands. Angioedema can also occur in areas of pressure, such as under clothing waistbands or straps. Angioedema is sometimes asymmetrical, such as swelling of only one half of an upper lip. When angioedema affects the upper airway, difficulty speaking, shortness of breath and even death from asphyxia may occur.

Angioedema without urticaria is unusual, and involves a specific differential diagnosis as will be discussed separately below. Angioedema without urticaria affects approximately 10% of patients and can involve the face, tongue, throat, extremities or genitals (Powell et al. 2007). The terms 'urticaria' and 'urticaria/angioedema' are used interchangeably within this chapter but the term 'angioedema' refers to angioedema without associated urticaria.

Urticaria

Clinical manifestations

The primary clinical manifestation of urticaria is the symptom of pruritus. Pruritus ranges in intensity from minimally inconvenient to intolerable. Pruritus may disrupt sleep, causing fatigue. The primary sign of urticaria is hives, and groupings of hives may appear and disappear episodically, several times per day. Secondary skin lesions from vigorous excoriation may also be observed.

Prevalence

The lifetime incidence of urticaria is estimated to be 15–20% affecting both genders and all ethnicities (Greaves and Tan 2007, Metz et al. 2008). Acute urticaria is more common in children and young adults. In contrast, chronic urticaria affects 0.5–1% of individuals, is more common in adults, and is more common in women (60–70% of cases) (Powell et al. 2007, Greaves and Tan 2007, Joint Task Force 2000, Baiardini et al. 2011).

Pathogenesis

The major effector cells of urticaria are mast cells, although basophils are also implicated (Powell et al. 2007, Greaves and Tan 2007, Metz et al. 2008, Mlynek et al. 2008, Saini 2009). Mast cells are found in the superficial dermis and sub-dermis in proximity of blood vessels as well on in mucosal surfaces of the mouth, nose, lungs and digestive tract. The allergic response of immediate hypersensitivity occurs when allergens cross-link immunoglobulin E (IgE) that is bound to high-affinity IgE receptors (FcεRI) on the surface of mast cells which leads to mast cell activation. However, mast cell activation may occur by IgE-independent means and this is called a pseudo-allergy. This phenomenon has been observed with physical stimuli such as heat or pressure, with medications such as NSAIDs, opioids and vancomycin, as well as with radiocontrast dye. Viral infections may also lead to urticaria that is likely not IgE-mediated.

The symptoms and signs of urticaria and some cases of angioedema (particularly in conjunction with urticaria) are due to multiple mediators that are released following activation of mast cells. Soon after activation of mast cells, mediators such as histamine, leukotriene C4 (LTC4), leukotriene D (LTD), prostaglandin GD2 (PGD2) as well as platelet activating factor (PAF) are released (Dreskin 2012, Greaves and Tan 2007, Mlynek et al. 2008, Brodell et al. 2008, Fonacier et al. 2010, Hiragun et al. 2013).

Histamine is released from preformed granules and is the primary contributor to hive formation. It leads to vasodilation and increased vascular permeability resulting in erythema and edema. Also the release of substance P, leukotrienes and PAF may potentiate the response by causing further vasodilation and stimulation of mast cells to release histamine (Greaves and Tan 2007, Hiragun et al. 2013).

Within 4 to 8 hours of activation of mast cells, the production and secretion of inflammatory cytokines results in a delayed inflammatory response. Chemokines such as monocyte chemotactic peptide 1 (MCP-1), cytokines such as interleukin-5 (IL-5) and Tumor Necrosis Factor α (TNF-α) promote inflammatory cell infiltrates that create lesions of greater temporal duration. As a result, lesions of chronic urticaria show a dense perivascular inflammatory cell infiltrate comprised of basophils, eosinophils, neutrophils and CD4- and CD8-positive T-lymphocytes, similar to that seen in late phase reactions (Greaves and Tan 2007, Hiragun et al. 2013).

Angioedema associated with urticaria is thought to have a similar pathogenesis of vasodilation and increased vascular permeability with plasma leakage in deeper tissue layers including the deep dermis and subcutaneous tissues, although additional mechanisms are likely at work (Powell et al. 2007, Grigoriadou and Longhurst 2009, Kaplan and Greaves 2005).

Etiology

Acute urticaria

The causes of acute urticaria (urticaria for < 6 weeks) include systemic allergic reactions, ingestion of allergens, skin contact with allergens, pseudo-allergic reactions, toxic reactions and viral infections (Dreskin 2012, Hiragun et al. 2013, Deacock 2008). The most frequent IgE-mediated reactions that cause acute urticaria are allergic reactions to foods and to medications. The most common culprit foods in children are milk, eggs and peanuts, whereas in adults, peanuts, tree nuts, shellfish and fin fish are most common. Ingestion of a medication to which a patient is allergic can also cause urticaria. Antibiotics, most typically penicillin or cephalosporins, are commonly implicated medications in acute urticarial reactions. Contact urticaria occurs after direct skin contact with an allergen, such as urticaria that appears on the extremities after sitting on grass in a grass-allergic patient. In addition to IgE mediated allergic reactions to medications, some medications activate mast cells through IgE-independent pathways, called pseudo-allergic reactions. The most frequently implicated medications in these pseudo-allergic reactions are nonsteroidal anti-inflammatory drugs (NSAIDs), opioids, contrast and vancomycin. A toxic reaction due to the ingestion of fish contaminated with histamine producing bacteria also results in hives, called scombroid food poisoning. Acute urticaria can also occur during or following an inflammatory process such as viral illness, as frequently observed in children.

Chronic urticaria

While most causes of acute urticaria can be identified by clinical history, approximately 75% of cases of chronic urticaria (urticaria for > 6 weeks) have no identifiable cause, and are classified as 'idiopathic' or 'spontaneous'. The remaining cases of chronic urticaria have specific physical triggers, most recently called 'inducible' urticaria, to reflect that these lesions can be induced by specific physical stimuli and can be elicited with specific testing (Zuberbier et al. 2018).

Physical stimuli activate mast cells by unknown mechanisms. Inducible urticaria/angioedema accounts for approximately 20% of chronic urticaria cases. The most common physical urticaria is dermatographism (also called dermographism) in which scratching or stroking of the skin leads to acute wheal production. Dermatographism affects 2–5% of the population (Hiragun et al. 2013). In patients with dermatographism, patterns or words can be 'written' on the patient's skin in wheals (Fig. 24.2). This is rarely a cause of chronic urticaria.

Many other physical stimuli have been reported for inducible urticaria, including exercise, heat, cold, solar radiation, water, pressure and vibration (Dice 2004).

Cholinergic urticaria is the most common cause of inducible urticaria accounting for up to 15% of cases. The mechanism is related to cholinergic stimulation of mast cells after exposure to exercise, heat or an increase in basal body temperature. Lesions are somewhat different from typical hives in that they are much smaller, even punctate in size (0.1–1 cm in diameter) although they can coalesce into larger lesions. In addition, they are markedly pruritic and are often surrounded by diffuse erythema. Cholinergic urticaria manifests on the neck and upper thorax initially, and may subsequently involve the entire body. Lesions that coalesce may have the appearance of angioedema.

Cold urticaria is characterized by erythema, pruritus and edema following exposure to a cold. Lesions typically develop on areas of the body exposed to cold-stimuli, and symptoms often peak as the cooled

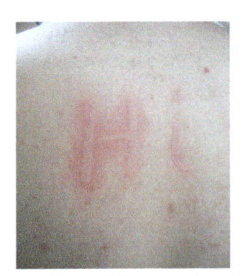

Figure 24.2. Example of dermographism with a greeting 'written' on the skin of a patient.

area is rewarmed. Cold urticaria can have localized findings with exposure to cold wind on the face, consumption of cold foods or contact with cold objects such as ice cubes. Symptoms can also be diffuse if the cold exposure is widespread, as with cold water exposure while swimming, which can potentially be fatal (Wanderer 1990). Swimming in cold water results in significant amount of mast cell activation that can lead to hypotension, which can be fatal due to resultant loss of consciousness and drowning; patients with cold urticaria should be informed of the increased risk of death by swimming in cold water. Cold urticaria must be distinguished from the cold auto inflammatory syndromes (see below).

Solar urticaria is a rare disorder that occurs after minutes of exposure to sunlight. Pruritus, erythema and swelling occur and are confined to UV light-exposed areas. With exposure of a large body surface area, systemic symptoms such as bronchoconstriction, hypotension and even death may occur.

Aquagenic urticaria occurs when water exposure results in the development of small hives. This is very rare and has been noted in only a small number of patients (Hiragun et al. 2013). Symptoms which occur after water exposure irrespective of temperature are characteristic of aquagenic urticaria and the disorder has been classified separately from the other forms of inducible urticarias.

Pressure-induced urticaria can occur independently or as a comorbid condition with chronic spontaneous urticaria. When it occurs independently, it is characterized by symptoms which occur 4 to 6 hours after the application of pressure to localized areas. Due to the time elapsed between exposure and symptoms, the condition is also termed 'delayed pressure urticaria' (Hiragun et al. 2013). Common sources of pressure include tight areas of clothing such as waistbands or straps and standing or sitting for prolonged periods of time. Manifestations of delayed pressure urticaria range from the sensation of edema in normal appearing skin, considered 'delayed pressure angioedema', to frank urticaria associated with marked swelling.

Only about 5% of chronic spontaneous urticaria/angioedema may have an identifiable cause. In rare cases, chronic urticaria/angioedema is associated with comorbid infection, environmental exposures or hormonal changes or systemic illness (Dreskin 2012). Appropriate management of these issues can result in resolution of the urticaria. In endemic areas, infections with multicellular parasites such as strongyloides or filaria elicit a significant IgE response and may result in chronic urticaria. Similarly, exposure to food, dietary supplements and medications may lead to chronic urticaria symptoms, however the exposure must be frequent, and would be considered a recurrent acute urticaria. Contact allergens such as detergents and soaps, latex, hair or nail products or other cosmetics may also cause contact hives, but exposure must be frequent and may also be better defined as contact urticaria. Food and environmental allergy are uncommon causes of chronic urticaria, and there is poor correlation with ingestion of suspected food triggers and provocation of urticaria in placebo controlled challenges. Some patients experience urticaria during menses or experience symptom flares during the menstrual cycle. These patients may have hypersensitivity to progesterone or autoimmune progesterone dermatitis. They may also have pseudoallergic reactions to analgesics such as NSAIDs taken for menstrual symptoms. Urticaria can rarely be due to systemic autoimmune illness. Cold-induced urticaria due to cryoglobulins has been rarely reported. There is no known association of urticaria with neoplasms, though acquired angioedema is associated with neoplastic disease, as discussed below.

Differential diagnosis

The differential diagnosis of urticaria varies based on the acute or chronic nature of the illness as discussed above. Conditions that may be mistaken for chronic urticaria/angioedema include infestations (scabies, bedbug bites and other insect bites), urticarial vasculitis, other skin diseases associated with intense pruritus (contact dermatitis, atopic dermatitis, bullous pemphogoid), flushing disorders (benign blushing, rosacea, pheochromocytoma, carcinoid syndrome), anaphylaxis (including idiopathic anaphylaxis, as well as exercise- and food-exercise induced anaphylaxis) and mastocytosis (urticaria pigmentosa and systemic mastocytosis).

Three important conditions that are on the differential diagnosis of urticaria are urticarial vasculitis, urticaria pigmentosa and systemic mastocytosis. Urticarial vasculitis is characterized by hives that are typically painful or burning. The lesions can be non-blanching, typically last longer than 24 hours and often have associated ecchymosis, and resolve with residual hyperpigmentation of the skin or frank scar formation (Davis and Brewer 2004). Urticaria pigmentosa presents with brownish-red cutaneous lesions that become erythematous, pruritic and edematous after gentle stroking, called 'Darier's sign'. This physical stimulation activates the nest of mast cells that comprise the lesions of urticaria pigmentosa and is pathognomonic for urticaria pigmentosa (Brockow 2004). Of note, this sign may be absent if a patient is taking antihistamines. Systemic mastocytosis is a rare disorder of mast cell hyperplasia and proliferation. Mast cells may infiltrate the skin, bone marrow and other organs. Classification and severity are based in part on the extent of mast cell burden. Patients may have urticaria pigmentosa but also may experience episodic flushing, urticaria, angioedema, gastrointestinal distress, anaphylaxis and neuropsychiatric abnormalities (Lim et al. 2009, Metcalfe 2008).

In patients with physical urticarias, systemic disorders must be further considered. For example, solar urticaria must be distinguished from other light-sensitive disorders including solar dermatitis, lupus, porphyria and photsensitivity reactions to medications (Dice 2004). Cold urticaria must be distinguished from the Familial Cold Autoinflammatory Syndrome (FCAS), an autosomal dominant disease (Wanderer 2004). Following cold exposure, individuals with FCAS experience papular dermatitis (not urticaria) with fever, chills, headache, arthralgia and myalgia and leukocytosis. Symptoms occurred at an average of 2.5 hours after cold exposure with average episodes lasting 12 hours (Hiragun et al. 2013). FCAS is a form of periodic fever with cold intolerance due to a defect in either of two genes, NLRPS or NLRP12 that regulate the inflammatory process (Hiragun et al. 2013).

Diagnosis and evaluation

The approach to diagnosis and evaluation of urticaria depends on the duration of hives. Acute and chronic urticaria are discussed separately below.

Acute urticaria

Due to the acute nature, a first episode of urticaria/angioedema may appear to occur without an identifiable stimulus. Initial evaluation should focus on the clinical history, specifically foods and medications ingested within the hours preceding the appearance of hives. It should also consider dietary supplements and contact exposures including occupational exposure, insect bites or stings and comorbid disease. Recent history of a viral infection should also be elicited as a potential trigger, particularly in children. A complete review of systems should be obtained as well as a complete physical examination (Joint Task Force 2000). Physician examination of the lesions and/or high quality photographs taken by the patient are helpful. A trial of discontinuation of non-critical medications and dietary supplements should be considered, or medications changed to structurally unrelated compounds if possible. If food is suspected as a trigger, but a specific food cannot easily be identified, patients should be instructed to keep a retrospective food diary, recording all food eaten up to 6 hours prior to each episode of urticaria. However, even if no etiology is evident, management of the acute hives for the next several days or weeks is based on symptomatic control, and no specific workup is required (Zuberbier et al. 2018).

292 Textbook of Allergy for the Clinician

Chronic urticaria

Chronic urticaria is characterized by hives that occur daily or almost daily for 6 weeks or more. Chronic Spontaneous Urticaria (CSU) is the most common type of chronic urticaria. CSU was previously called Chronic 'Idiopathic' Urticaria (CIU), but recent nomenclature has shifted to the term 'spontaneous' to reflect that urticaria occurs spontaneously without an apparent trigger. This lack of an identifiable cause of urticaria is sometimes difficult for both patients and health care providers to accept. Search for a cause of CSU can lead to expensive, potentially invasive and often fruitless investigations (Tarbox et al. 2011). The best diagnostic tool in the evaluation of chronic spontaneous urticaria is a thorough history and physical, performed by a board certified specialist knowledgeable in urticarial disease. Figure 24.3 outlines a diagnostic algorithm for chronic urticaria.

When embarking on an evaluation of chronic urticaria, it is first best to confirm that skin lesions are really hives. Direct observation and/or photographs of lesions are helpful. This is particularly true for chronic urticaria, as not all reported 'hives' are truly urticaria (Weldon 2005). It is important to ask the patient if they have associated fever with hive outbreaks, and if lesions last > 24 hours or leave residual skin discoloration, as these features are atypical for chronic urticaria and suggest other diagnoses (Zuberbier et al. 2018). Physical examination of the skin, lymph nodes and abdomen for organomegaly is also important in the differential diagnosis of chronic urticaria.

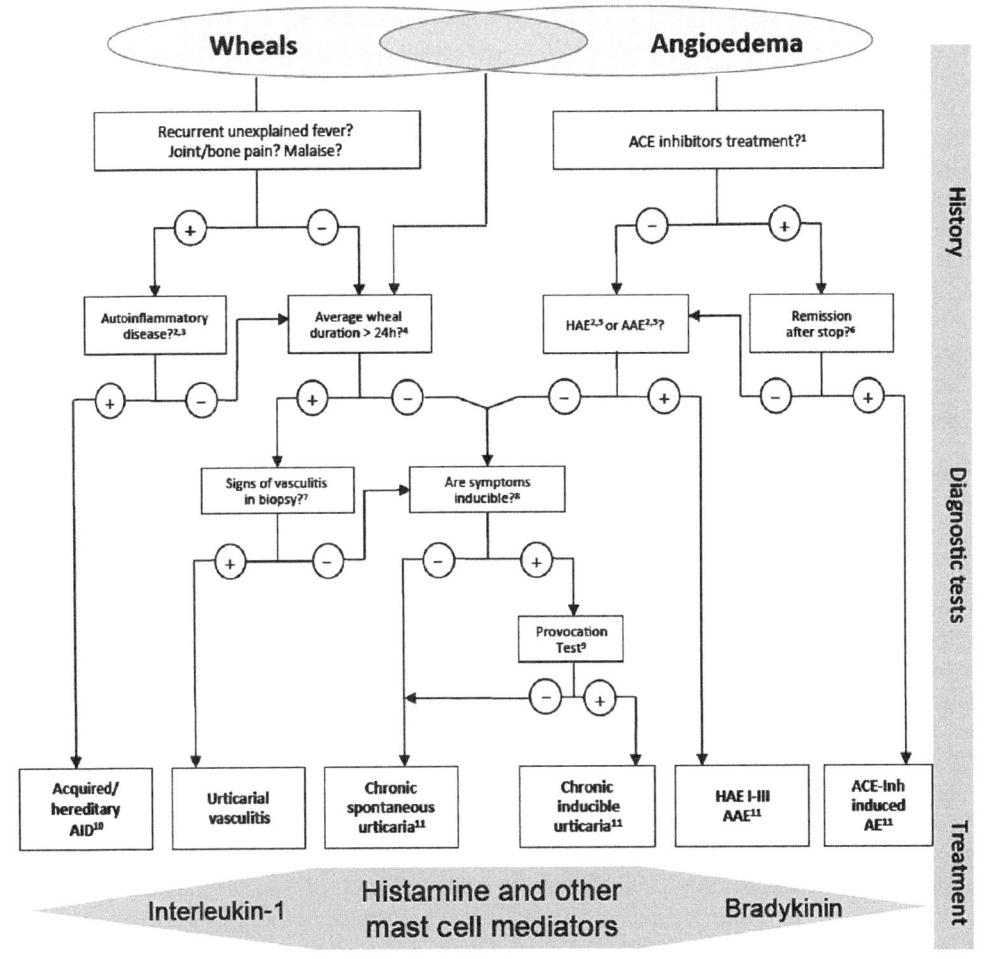

Figure 24.3. Recommended diagnostic algorithm for chronic urticaria (Reprinted with permission from Zuberbier, T. The EAACI/GA²LEN/EDF/WAO guideline for the definition, classification, diagnosis and management of urticaria. Allergy. 2018 Jul; 73(7): 1393–1414).

For the cases of chronic urticaria with a specific underlying cause, attention to physical triggers, foods, medications, supplements, contact exposures, autoimmune diseases and comorbid systemic illnesses is critical. If possible, medications which may cause pseudo allergic reactions such as non-steroidal anti-inflammatory medications (NSAIDS) should be discontinued, and consideration should be given to stop all other non-critical medications and supplements.

Testing for inducible urticarias

Once the diagnosis of chronic urticaria is established and a thorough history and physical examination completed, if chronic inducible urticaria is a consideration, in-office testing can be performed to verify the specific trigger(s).

Dermatographism can be elicited by stroking the skin with a tongue blade, wooden tip of a cotton applicator or a similar item. Testing for cold urticaria can be performed with the 'ice cube test' or with commercial devices like the TempTest. The ice cube test involves application of an ice cube to the volar forearm for 5 minutes, followed by removal and allowing the skin to rewarm for 5 minutes, after which the wheal is measured (Hiragun et al. 2013). An exercise challenge of running or bicycling in a 30 degree Celsius room for 10 to 15 minutes is a test for cholinergic urticaria. The hives of aquagenic urticaria may be evoked by application of room-temperature water compress directly to the skin. Testing for pressure-induced urticaria involves the application of pressure perpendicular to the plane of the skin. Usually sandbags are placed on the shoulders or slings with weights attached are placed on the forearm for 10 to 20 minutes; urticaria and/or angioedema will occur in 4 to 6 hours.

Solar urticaria has been classified into Types I through VI based on the wavelength of light that induces hives. Type I hives occur at 2800–3200Å, Type II at 3200–4000 Å, Type III and IV at 4000–5000Å, Type V at 2800–5000Å and Type VI at 4000 Å (Hiragun et al. 2013). Despite the rigorous classification of solar urticaria, screening can be performed by exposing patients to a broad, continuous light spectrum from fluorescent bulbs. If the screen is positive, various light filters can be used to isolate the causative light spectrum.

Allergy testing

While some patients with chronic urticaria will have positive skin tests to environmental allergens, there is little correlation between environmental aeroallergen skin test results and triggers of chronic urticaria (Kulthanan et al. 2008). Environmental allergens do cause contact urticaria, which is acute in nature, but as they are not major causes of chronic urticaria, and environmental allergen testing is of low utility in the evaluation of chronic urticaria.

Food allergens are 'often suspected but rarely implicated' in the etiology of chronic urticaria (Bernstein et al. 2008). While up to 40% of patients suspect food as triggers of their chronic urticaria, foods are implicated as the cause of urticaria in food challenges in 5% or less of suspected cases (Kobza Black et al. 1991, Hsu and Li 2012). Special diets which are 'pseudoallergen-free' or 'low histamine' have also been studied in urticaria and resulted in symptomatic improvement; however these studies have been short in duration and most patients with reported clinical improvement fail to have symptoms provoked in a food challenge (Zuberbier et al. 1995, Magerl et al. 2010, Wagner et al. 2017).

Neither environmental nor food allergy testing is routinely recommended in the latest international practice parameter on evaluation and treatment of chronic urticaria (Zuberbier et al. 2018).

Laboratory testing

In patients with uncomplicated chronic spontaneous urticaria, it may be appropriate to refrain from performing a laboratory workup or to limit investigation to a Complete Blood Count (CBC) and markers of inflammation such as Erythrocyte Sedimentation Rate (ESR) and C-Reactive Protein (CRP) (Zuberbier et al. 2018, Bernstein et al. 2014). Extensive laboratory investigations are unlikely to reveal a cause of urticaria and rarely lead to changes in management resulting clinical improvement in urticaria (Tarbox et al. 2011).

Although routine laboratory testing in chronic urticaria is not necessary, select laboratory testing may be indicated based on the history and physical examination. For example, if lesions are suggestive of urticaria pigmentosa a skin biopsy with specific staining for mast cells can be performed. If there is concern for mastocytosis, a serum tryptase level may be obtained, and if significantly abnormal, a bone marrow biopsy is indicated. A concern for carcinoid syndrome should prompt a 24 hour urine level measurement of 5-hydroxyindoleacetic acid (5-HIAA). For concerns of lupus or porphyria screening involves testing for anti-nuclear antibodies and measuring total plasma porphyrin respectively. Although few patients with Hashimoto's thyroiditis have urticaria, an increased incidence of elevated antibodies to thyroperoxidase or thyroglobulin have been found in multiple studies of patients with chronic urticaria (Dreskin and Andrews 2005). A TSH may be checked in those with symptoms or signs of hypothyroidism, which could potentially be treated. However, the utility of checking a TSH in all chronic urticaria patients is controversial.

Skin biopsy

A skin biopsy should be considered when there is concern for urticarial vasculitis, such as when urticaria lasts for more than 24 hours or leaves residual bruising. Biopsies should be sent for both standard Hemotaxolyn and Eosin (H&E) staining as well as immunofluorescence (IF) staining. Urticarial vasculitis lesions may demonstrate histologic evidence of vascular destruction and fibrinoid necrosis on H&E and they may demonstrate immune complex deposition on IF.

Treatment

Acute urticaria

Acute urticaria is typically self-limited and responds well to antihistamines. First generation antihistamines such as diphenhydramine and hydroxyzine cause sedation in many patients. Second generation antihistamines such as fexofenadine, cetirizine and loratadine are recommended as first line therapy as they cause minimal or no sedation due to less mobility across the blood-brain barrier. Third generation antihistamines can also be used, including desloratadine and levocetirizine. Superior results are achieved when these medications are taken on a scheduled basis and can block binding of histamine to the histamine receptor, rather than when they are taken to treat already existing hives. In some patients, it is useful to add a first generation antihistamine at night for breakthrough symptoms (Dreskin 2012, Hiragun et al. 2013). Ketotifen is an antihistamine-mast cell stabilizer and can also be used as an alternative agent (Egan and Rallis 1997). NSAIDs and opioids should be discontinued, at least temporarily, in all patients with urticaria if medically tolerable.

For some patients, a short course of corticosteroids may be required to achieve symptom control (Dreskin 2012, Kaplan 2009). For patients with a history of potentially life-threatening anaphylaxis or laryngeal edema, ready access to intramuscular epinephrine (1:1000 dilution) and education on indications, administration and the immediate medical care following epinephrine use is imperative.

Chronic urticaria

Histamine type 1 receptor blocking antihistamines are the mainstay of chronic urticaria treatment, and second generation antihistamines are preferred first-line agents (Dreskin 2012, Kaplan 2009, Morgan and Khan 2008a,b). However, H1 antihistamines at standard doses may not control symptoms in 25–50% of people affected. Guidelines on the treatment of urticaria (Fig. 24.4) state that if standard doses of second generation antihistamines do not control symptoms, then dosage can be increased 4-fold higher than standard doses (e.g., cetirizine 40 mg daily) (Zuberbier et al. 2018, Zuberbier 2012).

Increased doses of non sedating, second generation antihistamines may not control symptoms in up to 50% of those with chronic urticaria. If this occurs, some guidelines suggest the addition of sedating, first-generation H1 antihistamines such as hydroxyzine or doxepin (Bernstein et al. 2014). However, the side effect of sedation is significant, and more recent international guidelines do not recommend this

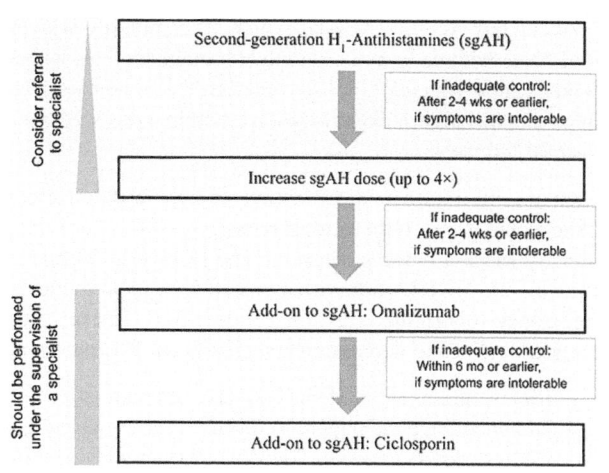

Figure 24.4. Recommended treatment algorithm for urticaria (Reprinted with permission from Zuberbier, T. The EAACI/GA²LEN/EDF/WAO guideline for the definition, classification, diagnosis and management of urticaria. Allergy. 2018 Jul; 73(7): 1393–1414).

(Zuberbier et al. 2018, Zuberbier and Bernstein 2018). As with acute urticaria, severe chronic urticaria symptoms may require a course of systemic corticosteroids to control symptoms. However, the deleterious effects of chronic systemic steroids limit their use, and there have been few controlled studies in chronic urticaria (Kaplan 2009, Loria et al. 2001).

If urticaria symptoms are refractory to antihistamines, international guidelines recommend initiation of omalizumab, a monocolonal antibody against IgE. If symptoms are refractory to omalizumab, immunomodulatory therapy can be initiated, with the best evidence supporting use of cyclosporine (Zuberbier et al. 2018).

Other treatments for antihistamine and omalizumab refractory chronic urticaria include anti-inflammatory medications such as hydroxychloroquine, sulfasalazine, dapsone and colchicine. Antimetabolites such as azathioprine, cyclophosphamide and methotrexate have also been used. Immunomodulators have shown similar benefit in some case series and small trials, including mycophenolate and tacrolimus (Grattan et al. 2000, Vena et al. 2006, Hollander et al. 2011).

Another aspect of the management of chronic urticaria involves prevention (Dreskin 2012, Kaplan 2009). For patients with physical urticaria, avoidance of triggers or minimization of trigger exposure is important. Additional modifiable exacerbating factors include medications such as NSAIDs or opioids, vasodilatory activities such as exercising, showering with hot water or vasodilatory compounds such as alcohol. Psychosocial stress is a common trigger for urticaria and should be managed as best as possible.

For most patients with chronic urticaria, the prognosis is good to excellent, with 20–80% of patients experiencing spontaneous resolution within 1 year (Maurer et al. 2011). However, many patients may have persistent symptoms for > 10 years and some of those who experience resolution of symptoms, may experience recurrence later in life (Maurer et al. 2011). Patients with physical urticaria, a component of pressure-induced urticaria or evidence of autoimmune associated urticaria tend to have more severe and persistent symptoms (Kozel et al. 2001).

Clinical pearls

Case: An 18 year-old girl presents to her primary care physician noting daily outbreaks of hives for the past 2 weeks. Her lesions are erythematous, raised and pruritic and occur on her trunk and extremities. Her mother stated that several days before her hives developed, the patient and several members of her family developed rhinitis, pharyngitis and nonproductive cough, all of which have since resolved. The patient is the only one in her household with urticarial lesions.

Teaching point. This patient has Acute Urticaria, which is commonly triggered by viral illnesses. Symptomatic treatment of hives with daily non sedating H1 antihistamines is the first line of treatment. If her symptoms are severe, a short course of oral steroids could also be prescribed. The patient and her mother should be reassured that lesions are likely to resolve within a few weeks and should be advised to follow up if symptoms persist > 6 weeks.

Case: A 28 year-old woman with a past medical history of hypothyroidism complains of a 4 month episode of daily hives. She experiences erythematous, raised, pruritic lesions that cover her entire body. The lesions also occasionally cause a burning sensation and resolve in 24 hours without residual scar. Tearfully, she recounts an episode 1 week prior with associated face and tongue swelling that prompted her to visit a nearby emergency room. She is unable to identify consistent triggers despite keeping a symptom diary. She expresses feelings of depression and significant frustration.

Teaching point. Chronic urticaria and/or angioedema can have dramatic effects on a patient's quality of life. A caring physician should encourage the patient to discuss how the disease affects their life, which may also enhance the patient-physician relationship. The physician should recommend first line treatment with daily, nonsedating H1 antihistamines and encourage follow up if symptoms do not improve.

Angioedema

Angioedema may occur without associated urticaria and is distinct from angioedema associated with urticaria. Patients with isolated angioedema fall into two broad categories (Dreskin 2012, Kaplan 2009, Grigoriadou and Longhurst 2009, Kaplan and Greaves 2005, Weldon 2006). The first group, which is due to bradykinin, includes hereditary angioedema (HAE), acquired angioedema (AAE) and angiotensin converting enzyme inhibitor (ACE-i) associated angioedema. The second group, idiopathic angioedema or histaminergic angioedema, appears to be mechanistically related to urticaria/angioedema and patients may respond to treatment with antihistamines and corticosteroids and the angioedema is likely due to mast cell activation.

Prevalence

Hereditary angioedema is an autosomal dominant disease that affects approximately 1 in 50,000 to 100,000 individuals across ethnic groups (Longhurst and Cicardi 2012). It is due to a decrease in the level or function of C1 esterase inhibitor. Although the disorder is inherited, a negative family history can occur in approximately 25% of cases. Acquired angioedema (AAE) has a clinical presentation and laboratory results similar to HAE, but is often due to an auto-antibody against C1-inhibitor which diminishes its level and function. AAE typically affects an older population in the setting of malignancies such as B-cell lymphoma, but it has also been noted in autoimmune diseases such as systemic lupus erythematosus (Hiragun et al. 2013). Angiotensin-converting enzyme (ACE) inhibitor associated angioedema occurs in 0.1 to 0.2% of patients treated with the medication and may develop over time even in patients who have tolerated the medication previously (Bernstein et al. 2008). While most patients with angioedema do not have a bradykinin mediated etiology for their angioedema, it is essential to identify patients with HAE, AAE and ACE-i induced AE, as the pathophysiology of their disease and treatments are different from other types of angioedema.

Pathogenesis

During episodes of angioedema of any cause, vasoactive mediators lead to vasodilation and increased vascular permeability resulting in plasma leakage in deeper tissue layers, including the deep dermis and subcutaneous tissues. Symptoms range from discomfort to the sensation of severe pressure, and in the case of laryngeal edema, angioedema can be fatal (Dreskin 2012, Hiragun et al. 2013, Longhurst and Cicardi 2012, Sardana and Craig 2011).

Symptoms of HAE include episodes of swelling that can be quite painful and can affect any part of the body (Dreskin 2012, Hiragun et al. 2013, Longhurst and Cicardi 2012, Sardana and Craig

2011). Angioedema episodes may be heralded by a faint erythematous rash (not urticaria) at locations unrelated to ensuing edema. Common areas of swelling include the face, tongue, hands, feet, genitals and abdomen. Patients also experience swelling of mucosal surfaces. Angioedema of the larynx or uvula and gastrointestinal tract have been observed. Gastrointestinal manifestations can lead to imaging and other diagnostic searches for an elusive cause of symptoms. Prior to the availability of effective treatment for HAE, there was a significant risk of death due to asphyxiation from laryngeal edema. This risk has been reduced by modern treatments, but still exists.

The symptoms of HAE may begin shortly after birth, but are typically mild until puberty (Longhurst and Cicardi 2012, Sardana and Craig 2011). Hereditary angioedema is often not diagnosed until the second and third decade, due in part to poor awareness of the disorder and because approximately 25% of cases are due to new mutations in patients without a family history. For 50% of patients, episodes of angioedema are due to trauma such as pressure-injury. Some patients experience episodes of angioedema post-operatively due to mucosal trauma from endotracheal intubation. Many patients with HAE also report increased symptom frequency during times of emotional stress. Acquired angioedema has a similar presentation to HAE due to the involvement of C1 inhibitor. Angioedema associated with angiotensin-converting enzyme inhibitors may present rapidly, with dramatic swelling including of the head and neck.

Idiopathic angioedema presents with sudden onset of swelling similar to HAE and AAE. Idiopathic angioedema is clearly a broad group with unclear pathogenesis. However, within the group of patients with idiopathic AE, most will respond, at least in part to corticosteroids and to anti-mast cell mediator drugs. For this reason, the disease is thought to be due to activation of mast cells in the subdermis and so these patients are considered to be like those with urticaria and angioedema, but without urticaria (see above).

Etiology

Hereditary angioedema types I and II are caused by deficient or defective C1 inhibitor, a regulatory protein which is involved in controlling the complement and kinin-generating pathways (Dreskin 2012, Hiragun et al. 2013, Longhurst and Cicardi 2012, Sardana and Craig 2011). C1 inhibitor inhibits proteins that promote bradykinin generation and activation of the classic complement cascade. Excess bradykinin, a vasoactive peptide, leads to plasma leakage and resultant angioedema.

The type I HAE variant includes 85% of patients and is caused by lack of production of C1 inhibitor by a defective gene. However, as two genes encode for C1 inhibitor, levels of C1 inhibitor are detectable but are not sufficient to allow regulation of the pathways discussed above. Type II HAE, which affects 15% of the patients, is characterized by a loss of function mutation where the defective gene produces non-functioning C1 inhibitor. Thus, normal levels of C1 inhibitor are produced, but C1 inhibitor function is reduced. In type I and II HAE the loss of C1 inhibitor regulation leads to decreased levels of C4 and C2 as well as increased levels of bradykinin (Dreskin 2012, Hiragun et al. 2013, Longhurst and Cicardi 2012, Sardana and Craig 2011).

HAE with Normal C1 Inhibitor, formerly called HAE type III is rare and does not involve C1 inhibitor. The level and function of C1 inhibitor are within normal limits, as are components of the complement pathway (e.g., C4) (Sardana and Craig 2011). The etiology of HAE with Normal C1 Inhibitor is unclear but may be related to a mutation in Factor XII, Hageman factor or other genes that may augment bradykinin formation (Dewald and Bork 2006). HAE with Normal C1 Inhibitor was initially reported in females and may be precipitated or worsened by increased estrogen such as during pregnancy or with certain contraceptive use (Bork et al. 2007). HAE with Normal complements C1 Inhibitor should only be diagnosed after careful consideration and evaluation of other etiologies of angioedema on the differential diagnosis.

Acquired angioedema involves a secondary immune process causing dysfunction or inactivation of C1 inhibitor. C1 inhibitor is unable to regulate the complement and kinin pathways due to inhibition by an autoantibody or immune complexes (Hiragun et al. 2013).

In those patients affected by angioedema associated with an angiotensin-converting enzyme inhibitor, the medication inhibits the normal inactivation of bradykinin (Hiragun et al. 2013, Bernstein et al. 2008). Thus bradykinin levels are elevated and lead to angioedema, however the complement pathway is unaffected unlike in HAE and AAE. For unknown reasons, the associated angioedema can occur days to years after initiation of the medication.

The etiology of idiopathic angioedema is often difficult to determine, and like chronic urticaria with angioedema, most cases of idiopathic angioedema will not have a specific etiology (see above).

Diagnosis

The diagnosis of HAE types I and II and AAE are made through strong clinical suspicion and appropriate laboratory testing (Dreskin 2012, Hiragun et al. 2013, Longhurst and Cicardi 2012, Sardana and Craig 2011). Initial screening for these disorders includes measurement of complement factor C4, which will be decreased at baseline and will be very low or absent during episodes of acute angioedema. After discovery of low C4 levels, the next step in diagnosis is to measure C1 inhibitor level and C1 inhibitor function (Figure 24.5).

In HAE type I, C1 inhibitor level and function will be decreased while in HAE type II, the C1 inhibitor function will be low. In AAE, C1 inhibitor level will be decreased, as will C4. AAE is unique in demonstrating a decreased C1q level, a component of the complement factor C1 complex. C1 inhibitor autoantibody may also be present in AAE, although it is not needed to make the diagnosis. ACE-i associated angioedema should be considered in any patient who develops angioedema while taking an ACE-i, but the diagnosis is only made after the suspected agent is discontinued and lasting resolution of symptoms occurs. ACE-i angioedema typically resolves with discontinuation of the medication, although this may take several weeks, and in rare cases, several months. HAE with normal complements should be diagnosed only after all other possible etiologies have been ruled out and the patient has failed to improve with a trial of antihistamines.

Idiopathic angioedema is also a diagnosis of exclusion, but is often aided by noting a clinical response to systemic corticosteroids and/or antihistamines and/or epinephrine which target histaminergic pathways. The differential of angioedema isolated to angioedema of the face and neck also includes superior vena cava syndrome. Rare patients may also present with factitious angioedema.

	C4 Level	C1 Inhibitor Level	C1 Inhibitor Function	Other tests
Hereditary Angioedema Type I (HAE I)	Low	Low	Low	
Hereditary Angioedema Type II (HAE II)	Low	Normal or High	Low	
Acquired Angioedema (AAE)	Low	Normal or High	Low	C1q (low) C1Inh Ab
Hereditary Angioedema with normal complements (HAE III)	Normal	Normal	Normal	FXII mutation
Ace-inhibitor induced Angioedema	Normal	Normal	Normal	
Histaminergic Angioedema	Normal	Normal	Normal	

Figure 24.5. Laboratory testing in Angioedema.

Treatment

Idiopathic/presumed histaminergic angioedema is typically treated similarly to chronic urticaria; however, bradykinin mediated angioedemas like HAE, AAE and ACE-associated AE do not respond to treatment with antihistamines, corticosteroids or epinephrine. Regardless of the etiology of angioedema, acute attacks of angioedema with laryngeal involvement should have supportive care including airway monitoring and intubation if indicated.

Acute attacks of HAE are most effectively treated with supplemental C1 inhibitor, a bradykinin B2 receptor antagonist (e.g., icatabant), or a kallikrein inhibitor (e.g., ecallantide) (Cicardi et al. 2010, Parikh and Riedl 2011, Zuraw et al. 2010, Antoniu 2011). The choice of medication is often based on availability. When these medications are not available, symptomatic care and airway monitoring for laryngeal edema should be provided. Administration of fresh frozen plasma, which contains C1 inhibitor, can also be considered; however there is significant concern that FFP may worsen ongoing AE in some patients (Dreskin 2012). The patient's airway should be monitored, and if there is concern for laryngeal edema and stridor or respiratory distress is evident, the patient should undergo endotracheal intubation. If intubation is unsuccessful due to angioedema, emergent cricothyroidotomy may need to be performed. Other supportive care measures may include intravenous fluids and antiemetics for gastrointestinal symptoms, as well as analgesics for pain.

Access to on demand therapy for acute attacks is effective and should be provided for all patients with HAE (Maurer et al. 2018). Prophylactic therapy should also be considered in HAE patients, particularly those with frequent or laryngeal attacks (Maurer et al. 2018). Androgens such as danazol, purified or recombinant C1 inhibitor and the kallekrein inhibitor lanedelumab have been shown to reduce the number of acute angioedema episodes in double-blind, placebo-controlled trials of HAE (Dreskin 2012, Hiragun et al. 2013, Maurer et al. 2018, Banerji et al. 2018) . Attenuated androgens do carry the risk of unwanted side-effects, and the lowest therapeutic dose should be targeted. Liver transaminases must be monitored at intervals and patients must be aware of possible masculinization (Dreskin 2012, Hiragun et al. 2013). C1 inhibitor preparations and lanadelumab have fewer side effects but are more costly (Maurer et al. 2018).

In addition to on-demand therapy and prophylactic therapy, patients with HAE should have prophylaxis prior to surgical or dental procedures. Individuals who are treated with supplemental C1 inhibitor have fewer post-surgical angioedema episodes (Maurer et al. 2018).

On-demand treatment of acute attacks of AAE is similar to that for HAE type I and II, given the involvement of C1 inhibitor. Prophylactic treatment with C1 inhibitor is often avoided in this population due to risk of development of resistance to C1 inhibitor and definitive treatment for AAE involves the discovery and treatment of the underlying disorder (Hiragun et al. 2013).

For patients with HAE with Normal C1 inhibitor, they should first have failed a trial of antihistamines to rule out idiopathic/histaminergic angioedema. They are then managed similarly to HAE types I and II, with the additional consideration that hormonal contraception should be avoided if possible. Patients with ACE inhibitor-associated angioedema must discontinue this type of medication. Given the usefulness of blocking the rennin-angiotensin pathway, it is worth noting that 90% of patients with ACEI-associated AE tolerate an Angiotensin Receptor Blocker (ARB) (Beavers et al. 2011).

Idiopathic angioedema is often a therapeutic dilemma. If the patient responds to antihistamines as in chronic urticaria, this should be continued. If corticosteroids are used, the course should be of a short duration and at the lowest doses needed. Attention should be given to possible steroid-induced side effects. Some patients need to carry self-injectable epinephrine in addition to antihistamines for acute attacks. For antihistamine refractory symptoms, omalizumab is effective (Staubach et al. 2018). Other immunomodulatory approaches as for chronic urticaria should also be considered if symptoms are refractory to omalizumab.

Prognosis

The prognosis for HAE depends on the frequency and severity of exacerbation (Dreskin 2012, Hiragun et al. 2013). Patients with frequent laryngeal edema are at higher risk of fatality. The use of newer medications has greatly improved the overall outlook. AAE improves with treatment of the underlying illness, and the prognosis is typically determined by the course of the underlying disease. Angioedema associated with angiotensin-converting enzyme inhibitor resolves after cessation of the offending agent. Idiopathic angioedema may persist for months to years and then spontaneously resolve.

Clinical pearls

Case: A 21 year-old male patient presents with complaints of chronic abdominal pain, episodic diarrhea and edema. He reports having episodes of abdominal pain associated with a lacy red rash on his arm and swelling of his hands and/or feet. The swelling is asymmetric and is painful and lasts for 1 to 3 days. He has previously had an appendectomy without improvement and exploratory laparotomy without abnormal findings. He does not have a family history of medical illness including inflammatory bowel disease. His symptoms do not improve with steroids or antihistamines, but narcotics do help manage his pain; he strongly denies narcotic abuse.

Teaching points. HAE can present as a new mutation in approximately 25% of cases. Abdominal pain due to edema of the bowel can be prominent and unfortunately, these patients often experience unnecessary laparoscopies and abdominal surgery. An 'acute' C4 level and C1 esterase inhibitor level and function should be obtained.

Conclusion

This chapter on Urticaria and Angioedema entails a comprehensive description of different types, differential diagnosis, varying pathophysiology as well as choice of treatment modalities available. The clinical scenarios have been included to provide a practical approach to this common yet perplexing clinical problem.

References

Antoniu SA. Therapeutic approaches in hereditary angioedema. Clin Rev Allergy Immunol 2011; 41: 114–122.
Baiardini I, Braido F, Bindslev-Jensen C, Bousquet PJ, Brzoza Z, Canonica GW, et al. Recommendations for assessing patient-reported outcomes and health-related quality of life in patients with urticaria: a GA(2) LEN taskforce position paper. Allergy 2011; 66: 840–844.
Banerji A, Riedl MA, Bernstein JA, Cicardi M, Longhurst HJ, Zuraw BL, et al. Effect of lanadelumab compared with placebo on prevention of hereditary angioedema attacks: A randomized clinical trial. Jama 2018; 320: 2108–2121.
Beavers CJ, Dunn SP, Macaulay TE. The role of angiotensin receptor blockers in patients with angiotensin-converting enzyme inhibitor-induced angioedema. Ann Pharmacother 2011; 45: 520–524.
Bernstein IL, Li JT, Bernstein DI, Hamilton R, Spector SL, Tan R, et al. Allergy diagnostic testing: an updated practice parameter. Ann Allergy Asthma Immunol 2008; 100: S1–148.
Bernstein JA, Lang DM, Khan DA, Craig T, Dreyfus D, Hsieh F, et al. The diagnosis and management of acute and chronic urticaria: 2014 update. J Allergy Clin Immunol 2014; 133: 1270–1277.
Bork K, Gul D, Hardt J, Dewald G. Hereditary angioedema with normal C1 inhibitor: clinical symptoms and course. Am J Med 2007; 120: 987–992.
Brockow K. Urticaria pigmentosa. Immunology and Allergy Clinics of North America 2004; 24: 287–316.
Brodell LA, Beck LA, Saini SS. Pathophysiology of chronic urticaria. Ann Allergy Asthma Immunol 2008; 100: 291–297; quiz 297–299, 322.
Cicardi M, Levy RJ, McNeil DL, Li H, Sheffer AL, Campion M, et al. Ecallantide for the treatment of acute attacks in hereditary angioedema. N Engl J Med 2010; 363: 523–531.
Davis MD, Brewer JD. Urticarial vasculitis and hypocomplementemic urticarial vasculitis syndrome. Immunol Allergy Clin North Am 2004; 24: 183–213, vi.
Deacock SJ. An approach to the patient with urticaria. Clin Exp Immunol 2008; 153: 151–161.
Dewald G, Bork K. Missense mutations in the coagulation factor XII (Hageman factor) gene in hereditary angioedema with normal C1 inhibitor. Biochem Biophys Res Commun 2006; 343: 1286–1289.
Dice J. Physical urticaria. Immunology and Allergy Clinics of North America 2004; 24: 225–246.
Dreskin SC. Urticaria and Angioedema. *In*: Goldman LaS AI (ed.). Cecil Medicine. 23rd ed. Philadelphia: Saunders 2012; 1628–1932.
Dreskin SC, Andrews KY. The thyroid and urticaria. Curr Opin Allergy Clin Immunol 2005; 5: 408–412.

Egan CA, Rallis TM. Treatment of chronic urticaria with ketotifen. Arch Dermatol 1997; 133: 147–149.
Fonacier LS, Dreskin SC, Leung DY. Allergic skin diseases. J Allergy Clin Immunol 2010; 125: S138–149.
Grattan CE, O'Donnell BF, Francis DM, Niimi N, Barlow RJ, Seed PT, et al. Randomized double-blind study of cyclosporin in chronic 'idiopathic' urticaria. Br J Dermatol 2000; 143: 365–372.
Greaves MW, Tan KT. Chronic urticaria: recent advances. Clin Rev Allergy Immunol 2007; 33: 134–143.
Grigoriadou S, Longhurst HJ. Clinical Immunology Review Series: An approach to the patient with angio-oedema. Clin Exp Immunol 2009; 155: 367–377.
Hiragun M, Hiragun T, Mihara S, Akita T, Tanaka J, Hide M. Prognosis of chronic spontaneous urticaria in 117 patients not controlled by a standard dose of antihistamine. Allergy 2013; 68: 229–235.
Hollander SM, Joo SS, Wedner HJ. Factors that predict the success of cyclosporine treatment for chronic urticaria. Ann Allergy Asthma Immunol 2011; 107: 523–528.
Hsu ML, Li LF. Prevalence of food avoidance and food allergy in Chinese patients with chronic urticaria. Br J Dermatol 2012; 166: 747–752.
Joint Task Force on Practice Parameters. The diagnosis and management of urticaria: a practice parameter part I: acute urticaria/angioedema part II: chronic urticaria/angioedema. Ann Allergy Asthma Immunol 2000; 85: 521–544.
Kaplan AP. Urticaria and Angioedema. In: Adkinson NF, Bochner BS, Busse WW, Holgate ST, Lemanske Jr. RF, Simons FER (eds.). Middleton's Allergy: Principles & Practice. Vol 2. 7th ed: Mosby/Elsevier; 2009: 1063–1081.
Kaplan AP, Greaves MW. Angioedema. J Am Acad Dermatol 2005; 53: 373–388; quiz 389–392.
Kobza Black A, Greaves MW, Champion RH, Pye RJ. The urticarias 1990. Br J Dermatol 1991; 124: 100–108.
Kozel MM, Mekkes JR, Bossuyt PM, Bos JD. Natural course of physical and chronic urticaria and angioedema in 220 patients. J Am Acad Dermatol 2001; 45: 387–391.
Kulthanan K, Jiamton S, Boochangkool K, Jongjarearnprasert K. Angioedema: clinical and etiological aspects. Clin Dev Immunol 2007; 26438.
Kulthanan K, Jiamton S, Rutnin NO, Insawang M, Pinkaew S. Prevalence and relevance of the positivity of skin prick testing in patients with chronic urticaria. J Dermatol 2008; 35: 330–335.
Lim KH, Tefferi A, Lasho TL, Finke C, Patnaik M, Butterfield JH, et al. Systemic mastocytosis in 342 consecutive adults: survival studies and prognostic factors. Blood 2009; 113: 5727–5736.
Longhurst H, Cicardi M. Hereditary angio-oedema. Lancet 2012; 379: 474–481.
Loria MP, Loria MP, Dambra PP, D'Oronzio L, Nettis E, Pannofino A, et al. Cyclosporin A in patients affected by chronic idiopathic urticaria: a therapeutic alternative. Immunopharmacol Immunotoxicol 2001; 23: 205–213.
Magerl M, Pisarevskaja D, Scheufele R, Zuberbier T, Maurer M. Effects of a pseudoallergen-free diet on chronic spontaneous urticaria: a prospective trial. Allergy 2010; 65: 78–83.
Maurer M, Weller K, Bindslev-Jensen C, Giménez-Arnau A, Bousquet PJ, Bousquet J, et al. Unmet clinical needs in chronic spontaneous urticaria. A GA(2)LEN task force report. Allergy 2011; 66: 317–330.
Maurer M, Magerl M, Ansotegui I, Aygören-Pürsün E, Betschel S, Bork K, et al. The international WAO/EAACI guideline for the management of hereditary angioedema-The 2017 revision and update. Allergy 2018; 73: 1575–1596.
Metcalfe DD. Mast cells and mastocytosis. Blood 2008; 112: 946–956.
Metz M, Bergmann P, Zuberbier T, Maurer M. Successful treatment of cholinergic urticaria with anti-immunoglobulin E therapy. Allergy 2008; 63: 247–249.
Mlynek A, Maurer M, Zalewska A. Update on chronic urticaria: focusing on mechanisms. Curr Opin Allergy Clin Immunol 2008; 8: 433–437.
Morgan M, Khan DA. Therapeutic alternatives for chronic urticaria: an evidence-based review, part 1. Ann Allergy Asthma Immunol 2008a; 100: 403–411; quiz 412–404, 468.
Morgan M, Khan DA. Therapeutic alternatives for chronic urticaria: an evidence-based review, Part 2. Ann Allergy Asthma Immunol 2008b; 100: 517–526; quiz 526–518, 544.
Parikh N, Riedl MA. New therapeutics in C1INH deficiency: a review of recent studies and advances. Curr Allergy Asthma Rep 2011; 11: 300–308.
Pickering RJ, Good RA, Kelly JR, Gewurz H. Replacement therapy in hereditary angioedema. Successful treatment of two patients with fresh frozen plasma. Lancet 1969; 1: 326–330.
Powell RJ, Du Toit GL, Siddique N, Leech SC, Dixon TA, Clark AT, et al. BSACI guidelines for the management of chronic urticaria and angio-oedema. Clin Exp Allergy 2007; 37: 631–650.
Saini SS. Basophil responsiveness in chronic urticaria. Curr Allergy Asthma Rep. 2009; 9: 286–290.
Sardana N, Craig TJ. Recent advances in management and treatment of hereditary angioedema. Pediatrics 2011; 128: 1173–1180.
Staubach P, Metz M, Chapman-Rothe N, Sieder C, Bräutigam M, Maurer M, et al. Omalizumab rapidly improves angioedema-related quality of life in adult patients with chronic spontaneous urticaria: X-ACT study data. Allergy 2018; 73: 576–584.
Tarbox JA, Gutta RC, Radojicic C, Lang DM. Utility of routine laboratory testing in management of chronic urticaria/angioedema. Ann Allergy Asthma Immunol 2011; 107: 239–243.
Vena GA, Cassano N, Colombo D, Peruzzi E, Pigatto P. Cyclosporine in chronic idiopathic urticaria: a double-blind, randomized, placebo-controlled trial. J Am Acad Dermatol 2006; 55: 705–709.
Wagner N, Dirk D, Peveling-Oberhag A, Reese I, Rady-Pizarro U, Mitzel H, et al. A Popular myth—low-histamine diet improves chronic spontaneous urticaria—fact or fiction? J Eur Acad Dermatol Venereol 2017; 31: 650–655.

Wanderer AA. Cold urticaria syndromes: historical background, diagnostic classification, clinical and laboratory characteristics, pathogenesis, and management. J Allergy Clin Immunol 1990; 85: 965–981.

Wanderer AA, Hoffman HM. The spectrum of acquired and familial cold-induced urticaria/urticaria-like syndromes. Immunol Allergy Clin of North America 2004; 24: 259–286.

Weldon D. When your patients are itching to see you: not all hives are urticaria. Allergy Asthma Proc 2005; 26: 1–7.

Weldon D. Differential diagnosis of angioedema. Immunol Allergy Clin North Am 2006; 26: 603–613.

Zuberbier T, Chantraine-Hess S, Hartmann K, Czarnetzki BM. Pseudoallergen-free diet in the treatment of chronic urticaria. A prospective study. Acta Derm Venereol 1995; 75: 484–487.

Zuberbier T, Bindslev-Jensen C, Canonica W, Grattan CEH, Greaves MW, Henz BM, et al. EAACI/GA2LEN/EDF guideline: definition, classification and diagnosis of urticaria. Allergy 2006; 61: 316–320.

Zuraw B, Cicardi M, Levy RJ, Nuijens JH, Relan A, Visscher S, et al. Recombinant human C1-inhibitor for the treatment of acute angioedema attacks in patients with hereditary angioedema. J Allergy Clin Immunol 2010; 126: 821–827 e814.

Zuberbier T. Pharmacological rationale for the treatment of chronic urticaria with second-generation non-sedating antihistamines at higher-than-standard doses. J Eur Acad Dermatol Venereol 2012; 26: 9–18.

Zuberbier T, Bernstein JA. A comparison of the united states and international perspective on chronic urticaria guidelines. J Allergy Clin Immunol Pract. 2018; 6: 1144–1151.

Zuberbier T, Aberer W, Asero R, Abdul Latiff AH, Baker D, Ballmer-Weber B, et al. The EAACI/GA(2)LEN/EDF/WAO Guideline for the Definition, Classification, Diagnosis and Management of Urticaria. The 2017 Revision and Update. Allergy. 2018.

25

Atopic Dermatitis

Luz Fonacier and *Amanda Schneider*

HISTORICAL PERSPECTIVE

Atopic Dermatitis (AD) is a chronic, relapsing inflammatory skin disorder. In the 1930s, the term atopic dermatitis was coined to describe the weeping eczema of children and the chronic, lichenified lesions of adults (Leung et al. 2004).

INTRODUCTION, DEFINITION, EPIDEMIOLOGY

The lifetime prevalence in children ranges from 6–12.98% in the United States, depending on the approach and study design used to analyze AD. The prevalence is increasing over time. More than 50% of patients with AD develop asthma, and nearly 75% develop allergic rhinitis usually after the AD has developed (referred to as the atopic march) (Eichenfield et al. 2003, Spergel and Paller 2003). Epidemiologic studies show wide variance in the prevalence from less than 1% in India and China and up to 22.5% in Ecuador. [PMID: 2857797].

Pathogenesis and pathology

Atopic dermatitis has a pathogenesis of complex immune dysregulation and interplay of genetic, environmental, epidermal and psychological factors. The stratum corneum of healthy skin functions as a barrier and provides water-retaining properties. It contains an extracellular lipid matrix including ceramides, cholesterol and free fatty acids (Leung 2001). When this layer becomes dry and fissured, it becomes a portal of entry for bacteria, mostly commonly *Staphylococcus aureus*. Disruption of the integrity of the stratum corneum exposes epidermal and dermal extracellular matrix proteins, such as fibronectin and collagen which can serve as anchors for *S. aureus* binding via adhesions (Cho et al. 2001). In AD, the stratum corneum lipid composition contains decreased levels of ceramides and sphingosine which normally act as water-retaining molecules. Deficient ceramide increases secretion of ceramidases, which leads to increased transepidermal water loss, resulting in dry, cracked skin of AD (Cardona et al. 2006, Arikawa et al. 2002). Sphingosine has been shown to normally possess antimicrobial properties, thus deficiencies may favor bacterial colonization (Arikawa et al. 2002).

NYU Long Island School of Medicine, Allergy & Immunology, Mineola, New York 11501.
  Email: Amanda.Schneider@nyulangone.org
* Corresponding author: Luz.Fonacier@nyulangone.org

Superantigen colonization results from defective skin barrier function, increased *S. aureus* adhesion to AD skin, and decreased innate immune responses resulting in failure to inhibit growth of *S. aureus* in the skin (Leung 2003). The skin of patients with atopic dermatitis (AD) exhibits a striking susceptibility to colonization with *Staphylococcus aureus* (Fig. 25.1).

This is in contrast to the skin flora of nonatopic patients in whom the colonization rate of *S. aureus* is less than 5% (Dahl 1983). Some strains of *S. aureus* secrete exotoxins with T-cell superantigen activity (toxigenic strains) (Bunikowski et al. 2000). Such bacterial superantigens can lead to activation and proliferation of T cells in AD skin, releasing cytokines and other inflammatory mediators and contribute to the pathogenesis and exacerbation of AD (Cardona et al. 2006).

The genetics of AD is complex. Most patients with AD have a predisposition to develop an IgE response to common environmental allergens. Loss-of-function mutations (R501X and 2282derl4) in the filaggrin gene (FLG) that cause ichthyosis vulgaris, one of the most common inherited skin disorders of keratinization, have been reported to be strong predisposing factors for AD. Filaggrin, which consolidates the keratin filaments into dense bundles at the granular layer–stratum corneum boundary, represents an integral part of the epidermis and is crucial for the development of the cornified envelope that maintains the barrier function of the uppermost layer of the skin (Weidinger et al. 2006). The skin lesions of AD are characterized by an infiltration of activated T cells, eosinophils and Langerhans cells (Akdis et al. 1999). Activated peripheral CD4+ T cells that preferentially secrete T helper (Th) 2 cytokines (IL-4, IL-5, IL-13, and IL-31) and stimulate B cells to produce large amounts of IgE have been reported to be associated with skin disease (Akdis et al. 1999).

Memory/effector T cells (CD45RO+) expressing the skin homing receptor, cutaneous lymphocyte associated Ag (CLA) has been demonstrated (Akdis et al. 1997). Almost all T cells that home to the skin express CLA on their surface and release IL-4 and IL-13. Activation and homing of peripheral blood memory/effector T cells followed by effector functions in the skin represent sequential immunological events in the pathogenesis of atopic dermatitis (AD). T cells infiltrating the skin use CLA and other receptors to recognize and traverse the vascular endothelium. In the peripheral blood of AD patients, both CD4+ and CD8+ subsets of CLA+CD45RO+ T cells are in an activated state with high CD25, HLA-DR and CD40-ligand expression. They express upregulated Fas and Fas-ligand and undergo activation-induced apoptosis. Keratinocyte apoptosis is induced by Fas-ligand, either soluble or expressed on the surface of T cells, leading to eczema formation. The dysregulated apoptosis of T cells, eosinophils and keratinocytes play a role in AD (Akdis et al. 2001).

IgE has a multifunctional role in the pathogenesis of allergic inflammation. Aside from involvement in IgE-mediated degranulation of mast cells and basophils, it is also involved in the activation of macrophage/monocytes and the stimulation of Th2 cells. The acute onset of skin inflammation in AD is

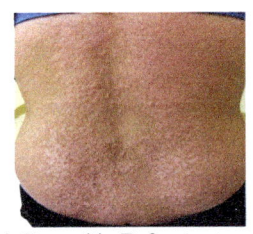

Figure 25.1. Atopic Dermatitis (Before treatment with Dupilumab).

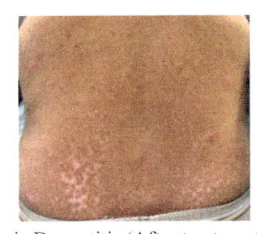

Figure 25.2. Atopic Dermatitis (After treatment with Dupilumab).

associated with a predominance of T lymphocytes and IL-4 gene expression. In chronic AD, macrophage and eosinophil activation dominate. These effector cells overexpress IL-5, IL-10, GM-CSF and PGE2, all of which may contribute to the persistence of this disease. In the case of AD, keratinocyte damage caused by scratching or microbial agents (e.g., *S. aureus*) is accompanied by the release of proinflammatory cytokines (Leung 1995).

Clinical features and diagnosis

AD typically appears in early childhood before 5 years of age and the diagnosis is based on characteristic signs and symptoms. In 1980, Hannifin et al. developed diagnostic criteria for AD. The major features include intense pruritus, facial and extensor involvement in infants and children, flexural lichenification in adults, a chronic and relapsing course and a personal or family history of atopic disease. Minor features include: xerosis, cutaneous infections, non-specific dermatitis of the hands or feet, ichthyosis, palmar hyperlinearity, keratosis pilaris, pityriasis alba, nipple eczema, white dermatographism and delayed blanch response, anterior subcapsular cataracts, elevated serum IgE levels and positive immediate-type allergy skin tests (Hanifin and Rajka 1980). Physical examination findings during infancy include involvement of the face, scalp and extensor surfaces of the extremities, with special care of the diaper area. In older patients, the flexural folds of extremities are predominantly involved. Acute AD lesions are intensely pruritic, erythematous papules associated with excoriation and serous exudation. Chronic lesions have undergone tissue remodeling from chronic inflammation and are associated with thickened plaques and increased skin markings (lichenification) and dry fibrotic papules (Akdis et al. 2006). Standardized signs and symptoms have been described and used mainly in research trials (i.e., SCORAD and EASI) (ETF 1993, Hanifin et al. 2001).

The atopic history of patient and family members are an essential part of the history to be obtained. Specific skin and blood tests and food challenge tests, can be utilized depending on the degree of the disease severity and on the suspected factors involved. Various studies suggest that allergens can impact the course of AD. Food triggers for clinical disease cannot be predicted by performing allergy testing alone; rather double-blinded, placebo-controlled food challenges have shown that foods may exacerbate disease in a subgroup of patients with AD. Elimination of these food allergens improves skin disease (Sampson and McCaskill 1985). Exacerbation of the disease can also occur with aeroallergen exposure such as pollen, dust mite or animal dander. A randomized, double-blind, placebo-controlled trial revealed development of cutaneous lesions after inhalation of household dust mite in asthmatics (Tupker et al. 1996). In addition, patients with AD may have higher levels of anxiety which can exacerbate the disease, in which they manage by scratching. Psychosocial factors in caregiver and patients are of grave importance in AD. Relaxation, behavioral modification (to break the scratching habit) have been shown to be beneficial (Koblenzer 1995).

Diagnostic Features of Atopic Dermatitis	

Major Features
• Pruritus
• Chronic, relapsing dermatitis
• Location:
   o Facial and extensor in infants and young children
   o Flexural in older children and adults
• Personal or family history of atopy
	Minor features
	• Xerosis
	• Elevated total IgE
	• Positive SPTs
	• Cutaneous infections
	• Dermatitis of the hands and/or feet
	• Early age of onset
	• Ichthyosis
	• Palmar hyperlinearity
	• Keratosis pilaris
	• Ichthyosis
	• Palmar hyperlinearity
	• Keratosis pilaris

Differential diagnosis

Several disorders may be mistaken for AD. Certain immunodeficiencies can present in infancy with dermatitis and must be considered. Immune dysregulation, polyendocrinopathy, enteropathy and X-linked (IPEX) syndrome, which is a rare condition associated with dermatitis, enteropathy, diabetes, thyroiditis, anemia and thrombocytopenia due to a mutation of FOXP3 (Chatila 2005). Wiskott-Aldrich syndrome, an X-linked recessive disorder is characterized by an eczematous rash, thrombocytopenia and severe bacterial infections. Hyper-IgE syndrome, also known as Job's Syndrome is an autosomal dominant disorder due to mutations in STAT3, with recurrent deep-seated bacterial infections due to *S. aureus* as well as diffuse eczematous dermatitis (Grimbacher et al. 1999). An autosomal recessive variant of Hyper IgE syndrome has been described due to loss of function of DOCK8 and is also characterized by atopic dermatitis and recurrent, potentially life threatening bacterial and viral infections (Dasouki et al. 2011). Omenn Syndrome is a combined immunodeficiency affecting both sexes and presents with generalized exudative erythroderma, eosinophilia, lymphadenopathy, in addition to severe respiratory infections, diarrhea and failure to thrive (Omenn 1965). Netherton syndrome is characterized by very high serum IgE levels, growth retardation, severe food allergies and typical hair finding of trichorrhexis invaginata. Diagnosis is confirmed by genetic analysis revealing a mutation in the SPINK5 gene. Netherton syndrome should be considered in the differential diagnosis in children who have generalized erythema with intractable eczematous lesions and elevated levels of IgE (Kilic et al. 2006).

In adult patients who develop an eczematous dermatitis without a history of childhood AD, other etiologies must be considered. Infectious diseases including scabies that can present as pruritic dermatitis, but can be differentiated by the distribution in skin folds of linear lesions with mites or ova on skin scrapings or biopsy and HIV are in the differential. Additionally cutaneous T cell lymphoma must be ruled out. Serial biopsy often from multiple sites could increase the yield in identifying abnormal cells. Contact dermatitis must also be considered; this can be identified given the distribution of the rash and confirmation with patch testing (Fonacier and Aquino 2010).

Differential Diagnosis	
Immunodeficiencies	• Wiskott Aldrich Syndrome • Omenn Syndrome • Job's Syndrome • DOCK8 Deficiency • Immune dysregulation, polyendocrinopathy, enteropathy, and X-linked (IPEX) syndrome
Neoplastic Disorders	• Cutaneous T cell lymphoma • Langerhans cell histiocytosis
Autoimmune disorders	• Dermatitis herpetiformis • Graft versus host disease • Dermatomyositis
Dermatologic diseases	• Seborrheic dermatitis • Contact dermatitis • Nummular eczema • Psoriasis
Infectious diseases	• HIV-associated dermatitis • Scabies
Congenital disorders	• Netherton's Syndrome
Metabolic disorders	• Acrodermatitis Enteropathica (zinc deficiency)

Treatment/management

An intact skin barrier provides the first line of defense against microbial infection (Imokawa et al. 1991). Maintaining this barrier via hydration, use of emollients and avoidance of irritants and known allergens is paramount in therapy of AD. Emollients are useful and important treatment adjuncts for patients with atopic dermatitis (AD) and may have a steroid-sparing effect (Lucky et al. 1997).

Soaking for 10 minutes in warm water followed immediately by application of an occlusive agent to prevent evaporation increases skin hydration. Baths with gentle cleansers can reduce *S. aureus* colonization (Boguniewicz et al. 2003). The addition of dilute bleach baths has been shown to be helpful in decreasing infection rates and disease severity. This is performed by the addition of 0.5 cup of 6% bleach to a full bathtub of water (40 gallons) and soaking for 5 to 10 minutes twice weekly (Huang et al. 2009). However, it is unclear whether clinical effect of bleach baths can be explained by Staph aureus reduction or the astringent effects of bleach baths. Some reviews concluded bleach baths are no more effective than water baths, alone and in combination with hydration. The use of emollients is crucial to maintain the skin barrier and has been shown to decrease the requirement for topical corticosteroids (Lucky et al. 1997). In addition to soaks, wet wrap dressings have been shown to reduce inflammation and pruritus by serving as a barrier to trauma, cooling the skin and improving penetration of topical therapies (Boguneiwicz and Nicol 2002). This involves wrapping damp cotton gauze over the affected skin, underneath a layer of dry gauze, usually overnight.

Topical Corticosteroids (TCS) are effective to decrease inflammation and pruritus in acute and chronic forms of AD. The underlying mechanism involves suppression of inflammatory genes. There is wide availability of various strengths and potency of TCS based on the vehicle in which the corticosteroid (CS) is formulated. The lowest effective potency should be used to avoid irreversible atrophy of the skin. For mild disease activity, small amounts of TCS in combination with liberal emollient use may be sufficient without producing adverse effects. Side effects of topical CS include skin atrophy, bruising, telangiectasias, acne, striae and secondary infections (Wollenberg and Shnopp 2010). More potent TCSs decrease inflammation faster, however they must be used with caution and for a short duration (especially if used under occlusion for more severe or chronic lesions). Once adequate control of AD has been achieved, long-term control can be maintained with twice-weekly use of the TCS or Topical Calcineurin Inhibitors (TCI) to areas previously affected even if they appear normal. Some studies show that patients on proactive treatment are less likely to flare, have significantly less disease relapse days and significantly more flare-free treatment days compared with a placebo (Van Der Meer et al. 1999, Breneman et al. 2008, Thaci et al. 2008).

Calcineurin inhibitors prevent T-cell activation, inhibit inflammatory cytokine release and down-regulate high affinity IgE receptor expression on Langerhans cells (Wollenberg et al. 2001). Topical tacrolimus (Protopic™) and pimecrolimus (Elidel™) have been approved for the treatment of AD in the United States and Europe (Hanifin et al. 2005). In a large (n:799) open-label study on the long-term safety and efficacy of 0.1% tacrolimus ointment in adult and pediatric patients, Hannifin, et al. found that with twice daily application in patients over 2 years of age was both safe and effective. Statistically significant improvement in AD was observed based on decreases in percent Body Surface Area (%BSA) affected and Eczema Area and Severity Index (EASI) scores as soon as the first week of application. These improvements were observed throughout the study period with no indication of loss of efficacy over time, and these benefits were noted over all age groups. The anti-inflammatory potency of 0.1% tacrolimus ointment is similar to a topical CS with intermediate potency whereas 1.0% pimecrolimus cream is less effective (Wollenberg and Schnopp 2010, Luger et al. 2001). Proactive therapy with topical tacrolimus ointment twice weekly to previously affected skin has also been shown to be effective (Wollenberg et al. 2008). In 2005, the FDA issued a black box warning suggesting that there may be a real risk of carcinoma based on reports of lymphoproliferative disease in selected post-transplantation patients, malignancies in animal models given amounts of calcineurin inhibitors exceeding that achievable by preparations of Topical Calcineurin Inhibitors (TCIs) approved for human use and rare cases of malignancies during the post-marketing surveillance period. However, current data do not show a causal relationship between these TCIs and lymphoma formation (Fonacier et al. 2006).

Another steroid free option but without the black box warning, crisaborole ointment (Eucrisa™), came on the market at the end of 2016 for children over 2 years of age and adults with mild to moderate AD. This agent works by inhibiting phosphodiesterase-4 (PDE-4), preventing breakdown of cyclic AMP (cAMP), ultimately leading to an increase in anti-inflammatory cytokines. The most common adverse side effect consists of pain (burning or stinging) at the site of application (Yang et al. 2019).

Occasionally AD lesions can become infected with Herpes Simplex Virus (HSV), which can be diagnosed via viral PCR, Tczank preps or culture from unroofed intact vesicles. These cases respond well to antiviral therapy (Boguniewicz and Leung 2006). In addition to bacterial and viral superinfections, *Malassezia* species infection can occur commonly in the seborrheic areas of the head and neck. Sensitization to *M. sympodialis* can be detected via ImmunoCAP assay. Antifungal therapy (topical or rarely systemic) has been effective in these patients (Boguniewicz et al. 2006). Since colonization with *S. aureus* can exacerbate acute AD and promote chronic skin inflammation, use of anti-staphylococcal therapy should be considered in poorly controlled AD with evidence of infection. Systemic antibiotics should be reserved for those that are heavily colonized or infected when it is clear that infection with *S. aureus* is a trigger. Erythromycin-resistant organisms are common, thus semi synthetic penicillins or first- or second- generation cephalosporins for 7 to 10 days can be effective (Boguniewicz et al. 2001). If Methacillin Resistant Staphylococcus aureus (MRSA) colonization exists, clindamycin, or trimethoprim-sulfamethoxazole and intranasal Mupirocin can be used. Topical Mupirocin three times daily for 7 to 10 days may be effective. The combination of topical corticosteroids and topical Mupirocin has been shown to be more effective than corticosteroids alone in achieving skin clearance and decreased colonization of *S. aurueus* (Lever et al. 1988).

Relieving the pruritus of AD is crucial in preventing the itch-scratching cycle of this disorder. Therapy with systemic antihistamines and anxiolytics are effective through their soporific effects used in the evening. The tricyclic antidepressant doxepin possesses both H1 and H2 receptor binding affinity. Doxepin can be given at low doses (10 mg to 50 mg) in the evening in adults. Second-generation antihistamines are often ineffective in relieving the pruritus of AD; however some studies have shown mild clinical benefit in a subgroup of patients with AD (Diepgen 2002). Topical antihistamines should generally be avoided because of irritation and possible sensitization (Shelley et al. 1996).

For severe disease that fails the above conventional topical therapy, compliance must first be confirmed before systemic therapies are used. Patients with uncontrolled moderate to severe atopic dermatitis over the age of 12 years, have the option of a monoclonal antibody, Dupilumab (Dupixent™). This targets the IL-4 receptor alpha subunit, which blocks both IL-4 and IL-13, leading to overall suppression of Th2 cytokines. It comes in two doses (200 mg and 300 mg) in pre-filled syringes intended for subcutaneous injection. Patients receive a loading dose (400 mg or 600 mg) and then continue with dosing every other week. The most common adverse reactions were similar in adult and adolescent patient populations, consisting of injection site reactions and the rarer, conjunctivitis and increased herpes simplex virus infection (Guttman-Yassky et al. 2019).

Additional options include brief courses of cyclosporine A which has been shown to be effective in randomized placebo-controlled studies in pediatric and adult patients. It can result in rapid and significant improvement in disease activity, however due to its multiple and sometimes persistent adverse effects (renal, hematologic and hepatic), no long term data exists. Other treatments may include phototherapy, mycophenolate mofetil, azathioprine and methotrexate, all of which have potential side effects and should be used with caution by experts well versed in use of these therapeutic agents (Boguniewicz and Leung 2006).

Case based problem solving

A 32 year old female presents with intensely pruritic eczematous rash on the face, neck, abdomen, back, extensors and flexural areas which is chronic and relapsing since childhood. On initial presentation she was receiving high dose topical corticosteroids and hydrocortisone injections every 3 months with uncontrolled pruritus. She also has a history of dust mite sensitization and food allergy. Skin examination is significant for diffuse, scaly, red eczematous lesions, in addition to generalized xerosis with lichenification (Fig. 25.1). There are overlying excoriations on her abdomen, arms and legs and areas of impetigo. Areas on her arms showed hypopigmentation and skin atrophy.

Initial therapies included high potency topical corticosteroids, tacrolimus, crisabole, oral and IM steroids, light therapy and cyclosporine. Despite these treatments, she continued to have frequent flares with significant impairment to her quality of life, including poor sleep and overall discomfort.

Given the recalcitrant nature of her disease she was started on Dupilumab 600 mg loading dose followed by 300 mg every 2 weeks. Over the next several months, she noted significant improvement in her skin with less severe and less frequent flares and overall improved quality of life (Fig. 25.2).

Key messages

- AD affects 10–20% of patients
- Proper skin hydration and moisturization repair and preserve adequate skin barrier
- Topical corticosteroids and/or calcineurin inhibitors can treat acute attacks and prevent relapse of disease
- Decreasing microbial colonization can improve disease
- Avoidance of allergens, education and psychosocial modifications can improve outcomes
- Dupilumab is an option for moderate to severe atopic dermatitis that has not responded to convention treatment.

Future direction

Future approaches aim at immunomodulation. Particular attention has focused on IL-31, which plays a role in both pruritis and perpetuation of the inflammatory response. Nemolizumab, an anti IL-31 receptor A monoclonal antibody has been shown to decrease pruritis and improve overall quality of life. Additionally, oral and topical JAK inhibitors are currently in Phase II and III trials and have shown promising results with favorable safety profiles. The JAK-STAT pathway is involved in the regulation of multiple AD related cytokines including IL-4, IL-13, IL-31, IL-33 and works via immunosuppressive and antiproliferative effects (Cotter et al. 2018).

References

Akdis CA, Akdis M, Simon D, Dibbert B, Weber M, Gratzl S, et al. T cells and T cell-derived cytokines as pathogenic factors in the nonallergic form of atopic dermatitis. J Invest Dermatol 1999; 113(4): 628–34.
Akdis CA, Akdis M, Bieber T, Bindslev-Jensen C, Boguniewicz M, Eigenmann P, et al. Diagnosis and treatment of atopic dermatitis in children and adults: European Academy of Allergology and Clinical Immunology/American Academy of Allergy, Asthma and Immunology/PRACTALL Consensus Report. J Allergy Clin Immunol 2006; 118(1): 152–69.
Akdis M, Akdis CA, Weigl L, Disch R, Blaser K. Skin-homing, CLA+ memory T cells are activated in atopic dermatitis and regulate IgE by an IL-13-dominated cytokine pattern: IgG4 counter-regulation by CLA-memory T cells. J Immunol 1997; 159(9): 4611–9.
Akdis M, Trautmann A, Klunker S, Blaser K, Akdis CA. Cytokine network and dysregulated apoptosis in atopic dermatitis. Acta Odontol Scand 2001; 59(3): 178–82.
Arikawa J, Ishibashi M, Kawashima M, Takagi Y, Ichikawa Y, Imokawa G. Decreased levels of sphingosine, a natural antimicrobial agent, may be associated with vulnerability of the stratum corneum from patients with atopic dermatitis to colonization by Staphylococcus aureus. J Invest Dermatol 2002; 119(2): 433–9.
Boguniewicz M, Sampson H, Leung SB, Harbeck R, Leung DY. Effects of cefuroxime axetil on Staphylococcus aureus colonization and superantigen production in atopic dermatitis. J Allergy Clin Immunol 2001; 108(4): 651–2.
Boguneiwicz M, Nicol N, Conventional therapy. Immunol Allergy Clin North Am 2002; 22: 107–124.
Boguniewicz M, Eichenfield LF, Hultsch T. Current management of atopic dermatitis and interruption of the atopic march. J Allergy Clin Immunol 2003; 112(6 Suppl): S140–50.
Boguniewicz M, Leung DY. Atopic dermatitis. J Allergy Clin Immunol 2006; 117(2 Suppl Mini-Primer): S475–80.
Boguniewicz M, Schmid-Grendelmeier P, Leung DY. Atopic dermatitis. J Allergy Clin Immunol 2006; 118(1): 40–3.
Breneman D, Fleischer Jr, AB, Abramovits W, Zeichner J, Gold MH, Kirsner RS, et al. Intermittent therapy for flare prevention and long-term disease control in stabilized atopic dermatitis: a randomized comparison of 3-times-weekly applications of tacrolimus ointment versus vehicle. J Am Acad Dermatol 2008; 58(6): 990–9.

Bunikowski R, Mielke ME, Skarabis H, Worm M, Anagnostopoulos I, Kolde G, et al. Evidence for a disease-promoting effect of Staphylococcus aureus-derived exotoxins in atopic dermatitis. J Allergy Clin Immunol 2000; 105(4): 814–9.

Cardona ID, Cho SH, Leung DY. Role of bacterial superantigens in atopic dermatitis : implications for future therapeutic strategies. Am J Clin Dermatol 2006; 7(5): 273–9.

Chatila TA. Role of regulatory T cells in human diseases. J Allergy Clin Immunol 2005; 116: 949–959.

Cho SH, Strickland I, Boguniewicz M, Leung DY. Fibronectin and fibrinogen contribute to the enhanced binding of Staphylococcus aureus to atopic skin. J Allergy Clin Immunol 2001; 108(2): 269–274.

Cotter DG, Schairer D, Eichenfield L. Emerging therapies for atopic dermatitis: JAK inhibitors. J Am Acad Dermatol 2018; 78(3 Suppl 1): S53–S62.

Dahl MV. Staphylococcus aureus and atopic dermatitis. Arch Dermatol 1983; 119(10): 840–846.

Dasouki M, Okonkwo KC, Ray A, Folmsbeel CK, Gozales D, Keles, et al. Deficient T Cell Receptor Excision Circles (TRECs) in autosomal recessive hyper IgE syndrome caused by DOCK8 mutation: implications for pathogenesis and potential detection by newborn screening. Clin Immunol 2011; 141(2): 128–132.

Diepgen TL. Long-term treatment with cetirizine of infants with atopic dermatitis: a multi-country, double-blind, randomized, placebo-controlled trial (the ETAC trial) over 18 months. Pediatr Allergy Immunol 2002; 13(4): 278–86.

Eichenfield LF, Hanifin JM, Beck LA, Lemanske Jr, RF, Sampson HA, Weist ST, et al. Atopic dermatitis and asthma: parallels in the evolution of treatment. Pediatrics 2003; 111(3): 608–16.

Fonacier LS, Charlesworth EN, Spergel JM, Leung DYM. The black box warning for topical calcineurin inhibitors: looking outside the box. Annals of Allergy, Asthma & Immunology 2006; 97(1): 117–120.

Fonacier LS, Aquino MR. The role of contact allergy in atopic dermatitis. Immunol Allergy Clin North Am 2010; 30(3): 337–50.

Grimbacher B, Holland SM, Gallin JI, Greenberg F, Hill SC, Malech HL, et al. Hyper-IgE syndrome with recurrent infections—an autosomal dominant multisystem disorder. N Engl J Med 1999; 340(692–702).

Guttman-Yassky E, Bissonnette R, Ungar B, Suarez-Farinas M, Ardeleanu M, Esaki H, et al. Dupilumab progressively improves systemic and cutaneous abnormalities in patients with atopic dermatitis. J Allergy Clin Immunol 2019; 143(1): 155–172.

Hanifin JM, Rajka G. Diagnostic features of atopic dermatitis. Acta Derm Venereol 1980; 92: 44–47.

Hanifin JM, Thurston M, Omoto M, Cherill R, Tofte SJ, Graeber M. The eczema area and severity index (EASI): assessment of reliability in atopic dermatitis. EASI Evaluator Group. Exp Dermatol 2001; 10(1): 11–8.

Hanifin JM, Paller AS, Eichenfield L, Clark RA, Korman N, Weinstein G, et al. Efficacy and safety of tacrolimus ointment treatment for up to 4 years in patients with atopic dermatitis. J Am Acad Dermatol 2005; 53(2 Suppl 2): S186–94.

Huang JT, Abrams M, Tlougan B, Rademaker A, Paller AS. Treatment of Staphylococcus aureus colonization in atopic dermatitis decreases disease severity. Pediatrics 2009; 123(5): e808–14.

Imokawa G, Abe A, Jin K, Higaki Y, Kawashima M, Hidano A. Decreased level of ceramides in stratum corneum of atopic dermatitis: an etiologic factor in atopic dry skin? J Invest Dermatol 1991; 96(4): 523–6.

Kilic G, Guler N, Ones U, Tamay Z, Guzel P. Netherton syndrome: report of identical twins presenting with severe atopic dermatitis. Eur J Pediatr 2006; 165(9): 594–7.

Koblenzer CS. Psychotherapy for intractable inflammatory dermatoses. J Am Acad Dermatol 1995; 32: 609–612.

Leung DY. Atopic dermatitis: the skin as a window into the pathogenesis of chronic allergic diseases. J Allergy Clin Immunol 1995; 96(3): 302–18; quiz 319.

Leung DY. Atopic dermatitis and the immune system: the role of superantigens and bacteria. J Am Acad Dermatol 2001; 45(1 Suppl): S13–6.

Leung DY. Infection in atopic dermatitis. Curr Opin Pediatr 2003; 15(4): 399–404.

Leung DY, Boguniewicz M, Howell MD, Nomura I, Hamid QA. New insights into atopic dermatitis. J Clin Invest 2004; 113(5): 651–7.

Lever R, Hadley K, Downey D, Mackie R. Staphylococcal colonization in atopic dermatitis and the effect of topical mupirocin therapy. Br J Dermatol 1988; 119(2): 189–98.

Lucky AW, Leach AD, Laskarzewski P, Wenck H. Use of an emollient as a steroid-sparing agent in the treatment of mild to moderate atopic dermatitis in children. Pediatr Dermatol 1997; 14(4): 321–4.

Luger T, Van Leent EJ, Graeber M, Hedgecock S, Thurston M, Kandra A, et al. SDZ ASM 981: an emerging safe and effective treatment for atopic dermatitis. Br J Dermatol 2001; 144(4): 788–94.

Omenn GS. Familial reticuloendotheliosis with eosinophilia. N Engl J Med 1965; 273: 427–32.

Sampson HA, McCaskill CC. Food hypersensitivity and atopic dermatitis: evaluation of 113 patients. J Pediatr 1985; 107(5): 669–75.

Shelley WB, Shelley ED, Talanin NY. Self-potentiating allergic contact dermatitis caused by doxepin hydrochloride cream. J Am Acad Dermatol 1996; 34: 143–144.

Severity scoring of atopic dermatitis: the SCORAD index. Consensus Report of the European Task Force on Atopic Dermatitis. Dermatology 1993; 186(1): 23–31.

Spergel JM, Paller AS. Atopic dermatitis and the atopic march. J Allergy Clin Immunol 2003; 112(6 Suppl): S118–27.

Thaçi D, Reitamo S, Gonzalez Ensenat MA, Moss C, Boccaletti V, Cainelli T, et al. Proactive disease management with 0.03% tacrolimus ointment for children with atopic dermatitis: results of a randomized, multicentre, comparative study. Br J Dermatol 2008; 159(6): 1348–56.

Tupker RA, De Monchy JG, Coenraads PJ, Homan A, van der Meer JB. Induction of atopic dermatitis by inhalation of house dust mite. J Allergy Clin Immunol 1996; 97(5): 1064–70.

Van Der Meer JB, Glazenburg EJ, Mulder PG, Eggink HF, Coenraads PJ. The management of moderate to severe atopic dermatitis in adults with topical fluticasone propionate. The Netherlands Adult Atopic DermatitisStudy Group. Br J Dermatol 1999; 140(6): 1114–21.

Weidinger S, Illig T, Baurecht H, Irvine AD, Rodriguez E, Diaz-Lacava A, et al. Loss-of-function variations within the filaggrin gene predispose for atopic dermatitis with allergic sensitizations. J Allergy Clin Immunol 2006; 118(1): 214–9.

Wollenberg A, Sharma S, von Bubnoff D, Geiger E, Haberstok J, Bieber T. Topical tacrolimus (FK506) leads to profound phenotypic and functional alterations of epidermal antigen-presenting dendritic cells in atopic dermatitis. J Allergy Clin Immunol 2001; 107(3): 519–25.

Wollenberg A, Reitamo S, Atzori F, Lahfa M, Ruzicka T, Healy E, et al. Proactive treatment of atopic dermatitis in adults with 0.1% tacrolimus ointment. Allergy 2008; 63(6): 742–50.

Wollenberg A, Schnopp C. Evolution of conventional therapy in atopic dermatitis. Immunol Allergy Clin North Am 2010; 30(3): 351–68.

Yang H, Wang J, Zhang X, Zhang Y, Qin ZL, Wang H, et al. Application of Topical Phosphodiesterase 4 Inhibitors in Mild to Moderate Atopic Dermatitis: A Systematic Review and Meta-analysis. JAMA Dermatol, 2019.

26

Contact Dermatitis

Luz Fonacier[1,*] and *Eleanor Feldman*[2]

HISTORICAL PERSPECTIVE

In the first century AD, Pliny junior made note of men who developed an itch associated with cutting pine trees (Lachapelle 2010). The Italian Bernardino Ramazzini from the 17th century is considered to be forerunner of occupational skin disease; in his text *De Morbis Artificum Diatriba* he urged medical personnel to be aware of the cutaneous adverse effects associated with work (Lachapelle 2010). Josef Jadassohn is believed to be the father of Patch Testing (PT); the first patch he performed was in September 1895 (Lachapelle 2010). Bruno Bloch continued and expanded the work of Josef Jadassohn; thus PT has been referred to as the Jadassohn-Bloch technique (Lachapelle 2010). In 1939, Dr. Paul Bonnevie published the first series for patch testing; this initial series includes some of the currently relevant culprits for allergic contact dermatitis (colophony, p-phenylenediame, nickel sulfate, potassium dichromate, Balsam of Peru and formaldehyde). In the 1970s, formation of societies for contact dermatitis (International Contact Dermatitis Research Group & North American Contact Dermatitis Group) lead to standardization of PT techniques (Cohen 2004).

INTRODUCTION

Contact Dermatitis (CD) is a common skin disorder marked by erythematous, vesicular, papular or lichenified pruritic skin lesions. It is caused by direct contact of an agent to the skin. It can be caused either by irritant triggers in 80% of patients versus allergic triggers in the remaining 20% of patients (Fonacier et al. 2010). It is estimated that more than 3,700 substances can act as contact allergens (Beltrani et al. 2006).

Definition, description of terminology/classification, epidemiology, prevalence and host features

Allergic Contact Dermatitis (ACD) is a cutaneous reaction caused by a type 4 cell-mediated reaction to an allergen; the reaction will recur with subsequent re-exposure to the same or cross-reacting allergen (Belsito 1989). The prevalence of ACD in children is generally comparable to the general adult population, with similar occurrences of nickel, fragrances, *Toxicodendron* and rubber chemicals. In patients with

---

[1] NYU Long Island School of Medicine, Head of Allergy and Immunology, NYU Langone Health. Mineola, New York 11501.
[2] NYU Langone Health, Mineola, New York 11501, Email: Eleanor.Feldman@nyulangone.org
* Corresponding author: Luz.Fonacier@nyulangone.org

Atopic Dermatitis (AD), the percent of positive patch test results varies from 23 to 49.4% which may be due to already impaired skin barrier in these patients (Giordano-Labadie et al. 1999, Ingordo et al. 2001, Sharma 2005, Belhadjali et al. 2008, Czarnobilska et al. 2009). A cross-sectional study of 1501 children aged 12 to 16 years using questionnaires, examination and patch testing found that the point prevalence of contact allergy was 15.2% (girls (19.4%) > boys, (10.3%); $P < 0.001$) and present or past ACD was found in 7.2% (girls (11.3%) > boys (2.5%) (Mortz et al. 2001). A recent systematic review looking at over 20,000 patients found the overall prevalence of contact allergy to be 20.1%. Of note, children had a lower prevalence than adults (16.5%) and women (27.9%) had a significantly higher prevalence than men (13.2%) (Alinaghi et al. 2019). Risk factors in patients with occupational dermatitis that confer a worse prognosis include ACD to nickel or chromium, delay of adequate treatment and a history of AD (Fonacier et al. 2010).

Pathogenesis & pathology

Irritant Contact Dermatitis (ICD) is caused by non-immunologic direct tissue activation. T-cells are stimulated to release inflammatory Th1 cytokines such as TNF-a, IL-1, IL-8 and GM-SCF via non-immune mechanisms (Pedersen et al. 2004), thus no immunologic memory or sensitization period is necessary for these reactions. In these irritant reactions there tends to be a higher concentration of the agent needed to provoke a response; it may also produce burning and stinging sensation in the patient as opposed to itching. The area of involvement is usually limited to the area that comes into contact with the involved agent and is a dose dependent response. Common agents that produce ICD include water, soap, detergents, acids/bases and bodily fluids including urine, saliva and stool.

ACD is mediated via type IV cell-mediated hypersensitivity. The allergens conjugate with proteins in the skin to induce activated epidermal keratinocytes to release inflammatory cytokines (Fonacier et al. 2010). Langerhans cells process peptides from these allergens in conjunction with HLA class I molecules. After migration to regional lymph nodes, the Langerhans cells present to naive T-cells. Once activated, T-cells produce regulatory and effector cells (primarily CD8+ cells with Th1 profile). These effector cells release proinflammatory cytokines that cause intense perivascular inflammation (interleukin [IL] 1, IL-6, IL-8, IL-17 and granulocyte-macrophage colony-stimulating factor [GM-CSF]). IL-17 has increasingly been shown to have a significant role in ACD (Peiser 2013). In addition, recent studies have shown hapten specific responses with allergens like nickel inducing a Th1/Th17 response while fragrances appear to induce Th2/Th22 responses (Dhingra et al. 2014). This hapten specific response may have significant implications with targeted therapy.

While ACD from a pathophysiologic standpoint is separate from AD, studies suggest a possible association. This may be in part due to the increases in skin barrier defects allowing for entrance of particles inducing ACD. A recent study in Vietnam found a significant association between hand eczema with AD where ACD accounted for 72.7% of patients (Minh et al. 2019).

Clinical features (Table 26.1)

Skin lesions can vary from erythematous papules, vesicles or bullae in acute reactions to more subtle lesions featuring lichenification, scaling, crusting and excoriations in chronic or sub-acute forms. Areas of the body where the skin is thinner (eyelids) are more susceptible to damage from irritant and contact allergens whereas skin that is thicker (palms, soles) see less involvement.

Eyelid dermatitis (Fig. 26.1) is most commonly due to ACD in one-half to two thirds of cases; culprits include fragrances (from facial tissues, cosmetics), preservatives, nickel (eyelash curlers), thiuram (rubber sponges, masks, balloons, toys), cocamidopropylbetaine and amidoamine (shampoos), tosylamide formaldehyde resin (nail polish) and gold (Rietschel et al. 2007). ICD accounts for 15% of eyelid dermatitis, AD accounts for less than 10%, and approximately 4% is attributed to seborrheic dermatitis (Ayala et al. 2003). Facial dermatitis can also be caused by allergens transferred from other parts of the body or from partners and caregivers. Rarely, facial dermatitis may also result from airborne allergens including pollens (Beltrani et al. 2006).

Table 26.1. Comparison of allergic and irritant contact dermatitis.

	Irritant CD	**Allergic CD**
Etiology	Non immune mediated tissue damage	Type IV mediated delayed hypersensitivity reaction
Symptoms	Burning, stinging	Itch
Causative agents	Water, acids/bases, body fluids (urine, stool, saliva), solvents, detergents	Plants (poison ivy/oak), cosmetics (fragrance, hair dye), metals, rubber
Lesion morphology	Erythema, edema, fissures	Erythema, edema, vesicles, papules, lichenification
Histology	Lymphocytic spongiosis	Neutrophilic spongiosis
Patch tests	Negative	Positive

*Adapted from (Fonacier 2010, Nosbaum et al. 2009).

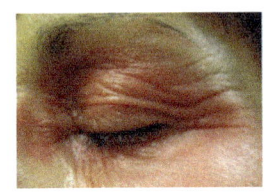

Figure 26.1. Patient with CD of eyelids.

Hand dermatitis (Figs. 26.2 and 26.3) is a common site for CD; in this location it is often difficult to distinguish between ICD and ACD and other skin diseases including AD and psoriasis. ICD commonly presents as a localized dermatitis without vesicles in webs of fingers, the dorsal and ventral surfaces of the hand including the palms and the ball of the thumb. ACD often has vesicles; locations include the fingertips, nail folds and dorsum of the hands (Fonacier et al. 2010). Often ICD can precede development of ACD and can manifest as increasing dermatitis from web spaces to fingertips or from palms to dorsal surfaces (Warshaw et al. 2003). Hand dermatitis is seen more commonly in patients with AD than the general population; it is also more common in older patients, specifically occupational hand dermatitis likely due to the frequent and repeated hand washing and other occupational insults (Fonacier et al. 2010).

Foot: Predisposing factors for foot dermatitis include heat, humidity and friction (Fonacier et al. 2010). Like hand dermatitis, patients with AD are also predisposed to foot dermatitis. Other causes of foot dermatitis include tineapedis, psoriasis, dyshidrosis and nummular eczema (Lazzarini et al. 2004). Foot dermatitis secondary to ACD frequently has lesions located on the dorsum of the feet and toes but can also have involvement of the sole and calcaneus (Fonacier et al. 2010). The interdigital areas are rarely involved. In a series of patients with foot dermatitis undergoing patch testing 70% of patients (37 out of 53) had at least one positive allergen on a patch test; nickel sulfate and mercaptobenzothiazole had the most number of positives (Lazzarini et al. 2004). Allergens pertinent to ACD of the foot include rubber compounds, leather, adhesives or glues, textile dyes and nickel used in buckles (Lazzarini et al. 2004).

Perioral dermatitis may result from habits such as lip licking, lip chewing or thumb sucking (Fonacier 2010). Allergens in dental care products (toothpastes and mouth washes) or chewing gum include cinnamon and peppermint. Balsam of Peru and cinnamic aldehyde are often used as a flavoring in food products, lipstick, mouthwash and dentifrices (Fonacier 2010). Patients may also have contact dermatitis in mucous membranes to orthodontics/dental implants that contains metals such as nickel, cobalt, chromate, mercury and gold. Thus PT for oral dermatitis should also include metals, fragrances and preservatives.

Systemic contact dermatitis refers to a condition where a patient sensitized to an allergen from contact of the skin develops symptoms after subsequent exposure from a different route, such as orally or intravenously (Aquino and Rosner 2019). Patients often present with generalized or localized dermatitis, the Baboon syndrome (well demarcated erythema of the buttocks, upper inner thighs, and axillae), flare

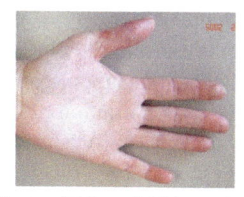

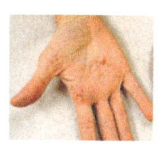

Figures 26.2 and 26.3. Patients with hand dermatitis.

of a previous site of dermatitis (recall reaction), flare of a previous positive PT, dyshidrotic hand eczema, flexural dermatitis or an exanthematous rash. This usually appears within hours to 2 days after systemic exposure to allergen. Common responsible agents include nickel and Balsam of Peru.

Diagnosis: Clinical/Laboratory (Table 26.2)

History is an important aspect to consider in evaluating patients with contact dermatitis. Particular attention should be paid to exposures at work (specific chemicals, vapors, fumes, food exposures, frequent hand washing), hobbies at home (gardening, painting, photography), and exposures at home (pets/pet products) (Beltrani et al. 2006). Alleviating and aggravating factors should be addressed as well; suspicion for corticosteroid allergy should be raised in patients with initial efficacy to corticosteroids then subsequent worsening of symptoms or non-responsiveness. However, history alone will not be able to predict the causative agent in the majority of patients.

Patch Testing (PT) (Fig. 26.4) is the gold standard for identification of a contact allergen and is indicated in any patient with acute and chronic pruritic, eczematous dermatitis if underlying or secondary ACD is suspected. Allergens are placed in chambers that are applied to the skin (particularly the back away from the spine) and good adhesion between the allergens and the skin is necessary. The back should be free of hair, emollients and other dermatitis. Due to the potential inhibition of response, topical corticosteroids and calcineurin inhibitors should be discontinued to the area of patch testing 1 week prior to placement. Oral corticosteroids greater than 20 mg of prednisone daily (or equivalent) should be discontinued 3–4 weeks prior to patch placement to avoid false negative results. Oral antihistamines need not be discontinued during PT.

Commercially available panels include T.R.U.E.® (thin layer rapid use epicutaneous test) where a panel of 35 allergens and a negative control are affixed to tape that is directly applied to the patient's back. More extensive series include the North American Contact Dermatitis (NACD) group panel and the American Contact Dermatitis Society (ACDS) series, the European standard series, the International standard series and specific occupation or exposure panels from Smart Practice Canada®, and Dormer®

Table 26.2. Grading/Interpretation of Patch Results.

0	no reaction	negative patch test
+/–	Faint non palpable erythema only	Doubtful positive patch test
1+	Palpable Erythema, possible papules	Weakly positive patch test
2+	Erythema, infiltration, papules, vesicles	Strongly positive patch test
3+	Intense Erythema and infiltration and coalescing vesicles	Extreme positive patch test

(Spiewalk 2008)

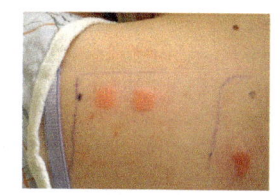

Figure 26.4. Positive results of Patch testing.

(www.dormer.com; www.allergeaze.com). Increasing the numbers of antigens tested may yield more positive results and testing with personal products is especially helpful in patients with facial, eyelid and lip dermatitis. Personal products that are washed off (shampoo, conditioner, detergents, body/facial washes) need to be diluted prior to placement (1:10–1:1000 dilution). If the patient does not know what the substance is, it should not be tested. Never apply unlabeled products with unknown ingredients as they may induce severe irritant reactions when placed on the skin. Supplementary allergens can also be used for PT based on profession (cosmetics, hairdresser, baker), medications (corticosteroid, antimicrobials, antibiotics) and specific exposures (shoes, plants, photoallergens).

Patch tests should be removed and read in 48 hours. Tests are read 30 minutes after removal of the patch to allow resolution of erythema due to the occluding pressure of the tape and/or chamber. Since 30% of reactions may be negative at 2 days, additional reading(s) should be performed at 72–96 hours and sometimes 7–10 days after the initial application. Metals, topical corticosteroids, p-phenylenediamine and topical antibiotics typically require a delayed reading (Davis et al. 2008).

Patch testing is graded on a scale from no reaction, designated as '–' up to a maximum of '+++' based on the presence of erythema, papules and vesicles in response to the patch (Uyesugi and Sheehan 2019). '±' is given to denote a doubtful response, while IR is given to denote an irritant response and not a truly positive reaction (Table 26.2). Relevance of a positive patch test must be part of its interpretation. A result is considered definite if the result of the 'use test' of a suspected item was positive or the reaction of PT with the object/product is positive. A probable response can be considered if the suspected allergen is verified in patient's skin contactants along with a consistent clinical presentation. A possible response can be considered when the patient's skin is in contact with materials that likely contain the suspected allergen. Past relevance is when the patient no longer has the exposure to the patch test positive allergen.

Other techniques which can be helpful include Repeat Open Application Test (ROAT) that involves the application of a suspected allergen to the antecubital fossa twice daily up to 1 to 2 weeks and observing for dermatitis or the 'use test' where the product is applied the same way as when the dermatitis developed (for example, facial cream on 1 × 1 cm area of the face) (Rietchel 2008). This is most useful for leave-on products intended for use on the skin. Skin biopsy may be helpful in differentiating contact dermatitis from other eczematous diseases.

Differential Diagnosis: The differential diagnosis of contact dermatitis includes other eczematous diseases such as atopic dermatitis, nummular eczema, psoriasis, lichen planus and seborrheic dermatitis. Other causes of eczema such as those associated with immunodeficiencies (Severe combined immunodeficiency (SCID), Wiskott Aldrich syndrome, and Hyper IgE syndrome) mycosis fungoides, erythroderma, dermatophytosis, and urticarial vasculitis should also be kept in mind (Fonacier 2010).

Treatment/Management: Identification of the relevant antigens causing disease in ACD is essential in treatment (Table 26.3). Once these are identified a topical skin care product list devoid of these allergens can be given to the patient. The American Contact Dermatitis Society (info@contactderm.org) maintains a database called the Contact Allergen Management Program (CAMP) for its members, which can generate a list of safe products for patient use including topical medicaments, cosmetics and personal products. In addition, SkinSAFE (formerly CARD or the contact allergen replacement database) provides an electronic application which is regularly updated and details the safety of skin products for use (www.allergyfreeskin.com).

Topical Corticosteroids (CS) are useful in the treatment of patients with CD; the potency of the CS needed for treatment depends both on the location and chronicity of the dermatitis. Non-medical interventions to aid in relief include cold compresses and oatmeal baths in oozing dermatitis. Oral antihistamines may decrease some of the associated pruritus. In severe cases of ACD, oral immunomodulators such as corticosteroids are often necessary. However, the continued use of oral CS is discouraged in patients with chronic CD. Patients with recalcitrant disease may require other modalities including phototherapy and medications including cyclosporine, methotrexate, azathioprine and mycophenolate mofetil. Barriers for nickel dermatitis and protective gloves in plant dermatitis can also be used.

Table 26.3. Common allergens.

Allergen	Found In	% Positive PT*	General Info
Nickel	Metals, jewelry, musical/surgical instruments, kitchen utensils, implants, bra hooks/underwire.	17.5%^	Greater in females; piercing is a risk factor. To check for nickel content: swab with dimethylglyoxime and ammonium hydroxide. A bright pink shows nickel is present.
Gold	Anti-inflammatory medications, electroplating industry, dental appliances, jewelry, ceramic paints, coins.	8.2 %^^	Relevance of a positive patch test to gold is low. Possible relevance may be seen in patients suspected of jewelry allergy, patients with facial or eyelid dermatitis and those with gold dental restorations. A trial of gold avoidance may be warranted if with + PT to gold. Avoidance period for benefit is long and may only be partial.
Fragrance	Cosmetics, personal products, household products, food flavorings, painting products and medicaments.	Fragrance mix I 11.3%^ Balsam of Peru 7.0%^ Fragrance mix II 5.3%^	Most common cause of ACD from cosmetics. Fragrance mix I will pick up 75–85% of fragrance allergic patients.
Paraphenylene-diamine PPD	Tattoo, hair dyes, darkly colored makeup/lipstick, textile dyes, printing ink	6.4%^	Most often affects hairline, eyelids and neck; common cause of occupational dermatitis in hairdressers. Theoretically, once fully oxidized, PPD will no longer precipitate contact reactions.
Formaldehyde	Disinfectant and preservative found in personal products, household products, newspapers, hygiene products, textiles, paint, fertilizer and building supplies/flooring.	6.4%^	Patients may flare if eating/drinking the following: artificial sweeteners, coffee, maple syrup. Patients need to avoid all formaldehyde releasers as well (quaternium-15, diazolidinyl urea, DMDM hydantoin and imidazolidinyl urea).
Paraben	Cosmetics and personal products; non-formaldehyde releaser. Used as a preservative.	0.6%^	Foods that may contain parabens include: salad dressings, condiments, soft drinks, fruit juices, and sauces. Rarely patients may cross react to paraphenylene diamine (hair dye), PABA sunscreens, benzocaine, disperse dyes, hydrochlorothiazide, and sulfa drugs.
Lanolin	Personal products including cosmetics, sunscreens and shaving creams, clothing, shoe/furniture polish and medicaments	4.1%^	Complex mixture therefore test actual lanolin used in wool alcohol sensitive patients Lanolin Paradox: sensitivity low in normal skin, moderate in atopic, high in stasis eczema and ulcers.
Rubber Accelerators: Carba mix, thiuram mix, thioureas, and benzothiazoles	Rubber gloves/shoes, clothing including swimsuits, hair/tooth brushes, baby bottles, condoms, kitchen utensils, balloons, pesticides/fungicides, and disinfectants.	Carba mix: 4.6%^ Thiuram mix: 3.4%^	Cross reactivity present between carbamates and thiuram.

Table 26.3 contd. ...

...Table 26.3 contd.

Toxicodendron (Poison Ivy)	plant		Most common plant allergy in children. Acute cases typically present with vesicles/bullae in linear pattern. PT is not recommended due to its sensitizing potential.
Neomycin	Antibiotic creams/lotions, bandaids/bandages, ear/eye/nose drops	6.9%^	Higher risk patients include those who suffer from stasis dermatitis, leg ulcers and patients with anogenital dermatitis. Patients may cross react to other antibiotics including: Tobramycin, Gentamicin, Streptomycin and Paromomycin. Mupirocin and silver sulfadiazine may be tolerated. The Committee on Infectious Diseases of the American Academy of Pediatrics no longer considers contact hypersensitivity to neomycin a contraindication to vaccination.
Corticosteroids (CS)	In gels, foams, ointments, creams, pills, inhalers or injections.	Hydrocortisone-17-butyrate: 0.2%^	Risk factors for development of CS allergy include patients with chronic venous leg ulcers, stasis dermatitis, and CD. CS is grouped into 5 classes whose cross reactivity is based on 2 immune recognition sites—C 6/9 & C16/17. Patients may be allergic to members within the same class.

^ = Reference: (De Koven et al. 2018)
^^ = reference (Sundquist et al. 2019)

Prognosis/natural history

The prognosis of CD depends on a multitude of factors including identification of the relevant allergen and ease of avoidance of that allergen. Allergens such as fragrance and preservatives are encountered frequently in daily life and are more difficult to avoid. Products labeled as 'fragrance free' are generally safe to use in patients with fragrance allergy; unscented and hypoallergenic products may still include low levels of fragrance used to mask an odor (Marks et al. 2002).

In patients with occupational contact dermatitis, prognosis also takes into account the effect on the patient's quality of life at home and at work and financial costs incurred by the patient, employer and community; early diagnosis and treatment of occupational CD and patient's understanding of their disease can improve prognosis (Cahill et al. 2004).

A long term follow up study in patients with occupational hand eczema in Finland via a questionnaire found that hand dermatitis had healed in 40% of patients; the duration of the disease prior to diagnosis and a history of atopic disease strongly correlated to the continuation of disease (Malkonen et al. 2010).

Case based problem solving

- *A 49-year-old female with history of atopic dermatitis presents with new onset hand dermatitis (Fig. 26.5).*
- *She works as a gardener and reports hand swelling with planting of marigolds.*
- *Topical corticosteroids and immunomodulators offer only minimal relief.*
- *Patch testing with TRUE® test, supplemental allergens (cosmetics) and plant parts (marigold, petunia, dalia and mum) was applied.*
- *Positive results to caine mix and marigold (Fig. 26.6).*

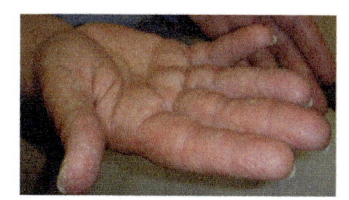

Figure 26.5. Picture of patient with hand dermatitis.

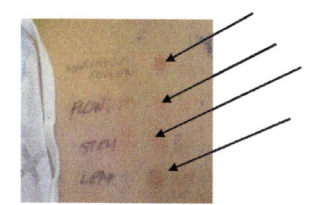

Figure 26.6. Results of patch testing with marigold.

- *Teaching Points:*
  - *Sesquiterpene lactone is an important allergen in the compositae family responsible for ACD to plants.*
  - *These plants are used readily in herbal medicaments and cosmetics.*
  - *Compositae sensitization is highly prevalent in florists, farmers and gardeners and in cosmetic dermatitis.*

Key messages or summary

- CD is due to irritation in the majority of patients.
- Identification of relevant antigens in the diagnosis of ACD is of upmost importance to the resolution of disease and quality of life.
- The diagnosis of ACD is made from history, physical examination and results of patch testing.
- The use of supplemental allergens including personal products and allergens related to specific exposures and/or occupations increases the positive yield of patch testing.
- Nickel sulfate is the most common allergen from PT results. Fragrances are most common cause of ACD from cosmetics.

Future directions/further study: Genotyping and risk modification

Filaggrin gene mutations and contact dermatitis: Filaggrin functions to aggregate keratin filaments leading to formation of the stratum corneum (Novak et al. 2008).

Impaired skin barrier formation may lead to allowance of allergens through the epidermis. In a population cohort study looking at two loss of function mutations in the filaggrin gene (R501X and 2282del4) an association with contact sensitization to nickel and an intolerance to costume jewelry via PT in patients was found (Novak et al. 2008). A recent study looked at 160 patients with three or more non cross-reacting patch tests.

They found a significant association with a loss of function filaggrin mutation and polysensitivity (Elhaji et al. 2009). In looking at patients with polymorphisms to N-acetyltransferases, those with a specific genotype may have less risk to sensitization with p-phenylenediamine (Blomeke et al. 2009).

References

Alinaghi F, Bennike NH, Egeberg A, Thyssen JP, Johansen JD. Prevalence of contact allergy in the general population: A systematic review and meta-analysis. Contact Dermatitis 2019; 80(2): 77–85.

Aquino M, Rosner G. Systemic contact dermatitis. Clin Rev Allergy Immunol 2019; 56(1): 9–18.
Ayala F, Fabbrocini G, Bacchilega R, Berardesca E, Caraffini S, Corazza M, et al. Italiano di Ricerca sulle Dermatiti da Contatto e Ambientali della Societa Italiana di Dermatologia e, Eyelid dermatitis: an evaluation of 447 patients. Am J Contact Dermat 2003; 14(2): 69–74.
Belhadjali H, Mohamed M, Youssef M, Mandhouj S, Chakroun M, Zili J. Contact sensitization in atopic dermatitis: results of a prospective study of 89 cases in Tunisia. Contact Dermatitis 2008; 58(3): 188–9.
Beltrani VS, Bernstein L, Cohen D, Fonacier L. Contact Dermatitis: A practice parameter. Annals of Allergy, Asthma & Immunology 2006; 97: S1–S38.
Belsito DV. The immunologic basis of patch testing. J Am Acad Dermatol 1989; 21(4 Pt 2): 822–9.
Blomeke B, Brans R, Coenraads PJ, Dickel H, Bruckner T, Hein DW, et al. Para-phenylenediamine and allergic sensitization: risk modification by N-acetyltransferase 1 and 2 genotypes. Br J Dermatol 2009; 161(5): 1130–5.
Cahill J, Keegel T, Nixon R. The prognosis of occupational contact dermatitis in 2004. Contact Dermatitis 2004; 51(5-6): 219–26.
Cohen DE. Contact dermatitis: a quarter century perspective. J Am Acad Dermatol 2004; 51(1 Suppl): S60–3.
Czarnobilska E, Obtulowicz K, Dyga W, Wsolek-Wnek K, Spiewak R. Contact hypersensitivity and allergic contact dermatitis among school children and teenagers with eczema. Contact Dermatitis 2009; 60(5): 264–9.
Davis MD, Bhate K, Rohlinger AL, Farmer SA, Richardson DM, Weaver AL. Delayed patch test reading after 5 days: the Mayo Clinic experience. J Am Acad Dermatol 2008; 59(2): 225–33.
DeKoven JG, Warshaw EM, Zug KA, Maibach HI, Belsito DV, Sasseville D, et al. North american contact dermatitis group patch test results: 2015–2016. Dermatitis 2018; 29(6): 297–309.
Dhingra N, Shemer A, Correa da Rosa J, Rozenblit M, Fuentes-Duculan J, Gittler JK, et al. Molecular profiling of contact dermatitis skin identifies allergen-dependent differences in immune response. J Allergy Clin Immunol 2014; 134(2): 362–72.
Elhaji Y, Sasseville D, Pratt M, Asai Y, Matheson K, McLean WHI, et al. Filaggrin gene loss-of-function mutations constitute a factor in patients with multiple contact allergies. Contact Dermatitis 2019; 80(6): 354–358.
Fonacier L. Pediatric Allergy: Principles and Practice, ed. Elsievier. 2010: Saunders.
Fonacier LS, Dreskin SC, Leung DY. Allergic skin diseases. J Allergy Clin Immunol 2010; 125(2 Suppl 2): S138–49.
Giordano-Labadie F, Rance F, Pellegrin F, Bazex J, Dutau G, Schwarze HP. Frequency of contact allergy in children with atopic dermatitis: results of a prospective study of 137 cases. Contact Dermatitis 1999; 40(4): 192–5.
Ingordo V, D'Andria G, D'Andria C, Cusano F. Clinical relevance of contact sensitization in atopic dermatitis. Contact Dermatitis 2001; 45(4): 239–40.
Lachapelle J. Giant Steps in Patch Testing: A historical Memoir, ed. S. Practice. 2010, Phoenix, AZ.
Lazzarini R, Duarte I, Marzagao C. Contact dermatitis of the feet: a study of 53 cases. Dermatitis 2004; 15(3): 125–30.
Malkonen T, Alanko K, Jolanki R, Luukkonen R, Aalto-Korte K, Lauerma A, et al. Long-term follow-up study of occupational hand eczema. Br J Dermatol 2010; 163(5): 999–1006.
Marks JE, Elsner P, DeLeo, V. Contact & Occupational Dermatology, ed. Mosby. 2002, St Louis, Missouri.
Minh PPT, Minh TT, Huu DL, Van TN, Huu SN, Thanh TV, et al. Using patch testing to improve therapeutic outcome in the treatment of hand eczema in vietnamese patients. Open Access Maced J Med Sci 2019; 7(2): 204–207.
Mortz CG, Lauritsen JM, Bindslev-Jensen C, Andersen KE. Prevalence of atopic dermatitis, asthma, allergic rhinitis, and hand and contact dermatitis in adolescents. The Odense Adolescence Cohort Study on Atopic Diseases and Dermatitis. Br J Dermatol 2001; 144(3): 523–32.
Nosbaum A, Vocanson M, Rozieres A, Hennino A, Nicolas JF. Allergic and irritant contact dermatitis. Eur J Dermatol 2009; 19(4): 325–32.
Novak N, Baurecht H, Schafer T, Rodriguez E, Wagenpfeil S, Klopp N, et al. Loss-of-function mutations in the filaggrin gene and allergic contact sensitization to nickel. J Invest Dermatol 2008; 128(6): 1430–5.
Pedersen LK, Johansen JD, Held E, Agner T. Augmentation of skin response by exposure to a combination of allergens and irritants—a review. Contact Dermatitis 2004; 50(5): 265–73.
Peiser M. Role of Th17 cells in skin inflammation of allergic contact dermatitis. Clin Dev Immunol 2013; p. 261037.
Rietschel RL, Warshaw EM, Sasseville D, Fowler JF, DeLeo VA, Belsito DV, et al. North American Contact Dermatitis, Common contact allergens associated with eyelid dermatitis: data from the North American Contact Dermatitis Group 2003–2004 study period. Dermatitis 2007; 18(2): 78–81.
Rietschel RL. Fischer's Contact Dermatitis, ed. B. Becker. Vol. 6. 2008, Lewiston, NY.
Sharma AD. Allergic contact dermatitis in patients with atopic dermatitis: A clinical study. Indian J Dermatol Venereol Leprol 2005; 71(2): 96–8.
Spiewak R. Patch testing for contact allergy and allergic contact dermatitis. The Open Allergy Journal 2008; 1: 42–51.
Sundquist BK, Yang B, Pasha MA. Experience in patch testing: A 6-year retrospective review from a single academic allergy practice. Ann Allergy Asthma Immunol 2019; 122(5): 502–507.
Uyesugi BA, Sheehan MP. Patch Testing Pearls. Clin Rev Allergy Immunol 2019; 56(1): 110–118.
Warshaw E, Lee G, Storrs FJ. Hand dermatitis: a review of clinical features, therapeutic options, and long-term outcomes. Am J Contact Dermat 2003; 14(3): 119–37.

27

Food Allergy
Introduction, Epidemiology Pathogenesis and Clinical Presentation

PA Mahesh,[1] *Hugo Van Bever*[2,*] *and Pudupakkam K Vedanthan*[3]

INTRODUCTION

Food related symptoms are an important cause of morbidity and occasionally mortality in the western world (Sicherer and Sampson 2010) and is likely to be important in other countries in the coming decades(Leung et al. 2018). In most of the countries in the western world, there has been documented increase in the prevalence of allergies such as allergic rhinitis and asthma and there is evidence that prevalence of food allergies may be increasing (Koplin et al. 2015). Usually the increase in food allergies in the general population occurs a couple of decades after the increase in asthma and allergic rhinitis.

Food Allergy (FA) should be approached scientifically. Only this approach will help children and parents suitably and will avoid useless testing, useless and dangerous interventions (diets) and useless spending of money. Concepts of FA are often understood wrongly, and therefore, approached wrongly. Often parents come to the clinic with the request to test their child for a food allergy, because the child has symptoms such as bad school results, sleep problems or tummy pain, and they suspect that the cause is a food allergy. Most of these children are not food allergic, and other causes (often psychological causes) are involved. Sometimes parents persist in their search for FA, use the Internet, and end up with all kinds of non-scientific diagnostic tests and extensive diet restrictions, which can lead to malnutrition and to even more psychological distress in child and family.

Epidemiology

The true prevalence of FA has been difficult to establish. Although more than 170 foods have been reported to cause IgE mediated reactions, most of the prevalence studies have focused on a few common foods (Table 27.1). However, there seems to be a rise in prevalence of FA over the past 10–20 years (Branum and Lukacs 2009). Challenges to determining true prevalence include misclassification, bias, lack of simple diagnostic tests, large number of potential triggers and varied clinical presentations. Nonetheless this is a common problem affecting approximately 3–6% of the population impacting the quality of

---

[1] J S S Medical College, JSSAHER, Mysore. INDIA, Email: mahesh1971in@yahoo.com
[2] National University of Singapore, Singapore.
[3] University of Colorado, Denver, Colorado USA, Email: pkv1947@gmail.com
* Corresponding author: paevbhps@nus.edu.sg

Table 27.1. Prevalence of food allergy to common foods.

Food	Children	Adults
Milk	0.5–3.8%	0.5%
Egg	2–8.9%	0.2%
Peanut	0.2–1.9%	0.7%
Tree nuts	1.1–1.6%	0.5–1%
Fish	0.2–0.5%	0.6%
Shell fish	0.5–5.2%	1.7–2.5%

Adapted from the following references:
Epidemiology of cow's milk allergy, Flom and Sicherer Nutrients 2019, 11, 1051

life significantly. There are a few landmark population-based studies by Bock (1987) and (Young et al. 1994) with reported prevalence of adverse reactions to foods in the range of 1–8%. Since then there have been several meta-analyses and large-scale reviews on this subject. Two meta-analyses, highlight the global prevalence of food allergies. The studies by (Rona et al. 2007) include 51 publications and have evaluated the prevalence of food allergies to milk, eggs, peanuts, fish and shell fish (the big five) and have estimated the prevalence of self-reported food allergies in children to be 12% and the prevalence of objectively documented food allergy in adults and children combined to be around 3%. Zuidmeer et al. 2008 estimated the prevalence of food allergies to fruits, vegetables and legumes and objectively confirmed food allergies to these foods were less common than that for the big five foods. Though any food can cause food allergy, the most common food allergens include milk, eggs, peanuts, tree nuts, shell fish, fish, wheat and soy (Sicherer and Sampson 2010). Recent epidemiological studies of food allergy prevalence in the United States estimated that approximately 8% of American children (Gupta et al. 2018) and 11% of American adults (Gupta et al. 2019) have a food allergy, based on self-report with convincingly IgE-mediated reaction symptoms. This has shown that prevalence varies by age, specific food, geographic location and race/ethnicity. Many food allergies resolve spontaneously. Recent studies (Chafen et al. 2010) have also generated novel theories and possible risk factors for the development of food allergy which include components like maternal and infant diet, obesity and timing of food introduction.

Definition of food allergy

Classification

Any aberrant reaction after consumption of a food or food additive is classified as an adverse food reaction, which may be immune mediated or non-immune mediated (Fig. 27.1). Immune mediated adverse food reactions are called food allergy or food hypersensitivity and non-immune mediated adverse food reactions are called food intolerance such as lactose intolerance. Immune mediated reactions can be IgE mediated, the classical food allergy or non-IgE mediated is now gaining in importance especially, gastrointestinal (GI) reactions.

A. IgE-mediated food allergy

This type of reaction has been extensively studied and described. In short, these reactions occur in genetically predisposed patients and are the result of an excessive production of food-specific IgE antibodies. These antibodies bind (through receptors) on different cells, such as mast cells and basophils (Wang and Sampson 2011). After the food allergens reach the food-specific IgE antibodies on mast cells and basophiles, various mediators (such as histamine) are released. These mediators then induce different symptoms of immediate hypersensitivity. The activated mast cells may also release various other mediators, called cytokines or chemokines, that play a part in inflammatory reactions (Wang and Sampson 2011).

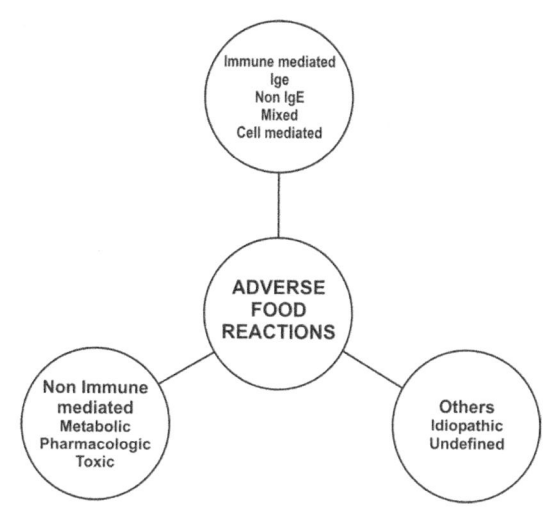

Figure 27.1. Types of adverse reactions to foods.

The prevalence of food allergy has been increasing at a far more rapid pace than changes observed in the human genome. Therefore, it is likely that the increase in food allergy noted the world over is due a gene-environment interaction, where different environmental influences switch on the allergy genes. Filaggrin null mutations are associated with a higher risk of peanut allergy on exposure to peanuts as explained by the transcutaneous sensitization through the defective epidermal barrier. HLA (DR and DQ) are associated with higher rates of peanut allergy. The hygiene hypothesis remains relevant with a lower environmental microbial load being associated with higher occurrence of food allergy. Lower levels of Vitamin D are associated with increased food allergy (Koplin et al. 2015).

B. Non-IgE-mediated food allergy

A large variety of non-IgE-mediated types of FA have been described (Kim and Burks 2015). However, these types are less well documented than the IgE-mediated type, and, therefore, the scientific evidence supporting these mechanisms is limited and not generally accepted. Certain types of cow's milk allergy are an example of non-IgE-mediated food allergy. It is generally believed that about 40% of cow's milk allergy in young children is non-IgE-mediated (60% is through IgE), although the debate on this still remains (Flom and Sicherer 2019). A role of (too) early administration of cow's milk-based formula (from day 1 of postnatal life) is suspected in non-IgE-mediated allergy, at a time that the intestine is not ready (immature) to digest cow's milk, inducing a non-IgE-mediated immunological response in the intestinal tract that persists for many months (Agyemang and Nowak-Wegrzyn 2019).

Sensitization to food

Sensitization to food allergens usually occurs through the oral route (drinking, eating), as well as through inhaling. However, recent studies in children with eczema (not in children who do not suffer from eczema) have shown that sensitization to food can also occur through the skin, called transcutaneous sensitization or epicutaneous sensitization (García-Boyano et al. 2016) (Comberiati et al. 2019).

Pathophysiology

Tolerance

Although FA poses a growing concern, large portions of the population do not have a food allergy. This is due to a few important properties of the gastrointestinal tract. A normal gastrointestinal tract protects us from developing an allergy to multiple food antigens which we ingest daily. Glycocalyx is an important lining along the mucosal surface providing the seal between the enterocytes (intestinal cells) as well as a cementing barrier capable of trapping food particles. This is a very efficient barrier system to the outside environment and is able to discriminate between pathogens and harmless foreign proteins or commensals. Despite the efficient barrier system, about 2% of ingested food antigens gets absorbed in an immunologically stable form (Cardoso-Silva et al. 2019).

The ingested food antigens are not generally immunogenic in most individuals due to the development of 'oral tolerance'. Intestinal epithelial cells play a major role in inducing food tolerance acting as 'non professional' antigen presenting cells (Allaire et al. 2018). The antigen presenting cells in the GI tract are said to be 'non professional' and are not capable of eliciting a T cell response and hence 'anergic'. The dendritic cells in the Peyer's patches along the gut also produce IL-10 and TGF-β, which favor oral tolerance. The regulatory T (T reg) cells as well as the gut flora also play a role in the propagation of the oral tolerance. Recent research has attributed a healthy gut microbiome as an important factor in maintaining immune homeostasis and tolerance in the gastrointestinal tract (Million et al. 2018). Breast feeding also promotes the development of oral tolerance and prevents food allergy to some extent (Dawod and Marshall 2019). An important issue is when to introduce the potentially allergenic foods in the infant's diet. Should exclusive breast feeding be advised for at least 6 months or should early introduction after 3 months of age be recommended? Two important studies, which were randomized control trials and thus had the power to answer this question were the Learning Early About Peanuts (LEAP) and the Enquiring About Tolerance (EAT) studies (Du Toit et al. 2018). Both showed that early introduction of allergenic foods such as Peanut (LEAP), and Egg, peanut, cow's milk, wheat, fish and sesame (EAT) along with breast feeding was beneficial. Many other studies for the early introduction of hen's egg into the infant's diet found it reduced the risk of hen's egg allergy; Solids Timing for Allergy Research (STAR), Starting Time for Egg Protein (STEP), Beating Egg Allergy (BEAT), Prevention of Egg Allergy in High-risk Infants with Eczema (PETIT) (Du Toit et al. 2018). All these were randomized control trials and showed a benefit of early introduction of hen's egg in the diet from 3 months of age onwards. Only the Hen's Egg Allergy Prevention (HEAP) study observed a higher risk of hen's egg food allergy when it was introduced from 4 months of age. While the dose of hen's egg protein in the other beneficial studies ranged from 0.175 grams to 6.3 grams per week, the HEAP study used 7.5 grams per week (Du Toit et al. 2018).

Sensitization

Sensitization to food allergens can occur in two different ways: 1. Traditional ingestion route or Class 1 food allergy 2. Inhalation of airborne allergen that cross reacts with a specific food item or Class 2 food allergy. Class 1 food antigens are water soluble glycoproteins, and are stable towards heat, acid and enzymes. Most of the Class 2 antigens are plant-derived proteins, which are heat labile and difficult to isolate. In children, cow's milk, eggs, groundnuts, soy, wheat and fish account for 85% of the documented food allergies. In adults, groundnuts, tree nuts, fish and shellfish account for the majority of the allergic reactions. In genetically predisposed individuals, typical IgE-mediated reactions will take place when food specific IgE antibodies, residing on the mast cells and basophils in the gut, bind the ingested food allergens. This leads to the release of several mediators and cytokines (described elsewhere in this chapter).

In genetically predisposed individuals, when the barrier mechanism and oral tolerance breaks down, IgE mediated reactions do develop.

Cross reactivity

Cross reactivity among homologous proteins conserved across families is an important problem for the clinician called upon to explain clinical symptoms in a patient. Some of the common cross-reactive proteins are profilin and lipid transfer proteins in plants and tropomyosin and casein in animals. It is important to realize that serological cross reactivity is far greater than clinical cross-reactivity (Faber et al. 2018). There is a need for further research to identify the reasons why some cross-reactive foods elicit a greater frequency and more severe reactions than others. Generally, more than 70% similarity in protein structure is necessary to induce cross-reactivity. The source of the first sensitization can be either as an inhalant as in the case of birch pollen sensitization leading to clinical symptoms on consumption of foods such as apple, peach or celery or as an ingestant as in the case of peanut allergy causing cross-reactive allergies on consumption of legumes or soy. Lipid transfer proteins are highly stable to acid digestion, heating and fermentation and are increasingly recognized as both an important allergen in foods and inhalants. Cross-reactive LTP's are present in pollens (weeds—mugwort, trees—plane tree) as also in various foods (grapes, lettuce, apple, hazelnut, sunflower seeds and cereals) and are an important allergen in latex. Some of the seed storage proteins such as 2S albumin, 7S Vicillin and 11S Legumin could be important in cross-reactivity among different legumes, but need further confirmation. Component resolved diagnostic evaluation (see below) can help to understand the role of cross-reactive proteins better, but is not readily available to the clinician especially in developing countries. Highly soluble proteins are more likely to elicit cross-reactivity than poorly soluble proteins (Fig. 27.2). Some of the common cross reactivities among different food groups are listed in Table 27.2.

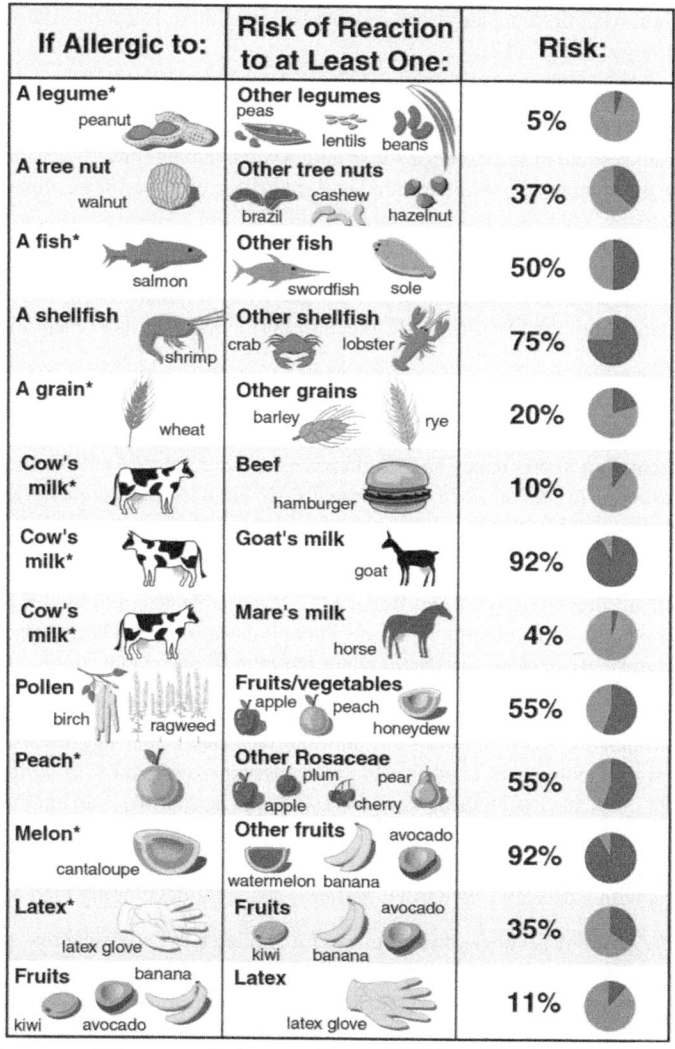

If Allergic to:	Risk of Reaction to at Least One:	Risk:
A legume* peanut	Other legumes peas lentils beans	5%
A tree nut walnut	Other tree nuts cashew brazil hazelnut	37%
A fish* salmon	Other fish swordfish sole	50%
A shellfish shrimp	Other shellfish crab lobster	75%
A grain* wheat	Other grains barley rye	20%
Cow's milk*	Beef hamburger	10%
Cow's milk*	Goat's milk goat	92%
Cow's milk*	Mare's milk horse	4%
Pollen birch ragweed	Fruits/vegetables apple peach honeydew	55%
Peach*	Other Rosaceae plum pear apple cherry	55%
Melon* cantaloupe	Other fruits avocado watermelon banana	92%
Latex* latex glove	Fruits avocado kiwi banana	35%
Fruits kiwi avocado banana	Latex latex glove	11%

Figure 27.2. Clinical cross reactivity among food groups. Source: JACI Dec. 2001 issue Vol 6. 881–890 with permission from Elseiver.

Table 27.2. Cross reactivity between different foods (Scott H Sicherer (J Allergy Clin Immunol 2001; 108: 881–90) and Scot H Sicherer J Allergy Clin Immunol 2018; 141: 41–58.

- Beef/veal: lamb = 50%;
- Fish: other fish > 50% (likewise for shellfish, especially amongst crustaceans)
- Cow milk : goat milk = 90%
- Egg: chicken meat < 5%;
- Cow milk: beef/veal = 10%
- Tree nuts: other nuts = > 50% (Among tree nuts, cashew and pistachio are clearly cross-reactive as are walnut and pecan).
- Peanuts: tree nuts = 35%
- Wheat: other grains = 25%
- Peanut: legumes < 10%; soybean: legumes < 5%

Risk factors

Family history—Family history of food allergy is an important risk factor for food allergy. If one of the parents or siblings has a peanut allergy, the child has a seven-fold higher risk of developing a peanut allergy. If one of monozygotic twins develops a peanut allergy, there is a 64% risk for the other twin to develop a peanut allergy (Lack 2012).

Gender—Endocrine influences can affect the development of food allergy. In children less than 4 years, males have a much higher risk of developing food allergy, nearly five times higher prevalence has been noted. The risk becomes equal in adolescence and in adults when females have twice the risk of developing food allergy. These differences in prevalence are similar to those observed for asthma (Lack 2012).

Genetic polymorphisms—The most important mutations associated with food allergy that are replicated in different populations is the Filaggrin loss of function mutations. Many other polymorphisms have been associated with food allergy. The most important are polymorphisms in IL-10, STAT-6, IL-13, CD-14, Thymic Stromal Lymphopoietin (TSLP), IL-12 receptor beta 1 and Toll like receptor 9 (Lack 2012).

Vitamin D—Data is conflicting about the role of Vitamin D in food allergies. The farming communities in Germany that had low prevalence of food allergies found an increasing prevalence of food allergies after Vitamin D supplementation to reduce rickets. A conflicting observation was that mothers who took a Vitamin D supplementation in pregnancy had children with a lower risk of food allergy. On the other hand, children who are exposed to less sunlight and consequently have lower Vitamin D levels have a higher prevalence of food allergy. Children born in winter have higher prevalence of food allergy (Lack 2012).

Hygiene hypothesis—This proposes that western lifestyles are associated with allergies. Lack of exposure to microbes, altered gut flora (Blázquez and Berin 2017) and parasites could hinder immune maturation and increase the likelihood of developing allergies. Though there is a large body of evidence for asthma, convincing evidence for association of the hygiene hypothesis and food allergy is currently lacking (Lack 2012).

Food allergen environmental exposure—This is an important area of current research. There is enough evidence to suggest that cutaneous exposure to food allergens, especially in children with impaired epidermal barrier function due to filaggrin mutations and atopic dermatitis, is an important mechanism for developing sensitization and food allergy. Studies have confirmed that food proteins are very commonly found in house dust. Currently, it is thought that oral exposure induces tolerance whereas cutaneous exposure in subjects with a defective epidermal barrier is a risk for developing food allergy (Lack 2012).

Severity of food allergy—The severity of reactions to FA is related to coexistence of asthma (Vogel et al. 2008). Some of the risk factors for severe food reactions are the presence of severe uncontrolled asthma, long term oral glucocorticoid use, younger age, severe sensitization to food allergens, consumption of food on an empty stomach, consumption of raw food rather than cooked food to which the person is sensitized and whether the person has co-consumed other foods along with the food to which they are sensitized. Inappropriate diagnosis and management of food allergies are important risk factors as well.

The severity of reactions to the food varies based upon: amount of food, food form, co-ingestion of other foods, age of the patient, degree of sensitization, rapidity of absorption, concomitant asthma, concomitant ingestion of alcohol, delayed administration of epinephrine, lack of skin symptoms, denial of symptoms and reliance on oral antihistamines.

Co-morbid conditions

Asthma: Asthma and FA seem to coexist in both children and adults. For example, a recent US population-based study of food allergy prevalence found that 1 in 3 food-allergic children and 1 in 4 food-allergic adults reported comorbid physician-diagnosed asthma. While FA is not a causal factor for asthma, both conditions fall along the so-called 'allergic march' and presence of FA seems to correlate directly with severity of asthma. Generally asthma in patients who have concomitant FA is more severe, more prone to hospitalizations and results in more ER visits (Vogel et al. 2008). This is also true in the case of children, where sensitivity to milk, wheat, peanuts or eggs have higher rates of hospitalization as well as requiring frequent steroid usage (Wang et al. 2005).

Atopic dermatitis: In population based studies up to 53% of children with Atopic Dermatitis (AD) have food specific IgE and 17% have challenge confirmed food allergy (Tsakok et al. 2016). Conversely, recent data indicate that nearly 20% of food-allergic children (ages 0–17 years) have AD, with this figure increasing to nearly 30% among infants (0–2 years). Milk, peanuts and eggs have been identified as the main culprit foods causing a flare-up of AD. There has been correlation noted with severity of AD and likelihood of FA.

Eosinophilic esophagitis (EOE): is generally associated with sensitization to foods. There is not enough data to judge the impact of FA on the natural course of EOE, however, recent epidemiological data suggest that roughly 1 in 3 EoE patients also have a comorbid IgE-mediated food allergy. The most common foods that are incriminated in food allergy and EOE are milk, soy, eggs, grains and meats (Hill et al. 2017). The prevalence of EOE is nearly 5% among patients with IgE mediated food allergy and it is seen in 0.04% of the subjects in the general population (Hill et al. 2017). In a birth cohort of more than 130,000 children, EOE was seen as part of the late progression of the atopic march (Hill et al. 2018). EOE can also be associated with non-IgE mediated food hypersensitivity (Simon et al. 2016) and with food pollen allergy syndrome (Mahdavinia et al. 2017). Patients with EOE respond well to food elimination diet (Simon et al. 2016). Oral immunotherapy to foods can in some cases cause EOE (Hill et al. 2017). There is a need for further research into the pathogenesis of EOE and some investigators have observed that EOE pathogenesis is independent of IgE mediated food allergy (Simon et al. 2016).

Food Dependent Exercise induced anaphylaxis (FDEIA): Exercise dependent food induced anaphylaxis is a form of IgE mediated food allergy that does not occur independently with either exercise or consumption of the said food, but when the subject exercises after consumption of the food, they may develop anaphylaxis. Usually the food has to be ingested up to 1–4 hours before exercise and rarely immediately after the exercise. Any level of exertion can trigger FDEIA (Feldweg 2017). Usually it is high levels of exertion such as aerobics or jogging, but sometimes it can be triggered by lower levels of exertion such as a brisk walk or some household work (Feldweg 2017). Symptoms can be sudden and rapid onset of abdominal pain, nausea, cramps, vomiting and/or diarrhea. Occasionally fainting due to hypotension can occur. EIA is triggered in adults by foods in about 30% of the patients. There are no studies in pediatric age group regarding EIA. A US survey (Shadick et al. 1999) showed 37% of the patients reported a food trigger, most commonly shellfish, alcohol, tomatoes, cheese and celery. The majority of the patients were female (75%). Mean age of symptoms was 37 years and the most frequent symptoms were pruritus (92%), urticaria (86%), angioedema (72%), flushing (70%) and shortness of breath (51%). Around 50% of such patients also reported seasonal allergies, 20% had asthma and 10% had eczema. In EIA, foods can be ingested without symptoms in the absence of exercise. EpiPen and observing a 'buddy' system as well as avoidance of ingestion of any food items 30 minutes before and after physical activity will control as well as prevent these episodes.

Allergic rhinitis (AR): is not considered to be a risk factor for development of FA (Comberiati et al. 2019).

Clinical features

In general, the most common clinical presentation of an IgE-mediated FA is the sudden appearance of urticaria (hives), within minutes after intake of a food, such as peanuts, seafood or fish. In more severe cases there is also the presence of swelling of the eyes or lips (angioedema). When the FA is very severe symptoms of difficult respiration (asthma, difficulty in breathing) and even shock (drop in blood pressure and coma) can appear, being potentially fatal and requiring urgent treatment. Shock caused by an allergic reaction is called anaphylactic shock.

A. Symptoms of IgE-mediated food allergy

1. Skin and respiratory food allergic reactions

   The skin is the most frequent target organ in IgE-mediated FA. The ingestion of food allergens can induce either immediate skin symptoms, mainly rash, itch or urticaria, or aggravate chronic skin symptoms, such as eczema. Acute urticaria and angioedema are the most common manifestations of FA, generally appearing within minutes of ingestion of the food allergen.

   Respiratory symptoms usually appear in association with skin symptoms and rarely as isolated symptoms of FA. Symptoms may include itchy eyes, tearing, blocked nose, sneezing, runny nose, coughs, changes in the voice and wheezing (whistle in the chest) and difficulty in breathing.

   A well-described entity in this group is The Oral Allergy Syndrome (OAS).

   OAS is considered a form of contact urticaria induced by exposure of the oral and pharyngeal mucosa to food allergens, being a consequence of a cross-reactivity between certain foods and pollen allergens (Carlson and Coop 2019). The syndrome is classified by some researchers under the group of gastrointestinal symptoms of FA. Affected patients may present with rapid onset of symptoms with increasing severity, from mild itching of the lips, mouth and throat, to lip and tongue swelling, to severe swelling of the throat, up to life-threatening emergencies, such as anaphylaxis. OAS is an important alarm manifestation in subjects at risk for severe allergic reactions. The triggering food may be dependent on geographically different nutritional habits and may thus vary from place to place. Patients with allergic rhinitis to certain airborne pollen (especially birch, mugwort and ragweed) are frequently afflicted with OAS (Europe, USA, seldom in Asia). Patients with birch pollen sensitization often have symptoms following the ingestion of stone fruits or after ingestion of vegetables such as carrots or celery, nuts and legumes. Patients with ragweed pollen sensitization may experience allergic symptoms following contact with certain melons (watermelon, cantaloupe, honeydew, etc.) and bananas.

   Other examples are:
   - Allergy to seafood in patients with house dust mite allergy.
   - Allergy to vegetables and fruits in patients with latex allergy (such as in children with spina bifida).

2. Gastrointestinal symptoms of FA

   IgE-mediated gastrointestinal symptoms of FA include immediate gastrointestinal hypersensitivity and allergic eosinophilic gastroenteritis (Vandenplas et al. 2015).

   - Immediate gastrointestinal hypersensitivity

     This type of hypersensitivity may accompany allergic symptoms in other organs. The symptoms vary but may include nausea, abdominal pain, abdominal cramping, vomiting and/or diarrhea. Symptoms may resemble those of a gastrointestinal infection and need to be distinguished from it. Complete elimination of the suspected food allergen for up to 2 weeks will lead to resolution of symptoms. Diagnosis is usually made by a food challenge, although positive skin prick tests suggest FA. Foods that have been associated with immediate gastrointestinal hypersensitivity are milk, eggs, peanuts, soy, cereal and fish.

- Allergic eosinophilic gastroenteritis

  This type of FA is a mixed IgE-mediated and non-IgE-mediated type of FA. It is a disorder characterized by infiltration of the gastric and/or intestinal wall with eosinophils and raised numbers of eosinophils in the blood. Patients presenting with this syndrome frequently have nausea and vomiting, abdominal pain, diarrhea, failure to thrive or weight loss. Diagnosis is difficult and is usually based upon an appropriate history and a gastrointestinal biopsy demonstrating a characteristic eosinophilic infiltration. However, multiple biopsies may be needed because the eosinophilic infiltrates may be quite patchy. Patients with this disease usually have other symptoms of allergy, such as eczema, and elevated IgE levels can be found in the blood. They also often have positive skin prick tests to food allergens. In patients with severe disease anemia and hypoalbuminemia can be found. An elimination diet of up to 12 weeks may be necessary before complete resolution of symptoms occurs.

A separate entity, related to eosinophilic gastroenteritis, is the eosinophilic esophagitis (sometimes with gastritis), which is a chronic allergic inflammatory condition of the esophagus, which most often results in difficulty in swallowing or the feeling that the food is stuck in the chest, heartburn or chest pain. Of importance is the differentiation from other inflammatory diseases of the esophagus, especially gastro-esophageal reflux disease. Biopsies from the proximal to the distal esophagus demonstrating > 15–20 eosinophils per field favor the diagnosis. Besides avoidance of the responsible food allergens, common treatment regimens involve the ingestion of topical corticosteroids (Martin et al. 2018).

B. Symptoms of non-IgE-mediated food allergy

Usually, these disorders are less well documented than the IgE-mediated type of FA (Agyemang and Nowak-Wegrzyn 2019, Nowak-Węgrzyn et al. 2015). Among the many disorders, the most important are:

1. Dietary protein enterocolitis (also called protein intolerance)

   This is a rare disease of young infants, usually starting between the age of 1 week to 3 months. The typical symptoms are isolated to the gastrointestinal tract and consist of recurrent vomiting and/or diarrhea. The symptoms can be severe, causing dehydration. The disease is usually associated with a non-IgE-mediated allergy to cow's milk or soymilk, while in older infants (older than 6 months) eggs have been reported to be responsible for the disease. Elimination of the offending food allergen generally will result in improvement or resolution of symptoms within 72 hours. Skin prick tests or determination of specific IgE in the blood are negative. Diagnosis is based on an oral food challenge, which can result in severe symptoms. The disease usually resolves by the age of 18–24 months.

2. Dietary protein proctitis—colitis

   This disease usually presents during the first months of life and is often caused by cow's milk or soy protein hypersensitivity, affecting the large intestine (or colon) and its terminal part. Infants with this disorder often do not appear ill, have normally formed stools and generally are discovered because of the presence of blood in their stools. It is accepted, without well-controlled studies, that the disease resolves by age 6 months to 2 years.

3. Celiac disease

   Celiac disease is a severe disease of the intestine (enteropathy) leading to malabsorption and failure to thrive. Total villous atrophy (destruction of the wall of the small intestine) and an extensive inflammation of the intestinal mucosa are associated with a specific sensitivity to the alcohol-soluble portion of gluten found in wheat, oat, rye, and barley, also called gluten intolerance. Gluten is found mainly in foods but may also be found in products we use every day, such as stamps, envelopes, adhesives, medicines and vitamins. Because the body's own immune system causes the damage, celiac disease is considered an autoimmune disorder, not as an allergy.

Celiac disease is a genetic disease, meaning it runs in families. Sometimes the disease is triggered—or becomes active for the first time—after surgery, pregnancy, childbirth, viral infection or severe emotional stress. Patients often present symptoms of diarrhea or steatorrhea, abdominal distention and flatulence, weight loss and occasionally nausea and vomiting. However, a person with celiac disease may have no symptoms. People without symptoms are still at risk for the complications of celiac disease, including malnutrition. The longer a patient goes undiagnosed and untreated, the greater the chance of developing malnutrition and other complications. Anemia, delayed growth and weight loss are signs of malnutrition: the body is just not getting enough nutrients.

C. Symptoms that are not caused by food allergy

FA usually manifests itself through reactions from the skin (urticaria, eczema), the respiratory tract (rhinitis, asthma) or the gastrointestinal tract (vomiting, diarrhea). Diseases from other organs (kidney, brain, heart, etc.) are usually not due to food allergy, especially neurological or psychological disorders. However, often parents believe that FA is involved in their child's problems. Neurological, psychological or psychiatric diseases are usually not caused by FA. These include sleep or learning problems, hyperactivity, autism and migraine.

Conclusion

Food allergy is a rapidly evolving field especially in the past 2 decades. Significant increase in the prevalence has been noted around the globe, especially in developed countries. This chapter has covered the different manifestations of adverse reactions to foods and related issues to be considered by the allergy specialist.

References

Agyemang A, Nowak-Wegrzyn A. Food protein-induced enterocolitis syndrome: a comprehensive review. Clin Rev Allergy Immunol 2019; https://doi.org/10.1007/s12016-018-8722-z.

Allaire JM, Crowley SM, Law HT, Chang S-Y, Ko H-J, Vallance BA. The intestinal epithelium: central coordinator of mucosal immunity. Trends Immunol 2018; 39(9): 677–696. https://doi.org/10.1016/j.it.2018.04.002.

Blázquez AB, Berin MC. Microbiome and food allergy. Transl Res 2017; 179: 199–203. https://doi.org/10.1016/j.trsl.2016.09.003.

Bock SA. Prospective appraisal of complaints of adverse reactions to foods in children during the first 3 years of life. Pediatrics 1987; 79(5): 683–688.

Branum AM, Lukacs SL. Food allergy among children in the United States. PEDIATRICS 2009; 124(6); 1549–1555. https://doi.org/10.1542/peds.2009-1210.

Cardoso-Silva D, Delbue D, Itzlinger A, Moerkens R, Withoff S, Branchi F, et al. Intestinal barrier function in gluten-related disorders. Nutrients 2019; 11(10): 2325. https://doi.org/10.3390/nu11102325.

Carlson G, Coop C. Pollen food allergy syndrome (PFAS): A review of current available literature. Ann Allergy Asthma Immunol 2019; 123(4): 359–365. https://doi.org/10.1016/j.anai.2019.07.022.

Chafen JJS, Newberry SJ, Riedl MA, Bravata DM, Maglione M, Suttorp MJ, et al. Diagnosing and managing common food allergies: a systematic review. JAMA 2010; 303(18): 1848. https://doi.org/10.1001/jama.2010.582.

Comberiati P, Costagliola G, D'Elios S, Peroni D. Prevention of food allergy: the significance of early introduction. Medicina 2019; 55(7): 323. https://doi.org/10.3390/medicina55070323.

Dawod B, Marshall JS. Cytokines and soluble receptors in breast milk as enhancers of oral tolerance development. Front Immunol 2019; 10: 16. https://doi.org/10.3389/fimmu.2019.00016.

Du Toit G, Sampson HA, Plaut M, Burks AW, Akdis CA, Lack G. Food allergy: Update on prevention and tolerance. J Allergy Clin Immunol 2018; 141(1): 30–40. https://doi.org/10.1016/j.jaci.2017.11.010.

Faber MA, Van Gasse AL, Decuyper II, Sabato V, Hagendorens MM, Mertens C, et al. Cross-reactive aeroallergens: which need to cross our mind in food allergy diagnosis? J Allergy Clin Immunol: In Practice 2018; 6(6): 1813–1823. https://doi.org/10.1016/j.jaip.2018.08.010.

Feldweg AM. Food-dependent, exercise-induced anaphylaxis: diagnosis and management in the outpatient setting. J Allergy Clin Immunol: In Practice 2017; 5(2): 283–288. https://doi.org/10.1016/j.jaip.2016.11.022.

Flom JD, Sicherer SH. Epidemiology of cow's milk allergy. Nutrients 2019; 11(5); 1051. https://doi.org/10.3390/nu11051051.

García-Boyano M, Pedrosa M, Quirce S, Boyano-Martínez T. Household almond and peanut consumption is related to the development of sensitization in young children. J Allergy Clin Immunol 2016; 137(4): 1248–1251.e6. https://doi.org/10.1016/j.jaci.2015.09.006.

Gupta RS, Warren CM, Smith BM, Blumenstock JA, Jiang J, Davis MM, et al. The public health impact of parent-reported childhood food allergies in the United States. Pediatrics 2018; 142(6): e20181235. https://doi.org/10.1542/peds.2018-1235.

Gupta RS, Warren CM, Smith BM, Jiang J, Blumenstock JA, Davis MM, et al. Prevalence and severity of food allergies among US Adults. JAMA Network Open 2019; 2(1): e185630. https://doi.org/10.1001/jamanetworkopen.2018.5630.

Hill DA, Dudley JW, Spergel JM. The prevalence of eosinophilic esophagitis in pediatric patients with ige-mediated food allergy. J Allergy Clin Immunol: In Practice 2017; 5(2): 369–375. https://doi.org/10.1016/j.jaip.2016.11.020.

Hill DA, Grundmeier RW, Ramos M, Spergel JM. Eosinophilic esophagitis is a late manifestation of the allergic march. J Allergy Clin Immunol: In Practice 2018; 6(5); 1528–1533. https://doi.org/10.1016/j.jaip.2018.05.010.

Kim EH, Burks W. Immunological basis of food allergy (IgE-Mediated, Non-IgE-Mediated, and Tolerance). In: Ebisawa M, Ballmer-Weber BK, Vieths S, Wood RA (eds.). Chem Immunol Allergyy 2015; 101: 8–17. S. Karger AG. https://doi.org/10.1159/000371646,

Koplin JJ, Mills ENC, Allen KJ. Epidemiology of food allergy and food-induced anaphylaxis: Is there really a Western world epidemic? Curr Opin Allergy Cl 2015; 15(5): 409–416. https://doi.org/10.1097/ACI.0000000000000196.

Lack G. Update on risk factors for food allergy. Journal of Allergy and Clinical Immunology 2012; 129(5): 1187–1197. https://doi.org/10.1016/j.jaci.2012.02.036.

Leung ASY, Wong GWK, Tang MLK. Food allergy in the developing world. Journal of Allergy and Clinical Immunology 2018; 141(1): 76–78.e1. https://doi.org/10.1016/j.jaci.2017.11.008.

Mahdavinia M, Bishehsari F, Hayat W, Elhassan A, Tobin MC, Ditto AM. Association of eosinophilic esophagitis and food pollen allergy syndrome. Ann Allergy Asthma Immunol 2017; 118(1): 116–117. https://doi.org/10.1016/j.anai.2016.10.012.

Martin LJ, He H, Collins MH, Abonia JP, Biagini Myers JM, Eby M, et al. Eosinophilic esophagitis (EoE) genetic susceptibility is mediated by synergistic interactions between EoE-specific and general atopic disease loci. J Allergy Clin Immunol 2018; 141(5): 1690–1698. https://doi.org/10.1016/j.jaci.2017.09.046.

Million M, Tomas J, Wagner C, Lelouard H, Raoult D, Gorvel J-P. New insights in gut microbiota and mucosal immunity of the small intestine. Human Microbiome Journal 2018; 7–8, 23–32. https://doi.org/10.1016/j.humic.2018.01.004.

Nowak-Węgrzyn A, Katz Y, Mehr SS, Koletzko S. Non–IgE-mediated gastrointestinal food allergy. J Allergy Clin Immunol 2015; 135(5): 1114–1124. https://doi.org/10.1016/j.jaci.2015.03.025.

Rona RJ, Keil T, Summers C, Gislason D, Zuidmeer L, Sodergren E, et al. The prevalence of food allergy: A meta-analysis. J Allergy Clin Immunol 2007; 120(3): 638–646. https://doi.org/10.1016/j.jaci.2007.05.026.

Shadick NA, Liang MH, Partridge AJ, Bingham C, Wright E, Fossel AH, Sheffer AL. The natural history of exercise-induced anaphylaxis: Survey results from a 10-year follow-up study☆☆☆★. J Allergy Clin Immunol 1999; 104(1): 123–127. https://doi.org/10.1016/S0091-6749(99)70123-5.

Sicherer SH, Sampson HA. Food allergy. J Allergy Clin Immunol 2010; 125(2): S116–S125. https://doi.org/10.1016/j.jaci.2009.08.028.

Simon D, Cianferoni A, Spergel JM, Aceves S, Holbreich M, Venter C, et al. Eosinophilic esophagitis is characterized by a non-IgE-mediated food hypersensitivity. Allergy 2016; 71(5): 611–620. https://doi.org/10.1111/all.12846.

Tsakok T, Marrs T, Mohsin M, Baron S, du Toit G, Till S, et al. Does atopic dermatitis cause food allergy? A systematic review. J Allergy Clin Immunol 2016; 137(4): 1071–1078. https://doi.org/10.1016/j.jaci.2015.10.049.

Vandenplas Y, Marchand J, Meyns L. Symptoms, diagnosis, and treatment of cow's milk allergy. Curr Pediatr Rev 2015; 11(4): 293–297.

Vogel NM, Katz HT, Lopez R, Lang DM. Food allergy is associated with potentially fatal childhood asthma. Journal of Asthma 2008; 45(10): 862–866. https://doi.org/10.1080/02770900802444195.

Wang J, Visness C, Sampson H. Food allergen sensitization in inner-city children with asthma. J Allergy Clin Immunol 2005; 115(5): 1076–1080. https://doi.org/10.1016/j.jaci.2005.02.014.

Wang J, Sampson HA. Food allergy. J of Clin Invest 2011; 121(3): 827–835. https://doi.org/10.1172/JCI45434.

Young E, Stoneham MD, Petruckevitch A, Barton J, Rona R. A population study of food intolerance. Lancet (London, England) 1994; 343(8906): 1127–1130. https://doi.org/10.1016/s0140-6736(94)90234-8.

Zuidmeer L, Goldhahn K, Rona RJ, Gislason D, Madsen C, Summers C, et al. The prevalence of plant food allergies: A systematic review. J Allergy Clin Immunol 2008; 121(5): 1210–1218.e4. https://doi.org/10.1016/j.jaci.2008.02.019.

28

Food Allergy
Diagnosis and Management

Neha T Agnihotri,[1] Jialing Jiang,[1] Christopher M Warren[2] and Ruchi S Gupta[3],*

INTRODUCTION

Adverse food reactions such as intolerance, pollen food allergy syndrome, and food allergy (FA) vary in symptom presentation and duration. A proper physician diagnosis for food-related conditions is essential to ensure appropriate management. Immunoglobulin E (IgE) -mediated FA, in particular, can result in anaphylaxis and requires strict allergen avoidance.

This chapter outlines steps for diagnosing IgE-mediated FA which includes collecting the patient's medical history, conducting a physical examination, and administering diagnostic tests including skin prick tests, serum IgE testing, and oral food challenges. Additionally, this section discusses developing FA treatments, prevention, patient and parent education, as well as the natural history of FA.

Diagnosis of food allergy

A. Medical history and physical examination

The evaluation of a patient with suspected Food Allergy (FA) must begin with a careful, focused medical history and physical examination. The true value of a medical history is largely dependent on the parent's (or child's) recollection of symptoms and the examiner's ability to differentiate disorders provoked by FA and other food-induced conditions. The history may be directly useful in diagnosing FA in acute events (such as acute anaphylaxis or acute urticaria). However, problems arise when the reaction is delayed (such as in some non-Immunoglobulin E (IgE)-mediated reactions) or occurs after several foods are ingested.

---

[1] Northwestern University Feinberg School of Medicine, Chicago, IL, USA.
  Emails: nagniho2@uic.edu; jialing.jiang@northwestern.edu
[2] Northwestern University Feinberg School of Medicine, Stanford University School of Medicine, Chicago, IL/Stanford, CA, USA, Email: christopher.warren@northwestern.edu
[3] Northwestern University Feinberg School of Medicine, Ann & Robert H. Lurie Children's Hospital of Chicago, Chicago, IL, USA.
* Corresponding author: r-gupta@northwestern.edu

Key information that should be elicited from the history to establish the likelihood that the reported reaction is related to a food allergy includes the following:

1. Identification of the food that has provoked the reaction. If multiple food items were ingested within a short time frame, these should be noted.
2. The amount of the food ingested (FA can occur after minimal amounts were ingested).
3. The length of time between ingestion and development of symptoms (FA usually manifests within minutes but can occur up to 1–2 hours after ingestion).
4. A detailed description of all the symptoms.
5. If similar symptoms developed on other occasions when the food was eaten (with FA, symptoms occur on every exposure). Note whether any of the foods that were ingested in the concerning time frame for a reaction have been eaten since and if they were tolerated.
6. If other co-factors may have contributed to the reaction (e.g., some types of FA occur preferentially after exercise).
7. Was treatment administered and what was the response to treatment?
8. What foods are currently being avoided? Even if only one food may have been the culprit for a reaction, families may avoid other classes of food prior to seeing the clinician.
9. It is helpful to keep an idea of roughly when the reaction(s) occurred relative to the clinician's visit.

When the history is less clear to explicitly suggest a food allergy and may be more concerned for a food intolerance, a diet diary can be used as an adjunct to the medical history. Parents (or children) are asked to keep a chronological record of all foods ingested over a specified period and to record any symptoms the child experiences during this time. The diary can then be reviewed to determine if there is any relationship between the foods ingested and the symptoms experienced. Remarkably this method will detect an unrecognized association between a food and a patient's symptoms, but as opposed to the medical history, information can be collected on a prospective basis that is less dependent on a patient's or parent's memory.

When a patient initially presents with any concern for a food allergic reaction, even before the diagnosis is formally established, it is important to determine whether and to what extent they are currently avoiding the suspected allergens. This is important as allergen avoidance is linked to increased risk of food allergy development among non-allergic patients (Du Toit et al. 2015, Perkin et al. 2016), as well as impaired food allergy-related quality of life of both patients and their caregivers (Warren et al. 2016). For example, data suggest that, while most individuals with cow's milk (Nowak-Wegrzyn et al. 2008) and egg allergy (Lieberman et al. 2012, Peters et al. 2014) can extensively tolerate baked dairy products, many patients nevertheless avoid baked products, leading to greater psychosocial burden and possibly greater risk of persistent allergy (Dang et al. 2016, D'Auria et al. 2019).

B. Skin prick and serum specific IgE testing

Once the history is suggestive of a FA, additional diagnostic testing is used to capture sensitization and clinically interpret the likelihood of a true food allergy. Skin Prick Testing (SPT) and IgE determination in the blood (by RAST or ImmunoCAP) assess IgE-mediated mechanisms but are not informative in the diagnosis of non-IgE-mediated food allergic reactions. Testing should ideally be limited to potential allergens or if there is concern for specific cross-reactivity, as positive testing otherwise in the absence of a clinical history can be non-specific and is not sufficient for a diagnosis of a food allergy.

Skin prick test: SPT is highly reproducible and is often the initial technique used to detect the presence of IgE and screen patients for suspected IgE-mediated FA. A positive SPT to food indicates sensitization but should be interpreted within the clinical context of the child to determine if it is concerning an allergy. A negative SPT has a strong negative predictive value and generally is sensitive enough to rule out an IgE-mediated allergy. However, in some cases, SPT can be negative in patients with IgE mediated reactions and if the clinical suspicion is high, it should be followed with serum specific IgE testing as described below. A negative test does not mean that the food cannot induce non-IgE-mediated symptoms. SPT can be confounded by recent antihistamine use and dermatographism. Finally, the reliability of SPT is further justified if appropriately standardized and good quality food extracts are utilized.

Prick on Prick (also known as 'fresh prick') skin test: Although there are several commercial preparations for SPT for vegetables and fruits (apple, banana, potato, carrot, celery), commercially available SPT materials are often inadequate due to lability of the antigens. In these instances, fresh antigen obtained by pricking the fruit or vegetable is then used to prick the patient's skin. This method of testing yields more reliable results, although the technique used is crude and non-standardized. To rule out non-specific reactivity, a control subject may also undergo prick on prick testing with the same food at the same time as the suspected food allergy case, although this method is not often used.

Intradermal testing, which involves injecting a minimal amount of allergen into the dermis of the skin should not be used in food allergy testing. It involves an increased risk of inducing a systemic reaction, has a high false positive rate, and is not known to be more reliable or useful than SPT or prick on prick testing as above (Kattan and Sicherer 2015).

Serum specific IgE test: Determination of specific IgE (by RAST or ImmunoCAP method) in the blood is often used to screen for IgE-mediated FA. In general, these measurements performed in high quality laboratories provide information similar to SPT. Without a clinical history, identification of serum IgE alone suggests sensitization but is not diagnostic of a food allergy. General food panels are not recommended in the absence of a history suggestive of a reaction given the high false positive rates. Comparison of SPT and specific IgE determination is shown in Table 28.1. Additionally, Table 28.2 provides diagnostic levels of food-specific IgE for a variety of foods. When a patient has a food-specific serum IgE level exceeding any of these values, they are greater than 95% likely to experience an allergic reaction if they ingest the specific food (Sampson et al. 2014). In general, if the clinical history is reassuring that symptoms are not consistent with an immediate food allergy, and testing include SPT and/or serum IgE is negative, gradual home introduction of the food can be considered (Nowak-Węgrzyn et al. 2009). This however should be determined by the clinician and discussed thoroughly with families to determine their comfort level and likelihood of introduction and continuance of the food in the diet.

Table 28.1. Comparison between skin prick test (SPT) and serum specific Immunoglobulin E (IgE) in the diagnosis of food allergy.

SPT	IgE
*Sensitive, excellent negative predictive value, low specificity, poor positive predictive value	*Sensitive, excellent negative predictive value, low specificity, poor positive predictive value
Moderate Cost- Less expensive than IgE	High Cost-More expensive
Generally need normal skin	for all patients, even with extensive skin disease in patients with severe dermatographism
Antihistamines suppress SPT	Not affected by medications
Must be delayed for 4–6 weeks after an anaphylactic reaction as the results may not be reliably interpretable	Can be performed in the setting of recent anaphylaxis
Irritating (may be itchy)	Painful (involving blood draw)
Requires specialty expertise to perform	Does not require specialty expertise
Visible results can immediately be seen by patient (allergen response on skin)	Patient must be informed of results by their doctor where the length of result reporting depends on the laboratory

*Note: Without a history of an allergic reaction, neither SPT nor IgE should be used for screening. If assessing an infant for risk of food allergy, specifically peanut allergy, these tests may be considered for infants at high-risk (4- or 6-month old infants with severe eczema and/or egg allergy).

Table 28.2. ImmunoCAP levels that predict likelihood of a food allergy (Perry et al. 2004, Sampson et al. 2014).

Food	> 95% positive sIgE	~ 50% negative sIgE
Egg white	≥ 7	≤ 2
	≥ 2 if age < 2 y	
Cow's milk	≥ 15	≤ 2
	≥ 5 if age < 1 y	
Peanut	≥ 14	≤ 2 (if clear history of reaction)
		≤ 5 (if no history of prior reaction)
Tree nut	≥ 15	≤ 5
Fish	≥ 20	
Soy	≥ 30	≤ 5
Wheat	≥ 26	≤ 10

Oral food challenge

Oral Food Challenges (OFC): OFC are recommended for more definitive diagnosis of FA particularly when the history and testing are not conclusive. Such challenges are not advisable if there is a very recent history of anaphylaxis and/or evidence of high serum IgE which serves as a guideline for risk stratification. More recent studies have tried to characterize IgE thresholds that are low enough to warrant an OFC with a > 50% likelihood of passing (Table 28.2) (Perry et al. 2004). Moreover, despite a food allergy to raw eggs and milk, a lot of research has shown the majority of these patients may still be able to largely tolerate baked eggs and baked milk products. As such, it is imperative to discuss with families to test extensively heated or baked egg or milk; this allows not only for expansion of the diet with social and nutritional benefits, but moreover may accelerate development of tolerance to raw eggs or milk (Lieberman et al. 2012, Kim et al. 2011, Dunlop 2018).

The gold standard for the diagnosis of food allergy is the Double-Blind Placebo-Controlled Food Challenge (DBPCFC) (Nowak-Węgrzyn et al. 2009). DBPCFC markedly reduces the potential bias of patients as well as the health personnel. This procedure can, however, be difficult to perform as it is time and labor intensive. Standardized protocols are available only for a few foods and it is very difficult to find an appropriate placebo to mask the food flavor. Due to the aforementioned limitations of the DBPCFC, other types of oral challenges like single-blind or open-food challenge may be considered for diagnosis. Open food challenges are more frequently used in the clinical setting for screening purposes and negative challenges can effectively rule out FA. When an OFC is positive, it may be considered diagnostic with supportive medical history and laboratory data.

Procedure of oral food challenge (Nowak-Węgrzyn et al. 2009):

The decision to perform OFC is complex and is influenced by several factors including past medical history, age, past adverse reactions, skin prick test results, food specific serum IgE levels and concomitant food allergies. The importance of OFC is significant in determining the nutritional value of eliminated food items, addressing patient and family preferences as well as, relieving parental or patient anxiety in relation to certain common food items that have the potential to cause life threatening reactions.

When do you not do the OFC?

If there is a high likelihood of reaction to the food item chosen, food challenges are typically not performed. Determining factors include high levels of food specific IgE and/or SPT wheal size and recent history of anaphylaxis. Other confounding medical conditions include unstable cardiovascular disease, pregnancy, treatment with beta blockers, uncontrolled eczema, allergic rhinitis or asthma. Concurrent illnesses, fever and active respiratory symptoms are other reasons to postpone OFC.

Who is the ideal patient for OFC? (Nowak-Węgrzyn et al. 2009):

Young patients with an estimated 50% or less likelihood of reacting to a food based upon Immunocap grading (Table 28.2) or negative SPT or values considered to be a low likelihood for reaction (Samson et al. 2014). These patients generally have the best risk to benefit ratio of having a negative OFC and are the optimal candidates for OFC performed in an allergist's office. However, absolute values of diagnostic testing do not correlate with or predict the severity of reaction. It is important to understand the patient and family, including social factors that may impact whether food will be incorporated into the diet if they pass. Generally, it is explained to the family that if an OFC is passed, the food should be maintained in the diet at least few times a week to maintain tolerance.

Types of OFC:

1. Open OFC: This is the simplest of OFCs, but has certain limitations. It is an unmasked, unblended feeding of the food item and is generally done for screening purposes. It is simple and reproduces a more natural setting. Compared to other approaches, it is easier to perform in the allergist's office and is cost-effective, and particularly useful if objective symptoms are anticipated. A clearly negative test will effectively rule out sensitivity to the food item. A positive test with only subjective symptoms may need to be confirmed by a blinded challenge but it is left to the clinician's discretion regarding how to proceed.

2. Blinded OFC: In this method, the food item is mixed with a masking vehicle (Table 28.3) or the item is placed in an opaque capsule to reduce the bias. In the single blind OFC, the observer, but not the patient, knows the food being tested. In the double-blind OFC, both the patient as well as the observer is unaware of the food being supplied; the dietician or a third party who supplies the food material is aware of it hence bias is minimized. Placebo-controlled challenges may also be administered in both methods. The PRACTALL consensus report describes ongoing efforts to standardize the administration of such placebo-controlled OFCs including pre-challenge assessment, challenge protocols and stopping criteria (Sampson et al. 2012). More recently, a European expert panel published a set of recommended practices to identify participants in population-based and clinical studies with suspected FA who should receive food challenges as well as harmonize the reporting of OFC results in these studies (Grabenhenrich et al. 2017).

Table 28.3. Suggested materials for preparing office-based blind OFCs (P.A. and Vedanthan 2016).

Vehicles	Spices/Flavors
Opaque Capsule	Sugar
Hamburger	Salt
Infant Formula	Black Pepper
Canned Tuna Fish	Corn Syrup
Applesauce	Mint Sauce
Ice Cream	
Grape Juice	
Popsicle	
Milk Smoothie	
Lentil Soup	
Chocolate Pudding	
Mashed Potato	
Oatmeal	
Fruit Smoothie	
Tapioca Fruit	
Amino Acid-Based Elemental Infant Formula	

1. Procedure for OFC:

   a. Preparation of patients: Documentation of verbal or written consent. Detailed discussion of the procedure, risks, benefits, outcome and limitations of the test.

   Patients need to be in good health and their allergic status under optimal control at the time of the OFC. Certain medications may need to be discontinued before the challenge (such as antihistamines if a repeat skin prick test is planned prior to challenge, short acting bronchodilators the day of challenge, or beta blockers if deemed safe by the primary physician). Patients should avoid eating for 2–4 hours prior to the challenge. In small children or infants, a light meal 2 hours before the challenge is allowed. Ideally, start the challenge at the normal breakfast time.

   b. Baseline vital signs should be recorded which include: respiratory rate, heart rate, blood pressure, temperature and basic physical findings (with special attention to the oropharynx, skin and respiratory exam). Emergency treatment should be readily accessible which includes epinephrine, antihistamines and possibly steroids, with doses calculated based on the patient's weight prior to the start of the OFC. Equipment for IV access and oxygen is also helpful. Recording pulse oximetry, peak flow or spirometry in asthmatics may be useful.

   c. The OFC needs to be conducted in a location where food may be measured. A small food scale might be required for graduated challenges. While there is no standardized protocol for dose increments, typically OFC is started at 5–10% of the goal dose, then given 20%, 30% and then 40% (which equal a total dose of 100%), monitoring 20 minutes between each step. Smaller initial doses (0.1–1%) may be indicated depending on the risk and reaction history.

   Throughout the OFC procedure, the patient needs to be under the supervision of a physician or a nurse. The patient needs to be re-examined before each dose of the food item is administered. At the first symptom or sign of an allergic reaction, examination of the skin, oropharynx and cardiovascular/respiratory tract should be done. The challenge should be stopped at any objective finding of an allergic reaction and treatment should be initiated immediately. Consider access to emergency medical services or transport to higher level facility when planning for OFC.

2. Interpretation of OFC:

   a. OFC is considered negative if the patient tolerates the entire procedure up to the goal dose of food (i.e., consumes 100%). Patients should still be observed for 1–2 hours prior to discharge. Families should be instructed to continue the food in the diet at least three times per week. The goal dose is determined by the physician based on the patient's age and the volume that they can consume, but should also take into account the total protein content in the food. A study by Nowak-Węgrzyn et al. offers some examples for portion sizes and OFC preparation (Nowak-Wegrzyn et al. 2009). If a patient consumes a notable portion (e.g., at least 50%) of the food without a reaction but is unable to consume additional amounts due to volume or lack of interest in eating, the clinician may consider discussing with families incorporating the dose achieved during the OFC into the patient's diet at home, and make a plan for gradual up-dosing at home over the course of the next few weeks to months.

   b. Positive OFC: For a positive OFC dose in a graded, monitored setting in clinic, patients should be observed for at least 2 hours after treatment is given provided symptoms have resolved (Sampson et al. 2012). For any acute evaluation that warrants higher level of care, patients should be sent to the emergency department for intervention. Patients presenting to the hospital directly for evaluation after consuming food outside of a monitored clinical setting with concern for anaphylaxis should be observed for at least 4 hours after the reaction; there is a risk for biphasic reactions in some cases (Lee et al. 2018). Written instructions, often in the form of an 'emergency action plan' should be given regarding how to identify and treat future food-allergic reactions. Ideally, patients should be prescribed auto-injectable epinephrine devices and taught appropriate use with a trainer device.

   In summary, OFC are extremely useful in the diagnosis of adverse food reactions, both immunologic as well as non-immunologic. They are generally safe if conducted under a physician's supervision.

Allergists/immunologists are particularly well-qualified to conduct these procedures and assist their patients in the correct identification of foods causing adverse reactions. If conducted appropriately, these procedures can improve the patient's quality of life and remove unnecessary dietary restrictions.

Clinical scenario

A 2 year-old Caucasian female, referred by her primary care physician, presents to the allergy clinic with symptoms of a rash on her face and vomiting after eating cake, brownies, pizza and peanut butter cookies at a birthday party two weeks ago. She has a medical history of eczema, currently well controlled with over the counter hydrocortisone cream. A month prior to her visit, she had pistachio ice cream which resulted in rashes on her face. An antihistamine was administered and symptoms subsided. She has previously consumed peanut containing foods with no history of an allergic reaction. She has never consumed pistachio before, but has had hazelnut and walnut with no history of reactions. Currently, she regularly eats wheat, eggs, soy, and milk with no complaints.

Her parents do not have a history of allergy or any other atopic disease. The patient lives with her mother and father. No pet exposure. No smoke exposure.

Physical examination was unremarkable except for mild erythematous dry patches in the flexures.

Laboratory data

In light of clinical history, skin prick testing was performed for peanuts and pistachios. SPT for peanuts was 3 mm and 1 mm for pistachios. sIgE results were elevated for peanuts (1.8 kU/L) and negative for pistachios (0.1 kU/L). Due to equivocal results (without availability of component testing for peanuts) with a suspicious reaction history, an oral food challenge is recommended for peanuts. Pistachio allergy was thought to be unlikely.

Oral food challenge was later administered for peanuts with a positive result.

Differential diagnoses

Food poisoning, viral gastroenteritis, food intolerance, oral allergy syndrome, food protein induced enterocolitis syndrome

Treatment plan and follow-up

The patient should avoid peanut consumption but may continue introducing tree nuts at home. The patient's parents were counseled on the prognosis of food allergy, signs and symptoms, treatment of allergic reactions and anaphylaxis and lifestyle modifications including dietary avoidance. An epinephrine auto-injector was prescribed. A food allergy action plan was developed and discussed along with the use of an epinephrine auto-injector. A follow-up visit was scheduled in one year.

Component-resolved diagnostics

Novel methods to improve diagnostic measures continue to remain under investigation. Component Resolved Diagnostics (CRD) are being used more as emerging literature shows their potential to improve diagnosis of a specific food allergy and even the predictive value in deciding to offer an OFC compared with standard testing. In allergen-specific IgE testing, the extract from the whole food is tested which contains a complex mixture of proteins, including both allergenic and non-allergenic molecules. CRD or component-based IgE testing uses individual proteins (purified or recombinant) within that food to detect specific IgE-binding epitopes. This allows for better means of distinguishing sensitization to proteins that are clinically relevant and may help determine risk of severity with some components better correlating with clinical reactivity. For example, sensitization to a heat-resistant protein is more likely to yield systemic reactions whereas sensitization to a heat-labile protein component may be less clinically relevant or allow for identification of cross-reactivity with similar pollen species (given the homologous nature

Table 28.4. Components of common allergens that are associated with severe reactions (Sampson et al. 2014, Borres et al. 2016).

Food	Higher risk for systemic reactions (CRD)
Peanut	Ara h 1, 2, 3, (6), 9
Hazelnut	Cor a 8, 9, 14
Walnut	Jug r 1, 2, 3
Pecan	Car i 1, 2
Pistachio	Pis v 1, 2
Cashew	Ana o 3
Soy	Gly m (4), 5, 6, 8
Wheat	Tri a (14), 19
Rosaceae fruits (peach, apple)	Pru p 3, Mal d 3

of some proteins to aeroallergens causing the classic pollen-food or oral allergy syndrome). Predicative capabilities of these components do vary, however, according to population background.

The components of peanuts are most well studied in CRD, specifically Ara h 2, which has been shown to increase the accuracy of diagnosing a peanut allergy. Compared to PST and whole peanut IgE, Ara h 2 sIgE appears to correctly identify more patients with true peanut allergy with better sensitivity and specificity (Dang et al. 2012). Seed-storage proteins Ara 1 and 3 as well as Ara h 6, which is closely related to Ara h 2, have also been shown to be associated with severe allergic reactions (Klemans et al. 2015, Lieberman et al. 2013). Sensitization to the heat labile protein Ara h 8 in peanuts is generally associated with mild symptoms, typically oral allergy, as it is commonly driven by Bet v 1 (birch pollen) sensitization. Ara h 9 sensitization is particularly linked to the Mediterranean population, also suggesting the role of CRD in investigating regional differences. Table 28.4 outlines components of common allergens that are associated with severe reactions (Sampson et al. 2014, Borres et al. 2016). Most frequently used CRD in practice currently are for peanuts, hazelnuts, cashews, walnuts and occasionally soy.

The conditions to use CRD need to be carefully considered. While no one diagnostic test is accurate, implementing CRD alongside SPT and IgE may further help differentiate true food allergy from positive testing due to cross-reacting antibodies. For example, for patients with peanut sIgE < 15 kU/L, to more accurately predict challenge outcomes, CRD may be used to further risk-stratify patients who could be safely challenged to determine tolerance (Lieberman et al. 2013). It may also be beneficial in patients with multiple hypersensitivities such as pollen and plant food allergens. It is important to note that even sIgE related to whole extract or CRD that is less than the limit of detection does not guarantee a successful challenge outcome. As further CRD studies are conducted, both regionally as well in the identification of additional relevant proteins, diagnostic utility may continue to evolve. As with all testing, CRD should be used in the context of clinical history.

Basophil activation test

Another emerging diagnostic modality for clinical food allergy testing is the Basophil Activation Test (BAT), which is a functional assay where the expression of activation markers is quantified on the surface of basophils following *in vitro* stimulation with food allergen extracts (Hemmings et al. 2018). The BAT, which relies on flow cytometry of either fresh whole blood or isolated peripheral blood mononuclear cells, has been compared to an OFC in a test tube (Santos and Lack 2016). While the BAT has yet to be widely adopted in the clinical setting, a recent study found it to be more accurate in diagnosing clinical peanut allergy than sIgE, SPT or CRD to peanuts (Santos et al. 2014). Remarkably, preliminary data also indicate that BAT results may predict food allergy severity, given that studies show that patients with more severe reaction histories have more reactive basophils. (Song et al. 2015, Santos et al. 2015) In contrast to SPT and sIgE, the BAT has a very high positive predictive value, with reported specificity exceeding 95% (Santos and Lack 2016). Consequently, its adoption has the potential to substantially reduce the need for OFC, with one study estimating that two of three confirmatory OFCs to peanut could be avoided (Santos et al. 2014). These authors concluded that based on their data, the most accurate and cost-effective potential diagnostic workflow would be to use a 2-step sequential approach in which SPT or Arah2-sIgE testing would be followed by BAT in equivocal cases. While the aforementioned study only addressed peanut allergy diagnosis, other researchers have found the BAT to be highly sensitive and specific for diagnosis of other major allergens, including hazelnut (Brandström et al. 2015), eggs (Ocmant et al. 2009), milk (Sato et al. 2010), wheat (Tokuda et al. 2009), and sesame (Appel et al. 2018). However, while BAT testing appears promising, especially for patients whose clinical history, SPT and/or sIgE results do not permit a definitive diagnosis, further standardization of laboratory workflows, data analysis pipelines, clinical validation studies and evaluation of cost-effectiveness are still needed (Santos and Shreffler 2017).

Treatment of food allergy

Acute management of food allergy typically involves recognition of an allergic reaction and appropriate pharmacotherapy is based on the severity of the clinical reaction (see also Chapter 10 on Severe allergic reactions and on anaphylaxis). Mild reactions (few hives, itching or flushing) can typically be managed with antihistamines. For more severe symptoms or concern for anaphylaxis, epinephrine (1:1000 dosed at 0.01 mg/kg, max 0.5 mg, given intramuscularly) is the first-line treatment and the only life-saving medication. Pediatric and adult dosing for pre-filled epinephrine auto-injectors are available readily in developed countries. Patients should seek immediate care after use of epinephrine. Adjunct therapy includes antihistamines, albuterol if indicated for bronchospasm, and at times oral corticosteroids, but should not replace epinephrine as the first line. If there is an inadequate response or an immediate life-threatening situation, a repeat IM epinephrine injection can be given in 3 to 5 minutes as needed. Before discharge from the clinic or the emergency room, the patient should be provided with an 'emergency action plan' that lists common symptoms and signs of an allergic reaction and how to treat. This should be regularly updated, particularly after any reaction or after food challenges.

There is as yet no approved long-term treatment of food allergy but there are many ongoing clinical trials surrounding immunotherapy with promising results, such as oral immunotherapy (OIT), sublingual immunotherapy (SLIT) and epicutaneous immunotherapy (EPIT). These forms vary in terms of their dosing, frequency and immunologic effects. The most studied is OIT which is outlined below. Notably, a recent multicenter, randomized, double-blind placebo-controlled phase 2a clinical trial in peanut-allergic adults found that a single dose of Etokimab, an anti–IL-33 biologic, significantly improved desensitization in peanut-allergic participants. Specifically, 73 and 57% increases in the tolerated threshold peanut allergen dose were observed via OFC days 15 and 45 post-treatment, compared to 0% increases among controls receiving placebo injections (Chinthrajah 2019). However, further, longer-term trials are clearly warranted given that only 20 patients participated in this pilot study.

Oral immunotherapy

Oral immunotherapy (OIT) consists of feeding an allergen to an allergic individual regularly in gradually increased amounts to achieve oral desensitization (when an individual can consume a specified quantity of an allergen without a reaction while undergoing therapy; clinical reactivity may return after ceasing treatment). In general, this exposure aims to increase the threshold that triggers an allergic reaction. Sustained Unresponsiveness (SU) may be achieved and refers to an individual temporarily or permanently tolerating the food without a reaction after ceasing treatment.

The mechanism to achieve desensitization is unclear but has been suggested to prompt immunologic changes including suppression of basophil and mast cell reactivity and interleukin-10 production which increases production of the IgG4 antibody (Jones et al. 2009). Additionally, antigen-specific IgA, IgG1, IgG4 and IgE production increases (Kulis et al. 2018, Patil et al. 2015). It is important to note that

12–18 months into therapy, IgE levels decrease below baseline levels. These immunologic changes prompt a decrease in tissue mast cells and eosinophils.

A common protocol for OIT consists of starting the patient with a small dose of food lower than the amount known to start a reaction or an amount that is expected to result in an allergic reaction. Protocols for the initial dose escalation phase vary, but generally begin OIT with very low doses (≤5 mg, often 0.01–0.1 mg) and is gradually increased in the initial treatment escalation day to a maximum goal dose (Jones et al. 2009). Doses are then consumed daily and increased every 1–2 weeks by 50% during the dose escalation phase until maintenance dose is reached (300 mg–4000 mg). At larger doses, dose increment changes are made by 20–25% every 2–4 weeks. The increase in dosage is conducted under strict supervision of a healthcare professional. The new dosage is consumed daily. While these percentages serve as rough guidelines, they are very individualistic to a patient and their clinical history. Oral food challenges may be performed at baseline and after 6 months of consistent therapy to assess efficacy.

Adverse events may occur during OIT administration but rates vary in each trial of different allergens and adverse event categorization also may differ by trial. Rates range from 69–92% of subjects experiencing an adverse event and 5–12% patients undergoing OIT needed intramuscular epinephrine administered (Romantsik et al. 2014, Virkud et al. 2017, Yeung et al. 2012). Additionally, in a randomized, placebo-controlled OIT study, adverse events were considerably more common among the active treatment group compared to the placebo group (Burks et al. 2012, Skripak et al. 2008). Some possible risk factors associated with adverse events include presence of baseline allergic rhinitis, baseline SPT wheal size, higher specific serum IgE levels (greater than 50 kU/L), asthma and lower thresholds of food consumption (Elizur et al. 2015, Vazquez-Ortiz et al. 2014a, Vazquez-Ortiz et al. 2014b, Vazquez-Ortiz et al. 2013, Virkud et al. 2017). Additionally, concurrent illness, consuming doses on an empty stomach, exercise/physical exertion after dosing and consuming doses during menses may also contribute to adverse events during doses formerly tolerated (Staden et al. 2008, Varshney et al. 2009). Gastrointestinal (GI) symptoms are commonly reported in OIT patients for all foods (Goldberg et al. 2017).

Single-food OIT trials on milk, eggs and peanuts are the most common. It is important to consider that these trials varied in maintenance doses. Meglio et al. in the earliest milk OIT study, demonstrated that 71% of subjects with a positive baseline double-blind placebo-controlled food challenge tolerated a daily dosage of 200 mL of cow's milk following a 6 month desensitization protocol (Meglio et al. 2004). Other studies have also demonstrated that the majority of subjects (67–100%) were able to complete protocol and consume the goal milk dosage daily (Keet et al. 2012, Martorell et al. 2011, Pajno et al. 2010, Salmivesi, et al. 2013, Skripak et al. 2008). Egg and peanut OIT trials have also demonstrated that desensitization can be accomplished among the majority of subjects, approximately 56–100% for eggs (Burks et al. 2012, García Rodríguez et al. 2011, Itoh et al. 2010, Jones et al. 2016, Pérez-Rangel et al. 2017, Vickery et al. 2010) and 62–93% for peanuts (Blumchen et al. 2010, Jones et al. 2009, Anagnostou et al. 2014). Other studies have examined wheat OIT and it also appears to lead to successful desensitization, although these studies were not placebo controlled and some did not have a post-treatment challenge (Kulmala et al. 2018, Pacharn et al. 2014, Rodríguez del Río et al. 2014). While to date OIT has been mostly administered in the private practice setting or via clinical trials of experimental therapies, FDA-approved immunotherapies may be on the horizon, given the completion of phase 3 trials of AR101 (The PALISADE Group of Clinical Investigators 2018) (proposed trade name PALFORZIA™), and recent vote from the FDA Allergenic Products Advisory Committee who found the efficacy and safety data to support its use in peanut allergy OIT.

Since nearly 40% of food allergic children in the US have multiple food allergies, multi-food OIT may be warranted in this context (Gupta et al. 2018). Previous literature has suggested that multi-food OIT is safe and feasible (Bégin et al. 2014), however there is a paucity of long-term data regarding its efficacy. One recent study found that patients given a monoclonal anti-IgE antibody (Omalizumab) in conjunction with multi-allergen OIT, were much more likely to achieve desensitization to two or more of their allergens at 36 weeks relative to OIT participants randomized to receive a sham injection (83 vs 33%) (Andorf et al. 2018). This biologic therapy is currently being studied both as an adjunct to solo and multi-food OIT, as well as a monotherapy, after receiving the FDA's Breakthrough Therapy Designation for prevention of severe food-allergic reactions.

Prevention of food allergy

Previously, delayed introduction of highly allergenic food was recommended; however, more recent evidence has strongly supported early introduction of highly allergenic foods, specifically peanuts, prompting changes in guidelines. The Learning Early About Peanut Allergy trial (Du Toit et al. 2015) showed an impressive reduction in the prevalence of peanut allergy from 17.2% in the avoidance group to 3.2% in the early consumption group, with 86.1% relative reduction at 5 years with early introduction of peanuts to high risk infants and regular consumption. Based on this study, the 2017 National Institute of Allergy and Infectious Diseases addendum guidelines were published (Togias et al. 2017) which recommend: (1) infants with a known egg allergy and/or severe eczema should be evaluated for peanut sensitization (via SPT or serum sIgE) before the decision of peanut introduction, which should occur at 4–6 months of age; (2) infants with mild to moderate eczema should be introduced to age-appropriate peanut products by 6 months; (3) infants without any history of atopy can be fed peanut based on family preferences. Although there have been several trials regarding early introduction of other highly allergic foods, some of which have been promising such as with eggs, there are not established guideline recommendations for these.

Breastfeeding until 6 months, if possible, has been associated with many positive outcomes. The American Academy of Pediatrics recommends breastfeeding for at least 6 months, or if not feasible to use extensively hydrolyzed formula, for the prevention of atopic dermatitis and cow's milk allergy (Sampson et al. 2014). At this time, there are no changes advised to the maternal diet during pregnancy or lactation for the prevention of FA.

Role of patient-parent education

Patient and parent education and support are essential for families with FA. Parents and older children must be informed of symptoms of a food allergic reaction and how to manage the reaction in the moment. Providing and reviewing an 'emergency action plan' can be beneficial for families. Children older than 7 years can usually be taught to inject themselves with an epinephrine auto-injector and for younger children parents and caregivers should be appropriately instructed. Preventative management chiefly consists of identification of the offending food and planning strict food avoidance, which can be particularly difficult for children. Standardization of food labeling is poor in countries like India and can add further challenges. Meal preparations at home should be done with efforts to avoid cross-contact. In addition to good hand washing, utensils, cookware, storage containers and tabletops should be thoroughly cleaned with soap and water. Vigilance should also be maintained when dining out or traveling on public transportation. In addition, when eating away from home (in schools or restaurants), food-sensitive children should feel comfortable to request information about the contents of prepared foods. Schools should also be equipped to treat anaphylaxis in allergic students (which has already been recommended by the American Academy of Pediatrics Committee of School Health in USA). Physicians must be willing to explain, and with the parents' help, instruct school personnel about these issues. A variety of organizations and support groups, including parent groups of children with FA, can help provide information, advocacy and education.

Natural history of food allergy

The natural course of food allergies depends typically on the food causing the allergy. It is generally believed that clinical allergy to peanuts and tree nuts have a lower likelihood of resolution compared to eggs and milk which have a higher likelihood of resolution with age (Savage et al. 2016). A large cohort of egg allergic children showed that 4% of the children developed tolerance by age 4 years, 12% by 6 years, 37% by 10 years and 68% by age 16 years (Savage et al. 2007). The key associations in this study that corresponded to persistence of egg allergies was high levels of egg specific IgE > 50 kU/L and the presence of other food allergies. A large study that evaluated the natural history of cow's milk allergy observed that the rates of resolution of the allergy were 19% by 4 years, 42% by 8 years, 64% by 12 years, and 79% by 16 years of age (Skripak et al. 2007). Similar to the study on egg allergy, the predictors for persistence of cow's milk allergy were high levels of cow's milk specific IgE, coexisting asthma and allergic rhinitis. As previously mentioned, extensively heated milk and eggs are likely to be tolerated before cooked or raw egg or uncooked milk and should be incorporated into the diet as soon as safely determined as it may also accelerate development of tolerance to uncooked forms of egg and milk (Savage et al. 2007). In contrast, typically, only 20–25% of patients with peanut allergy are likely to develop tolerance (Savage et al. 2016). Tree nuts have been found to have a similar trajectory. Wheat and soy appear to have more rapid resolution rates where nearly two-thirds of children outgrow the allergy by age 10–12 years (Savage et al. 2007). It is important to continue to reassess patient's clinical history every year, particularly during childhood and adolescence, with repeat testing every 1–3 years as feasible to monitor trends and consideration of oral food challenge.

Interestingly, recent epidemiological data indicate that adult-onset food allergies are remarkably common—with approximately half of food-allergic adults reporting at least 1 adult-onset FA (Gupta et al. 2019). Shellfish allergy is the most frequently developed adult-onset allergy, as well as the most common FA among adults in general. However, rates of physician-diagnosis and report of current epinephrine prescriptions are far lower among adults who report convincingly IgE-mediated food allergies, relative to their pediatric counterparts (Gupta et al. 2019). Given that the burden of disease is likely to increase among adult populations, as food-allergic adolescents age into adulthood and adults increasingly develop new allergies (Tang and Mullins 2017), efforts to ensure that all FA patients—regardless of their age—receive appropriate clinical diagnoses and management have never been more critical.

Conclusion

The diagnosis of a suspected FA begins with a detailed assessment that includes a focused history, physical exam, and differential diagnosis. Diagnostic testing can capture sensitization and help the clinician interpret the likelihood of a true IgE-mediated FA. Common FA tests include the SPT, IgE blood test, and OFC (the most definitive diagnostic tool). Research suggests early introduction of highly allergenic food as early as 4–6 months might prevent the development of FA, but guidelines to do so currently only exist for peanut in the US (Togias et al. 2017). There currently exists no approved, long-term treatment for FA, although encouraging immunotherapy trials are underway. Management of FA relies on avoidance, early recognition of an allergic reaction, and appropriate pharmacotherapy. It is comprised of comprehensive patient-parent education, the development of an individualized emergency action plan, and epinephrine auto-injector prescriptions.

References

Anagnostou K, Islam S, King Y, Foley L, Pasea L, Bond S, et al. Assessing the efficacy of oral immunotherapy for the desensitisation of peanut allergy in children (STOP II): a phase 2 randomised controlled trial. The Lancet 2014; 383(9925): 1297–1304.

Andorf S, Purington N, Block WM, Long AJ, Tupa D, Brittain E, et al. Anti-IgE treatment with oral immunotherapy in multifood allergic participants: a double-blind, randomised, controlled trial. Lancet Gastroenterol Hepatol 2018; 3(2): 85–94.

Appel MY, Nachshon L, Elizur A, Levy MB, Katz Y, Goldberg MR. Evaluation of the basophil activation test and skin prick testing for the diagnosis of sesame food allergy. Clin Exp Allergy 2018; 48(8): 1025–1034.

Bégin P, Winterroth LC, Dominguez T, Wilson SP, Bacal L, Mehrotra A, et al. Safety and feasibility of oral immunotherapy to multiple allergens for food allergy. Allergy Asthma Clin Immunol 2014; 10(1): 1.

Blumchen K, Ulbricht H, Staden U, Dobberstein K, Beschorner J, de Oliveira LCL, et al. Oral peanut immunotherapy in children with peanut anaphylaxis. J Allergy Clin Immun 2010; 126(1): 83–91.e1. https://doi.org/10.1016/j.jaci.2010.04.030.

Borres MP, Maruyama N, Sato S, Ebisawa M. Recent advances in component resolved diagnosis in food allergy. Allergol Int 2016; 65(4): 378–387.

Brandström J, Nopp A, Johansson SGO, Lilja G, Sundqvist AC, Borres MP, et al. Basophil allergen threshold sensitivity and component-resolved diagnostics improve hazelnut allergy diagnosis. Clin Exp Allergy 2015; 45(9): 1412–1418.

Burks AW, Jones SM, Wood RA, Fleischer DM, Sicherer SH, Lindblad RW, et al. For the Consortium of Food Allergy Research (CoFAR). Oral immunotherapy for treatment of egg allergy in children. New Engl J Med 2012; 367(3): 233–243. https://doi.org/10.1056/NEJMoa1200435.

Chinthrajah RS, Purington N, Andorf S, Long A, O'Laughlin KL, Lyu SC, et al. Sustained outcomes in oral immunotherapy for peanut allergy (POISED study): a large, randomised, double-blind, placebo-controlled, phase 2 study. The Lancet 2019; 394(10207): 1437–1449.

Dang TD, Tang M, Choo S, Licciardi PV, Koplin JJ, Martin PE, et al. Increasing the accuracy of peanut allergy diagnosis by using Ara h 2. J Allergy Clin Immun 2012; 129(4): 1056–1063. https://doi.org/10.1016/j.jaci.2012.01.056.

Dang TD, Peters RL, Allen KJ. Debates in allergy medicine: baked egg and milk do not accelerate tolerance to egg and milk. World Allergy Organ J 2016; 9: 2.

D'Auria E, Salvatore S, Pozzi E, Mantegazza C, Sartorio MUA, Pensabene L, et al. Cow's milk allergy: immunomodulation by dietary intervention. Nutrients 2019; 11(6).

Du Toit G, Roberts G, Sayre PH, Bahnson HT, Radulovic S, Santos AF, et al. Randomized trial of peanut consumption in infants at risk for peanut allergy. New Engl J Med 2015; 372(9): 803–13.

Du Toit G, Sampson HA, Plaut M, Burks AW, Akdis CA, Lack G Food allergy: Update on prevention and tolerance. J Allergy Clin Immun 2018; 141(1): 30–40. https://doi.org/10.1016/j.jaci.2017.11.010.

Dunlop JH, Keet CA, Mudd K, Wood RA. Long-term follow-up after baked milk introduction. J Aller Cl Imm-Pract 2018; 6(5): 1699–1704.

Eigenmann PA, Beyer K, Lack G, Muraro A, Ong PY, Sicherer SH, et al. Are avoidance diets still warranted in children with atopic dermatitis? Pediatr Allergy Immunol 2019; https://doi.org/10.1111/pai.13104.

Elizur A, Goldberg MR, Levy MB, Nachshon L, Katz Y. Oral immunotherapy in cow's milk allergic patients: Course and long-term outcome according to asthma status. Ann Allerg Asthma Im 2015; 114(3): 240–244.e1. https://doi.org/10.1016/j.anai.2014.12.006.

García Rodríguez R, Urra JM, Feo-Brito F, Galindo PA, Borja J, Gómez E, et al. Oral rush desensitization to egg: Efficacy and safety: Rush desensitization to egg. Clin Exp Allergy 2011; 41(9): 1289–1296. https://doi.org/10.1111/j.1365-2222.2011.03722.x.

Goldberg MR, Elizur A, Nachshon L, Appel MY, Levy MB, Golobov K, et al. Oral immunotherapy–induced gastrointestinal symptoms and peripheral blood eosinophil responses. J Allergy Clin Immun 2017; 139(4): 1388–1390.e4. https://doi.org/10.1016/j.jaci.2016.09.053.

Grabenhenrich LB, Reich A, Bellach J, Trendelenburg V, Sprikkelman AB, Roberts G, et al. A new framework for the documentation and interpretation of oral food challenges in population-based and clinical research. Allergy 2017; 72(3): 453–461.

Gupta RS, Warren CM, Smith BM, Blumenstock JA, Jiang J, Davis MM, et al. The public health impact of parent-reported childhood food allergies in the United States. Pediatrics 2018; 142(6): e20181235. https://doi.org/10.1542/peds.2018-1235.

Gupta RS, Warren CM, Smith BM, Jiang J, Blumenstock JA, Davis MM, et al. Prevalence and severity of food allergies among US adults. JAMA Netw Open 2019; 2(1): e185630–e185630.

Hemmings O, Kwok M, McKendry R, Santos AF. Basophil activation test: old and new applications in allergy. Curr Allergy Asthm R 2018; 18(12): 77.

Itoh N, Itagaki Y, Kurihara K. Rush specific oral tolerance induction in school-age children with severe egg allergy: one year follow up. Allergol Int 2010; 59(1): 43–51. https://doi.org/10.2332/allergolint.09-OA-0107.

Iweala OI, Choudhary SK, Commins SP. Food allergy. Curr Gastroenterol Rep 2018; 20(5): 17. https://doi.org/10.1007/s11894-018-0624-y.

Jones SM, Pons L, Roberts JL, Scurlock AM, Perry TT, Kulis M, et al. Clinical efficacy and immune regulation with peanut oral immunotherapy. J Allergy Clin Immun 2009; 124(2): 292–300.e97. https://doi.org/10.1016/j.jaci.2009.05.022.

Jones SM, Burks AW, Keet C, Vickery BP, Scurlock AM, Wood RA, et al. Long-term treatment with egg oral immunotherapy enhances sustained unresponsiveness that persists after cessation of therapy. J Allergy Clin Immun 2016; 137(4): 1117–1127.e10. https://doi.org/10.1016/j.jaci.2015.12.1316.

Kattan JD, Sicherer SH. Optimizing the diagnosis of food allergy. Immunol Allergy Clin North Am 2015; 35(1): 61–76.

Keet CA, Frischmeyer-Guerrerio PA, Thyagarajan A, Schroeder JT, Hamilton RG, Boden S, et al. The safety and efficacy of sublingual and oral immunotherapy for milk allergy. J Allergy Clin Immun 2012; 129(2): 448–455.e5. https://doi.org/10.1016/j.jaci.2011.10.023.

Kim JS, Nowak-Węgrzyn A, Sicherer SH, Noone S, Moshier EL, Sampson HA. Dietary baked milk accelerates the resolution of cow's milk allergy in children. J Allergy Clin Immun 2011; 128(1): 125–131.

Klemans R, Meijer Y, Van Erp F, Van der Ent C, Bruijnzeel-Koomen C, Otten H, et al. SIgE to peanut components does not accurately predict the severity of allergy in subjects suspected of peanut allergy. Clin Transl Allergy 2015; 5(S3): P34, 2045-7022-5-S3-P34. https://doi.org/10.1186/2045-7022-5-S3-P34.

Kulis MD, Patil SU, Wambre E, Vickery BP. Immune mechanisms of oral immunotherapy. J Allergy Clin Immun 2018; 141(2): 491–498.

Kulmala P, Pelkonen AS, Kuitunen M, Paassilta M, Remes S, Schultz R, et al. Wheat oral immunotherapy was moderately successful but was associated with very frequent adverse events in children aged 6–18 years. Acta Paediatr (Oslo, Norway: 1992) 2018; 107(5): 861–870. https://doi.org/10.1111/apa.14226.

Lee J, Rodio B, Lavelle J, Lewis MO, English R, Hadley S, et al. Improving anaphylaxis care: the impact of a clinical pathway. Pediatrics 2018; 141(5): e20171616. https://doi.org/10.1542/peds.2017-1616.

Lieberman JA, Huang FR, Sampson HA, Nowak-Wegrzyn A. Outcomes of 100 consecutive open, baked-egg oral food challenges in the allergy office. J Allergy Clin Immunol 2012; 129(6): 1682–1684 e1682.

Lieberman JA, Glaumann S, Batelson S, Borres MP, Sampson HA, Nilsson C. The utility of peanut components in the diagnosis of IgE-mediated peanut allergy among distinct populations. J Allergy Clin Immun: In Practice 2013; 1(1): 75–82. https://doi.org/10.1016/j.jaip.2012.11.002.

Martorell A, De la Hoz B, Ibáñez MD, Bone J, Terrados MS, Michavila A, et al. Oral desensitization as a useful treatment in 2-year-old children with cow's milk allergy: Oral desensitization to cow's milk allergy. Clin Exp Allergy 2011; 41(9): 1297–1304. https://doi.org/10.1111/j.1365-2222.2011.03749.x.

Meglio P, Bartone E, Plantamura M, Arabito E, Giampietro PG. A protocol for oral desensitization in children with IgEmediated cow's milk allergy. Allergy 2004; 59(9): 980–987. https://doi.org/10.1111/j.1398-9995.2004.00542.x.

Nowak-Węgrzyn A, Bloom KA, Sicherer SH, Shreffler WG, Noone S, Wanich N, et al. Tolerance to extensively heated milk in children with cow's milk allergy. J Allergy Clin Immunol 2008; 122(2): 342–347, 347 e341–342.

Nowak-Węgrzyn A, Assa'adAH, Bahna SL, Bock SA, Sicherer SH,Teuber SS.WorkGroup report:Oralfood challenge testing. J Allergy Clin Immun 2009; 123(6): S365–S383. https://doi.org/10.1016/j.jaci.2009.03.042.

PA M, Vedanthan PK. Chapter 23. Food allergy. pp. 310–325. In: Vedanthan PK, Nelson HS, Agashe SN, PA M, Katial R (eds.). Textbook of Allergy for the Clinician 2016. CRC Press, Florida, USA.

Pacharn P, Siripipattanamongkol N, Veskitkul J, Jirapongsananuruk O, Visitsunthorn N, Vichyanond P. Successful wheatspecific oral immunotherapy in highly sensitive individuals with a novel multirush/maintenance regimen. Asia Pac Allergy 2014; 4(3): 180. https://doi.org/10.5415/apallergy.2014.4.3.180.

Pajno GB, Caminiti L, Ruggeri P, De Luca R, Vita D, La Rosa M, et al. Oral immunotherapy for cow's milk allergy with a weekly up-dosing regimen: A randomized single-blind controlled study. Ann Allerg Asthma Im 2010; 105(5): 376–381. https://doi.org/10.1016/j.anai.2010.03.015.

Patil SU, Ogunniyi AO, Calatroni A, Tadigotla VR, Ruiter B, Ma A, et al. Peanut oral immunotherapy transiently expands circulating Ara h 2–specific B cells with a homologous repertoire in unrelated subjects. J Allergy Clin Immun 2015; 136(1): 125–134.

Pérez-Rangel I, Rodríguez del Río P, Escudero C, Sánchez-García S, Sánchez-Hernández JJ, Ibanez MD, et al. Efficacy and safety of high-dose rush oral immunotherapy in persistent egg allergic children. Ann Allerg Asthma Im 2017; 118(3): 356–364.e3. https://doi.org/10.1016/j.anai.2016.11.023.

Peters RL, Dharmage SC, Gurrin LC, Koplin JJ, Ponsonby AL, Lowe AJ et al. The natural history and clinical predictors of egg allergy in the first 2 years of life: a prospective, population-based cohort study. J Allergy Clin Immunol 2014; 133(2): 485–491.

Peters RL, Allen KJ, Dharmage SC, Koplin JJ, Dang T, Tilbrook KP, et al. Natural history of peanut allergy and predictors of resolution in the first 4 years of life: A population-based assessment. J Allergy Clin Immun 2015; 135(5): 1257–1266. e1-2. https://doi.org/10.1016/j.jaci.2015.01.002.

Perkin, MR, Logan K, Tseng A, Raji B, Ayis S, Peacock J, et al. Randomized trial of introduction of allergenic foods in breast-fed infants. N Engl J Med 2016; 374(18): 1733–43.

Perry TT, Matsui EC, Kay Conover-Walker M, Wood RA. The relationship of allergen-specific IgE levels and oral food challenge outcome. J Allergy Clin Immunol 2004; 114(1): 144–149.

Rodríguez del Río P, Díaz-Perales A, Sanchez-García S, Escudero C, do Santos P, Catarino M, et al. Oral immunotherapy in children with IgE-mediated wheat allergy: Outcome and molecular changes. J Investig Allergol Clin Immunol 2014; 24(4): 240–248.

Romantsik O, Bruschettini M, Tosca MA, Zappettini S, Della Casa Alberighi O, Calevo MG. Oral and sublingual immunotherapy for egg allergy. Cochrane Database Syst Rev 2014; (11): CD010638. https://doi.org/10.1002/14651858.CD010638.pub2.

Salmivesi S, Korppi M, Mäkelä MJ, Paassilta M. Milk oral immunotherapy is effective in school-aged children: Oral immunotherapy in milk allergy. Acta Paediatr 2013; 102(2): 172–176. https://doi.org/10.1111/j.1651-2227.2012.02815.x.

Sampson HA. Food hypersensitivity and dietary management in atopic dermatitis. Pediatr Dermatol 1992; 9(4): 376–379. https://doi.org/10.1111/j.1525-1470.1992.tb00636.x.

Sampson HA, Gerth van Wijk R, Bindslev-Jensen C, Sicherer S, Teuber SS, Burks AW, et al. Standardizing double-blind, placebo-controlled oral food challenges: American academy of allergy, asthma & immunology–european academy of allergy and clinical immunology PRACTALL consensus report. J Allergy Clin Immun 2012; 130(6): 1260–1274. https://doi.org/10.1016/j.jaci.2012.10.017.

Sampson HA, Aceves S, Bock SA, James J, Jones S, Lang D, et al. Food allergy: a practice parameter update-2014. J Allergy Clin Immunol 2014; 134(5): 1016–1025 e1043.

Santos AF, Douiri A, Bécares N, Wu SY, Stephens A, Radulovic S, et al. Basophil activation test discriminates between allergy and tolerance in peanut-sensitized children. J Allergy Clin Immun 2014; 134(3): 645–652.

Santos AF, Du Toit G, Douiri A, Radulovic S, Stephens A, Turcanu V, et al. Distinct parameters of the basophil activation test reflect the severity and threshold of allergic reactions to peanut. J Allergy Clin Immun 2015; 135(1): 179–186.

Santos AF, Lack G. Basophil activation test: food challenge in a test tube or specialist research tool? Clin Transl Allergy 2016; 6(1): 1–9.

Santos AF, Shreffler WG. Road map for the clinical application of the basophil activation test in food allergy. Clin Exp Allergy 2017; 47(9), 1115-1124.

Sato S, Tachimoto H, Shukuya A, Kurosaka N, Yanagida N, Utsunomiya T, et al. Basophil activation marker CD203c is useful in the diagnosis of hen's egg and cow's milk allergies in children. Int Arch Allergy Imm 2010; 152(Suppl 1): 54–61.

Savage J, Johns CB. Food allergy: Epidemiology and natural history. Immunol Allergy Clin North Am 2015; 35(1): 45–59. https://doi.org/10.1016/j.iac.2014.09.004.

Savage, JH, Matsui, EC, Skripak JM, Wood RA. The natural history of egg allergy. J Allergy Clin Immun 2007; 120(6): 1413–1417.

Savage J, Sicherer S, Wood R. The natural history of food allergy. J Aller Cl Imm-Pract 2016; 4(2): 196–203; quiz 204. https://doi.org/10.1016/j.jaip.2015.11.024.

Skripak JM, Matsui EC, Mudd K, Wood RA. The natural history of IgE-mediated cow's milk allergy. J Allergy Clin Immun 2007; 120(5): 1172–1177.

Skripak JM, Nash SD, Rowley H, Brereton NH, Oh S, Hamilton RG, et al. A randomized, double-blind, placebo-controlled study of milk oral immunotherapy for cow's milk allergy. J Allergy Clin Immun 2008; 122(6): 1154–1160. https://doi.org/10.1016/j.jaci.2008.09.030.

Somanunt S, Chinratanapisit S, Pacharn P, Visitsunthorn N, Jirapongsananuruk O. The natural history of atopic dermatitis and its association with Atopic March. Asian Pac J Allergy Immunol 2017; 35(3): 137–143. https://doi.org/10.12932/AP0825.

Song Y, Wang J, Leung N, Wang LX, Lisann L, Sicherer SH, et al. Correlations between basophil activation, allergen-specific IgE with outcome and severity of oral food challenges. Ann Allerg Asthma Im 2015; 114(4): 319–326.

Spahn TW, Weiner HL, Rennert PD, Lügering N, Fontana A, Domschke W, et al. Mesenteric lymph nodes are critical for the induction of high-dose oral tolerance in the absence of Peyer's patches. Eur J Immunol 2002; 32(4): 1109–1113. https://doi.org/10.1002/1521-4141(200204)32:43.0.CO;2-K.

Staden U, Blumchen K, Blankenstein N, Dannenberg N, Ulbricht H, Dobberstein K, et al. Rush oral immunotherapy in children with persistent cow's milk allergy. J Allergy Clin Immun 2008; 122(2): 418–419. https://doi.org/10.1016/j.jaci.2008.06.002.

Tait C, Goldman RD. Dietary exclusion for childhood atopic dermatitis. Can Fam Physician 2015; 61(7): 609–611.

Tang ML, Mullins RJ. Food allergy: is prevalence increasing?. Intern Med J 2017; 47(3): 256–261.

Thalayasingam M, Lee BW. Fish and shellfish allergy. Chem Immunol Allergy 2015; 101: 152–161. https://doi.org/10.1159/000375508.

Togias A, Cooper SF, Acebal ML, Assa'ad A, Baker JR, Beck LA, et al. Addendum guidelines for the prevention of peanut allergy in the United States: report of the National Institute of Allergy and Infectious Diseases-sponsored expert panel. Allergy Asthma Clin Immunol 2017; 13(1): 1–20.

Tokuda R, Nagao M, Hiraguchi Y, Hosoki K, Matsuda T, Kouno K, et al. Antigen-induced expression of CD203c on basophils predicts IgE-mediated wheat allergy. Allergol Int 2009; 58(2); 193–199.

Varshney P, Steele PH, Vickery BP, Bird JA, Thyagarajan A, Scurlock AM, et al. Adverse reactions during peanut oral immunotherapy home dosing. J Allergy Clin Immun 2009; 124(6): 1351–1352. https://doi.org/10.1016/j.jaci.2009.09.042.

Vazquez-Ortiz M, Alvaro-Lozano M, Alsina L, Garcia-Paba MB, Piquer-Gibert M, Giner-Muñoz MT, et al. Safety and predictors of adverse events during oral immunotherapy for milk allergy: Severity of reaction at oral challenge, specific IgE and prick test. Clin Exp Allergy 2013; 43(1): 92–102. https://doi.org/10.1111/cea.12012.

Vazquez-Ortiz M, Alvaro M, Piquer M, Dominguez O, Machinena A, Martin-Mateos MA, et al. Baseline specific IgE levels are useful to predict safety of oral immunotherapy in egg-allergic children. Clin Exp Allergy 2014 a; 44(1): 130–141. https://doi.org/10.1111/cea.12233.

Vazquez-Ortiz Marta, Alvaro M, Piquer M, Giner MT, Dominguez O, Lozano J, et al. Life-threatening anaphylaxis to egg and milk oral immunotherapy in asthmatic teenagers. Ann Allergy Asthma Im 2014b; 113(4): 482–484. https://doi.org/10.1016/j.anai.2014.07.010.

Vickery BP, Pons L, Kulis M, Steele P, Jones SM, Burks AW. Individualized IgE-based dosing of egg oral immunotherapy and the development of tolerance. Ann Allerg Asthma Im 2010; 105(6): 444–450. https://doi.org/10.1016/j.anai.2010.09.030.

Virkud YV, Burks AW, Steele PH, Edwards LJ, Berglund JP, Jones SM, et al. Novel baseline predictors of adverse events during oral immunotherapy in children with peanut allergy. J Allergy Clin Immun 2017; 139(3): 882–888.e5. https://doi.org/10.1016/j.jaci.2016.07.030.

Warren CM, Otto AK, Walkner MM, Gupta RS. Quality of life among food allergic patients and their caregivers. Curr Allergy Asthma Rep 2016; 16(5): 38.

Yeung JP, Kloda LA, McDevitt J, Ben-Shoshan M, Alizadehfar R. Oral immunotherapy for milk allergy. Cochrane Database Syst Rev 2012; 11: CD009542. https://doi.org/10.1002/14651858.CD009542.pub2.

29

Immunodeficiency Diseases

Mandakolathur R Murali

INTRODUCTION

A functioning immune system is not only essential to successfully protect the host from foreign or 'non self' antigens such as various infectious pathogens but also to prevent immune responses to 'self' antigens and emergence of autoimmune diseases. In addition, its surveillance function is called upon to recognize the 'altered self' or tumor cells and eliminate or restrain them. Defects in this regulation results in a spectrum of immunodeficiency diseases, wherein recurrent infections, autoimmune diseases and malignancy are clinical features.

The function of normal innate and adaptive immune system

The recognition of self and -non- self-antigens is a function of both the inborn or innate immune system and the adaptive immune system (Flajnik 2018). The innate immune system has a limited repertoire of responses as its Pattern Recognition Receptors (PRR), such as the Toll like receptor, NOD, RIG-1, etc., are encoded in its germ line. These PRR recognize Pathogen Associated Molecular Patterns (PAMP) and Danger Associated Molecular Patterns (DAMP). While they do not have a memory of their interactions, they are instrumental in recruitment of the adaptive immune system by virtue of their location, cytokine profile and rapid response. The adaptive immune system, on the other hand, has considerable diversification of the cell types, such as the T and B cells. These cells acquire high affinity antigen specific receptors by virtue of their germ line gene recombination, somatic hyper-mutation, selection and receptor editing. This process also results in the generation of memory cells. This entire network is tightly regulated by natural T regulatory cells as well as the cytokine network (O'Shea and Paul 2010). It is therefore not surprising that subjects with an immunodeficiency syndrome may manifest increased susceptibility to infections, manifest autoimmune diseases, autoinflammatory disorders and even develop malignancy. A developmental defect in this system results in primary or congenital immunodeficiency while an acquired defect, such as due to systemic diseases or viral infections affect a hitherto normal immune system and hence is called secondary immunodeficiency disease. While secondary immunodeficiency is more common, primary immunodeficiency can be looked upon as 'experiments of nature' and dissecting the nature of the defect has been most productive in not only understanding the functions and therapeutic approaches to immunodeficiency states but also to autoimmune diseases and malignancy.

    A functioning immune system represents a sequential and organized maturation and differentiation of the Hematopoietic Stem Cell (HSC). The HSCs reside in the bone marrow and have the property of self-

---

Harvard Medical School, Massachusetts General Hospital, Boston, MA, Email: murali50@aol.com

renewal and differentiation facilitated by the stromal microenvironment. The human HSC is recognized by its cell surface markers—CD 34+, CD 38–, Thy lo, kit + and Lin –. This stem cell differentiates into either the hematopoietic lineage that gives rise to erythrocytes, myeloid cells as well as platelets or to the Common Lymphoid Progenitor (CLP) that gives rise to T and B cells as well as the Natural Killer (NK) cells. The orderly development and functional integrity of the innate as well as adaptive immune system is regulated by genes that control the critical enzymes and cytokines necessary for this process (Wilson and Trumpp 2015). This network of specific receptor-ligand associations activate a cascade of protein-protein interactions and post translational modification (e.g., phosphorylation, ubiquitination, etc.). These events lead to the activation of specific and critical transcriptional factors that modulate the expression of immunologic and inflammatory genes. Aberrations due to mutations of genes in these coordinated pathways results in disease states characterized by immunodeficiency, autoimmunity and malignancy.

Primary or congenital immunodeficiency can thus be looked upon as a defect or block in the development and maturation of the immune system. Defects at discrete steps in this process result in alteration of the numbers of the T and B cells or of their function leading to an immunodeficient state. The basis of this deficiency could be a monogenic defect that follows a Mendelian inheritance or it may be polygenic. The interaction of the genetic (such as consanguinity) and environmental factors leads to phenotypic diversity. Increased clinical awareness as well as more detailed immunological and molecular diagnostic testing has resulted in the description of new defects. Some of these mutations lead to defects in molecules essential for the development, survival, and/or function of regulatory T cells (T regs). These are now called 'Tregopathies' (Cepika et al. 2018). Further, advances in bone marrow and stem cell transplantation, coupled with genetic engineering and replacement therapy with cytokines and intravenous immunoglobulin (IVIG) therapy has altered the natural history of these diseases resulting in better quality of life.

- PID is classified based on the component of the immune system that is deranged (Geha et al. 2007). Defects of innate immunity comprise disorders of phagocytes, NK cells and complement system. Mutations in Pattern Recognition Receptors (PRR) like the Toll-Like Receptor (TLR) RIG-1 or complement proteins are associated with immunodeficiency as well as autoimmunity. Defects in adaptive immunity include antibody deficiency syndromes as well as cellular deficiencies. It is important to recognize that for a fully integrated and competent immune system both innate and adaptive immune systems are essential. Derangements contribute to PID.
- Classification based on the component of immune system that is primarily defective.

PID is classically divided into five main groups.

(1) Combined cellular and antibody deficiency diseases (CID)
(2) Cell mediated immunodeficiency
(3) Antibody deficiency syndromes
(4) Complement deficiencies
(5) Phagocytic cell deficiency

These defects lead to severe infections or recurrent infections with distinctive susceptibility to various types of pathogens Cunningham-Rundles 1989). They may also present with features of autoimmunity, autoinflammatory and malignancy.

When to suspect a primary immunodeficiency syndrome

A defect in the structure and/or function of the immune system results in a derangement of the host defensive system resulting in severe or recurrent infections. The pathogens causing the infections often provide a clue to the component of the immune system that is defective (see Table 29.1).

Some of the clinical clues to an immunodeficient state are rare but pathognomonic and others are very subtle but often lower the threshold for clinical suspicion (O'Sullivan and Cant 2012). These can be considered under three groups:

Table 29.1. Pathogens characteristically associated with specific immune defects.

Deficiency	Bacteria	Virus	Fungi	Protozoa
Cellular deficiency	S.pneumonia, H.Influenza, M.Catarrhalis, P.aeruginosa, S.aureus, Mycoplasma pneumonia. Also S.typhi, Listeria monocytogenes and enteric flora	CMV, RSV, EBV Parainfluenza Type 3, herpes viruses and others	Candida species, Aspergillus species, H.capsulatum, C.neoformans.	P. jiroveci, T. gondii, Cryptosporodium parvum
Antibody deficiency	S.pneumonia, H.Influenza, Catarrhalis, P.aeruginosa, S.aureus, Mycoplasma pneumonia.	Enterovirus	None	Giardia lamblia
Phagocytic	S.aureus, P.aeruginosa, Nocardia asteroides, S.typhi.	None	Candida species, Aspergillus species.	No
Complement	S.pneumonia, H.Influenza, Catarrhalis, P.aeruginosa, S.aureus, Mycoplasma pneumonia and Neisseria species	None	None	None

1. Those features that are rare but when present are pathognomonic of a PID.
   These include:
   (a) neonatal tetany with cardiac abnormalities (DiGeorge syndrome)
   (b) somatic abnormalities (DiGeorge, ADA, Job's syndrome)
   (c) eczema and generalized erythroderma (Omenn's)
   (d) thrombocytopenia (Wiscott-Aldrich syndrome)
   (e) ataxia and/or telangiectasia (ataxia-telangiectasia syndrome)
   (f) oculo-cutaneous albinism (Chediak-Higashi syndrome)

2. Those features that are often present and in the clinical context of recurrent infections or autoimmunity should raise a high index of suspicion of PID.
   These include:
   (a) skin rash such as eczema (Job's syndrome, Omenn's syndrome), Candidiasis (T cell defects, APECED)
   (b) diarrhea and failure to thrive (CVID)
   (c) recurrent sinusitis in absence of allergies, anatomical abnormalities or systemic diseases. Pneumonias in different regions of the lung in the absence of structural lung defects are a useful clue (CVID, B cells defects, CID)
   (d) recurrent abscesses (Job's syndrome, LAD)
   (e) unexplained hepatosplenomegaly (CVID, CGD, HLH)

3. Those that are subtle but need to be explored.
   These include:
   (a) frequent infections without a predisposing factor such as diabetes, alcohol excess, viral infections or anatomical causes such as bronchiectasis, aspiration pneumonia, etc.
   (b) infections with opportunistic pathogens such as P. jerovici and giardia
   (c) incomplete response to appropriate antimicrobials
   (d) incomplete clearance between episodes of infection
   (e) recurrent deep infections or infections in unusual areas (liver, bone as in CGD, CVID)

In addition, a family history of similar illness or a male preponderance or history of consanguinity lowers the threshold for consideration and exclusion of a PID.

The pathogenesis and clinical features of PID diseases

Tables 29.2–29.5—provide a summary of the pathogenesis and clinical features, while defects arising due to block in the pathways of T, B and NK cells are shown in Fig. 29.1.

Table 29.2. Spectrum of primary immunodeficiency disease Severe Combined Immunodeficiency (SCID) and cellular immunodeficiency disease.

Position of block/defect	Nature of defect	Clinical phenotype
1	AK2, ADA and PHP deficiency	SCID with T-B-NK-profile with hematological and somaticabnormalities (ADA 10–15% and PNP 1–2%)
2	γc(X linked or SCIDX1), JAK3 (autosomal recessive), IL7-Rα mutations	γc and JAK-3 are T-B+NK-SCID (about 40%) While IL-Rα is T-B+NK+SCID
3	RAG-1 and 2, Artemis, Cernunnos, DNA ligase 4, DNA-PKC's mutations	T–B - NK+SCID (4–20%)
4	Mutations in CD 3δ, CD 3ε, CD 3ζ and CD 45 tyrosine kinase	Generally T-B + NK + SCID except for CD 45 deficiency which is T-B-NK + variant
5	Defects in MHC class II expression	T – B + NK +CID with profound CD4 cytopenia
6	Mutation of ZAP-70	CD8–, CD4+ but deficient function, NK+
7	Mutations of TAP1, TAP2 and Tapasin and resulting MHC Class 1 deficiency	CD 8 deficiency, CD 4 normal. Midline granulomas and vasculitis common
8	Genetic defects in STIM1 and ORAII-calcium sensor and calcium-release activated channels	T cell receptor (TCR) mediated defects, Also associated with myopathy
9	γc (X linked or SCIDX1), JAK3 (autosomal recessive) mutations	NK cell deficiency as part of T – B + SCID

Table 29.3. Spectrum of primary immunodeficiency disease antibody deficiency diseases.

Position of block/defect	Nature of defect	Clinical phenotype
10	BTK and BLNK deficiency, mutations in IGHM, defects in λ5, Igβ, LRRC8. Also with mutations of RAG1, 2 DNA ligase 4, DNA PKC's, Artemis, Cernunnos	Congenital hypogammalobulinemia, BTK (85%) IGHM (5%), LRRC8 (1%)
11	Mutations in CD 40, CD 40L, AID, UNG, TACI, ICOS and CD 19	Hyper IgM syndrome, CVID
12	Mutations in AID, UNG	Hyper IgM syndrome
13	Mutations in TACI, BAFFR implicated	Specific antibody deficiency syndrome, IgG subclasses and IgA deficiency

(a) Defects in adaptive immunity—T and B cells

The defect in the development and maturation of T, B and NK cells at specific sites (1 to 9) are indicated in Fig. 29.1. The details of the defect, often genetic, leading to the clinical phenotype characteristics of SCID and cellular deficiencies (CID) are depicted in Table 29.2 (Fischer et al. 2005, Lagresle-Peyrou et al. 2009). Table 29.3 delineates the sites (10 to 13 in Fig. 29.1) of maturational block and the genetic and molecular basis that lead to quantitative and qualitative deficiencies of antibody system manifesting as distinct clinical phenotypes. While the majority is due to intrinsic defects in B cells, some are a reflection of defects in T and B cell interaction such as the Hyper IgM syndrome due to CD40-CD40L as well as defects in ICOS, TACI and BAFF pathways (Conley et al. 2009, Chapel and Cunningham-Rundles 2009, Chapel et al. 2008, Wehr et al. 2008).

Table 29.4. Spectrum of primary immunodeficiency disease. Syndromes with autoimmunity and immune dysregulation.

Entity	Molecular defect (Inheritance)	Clinical phenotype/Lab findings
Autoimmune lymphoproliferative syndrome (ALPS)	Defective apoptosis due to mutations in TNFRSF6 or Fas (AD & rarely AR) TNSF6 or FasL (AD and AR) Caspase 10 and 8 (AR) Neuroblastoma RAS viral oncogene homologue or NRAS (AD)	Lymphoproliferative disease often with immune thrombocytopenic purpura and immune hemolytic anemia. Lab: Increased CD3 +AB-CD4-CD8-cells, Hypergammaglobulinemia, increased Vit. B12 and IL-10, and Soluble Fas ligand levels
Autoimmune polyendocrinopathy Candidiasis Ectodermal Dystrophy APECED	Defective negative selection and failure of elimination of autoreactive T cells. Autoimmune regulator or AIRE gene defects on chromosome 21 (AR)	Autoimmune polyendocrinopathy with candidiasis, hypothyroidism, Addison's disease and less often diabetes mellitus Lab: organ specific autoantibodies
Immune dysregulation, polyendocrinopathy and entropathy (X linked) or IPEX	Defect in immune downregulation due to defective T regs Thgis is due to mutation and dysfunction of the transcriptional activator forkhead box protein 3 or FOXP3 on the X chromosome	Autoimmune diarrhea, early onset diabetes, thyroiditis, hemolytic anemia, thrombocytopenia and eczema Lab: Increased IgE levels, diminished Fox P3+CD4 T cell subpopulation
CD 25 deficiency	Defective IL-2 signaling needed for cell activation and T reg induction (AR)	Lymphoproliferation, autoimmunity, impaired T cell proliferation

Table 29.5. Spectrum of primary immunodeficiency disease immunodeficiency with impaired cell mediated cytotoxicity.

Entity	Molecular defect (Inheritance)	Clinical phenotype/Lab findings
Immunodeficiency with hypopigmentation (Chediak-Higashi syndrome)	Defects in LYST causing impaired lysosomal trafficking, failure of lysosome/phagosome fusion (AR)	Oculo-cutaneous albinism, severe bacterial infections, neurologic abnormalities and late onset lymphoma-like syndrome that is a form of hemophagocytic lymphohistiocytosis (HLH)
Familial hemophagocytic lumphohostiocytos is (FHL-1)	Unknown (AR)	Viral infections, enhanced macrophage activity and in 'accelerated phase' of disease with hemophagocytosis, due to high levels of γ interferon
FHL-2	Defects in Perforin 1 and hence cytolytic function (AR)	Same as in FHL-1
FHL-3	Defective UNC 13D required for priming vesicles for fusion (AR)	Same as in FHL-1
FHL-4	Defect in syntaxin 11, required for cytotoxic/target cell contact, vesicle trafficking and fusion (AR)	Same as FHL-1
FHL-5	Defect in suntaxin binding protein STXBP2 (AR)	Same as FKL-1

A normal immune system not only eliminates 'foreign or non-self' antigens but at the same time is tolerant to 'self-antigens'. Failure of tolerance leads to autoimmune diseases. This homeostatic immune balance is mediated by regulatory cells. They include the CD4+CD25+ T regs, regulatory NK cells as well as cytokines such as TGF-β and IL-10. The molecular and clinical features of immunodeficiency syndromes that manifest autoimmune features are summarized in Table 29.4 (Notarangelo 2006, Moraes-Vasconcelos et al. 2008, Caudy et al. 2007).

Table 29.5—represents syndromes resulting from a defect in cell mediated cytotoxic function, either due to structural protein defects or abnormality in fusion of phagosomes and lysosomes or defects in the granzyme or perforin functions. They may manifest as infections as in Chediak-Higashi syndrome or lymphoproliferative diseases (Huizing et al. 2008, Kaplan et al. 2008).

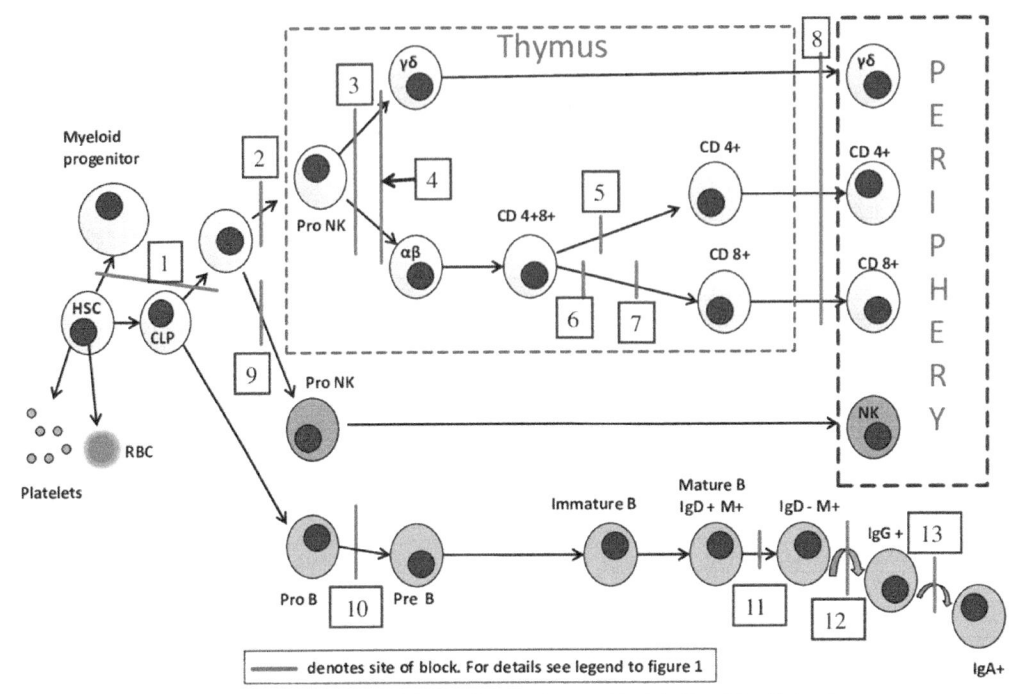

Figure 29.1. Primary Immunodeficiency diseases due to a block in T and B cell development.

While those described above reflect defects in adaptive immune system, the next group is immune deficiency diseases due to defects in innate pathways—complement, phagocytic cells as well as defects in toll like receptors and signaling pathways.

(b) Defects in innate immunity

(1) Complement

The complement system comprises a tightly regulated pathway that recognizes biochemical divergence between self-structures from structural pathogen associated molecular patterns such as the lipopolysaccharide of gram-negative bacteria, mannose of fungi, ficolins of some gram-positive bacteria. This leads to activation of distinct early complement proteins, generation of convertases that converge on C3 giving rise to the anaphylatoxins C4a and C3a as well as C3b. Beside its opsonic function C3b functions as an enzyme in generating C5a, a chemoattractant for phagocytic cells. Collectively, the anaphylatoxins (C3a, C4a and C5a) mediate the vascular phase of inflammation while C5a recruits the phagocytic cells resulting in integrating the vascular and cellular phase of immune defenses and inflammation. Derangements in this cascade of activating and regulatory proteins leads to either failure of complement mediated defenses and hence recurrent or severe infections or auto activation of complement proteins leading to immune inflammation, defects in complement mediated clearance of apoptotic cells causing autoimmune diseases. Figure 29.2 summarizes the clinical picture as well as the laboratory evaluation of the complement system that leads to a definition of the specific complement protein deficiency.

In Table 29.6—some of the congenital complement deficiency diseases and the resulting infections and/or autoimmune manifestations are depicted (Unsworth 2008).

(2) Phagocytic cells

Phagocytic cells play a pivotal role in the defense against bacteria and fungi. Thus, patients with defects in number, function or both are vulnerable to recurrent and severe infections caused by bacteria as

- Recurrent pyogenic infection with normal antibody function
- Disseminated Neisserial infection
- Autoimmune diseases with normal antibody function
- Family history of complement deficiency

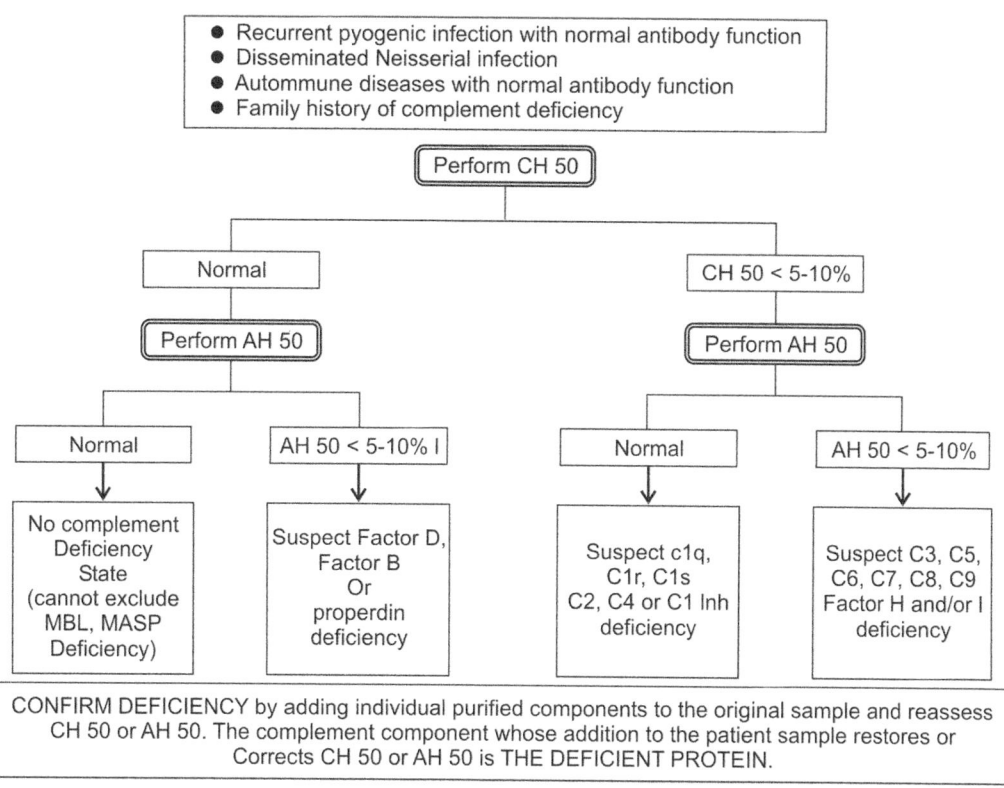

Perform CH 50

Normal → Perform AH 50
- Normal → No complement Deficiency State (cannot exclude MBL, MASP Deficiency)
- AH 50 < 5-10% → Suspect Factor D, Factor B Or properdin deficiency

CH 50 < 5-10% → Perform AH 50
- Normal → Suspect c1q, C1r, C1s C2, C4 or C1 Inh deficiency
- AH 50 < 5-10% → Suspect C3, C5, C6, C7, C8, C9 Factor H and/or I deficiency

CONFIRM DEFICIENCY by adding individual purified components to the original sample and reassess CH 50 or AH 50. The complement component whose addition to the patient sample restores or Corrects CH 50 or AH 50 is THE DEFICIENT PROTEIN.

Figure 29.2. Features and evaluation of inherited complement diseases.

Table 29.6. Complement deficiency diseases.

Complement deficiency	Disease association
C1q, C1r, C1s, C4, C2 and C3	Autoimmune manifestations like SLE
C2 and C3	Increased infections from encapsulated bacteria
Late components C5 to C8	Recurrent and invasive neisserial infections
Factor D and properdin	Recurrent and invasive neisserial infections
MBP and MASP-2	Increased risk of infections
Factor H and I and also MCP	Membranoproliferative glomerulonephritis and atypical hemolytic uremic syndrome
C1 inhibitor	Hereditary angioedema
DAF (CD55), Homologous restriction factor or Decorin (CD59)	Paroxysmal nocturnal hemoglobinuria

well as fungi, especially Candida and Aspergillus species. In general, subjects with phagocytic defects manifest respiratory tract and cutaneous infections. Recurrent and often erosive gingivitis and stomatitis is common. Deep seated subcutaneous abscesses are not uncommon (Lekstrom-Himes and Gallin 2000). Phagocytic defects are heterogeneous and will be described as

(a) Disorders of neutrophil production (Table 29.7)

Table 29.7. Disorders of neutrophil production.

Disease entity	Nature of defect	Clinical phenotype
Severe congenital neutropenia (SCN)	Commonly due to heterozygous mutation of Elastase-2 or ELA2 gene. Other mutations include HAX1, G6PC3, GFI1 and WAS gene	Absolute neutrophil count or ANC < 500/uL with severe neonatal pyogenic bacterial infections
Cyclic neutropenia	Sporadic or autosomal mutations of ELA2 gene	Approximately every 21 days the ANC < 500/uL resulting in periodicity of infections. Some develop MDS or AML
Shwachman-Bodian-Diamond syndrome (SBDS)	Autosomal recessive mutation of genes in 7q11 region regulating RNA metabolism	Anemia, failure to thrive, exocrine pancreatic deficiency, metaphyseal dysostosis and shortened ribs on X-rays

(b) Intrinsic defects in neutrophil granules (Table 29.8)

Table 29.8. Intrinsic defects in neutrophil granules.

Disease entity	Nature of defect	Clinical phenotype
Specific granule deficiency	Mutation in C/EBPε on 14q 11.2 blocks promyelocyte-myelocyte maturation	Neutrophils have bilobed nucleus and lack granules. Platelets lack HMW VWF, and fibrinogen resulting in bleeding. Bone marrow transplant useful when done early
Primary myeloperoxidase (MPO) deficiency	Misense mutation resulting in replacement of arginine 549 with tryptophan (R549W) in MPO precursor	Often asymptomatic as MPO independent oxidative pathway compensates for the defect. Aspergillus and candida infection occur if diabetes is associated with MPO deficiency
Secondary MPO deficiency	Somatic mutation of MPO seen in hematological malignancy, severe iron deficiency, lead and cytotoxic agent toxicity	Same as in primary MPO deficiency described above
Chediak-Higashi syndrome	Autosomal recessive defect in CHS 1 gene coding for lysosomal transporter resulting in abnormal (giant) neutrophil and melanocyte granules	Characterized by oculocutaneous albinism. Features include photophobia and infections. Biphasic immunodeficiency; infections early and lymphoproliferation later. Neurological deficits occur

(c) Defects in transcription factors (Table 29.9)

Table 29.9. Defects in transcription factors.

Disease entity	Nature of defect	Clinical phenotype
Hyper- IgE or Job's syndrome	Autosomal dominant disorder caused by mutations in STAT 3 located at 17q21	Recurrent infections of lower respiratory tract often with lung abscesses and pneumatoceles, chronic eczema and skin infections, extremely elevated IgE with eosinophilia. Facial, skeletal and dental abnormalities are common
Autosomal recessive Hyper-IgE syndrome	DOCK8 (located at 9p24) deficiency	Besides infections have food allergies, asthma, viral infections. Prone to cutaneous and lymphoid malignancy
MonoMAC syndrome (Monocytopenia and mycobacterial infections hence - MonoMAC	Haploinsufficiency of GATA2 (located on 3q21.3)	Late childhood or adult onset infections with disseminated nontuberculous mycobacterial or fungal infections. Monocytes, NK cell and B cell cytopenia are characteristic abnormalities

(d) Defects in leukocyte adhesion function (Table 29.10)

Table 29.10. Defects in leukocyte adhesion function.

Disease entity	Nature of defect	Clinical phenotype
Leukocyte adhesion deficiency 1 (LAD 1)	Mutation of the CD18 of Beta 2 integrin	Delayed separation of the umbilical cord, gingivitis and periodontitis, recurrent bacterial infections,-, skin ulcers, poor wound healing. Persistent leukocytosis is a feature even in absence of infection
Leukocyte adhesion deficiency 2 (LAD 2)	Hypofucosylation of CD 15s (sialyl Lewis^X) due to mutation in GDP-fucose transporter-1	Less severe infection but have dysmorphic features, hypotonia, mental retardation and seizures
Leukocyte adhesion deficiency 3 (LAD3)	Mutation in FERMT3 which encodes KINDLIN3 which regulates integrin activation	Besides bacterial infections have bleeding tendencies due to platelet integrin defects

(e) Defects in intracellular killing (Table 29.11)

Table 29.11. Defects in intracellular killing.

Disease entity	Nature of defect	Clinical phenotype
Chronic granulomatous disease (CGD)	- Commonest is membrane associated gp91 phox deficiency (X-linked) - Less common autosomal recessive deficiency of cytosolic p47, p67, p40 and p21rac1/p21rac2	Recurrent sino-pulmonary infections, skin abscesses, perianal abscesses, osteomyelitis, inflammatory bowel disease due to catalase- positive organisms such as S. aureus, Burkholderia cepacia, Serratia marcescens, Nocardia and Aspergillus species. Granulomas can cause luminal obstruction in gastrointestinal and genitourinary passages

(3) Toll like receptors (TLR's)

TLRs are Pattern Recognition Receptors (PRRs) expressed on cell surfaces or an endosomal membrane of immune and non-immune cells, they recognize Pathogen Associated Molecular Patterns (PAMPs) such as lipopolysaccharides of gram-negative bacteria, glycolipids from fungi and single or double stranded RNA and DNA. TLR activation involves the adaptor protein MyD88 and intracellular kinases such as IL-1 receptor associated kinase (IRAK) 4 and IRAK-1 resulting in the generation of NFκB and production of inflammatory cytokines such as IL-1, IL-6, TNF-α and IL-12. TLR 3, TLR7, TLR8 and TLR9 recruit other adaptor proteins such as TRIF and UNC-93B leading to generation of the Type 1 interferons—IFN α/β.

Autosomal recessive mutations of IRAK4 and MYD88 are associated with severe and invasive pyogenic infections early in life (Von Bernuth et al. 2008). Heterozygous mutations in TLR3 and biallelic mutations in UNC93B have been associated with reduced production of type 1 IFN and selective susceptibility to herpes simplex encephalitis (Casrogue et al. 2006).

(4) IL-12/IFN-γ signaling pathway (Al-Muhsen and Cassonova 2008)

Mendelian Susceptibility to Mycobacterial Disease (MSMD) has been associated with defects in IL-12/IFN-γ pathway. The immune response against mycobacteria is based on secretion of IL-12 by macrophages. IL-12 binds to its specific receptors expressed on T and NK cells and induces secretion of IFN-γ that triggers macrophage microbicidal function on binding to its receptor. Mutations of the IL-12 p40 subunit, the IL-12 receptor β1 chain, both chains of the INF-γ receptor and the STAT 1 gene (which encodes for the transcription factor downstream of INF-γ receptor) all contribute to MSMD. Table 29.12 summarizes the defects due to IL-12/IFN-γ signaling pathway.

Table 29.12. Defects in IL-12/IFN – γ signaling pathway.

Disease entity	Nature of defect	Clinical phenotype
NEMO	Mutations in IKBKG gene, encoding IKK-γ or NFκB essential modulator (NEMO) and defects in class switch recombination. X-linked trait	Increased susceptibility to mycobacterial infections, combined immunodeficiency, ectodermal dystrophy.
MSMD	IL-12RB 1 mutations	Increased susceptibility to mycobacteria, Salmonella, Listeria and Histoplasma
MSMD	Complete STAT 1 deficiency	Increased susceptibility to mycobacteria and viruses

Miscellaneous immunodeficiency syndromes

(A) Recurrent infections with unique and distinctive clinical features are the hallmark of this group and are depicted in Table 29.13. They represent defects at the gene level

Table 29.13. Miscellaneous immunodeficiency diseases.

Disease entity	Nature of defect	Clinical phenotype
Wiskott-Aldrich syndrome (WAS)	X-linked and is due to mutation of WASP gene, a regulator of actin cytoskeleton in hematopoietic cells	Eczema, thrombocytopenia, immunodeficiency, autoimmunity and lymphoid malignancies
Ataxia-telangiectasia	Autosomal recessive due to mutation of the ataxia-telangiectasia mutated gene (ATM) with defects in DNA breaks and repair	Ataxia, ocular telangiectasia, increased risk of infections and tumors
Nijmegen syndrome	Mutation of the Nibrin gene (NBS1)	Microcephaly, 'bird-like facies', short stature and malignancies
Omenn syndrome	Hypomorphic defects in RAG-1, RAG-2 and class switch recombination (CSR)	T and B cell deficiency, eosinophilia, erythroderma, lymphadenopathy and protein losing enteropathy.

(B) Monogenic diseases resulting in regulatory T-cell deficiency or 'Tregopathies'

Monogenic diseases affecting T regulatory cell biology, the role of T cell associated molecules and regulation of peripheral T cell tolerance are called Tregopathies (Cepka et al. 2018). They manifest with recurrent infections, autoimmunity and malignancy. In 2017 the International Union of Immunological Societies (IUIS) classified them as inborn errors of immunity. Each of these genes encode proteins that uniquely contribute to the function of thymus-derived forkhead box P3 *(FOXP3)* regulatory T cells or Tregs. They are caused by Loss-Of-Function (LOF) mutations in *FOXP3*, cytotoxic T lymphocyte-associated antigen 4 *(CTLA4)*, LPS- Responsive and Beige-like Anchor protein *(LRBA), CD25,* BTB domain and CNC homolog 2 *(BACH2)* and Gain Of Function (GOF) mutation in Signal Transducer and activator of Transcription 3 *(STAT3)*. A description of the specific entity, the molecular defect and clinical phenotype/lab findings are depicted below in Table 29.14.

(C) Spectrum of primary immunodeficiencies due to genetic mutations in pathways leading to formation of the transcription factor, NFκB.

For efficient production of NFκB, after the activation of T and B cell receptors, a coordinated sequence of events is necessary both at the level of the bilipid layer of immune cells (e.g., by PI3Kδ pathway) (Nunes-Santos et al. 2019) as well as a system of critical molecular bridge exemplified by CBM complexes (CARD-BCL10-MALT1) (Lu et al. 2019). Germ line mutations of PI3Kδ pathway lead to immune deficiency and immune dysregulation while germ line mutations of the CBM complex (termed CBM opathies) result in a wide spectrum of clinical phenotypes ranging from CID to disorders of B cell lymphocytosis. These are depicted in Table 29.15 for PI3Kδ defects and in Table 29.16 for CBM opathies.

Table 29.14. Regulatory T cell deficiencies or Tregopathies.

Disease entity	Nature of defect	Clinical phenotype/Lab findings
CTLA-4 deficiency (ALPS V; CHAI)	Mutation of *CTLA-4* gene, autosomal dominant	Enteropathy, type I diabetes, cytopenia, respiratory infections. Normal or increased circulating FOXP3 Tregs and reduced FOXP3 expression causing impaired Treg cell mediated immune suppression.
LRBA deficiency (LATAAIE)	Mutation in *LRBA* gene, autosomal recessive	Enteropathy, cytopenia, respiratory infections and lymphoproliferation. Normal or decreased circulating FOXP3 Tregs with reduced FOXP3 expression causing impaired Treg cell mediated immune suppression.
CD 25 deficiency	Mutation in *IL2RA* gene, autosomal recessive	Enteropathy, eczema, recurrent infections and lymphoproliferation. Normal or decreased circulating FOXP3 Tregs with reduced FOXP3 expression causing impaired Treg cell mediated immune suppression.
IPEX syndrome: Immune dysregulation, Polyendocrinopathy, Enteropathy, **X**-linked	*FOXP3* and X-linked defect	Enteropathy, type I diabetes, thyroiditis, hepatitis, eczema, cytopenia and failure to thrive. Normal or decreased circulating FOXP3 Tregs with reduced FOXP3 expression. High TSDR (regulatory T cell-specific demethylation region) demethylation
BACH 2 deficiency	Mutation in *BACH2* gene, autosomal dominant	Enteropathy, recurrent respiratory infections and lymphoproliferation. Decrease in FOXP3 expression level on Treg cells
STAT 3 GOF mutation or **A**utoimmune **D**isease, **M**ultisystem, **I**nfantile **O**nset or **ADMIO**	Gain of function mutation of *STAT3*, autosomal dominant	Enteropathy, cytopenia, type I diabetes, respiratory infections and lymphoproliferation. Normal or decreased circulating FOXP3 Tregs

PI3Kδ defects can result in either increased or decreased PI3Kδ activity and are shown in Table 29.15

(A) High PI3Kδ activity

Table 29.15. PI3Kδ defects.

High PI3Kδ activity

Clinical entity	Gene/molecular defect	Clinical phenotype/laboratory findings	Treatment
APDS 1	Monoallelic GOF mutation of *PIK3Cδ* gene	Recurrent mucosal infection, autoimmunity, enteropathy, hypogammaglobulinemia, lymphoproliferation. Increased transitional B cells and CD8 cells, decreased class switched memory B cells and naïve T cells.	IVGG Specific mTOR inhibitors PI3Kδ inhibitors HSCT
APDS 2	Monoallelic LOF mutation of *PIK3R1*	Same as above with addition of short stature and dysmorphisms	Same as above.
APDS 3	Monoallelic LOF mutation of *PTEN*	Lymphoproliferation, autoimmunity, enteropathy, with or without mucosal infections, increased transitional B cells and decreased class switched memory B cells with or without hypogammaglobulinemia.	Same as above

Note: APDS stands for **A**ctivated **P**hosphoinositide 3-kinase **δ** **S**yndrome
  GOF is Gain of Function and **LOF** is Loss of Function **HSCT** = Hematopoietic Stem Cell Transplant

(B) Low PI3Kδ activity

Low PI3Kδ activity

Clinical entity	Gene/molecular defects	Clinical phenotype/laboratory findings	Treatment
PIK3Cδ	Biallelic LOF	Recurrent sinopulmonary, enteropathy and autoimmunity. Dysmorphic features present. Hypogammaglobulinemia or hyper IgM syndrome. Reduced class switched memory B cells.	IVGG Antibiotics HSCT
PIK3R1	Biallelic LOF	Recurrent sinopulmonary, enteropathy and autoimmunity. Hypogammaglobulinemia or hyper IgM syndrome. Reduced class switched memory B cells.	Same as above

(C) CBM opathies

Table 29.16. CBM opathies.

CBM opathies

Clinical entity	Gene /Molecular defects	Clinical phenotype/laboratory features	Treatment
Combined immunodeficiency (CID)	Biallelic LOF mutation of CARD 11, BCL 10 and MALT1	Recurrent bacterial and fungal infections of CNS, respiratory and GI systems. Normal total lymphocytes, absent Tregs, increased naïve B and T cells and decreased memory B and T cells. Impaired T and B cell receptor mediated activation/proliferation, impaired NFκB activation and decreased specific antibody responses.	IVGG Antibiotics HSCT
Atopic dermatitis and cutaneous viral and respiratory infections	Hypomorphic mutations of CARD 11 and 14	Increased IgE and eosinophils, normal T and B cells, and decreased T cell proliferation.	Antimicrobials, dupilumab, Omalizumab

Laboratory tests to confirm clinical diagnosis

Before the tests are done it is imperative to exclude secondary immunodeficiency such as HIV infection, malignancy and effects of drugs and to compare the values with age matched healthy controls. Laboratory tests can be grouped under these five categories for purposes of methodical evaluation and ease of interpretation and to correlate with clinical presentation. This also permits the clinician to have a focused approach to genetic and molecular testing. The categories are

(1) Tests for T cell function
(2) Tests for B cell function
(3) Tests for complement function
(4) Test for phagocytic cell function
(5) Tests for Innate immunity

1—Tests for T cell function

(a) Complete blood count, differential count so as to determine absolute lymphocyte counts
(b) Chest X ray or a CT scan
(c) Flow cytometry for CD3, CD4. CD8, CD 45RO and CD 45RA T cells, CD 19 or 20, CD 27 and CD 16/56/57. Additional markers that are useful include CD 40L (CD154 0n activated T cells), IL-2 receptor γ chain (CD132), MHC class I and class II, IL-7 receptor α chain (CD127), CD3 λ and δ chains and WASP

(d) TRECs or T cell receptor excision circles
(e) Lymphocyte proliferation assays and cytokine production assays
(f) Miscellaneous such as Fluorescent *In Situ* Hybridization (FISH) for 22q11 deletion, enzyme assays, mutational analysis.

The panel of tests indicated in a, b and c above are excellent screening tests while panels d, e and f are for conformation and further characterization of the defect.

(a) Complete blood count, differential count and absolute lymphocyte counts. T cells are the major population, comprising 70–80% of the peripheral blood lymphocytes. Hence an absolute lymphopenia (< 3000 mm3 in an infant) is associated with T cell defect rather than a B cell deficiency disease. Maternal T cell engraftment or a residual autologous T cells in patients with CID might result in in a near normal lymphocyte count on differential count. This can be defined by flow cytometry as maternal cells are of the activated/memory phenotype CD45RO+ and there is often a paucity or absence of naïve CD45RA+ cells (Muller et al. 2001).

(b) Absence of thymic shadow or alterations of the vascular pedicle and cardiac silhouette can give a clue to clinical phenotype and diagnosis, e.g., complete DiGeorge syndrome, etc. Mediastinal and pulmonary nodules may be seen in CID and one then needs to exclude a lymphoma.

(c) Developments in flow cytometry for not only T, B and NK cells but also for subsets such as memory T cells, B cells and T regs has permitted better understanding of the defect as well as monitoring their development after immune replacement therapy. Flow cytometric analyses are an integral part of evaluation of PID. Flow cytometry for CD3, CD4. CD8, CD 45RO and CD 45RA T cells, CD 19 or 20, CD 27 and CD 16/56/57 define the various T and B cell subsets and this along with NK cell markers facilitate the diagnosis and classification of not only SCID but also many other PID syndromes. For evaluation of Hyper-IgM syndrome, flow cytometric evaluation of CD 40L on activated T cells is useful. CD 132 or the common γ chain of IL-2 receptor and CD 127, the α chain of IL-7 receptor help define genetic variants causing the SCID phenotype.

(d) TRECs or T cell receptor excision circles are circularized signal joints during VDJ recombination. They represent a byproduct of T cell maturation in the thymus. They are exported to the periphery by the newly generated T cells as they emigrate from the thymus and are enumerated by PCR. The level of TRECs in circulating lymphocytes is high in newborns and infants and indicates active thymic function. Levels decrease progressively with age and are absent or markedly decreased in SCID. Prematurity may be a confounding factor and hence TREC count has to be interpreted in the context of period of gestation. An abnormal TREC data is to be followed up with flow cytometric evaluation of T cell maturation and subsets as described above in c. The application of this as a newborn screening test from Guthrie samples is now a standard of care in many states in the US and has improved the opportunity for early stem cell/marrow transplantation with excellent outcomes. TREC data is also useful to monitor the arrival of new thymic emigrants following immune reconstitution (Routes et al. 2009).

(e) Lymphocyte proliferation to mitogens such as phytohemagglutinin (PHA), or by cross linking of T cell receptor using anti-CD3 or T cell dependent antigens such as tetanus toxoid are used to evaluate T cell function. B cell mitogens include pokeweed or antigens such as Staph. aureus Cowan strain. Proliferation assays are useful though they are limited by the number of cells available as in SCID as well as the need for age matched controls. Proliferation coupled to cytokine release assays or Cytokine ELISPOT is used to evaluate T and B cell function (Fleisher and Oliveira 2004).

(f) FISH analyses for 22q11 deletion in DiGeorge syndrome, analyses of adenosine deaminase (ADA) and Nucleoside Phosphorylase (NP), and mutational analyses of CD3 chains for T cell defects and T cell receptor (TCR) for oligoclonal expression of Vβ CDR3 is helpful in Omenn syndrome and atypical DiGeorge syndrome.

2—Tests for B cell function

The following is a cost-effective approach to evaluate B cell number and function. Panel a to e below defines the quantitative and functional aspects of B cell function, while panel f below is useful to elucidate the mechanism of the defect. They are:

(a) Review of comprehensive metabolic panel
(b) Serum protein electrophoresis (SPEP)
(c) Quantitative immunoglobulins
(d) Flow cytometry for CD 19 or 20 and CD 27. For switched memory B cells enumeration of IgD-IgM+ cells are useful. Also determinations of CD3, CD4, CD8, CD 45RO and CD 45RA T cells as they affect B cell function.
(e) Functional antibody responses are essential to determine integrity of B cell function. Specific antibodies to blood group antigens, the isohemagglutinins reflect IgM responses. Antibody titers pre- as well as post-vaccination to tetanus toxoid and pneumococcal polysaccharide and if needed H. influenza and bacteriophage Phi X 174 are useful to evaluate IgG responses (Ochs et al. 1992).
(f) B cell proliferation and assays to evaluate antibody secretion and cytokine production.

(a) Review of comprehensive metabolic panel often provides a clue to a B cell disorder. A normal serum albumin with a low total protein often draws attention to a B cell deficiency.

(b) Serum protein electrophoresis provides an integrated profile of albumen and various globulin fractions. It was the profile of a markedly decreased gamma globulin fraction on SPEP in a child with recurrent sino-pulmonary infections, which led Colonel Bruton to diagnose agammaglobulinemia and essentially integrate the laboratory basis for clinical immunodeficiency diseases. A monoclonal paraprotein or 'M spike' on an SPEP should suggest an acquired B cell disorder such as multiple myeloma or B cell lymphoma.

(c) Quantitation of serum immunoglobulins IgM, IgG, IgA and IgE and at times IgG subclasses is an integral part of the assessment of B cell functional integrity. Serum IgG and IgA levels need to be adjusted for age in infants and children. A normal or elevated level of immunoglobulins does not exclude functional defects of the B cell. Further, syndromes of B cell class switch such as Hyper IgM syndrome often manifest with an imbalance among the isotypes of immunoglobulins. IgG and IgA are often low with normal or increased IgM levels.

(d) Flow cytometry for CD 19 or 20 and CD 27 is essential for evaluating B cell diseases. Absence of class switch memory B cells that are CD27+ is associated with a more severe phenotype of CVID, often with granulomas in the lungs, lymph nodes, etc. Also useful are markers for CD3, CD4. CD8, CD 45RO and CD 45RA T cells as they affect B cell function and subtle phenotypes among B cell disorders.

(e) Antibody levels as enumerated by levels of IgG, IgA and IgM reflect the antigenicity of these molecules but not their avidity and affinity to interact with peptides as well as polysaccharide determinants of pathogens. This is best determined by evaluating functional antibody responses to T dependent as well as T independent antigens. In practice, titers for tetanus toxoid and for the 23 serotypes present in pneumovax are measured both before and 4–6 weeks after immunization with these vaccines. A fourfold rise in titer or a quantitative threshold defined for that serotype specific antibody is evaluated. Failure to achieve the threshold defined in normal subjects defines a B cell immunodeficient status.

(f) B cell proliferation as measured by pokeweed mitogen or S. aureus Cowan strain coupled to cytokine release assays or Cytokine ELISPOT is used to evaluate B cell synthesis and the secretory function. Studies of B cell signaling defects are still at the clinical research level.

3—Tests for complement function

The antigenic component of the individual complement proteins or their inhibitors is measured by nephelometry. This does not define the functional integrity of the cascade as well as do the dynamics of activation and regulation. The ability to generate molecules that activate the vascular and cellular phase of inflammation and destruction of pathogens by the terminal complement components are measured in a hemolytic assay using IgG coated sheep red cells for classical pathway (Classical CH50) or rabbit cells as the indicator cells for the alternate pathway (AH50) (Glovsky et al. 2004). Rabbit's red cells are deficient in sialic acid and hence serve as the activating surface for Factor B, Factor D and properdin. In both CH 50 and AH50 the terminal cascade beyond C3 is similar. Table 29.6 depicts the algorithm for evaluating complement deficiency.

4—Tests for phagocytic cell function

Tests to define disorders of phagocytic cells can be considered under
(1) Quantitative and morphological abnormalities and
(2) Functional abnormalities

(1) Quantitative and morphological abnormalities: It is essential to start with a complete white blood cell count, differential count and a morphological review of the peripheral smear. Multiple absolute neutrophil counts may be needed every 2 to 3 days for a 4 to 6-week period to establish a diagnosis of cyclic neutropenia. A diagnosis of Severe Congenital Neutropenia (SCN) or Kostmann syndrome is made with neutrophil counts of less than 0.5×10^6 cells per µL on several occasions. Nuclear abnormalities such as Pelger-Huet (sometimes associated with infections) or giant lysosomal granules (Chediak-Higashi syndrome) are important morphological observations. Bone marrow analysis is useful to exclude inadequate production because of neoplasia or other causes. Maturation arrest is seen in Kostmann syndrome.

(2) Functional abnormalities: Having excluded neutropenia, morphological abnormalities and bone marrow defects assays directed to determine neutrophil functions follow:

   (a) Tests for Leukocyte Adhesion Defects (LAD). LAD evaluation involves flow cytometric assessment of neutrophil adhesion molecules CD11a and CD 18 and CD 15 (sialyl—Lewis X). CD11a and CD18 are absent or reduced on neutrophils and other leukocytes in patients with LAD 1. While CD 15 is absent on neutrophils from those with LAD 2 (Oliveira et al. 2008). LAD 3 is very rare and resembles LAD 1 clinically with neurological defects as well as defects in platelet activation and bleeding tendencies due to defective activation of integrin activation. They have normal CD 18 and genetic analyses are necessary to define mutations in FERMT3 gene.

   (b) Tests for defects in oxidative burst and thus killing abnormalities. The integrity of neutrophil oxidative burst and pathways involved are best evaluated by dihydrorhodamine 123 (DHR) reduction assays by flow cytometry. The profile of flow cytograms of suspected CGD patients (and siblings) and their parents are useful to define both X-linked as well as autosomal recessive variants (Jirapongsananuruk et al. 2003). Complete G6PD deficiency also results in abnormal oxidative burst.

   (c) Tests for chemotaxis and phagocytic assays. Evaluation of directed migration of neutrophils or chemotaxis is not standardized and is only available in limited research laboratories. Historically it was studied *in vivo* by using the Rebuck skin window and *in vitro* using Boyden chamber or migration under agarose. Defects have been described in Chediak-Higashi syndrome, Pelger-Huet anomaly, LAD and rarely in juvenile periodontitis.

   (d) Tests to detect mutations in Hyper IgE and MonoMAC syndrome. Autosomal dominant mutations of STAT3 and autosomal recessive mutations of DOCK8 are associated with Hyper-IgE syndrome, while haploinsufficiency of GATA 2 is a feature of MonoMAC syndrome (Hsu et al. 2011).

5—Tests for Innate immunity

(a) Functional evaluation of NK cells.

NK cell defects manifest as recurrent herpes infection or as hemophagocytic lymphocytosis (HLH) or X linked lymphoproliferative syndrome. Testing involves immunophenotyping for CD16/CD56/57 cells and assaying for cytotoxicity against labeled K562 cells as the target. Patients with XLP1 have absent CD3+Vα24+Vβ11+ staining. Intracellular flow cytometry is used to evaluate expression of SAP (SLAM associated protein) XIAP (X-linked inhibitor of apoptosis), the proteins defective in XLP1 and XLP 2 respectively (Marsh et al. 2009).

Low intracellular perforin expression, as determined by flow cytometry, is useful to diagnose HLH2. Other HLH variants have decreased expression of CD 107a (LAMP1 or lysosomal associated membrane protein 1) on NK cells after activation and this indicates the presence of mutations in MUNC 13-14 and syntaxin.

(b) Evaluation of IL-12/23-IFN-γ pathways.

Defects in IL-12 production can be tested by evaluating IL-12 production in response to *ex vivo* stimulation of mononuclear cells with LPS and IFN-γ. Defects in genes coding for IFN-γ receptor 1 and 2 and IL-12 R can be evaluated by flow cytometry using monoclonal antibody for these receptors. Monocyte STAT 1 phosphorylation, either by flow cytometry or Western blotting, can be studied *ex vivo* in response to IFN-γ (Fleischer et al. 1999).

(c) Tests to evaluate Toll-like receptor and NFκB signaling defects.

Stimulating mononuclear cells with specific TLR ligands and measuring cytokine production is used as a screening test followed by direct sequencing of the suspected mutant gene involved in that pathway.

Laboratory features and genetic mutations causing distinctive immune dysregulation syndromes are indicated in Table 29.4. These defects are confirmed by sequencing the implicated gene and analyzing for mutations.

Treatment

Advances in genetic tests have facilitated identification of the molecular defects in many PID syndromes. However, it is important to recognize that in some cases (e.g., patients with SCID); the urgency of the condition might require that patients be treated in time and aggressively, to avoid complications and better outcomes, even if elucidation of the genetic is pending.

For SCID and CID: Infants with a suspicion of SCID or CID require the following prompt intervention to not only avoid infectious complications but also improve outcomes of more definitive immune reconstitution. These include:

(a) Use of cotrimoxazole to prevent Pneumocystis infection, appropriate antifungal therapy, antibiotics and immunoglobulin replacement therapy
(b) Only irradiated and filtered blood products should be used in SCID because of the high risk of Graft-Versus-Host (GVH) reaction and transmission of CMV infection
(c) Live attenuated viral vaccines must be avoided to prevent vaccine-associated infections
(d) Immune suppression mitigates the inflammatory reactions associated with Omenn syndrome
(e) Nutritional support and concomitant care of cardiac anomalies forms an integral part of care

Hematopoietic Cell Transplant (HCT) provides the opportunity for permanent cure in SCID and CID syndromes. When performed from an HLA-identical sibling, HCT can allow greater than 90% long term survival and sustained immune reconstitution (Antoine et al. 2003). HCT from a HLA-mismatched related donor provides excellent results when performed in the first 3.5 months of life. The outcome is less satisfactory in older infants (Buckley 2004). The results are less optimistic when the donor is HLA matched but unrelated.

In severe form of CID, other than SCID, such as Omenn syndrome, HLA class II deficiency, residual autologous T cells may cause immune dysregulation and need judicious use of immunosuppression.

Gene therapy has been effective in immune reconstitution in patients with ADA deficiency and X linked SCID, but clonal proliferative disease in some due to insertional mutagenesis has led to a reappraisal of the vectors for more safety (Aluti et al. 2009).

Enzyme replacement therapy for ADA, thymic transplants for DiGeorge syndrome has been successful (Notarangelo 2010).

Treatment of antibody deficiency syndromes

Since the observation of Bruton in 1952 that immunoglobulins are beneficial in decreasing infections and its attendant complications, therapy with gamma globulin preparations has seen great improvements in the preparation as well as mode of delivery. In fact, they continue to be the fulcrum in the management of antibody deficiency syndromes. Immunoglobulin replacement therapy can be performed with intravenous (IVIG) or subcutaneous (SCIG) preparations. Both are effective in reducing incidence of pyogenic, encapsulated bacterial infections. The usual dose of IVIG is 400–600 mg/kg every 3 weeks, but the dose has to be titrated so as to provide protection from infections. Higher doses are needed in those with bronchiectasis, viral meningoencephalitis or during an acute exacerbation or associated autoimmune diseases. SCIG is administered at the dose of 100 mk/kg/week and could be given 2 or 3 times a week and at 1 or 2 sites. SCIG has the advantage of sustaining more stable IgG levels, lower rate of systemic side effects and aseptic meningitis. IVIG can be used in acute infections to boost serum IgG levels as well as when larger doses are needed as in autoimmune cytopenia (Berger 2008). Newer preparations include 10% solutions, greater stability at room temperature and use of hyaluronic acid to facilitate subcutaneous administration of larger doses without local side effects. Continuous antibiotic prophylaxis has been used in those with severe bronchiectasis and refractory sinusitis.

Treatment of neutrophil defects

Disorders of neutrophils require appropriate use of antibiotics and antifungals. Cotrimoxazole and itraconazole are very useful in treating patients with CGD as they are prone to aspergillus infections. γ-interferon has reduced infections in CGD patients. Gene therapy and HCT have been used in treating CGD with varying outcome. For LAD HCT is the treatment of choice. Recombinant G-CSF has been used successfully in severe congenital neutropenia (Notarangelo 2010).

Treatment of rarer syndromes

Wiscott-Aldrich syndrome is treated with antibiotics, immunoglobulin replacement therapy and avoidance of trauma associated bleeding. HCT from a HLA-identical donor provides the best chance of correction of the defect. Familial forms of HLH and those with IPEX benefit from HCT. In the X-linked immunoproliferative syndrome immunosuppressive agents are useful while massive splenectomy may be needed in ALPS syndrome (Notarangelo 2010). Advances in gene therapy hold the promise for immune reconstitution in the future.

Conclusion

Understanding of immunobiology and advances in molecular diagnostics have resulted in earlier diagnoses of immunodeficiency syndromes. Understanding the pathogenesis and clinical recognition are the key to the evaluation and therapy of this large and heterogeneous group of diseases. This chapter explores this emerging field and lessons learnt will influence understanding and therapy of infectious, autoimmune and malignant diseases.

References

Aiuti A, Cattaneo F, Galimberti S, Benninghoff U, Cassani B, Callegaro L, et al. Gene therapy for immunodeficiency due to adenosine deaminase deficiency. N Engl J Med 2009; 360: 447–458.

Al-Muhsen S, Cassonova JL. The genetic heterogeneity of mendelian susceptibility to mycobacterial diseases. J Allergy Clin Immunol 2008; 122: 1043–1051.

Antoine C, Müller S, Cant A, Cavazzana-Calvo M, Veys P, Vossen J, et al Long-term survival and transplantation of hematopoietic stem cells for immunodeficiencies: report of the European experience 1968–1999. Lancet 2003; 361: 552–560.

Berger M. Subcutaneous administration of IgG. Immunol Allergy Clin North Am 2008; 28: 779–802.

Buckley RH. Molecular defects in human severe combined immunodeficiency and approaches to immune reconstitution. Annu Rev Immunol 2004; 22: 625–655.

Casrouge A, Zhang SY, Eidenschenk C, Jouanguy E, Puel A, Yang K, et al. Herpes simplex viral encephalitis in human UNC-93B deficiency. Science 2006; 314: 308–312.

Caudy AA, Reddy ST, Chatila T, Atkinson JP, Verbsky JW. CD 25 deficiency causes an immune dysregulation, polyendocrinopathy, enteropathy, X linked-like syndrome, and defective IL-10 expression from CD4 lymphocytes. J Allergy Clin Immunol 2007; 119: 482–487.

Cepika AM, Sato Y, Liu JM, Uyeda J, Bacchetti R, Roncarlo MG. Tregopathies: Monogenic diseases resulting in regulatory T cell deficiency. J Allergy Clin Immunol 2018; 142: 1679–1695.

Chapel H, Lucas M, Lee M, Bjorkander J, Webster D, Grimbacher B, et al. Common variable immunodeficiency disorders: division into distinct clinical phenotypes. Blood 2008; 112: 277–286.

Chapel H, Cunningham-Rundles C. Update in understanding common variable immunodeficiency disorders (CVIDs) and the management of patients with these conditions. Br J Haematol 2009; 145: 709–727.

Conley ME, Dobbs AK, Farmer DM, Kilic S, Paris K, Grigoriadou S, et al. Primary B cell immunodeficiencies: comparisons and contrasts. Ann Rev Immunol 2009; 27: 199–227.

Cunningham-Rundles C. Clinical and immunological analyses of 103 patients with common variable immunodeficiency. J Clin Immunol 1989; 9: 22–33.

Fischer A, Le Deist F, Hacein-Bey-Abina S, André-Schmutz I, Basile Gde S, de Villartay JP, et al. Severe combined immunodeficiency > A model disease for molecular immunology and therapy. Immunol. Rev 2005; 203: 98–109.

Flajnik M. A cold-blooded view of adaptive immunity. Nat. Rev. Immunol 2018; 18: 438–453.

Fleisher TA, Dorman SE, Anderson JA, Vail M, Brown MR, Holland SM. Detection of intracellular phosphorylated STAT-1 by flow cytometry. Clin Immunol 1999; 90: 425–430.

Fleisher TA, Oliveira JB. Functional and molecular evaluation of lymphocytes. J Allergy Clin Immunol 2004: 114: 227–235.

Geha RS, Notarangelo LD, Cassanova JL, Chapel H, Conley ME, Fischer A et al. Primary immunodeficiency disease: an update from the International Union of Immunological Societies Primary Immunodeficiency Diseases Classification Committee. J Allergy Clin Immunol 2007; 120: 774–794.

Glovsky MM, Ward PA, Johnson KJ. Complement determinations in human disease. Ann Allergy Asthma Immunol 2004; 93: 513–522.

Hsu AP, Sampaio EP, Khan J, Calvo KR, Lemieux JE, Patel SY, et al. Mutations in GATA2 is associated with the autosomal dominant and sporadic monocytopenia and mycobacterial infection (MonoMAC) syndrome. Blood 2011; 118: 2653–2655.

Huizing M, Helip-Wooley A, Westbroek W, Gunay-Aygun M, Gahl WA. Disorders of lysosome-related organelle biogenesis: clinical and molecular genetics. Annu Rev Genomics Hum Genet 2008; 9: 359–386.

Jirapongsananuruk O, Malech HL, Kuhns DB, Niemela JE, Brown MR, Anderson-Cohen M, et al. Diagnostic paradigm for evaluation of male patients with chronic granulomatous disease based on the dihydrorhodamine 123 assay. J Allergy Clin Immunol 2003; 111: 374–379.

Kaplan J, De Dominico I, Ward DM. Chediak-Higashi syndrome. Current Opin Hematol 2008: 15: 22–29.

Lagresle-Peyrou C, Six EM, Picard C, Rieux-Laucat F, Michel V, Ditadi A, et al. Human adenylate kinase 2 deficiency causes a profound hematopoietic defect associated with sensorineural deafness. Nat Genet 2009; 41: 106–111.

Lekstrom-Himes JA and Gallin J. N Engl J Med 2000; 343: 1703–1714.

Lu HY, Biggs C, Blanchard-Rohner G, Fung SY, Sharma M, Turvey SE. Germline CBM opathies: From immunodeficiency to atopy. J Allergy Clin Immunol 2019; 143: 1661–1673.

Marsh RA, Villanueva J, Zhang K, Snow AL, Su HC, Madden L, et al. A rapid flow cytometric screening test for X-linked lymphoproliferative disease due to XIAP deficiency. Cyometry B Clin Cytom 2009; 76: 334–344.

Moraes-Vasconcelos D, Costa-Carvalho BT, Torgerson TR, Ochs HD. Primary immune deficiency disorders presenting as autoimmune diseases: IPEX and APECED. J Clin Immunol 2008; 28(suppl 1): S11–19.

Müller SM, Ege M, Pottharst A, Schulz AS, Schwarz K, Friedrich W. Transplacentally acquired maternal T lymphocytes in severe combined immunodeficiency: a study of 121 patients. Blood 2001; 98: 1847–1851.

Notarangelo LD, Gambineri E, Badalato R. Immunodeficiencies with autoimmune consequences. Adv Immunol 2006; 89: 321–370.

Notarangelo LD. Primary immunodeficiencies. J Allergy Clin Immunol 2010; 125: S 182–194.

Nunes-Santos CJ, Uzel G, Rosenzweig BD. PI3K pathway defects in immunodeficiency and immune dysregulation. J Allergy Clin Immunol 2019; 143: 1676–1687.

Ochs HD, Buckley RH, Kobayashi RH, Kobayashi AL, Sorensen RU, Douglas SD, et al. Antibody responses to bacteriophage phi X174 in patients with adenosine deaminase deficiency. Blood 1992; 80: 1163–1171.

Oliveira JM, Notarangelo LD, Fleischer TA. Applications of flow cytometry for the study of primary immunodeficiencies. Curr Opin Allergy Clin Immunol 2008; 8: 499–509.

O'Shea JJ, Paul WE. Mechanisms underlying lineage commitment and plasticity of CD4+ T cells. Science 2010; 327: 1098–1102.

O'Sullivan MD and Cant A. The 10 warning signs: a time for a change. Curr Opin Allergy Clin Immunol 2012; 12: 588–594.

Routes JM, Grossman WJ, Verbsky J, Laessig RH, Hoffman GL, Brokopp CD, et al. State wide newborn screening for severe T cell lymphopenia. JAMA 2009; 302: 2465–2470.

Unsworth DJ. Complement deficiency and disease. J Clin Pathol 2008; 61: 1013–1017.

Von Boehmer H. Selection of the T cell repertoire: receptor-controlled checkpoints in T cell development. Adv Immunol 2004; 84: 201–238.

von Bernuth H, Picard C, Jin Z, Pankla R, Xiao H, Ku CL, et al. Pyogenic bacterial infection in humans with MyD88 deficiency. Science 2008; 321: 691–696.

Wehr C, Kivioja T, Schmitt C, Ferry B, Witte T, Eren E, et al. The EURO class trial: defining subgroups in common variable immunodeficiency. Blood 2008; 111: 77–85.

Wilson A, Trumpp A. Bone marrow hematopoietic stem cell niches. Nature Immunol Rev 205; 6: 93–107.

30

Integrative Allergy and Asthma for Traditional Practice

William S Silvers[1] *and Heidi Bailey*[2,*]

Experienced physicians and extended healthcare providers always consider the whole patient, not just the specific complaints or diseases they present. So goes the adage that a good physician knows the disease, but a great physician knows the patient. While this holistic approach incorporates the art and science of patient care, more tools are needed to care for our patients today given the popularity of the so called Complementary and Alternative Medicines (CAM). To address the spectrum of CAM available to the patient with allergies and asthma, health history intake forms have recently been developed and published. See Table 30.1 (George et al. 2018).

Treatment of allergy and asthma can drastically improve quality of life for patients. Although there are many very effective conventional treatments for allergies and asthma, people continue to seek out alternative methods of treatment due to lack of symptom control (Shen and Oraka 2012), therapy side effects or access and cost of medications. Whatever the reasons may be, it is important to know about these alternative modalities and which ones have an evidence basis of being safe and effective therapeutic approaches. Additionally, one should always keep in mind 'primum non-nocere'—'first, do no harm'. Ever mindful of the 'placebo effect' of any positive action for the patient, one should keep this benefit as a resourceful tool for patient care and monitor the effects of the complementary and alternative medicine (CAM) modalities separately.

This chapter is devoted to describing an 'integrative' approach to allergies and asthma, integrating complementary modalities with evidence based recommendations within a conventional western practice (Silvers 2003). By employing an integrative approach to treating your patients, you address their physical and emotional needs which are all fundamental to optimal health and wellness.

The National Center for Complementary Integrative Health (NCCIH) previously the National Center for Complementary and Alternative Medicine (NCCAM) at the US National Institutes of Health defines (CAM) as a group of diverse medical and health care systems, practices, and products that are not generally considered part of conventional medicine (Anon. 2017).

While there are numerous modalities that comprise complementary and alternative medicine, for simplicity, they can roughly be divided into six broad categories: lifestyle therapies/environmental factors, dietary management, mind-body interventions, energy therapies, manipulative/body-based methods and alternative medical systems.

---

[1] 6807 E. Archer Dr., Denver, CO 80230, Email: Skiersnoz@silversmd.com
[2] 7180 E. Orchard Rd. Suite 107, Greenwood Village, CO 80111.
* Corresponding author: Heidib@coloradoallergy.com

Table 30.1. The integrative medicine index of natural products. This is a patient-reported overview of common natural products highlighted on the NCCIH and NIH Medline Plus: Herbal Medicine websites.

Integrative Medicine Index of Natural Products (Patient Administered)		
Name:	Date of Birth:	
Allergies:		
☐ Acai	☐ Eucalyptus	☐ Pomegranate
☐ Alfalfa	☐ European elder/Elderberry	☐ Probiotics
☐ Aloe	☐ European mistletoe	☐ Propolis
☐ Aloe vera	☐ Evening primrose oil	☐ Pycnogenol
☐ Aristolochic acids	☐ Fenugreek	☐ Red Clover
☐ Asian ginseng	☐ Feverfew	☐ Red yeast or red yeast rice
☐ Astragalus	☐ Fish oil	☐ Roman chamomile
☐ Bacillus coagulans	☐ Flaxseed or flaxseed oil	☐ Saccharomyces boulardii
☐ Belladonna	☐ Folate or folic acid	☐ S-adenosyl L-methionine (SAMe)
☐ Bifidobacteria	☐ Garlic	☐ Sage
☐ Bilberry	☐ Ginger	☐ Saw palmetto
☐ Biotin	☐ Ginkgo	☐ Selenium
☐ Bitter orange	☐ Ginseng, American	☐ Senna
☐ Black cohosh	☐ Ginseng, Panax	☐ Soy
☐ Black psyllium	☐ Ginseng, Siberian	☐ St. John's Wort
☐ Black tea	☐ Glucosamine hydrochloride	☐ Sun's Soup (selected vegetables)
☐ Bladderwrack	☐ Glucosamine sulfate	☐ Tea tree oil
☐ Blessed thistle	☐ Goldenseal	☐ Thunder god vine
☐ Blond psyllium	☐ Grape seed extract	☐ Turmeric
☐ Blueberry	☐ Green tea	☐ Valerian
☐ Blue-green algae	☐ Hawthorn	☐ Vitamin A
☐ Boron	☐ Hoodia	☐ Vitamin B-1 (thiamine)
☐ Bromelain	☐ Horse chestnut	☐ Vitamin B-2 (riboflavin)
☐ Butterbur	☐ Horsetail	☐ Vitamin B-3 (niacin)
☐ Calcium	☐ Hydrazine sulfate	☐ Vitamin B-5 (pantothenic acid)
☐ Calendula	☐ Iodine	☐ Vitamin B-6 (pyridoxine)
☐ Cancell/Cantron/Protocel	☐ Iron	☐ Vitamin B12
☐ Cartilage (bovine or shark)	☐ Kava	☐ Vitamin C (ascorbic acid)
☐ Cassia	☐ Lactobacillus	☐ Vitamin D
☐ Cat's Claw	☐ Laetrile/amygdalin	☐ Vitamin E
☐ Chamomile	☐ L-arginine	☐ Vitamin K
☐ Chasteberry	☐ Lavender	☐ Wild Yam
☐ Chondroitin sulfate	☐ Licorice	☐ Yohimbe
☐ Chromium	☐ Licorice root	☐ Zinc
☐ Cinnamon	☐ Lycium	☐ 5-HTP (oxitriptan)
☐ Clove	☐ Lycopene	Other:
☐ Coenzyme Q10	☐ Magnesium	
☐ Colloidal silver products	☐ Manganese	

Table 30.1 contd. ...

...Table 30.1 contd.

☐ Cranberry	☐ Melatonin	
☐ Creatine	☐ Milk thistle	
☐ Dandelion	☐ Mistletoe extracts	
☐ Devil's clas	☐ Noni	
☐ DHEA	☐ Passionflower	
☐ Dong quai	☐ PC-SPES	
☐ Echinacea	☐ Pennyroyal	
☐ Ephedra	☐ Peppermint	
☐ Essiac/Flor-essence	☐ Phosphate salts	

Lifestyle therapies and environmental factors

There are environmental and lifestyle changes that can be made to help decrease the burden of asthma and allergy symptoms. Trying to provide modifications to the environment to limit exposure to triggers can be helpful for both asthma and rhinitis. Irritants that can worsen asthma and rhinitis symptoms include indoor and outdoor air pollution, smoking (cigarette, e-cigarette, hookah, bidi), animal dander, dust mites and pollen (Aggarwal et al. 2006, Clapp and Jaspers 2017).

Indoor air may be improved by using clean burning fuels. There are several studies that link an increased incidence of asthma and breathing symptoms with indoor cooking utilizing combustible biomass fuels (Aggarwal et al. 2006, Po et al. 2011, Barry et al. 2010, Mishra 2003). Smoke is an irritant and smoking, in any form, should be avoided for both prevention and treatment of asthma (Aggarwal et al. 2006, Diette et al. 2008, Clapp and Jaspers 2017). High-Efficiency Particulate Air (HEPA) filters may also useful for removing indoor air pollutants. There is some controversy on their effectiveness on impacting allergy and asthma symptoms (Reisman 2001, Sublett 2011, Warburton et al. 1994, Sulser et al. 2009, Wood et al. 1998). The cleaning of indoor surfaces with a dilute bleach solution can decrease mold and bacteria, denature allergenic proteins in dust, and was associated with improved quality of life scores in children with asthma (Barnes et al. 2008). The humidity of indoor environments would ideally be maintained at less than 50% (Evans 1992, German and Harper 2002).

Other environmental modifications are targeted at animal and pest control. Keeping animals out of the sleeping area can be beneficial for minimizing animal dander exposures (Bush 2008, Chapman and Wood 2001, Eggleston 2001). Encasements of bedding, pillows and mattresses in allergen proof material may be helpful for limiting dust mite exposure. Frequent washing of linen in hot water, greater than 58°C, can decrease exposure to dust mite antigen (Evans 1992, Eggleston 2001). Utilizing pest control measures to minimize cockroaches in indoor areas are also important for persons who are sensitized (German and Harper 2002, Bush 2008, Eggleston 2001).

Prolonged exposure to outdoor air pollution should be avoided. There is evidence that increases in particulates, nitrogen dioxide and ozone levels are related to increases in the incidence of asthma and asthma exacerbations (Bontinck et al. 2020). Minimizing cardiovascular activities on days of increased pollution and wearing a particulate filtering mask may also be helpful (German and Harper 2002, Laumbach 2010).

Nasal saline irrigation originates from the Hindu practice of Ayurveda. The use of nasal saline irrigation utilizing sterile, distilled or previously boiled water to make an isotonic or hypertonic saline solution for nasal washes may be helpful for moisturizing the nasal passages, removing nasal debris, thinning nasal mucus and increasing mucociliary clearance (Khianey and Oppenheimer 2012).

There is evidence that exercise can significantly benefit asthma patients (Eichenberger et al. 2013). There are also indications that it will benefit patients with seasonal allergies. Two-hundred-eighty clinicians participated in a WAO cross sectional worldwide survey, in which 40% strongly believed exercise improved allergic rhinitis control and 30% largely agreed that it reduces allergic rhinitis incidence (Moreira et al. 2014).

There is a connection between psychological stress and asthma. Although it is difficult to determine and study stress levels in patients, there are studies that have examined this connection (de Marco et al. 2012, Kozyrskyj et al. 2008, Quon and Goss 2012, Wright 2007, Ritz 2012, Dave et al. 2011, Kiecolt-Glaser et al. 2009, Marshall 2011a, Marshall 2011b, Marshall and Agarwal 2000, Marshall 2004a, Marshall 2004b). Studies examining maternal psychological stress, found that *in utero* stresses may increase future development of asthma. The pathophysiology of psychosocial stressors and their role in asthma have been studied, and although they are not entirely understood, there appears to be connections with asthma and the neuroendocrine pathway (Wright 2007, Marshall 2004a, Marshall and Agarwal 2000). Studies have demonstrated that stress causes changes in immune regulation including a shift from type-1 to type-2 cytokine predominance (Marshall and Agarwal 2000). Additionally, both vagal excitation and ventilation effects are involved as likely physiological pathways between stress and asthma (Marshall and Agarwal 2000, Ritz 2012). Since psychological stress seems to play a role in asthma, stress management via alternative methods may be helpful for patients.

Dietary management and supplementation

The effect of diet on the development of asthma and allergic diseases has been studied, such as maternal diets in pregnancy and associations with the later development of allergy and asthma in progeny (Castro-Rodriguez et al. 2008, Chatzi and Kogevinas 2009, Chatzi et al. 2008, Lange et al. 2010, Allan et al. 2015). Low levels of vitamin D and E in maternal diets were associated with an increased incidence of asthma by the age of 10 years-old in the offspring (Allan et al. 2015). Adherence to a Mediterranean diet, rich in fruits, vegetables, legumes, nuts, cereals, fish and low in red meat, margarine and junk food, may not only have general health benefits, but may also be protective against future atopic diseases in offspring (Chatzi and Kogevinas 2009, Chatzi et al. 2008, Lange et al. 2010). Children, adolescents, and adults all seem to benefit from decreased asthma symptoms and allergic rhinitis when a Mediterranean type diet is followed (Castro-Rodriguez et al. 2008, Ellwood et al. 2013, Scott et al. 2012).

There is evidence that breastfeeding may help prevent eczema and asthma in infants (Oddy 2017). In highly allergic families, having breast feeding mothers on a low allergenic diet or using extensively hydrolyzed formula may be helpful to decrease the risk of future asthma for infants (Protudjer et al. 2012). Water intake should be encouraged up to one-half to one ounce of water per pound body weight, depending on size, activity level and where you live. Keep the respiratory mucosal surfaces moist.

Gastroesophageal reflux disease (GERD) may be a confounding disorder with asthma. There is debate about the treatment of GERD with Proton Pump Inhibitors (PPI) in asthma, but it has been recommended that a trial of a PPI be used if asthma is not responding to standard treatment if GERD severity scores reach 10% or greater (Sopo et al. 2009). If there is no improvement in asthma symptoms after PPI treatment and no symptoms of regurgitation the PPI should be discontinued (Naik and Vaezi 2015).

Nutritional avoidance of highly processed foods and minimizing dairy intake to decrease mucus production are popular approaches with great anecdotal testimonial, even in patients without lactose intolerance. Elimination of wheat may be worth a trial with subsequent re-challenge.

Nutritional enhancement with foods high in omega-3 fatty acids (i.e., cold-water fish like salmon, mackerel), yogurt, fruits and vegetable may be helpful (Giovannini et al. 2007).

Patients with asthma have decreased levels of circulating antioxidants rendering them more susceptible to the damaging effects of oxidative stress (Wood and Gibson 2010). Therefore, integrative therapy has been aimed at supplementing and augmenting a patient's ability to negate the effects of free radical damage.

Supplements with good evidence to support their use are the probiotics-Lactobacillus GG given in pregnancy and infancy-1-10 billion units TID to QID 2–4 week's pre delivery and to continue 3–6 months during breastfeeding (Das 2012, Kalliomaki et al. 2003, Kalliomaki et al. 2007). There is also evidence to support the use of lactobacillus in the treatment of allergic rhinitis (Güvenç et al. 2016).

Multivitamins and Vitamin C have been recommended but there is conflicting evidence regarding their efficacy in treatment of asthma and allergic rhinitis.

The role of Vitamin D has received great attention recently, with low serum levels correlating with worsening asthma (Wu et al. 2012). A supplementation of Vitamin D has been shown to be of value in children with asthma, and evidence is accumulating in adults. Vitamin D3 2000+ IU daily can be given to achieve good serum levels.

The form of vitamin E found primarily in food (gamma-tocopherol) increased lung inflammation in induced asthma, while the form of vitamin E found primarily in dietary supplements (alpha-tocopherol) reduced inflammation, so while supplementation may be helpful, firm recommendations can not be made (Berdnikovs et al. 2009).

Potential therapies for asthma

- *Caffeine:* Is a natural bronchodilator, similar to the asthma medication theophylline, and can be found in coffee, tea, cocoa, and cola-drinks. Its use can improve lung functioning and symptomatic relief for several hours (Welsh et al. 2010).
- *Beta-carotene:* Gives orange coloring to many fruits and vegetables, most notably cantaloupe, mangos, papayas, orange root vegetables (i.e., carrots, yams, sweet potatoes) and can be protective against exercise-induced asthma (Neuman et al. 1999).
- *Choline:* Found in eggs, cauliflower, spinach, amaranth and soy products, and its supplementation was found to decrease asthma symptoms (Mehta et al. 2010) as well as reduce medication usage (Gupta and Gaur 1997). Choline's proposed mechanism of action is lower lysophosphatidylcholine levels, which has anti-inflammatory effects. Caution: May cause sweating, GI distress.
- *Fish Oil* (Fig. 30.1): Contains Omega 3 fatty acids which have anti-inflammatory properties that have been shown to have potential use in both treatment and prevention of asthma (Okamoto et al. 2000, Hodge et al. 1998, Mickleborough et al. 2004).
- *Magnesium sulfate:* Can be helpful as an adjunct to corticosteroids, inhaled beta-agonists in severe acute asthma exacerbations, but has not been shown to be helpful at baseline (Powell 2014).
- *Pycnogenol:* The active ingredient derived from the bark of Pinus pinaster tree when used as an adjunct to management in mild-to-moderate childhood asthma was shown to increase pulmonary functions, to decrease asthma symptoms including reduction or cessation of rescue inhaler use and decreased urinary levels of leukotrienes when compared to placebo (Lau et al. 2004). Caution: not recommended for patients with autoimmune disorders.

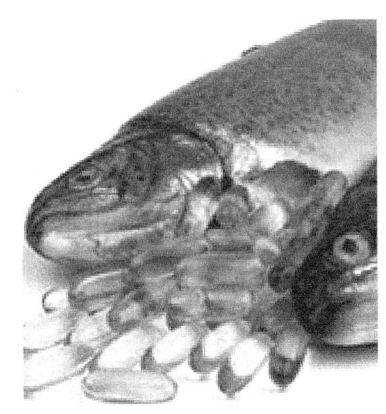

Figure 30.1 Fish oil.

Potential therapies for allergic rhinitis

- *Butterbur (Petasiteshybridus)* (Fig. 30.2): Has an inhibitory effect on leukotrienes and histamine synthesis (Thomet et al. 2002). Shown to be as effective as cetirizine (Schapowal 2002) and fexofenadine. Caution: may not be appropriate for patients Ragweed allergic.

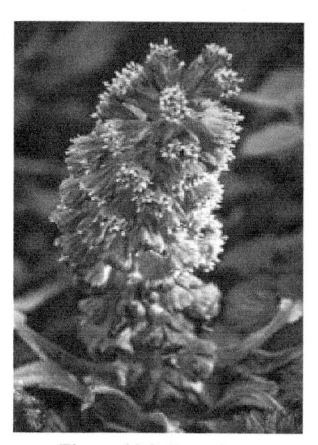

Figure 30.2 Butterbur.

- *Capsicum* (Fig. 30.3): Contains the active ingredient of capsaicin within its fruit of the chili pepper, which sensitizes mucus membrane and blocks substance P, a neuropeptide implicated in inflammation and bronchospasm (Valencia and Randazzo 1992) as well as pain. Effects of capsaicin include increased mucus production aiding the body to flush out bacteria and vasodilation of vessels. Caution: potential interaction with anticoagulants and theophylline. Oral use of capsaicin can cause sweating, flushing, salvation, lacrimation (Bernstein et al. 2011).
- *Other potential therapies: Milk thistle, Phleum pretense, Tinosporacordifolia*

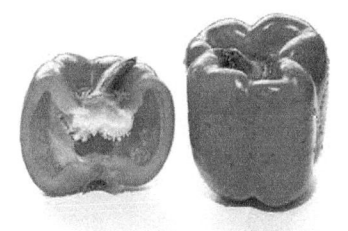

Figure 30.3 Capsicum.

Mind-body interventions

Mind body interventions use a variety of techniques to enhance the mind's capacity to affect bodily functions and symptoms, such as patient support groups, cognitive-behavioral therapy, meditation and yoga.

Meditation and yoga are examples used in asthma management. It is known that stress and anxiety can increase the skin tests wheal response, and therefore may enhance and prolong the allergic symptoms (Kiecolt-Glaser et al. 2009). Stress also increases morbidity in asthma patients and therefore is an important factor to address when treating patients (Turyk et al. 2008). Mind-body therapies are powerful tools for stress management.

When added to standard asthma management, yoga improved patients' sense of well-being and exercise tolerance, decreased rescue inhaler use, but did not improve pulmonary functions (Vedanthan et al. 1998). However, there is conflicting evidence and data is still lacking to support yoga as an effective treatment for asthma (Burgess et al. 2011).

Other mind and body practices include a review of research on specific breathing techniques—the Papworth Method and Buteyko Breathing Technique found a trend toward improvement in asthma symptoms (Holloway and West 2007) but not enough evidence to draw reliable conclusions.

Energy therapies

Energy medicine and therapies are other modalities of alternative medicine that manipulate unbalanced energy fields within the body in order to treat illness and restore health (Anon. 2017, Clinic 2010). Acupuncture, magnetic therapy, qi gong, reiki and therapeutic touch are some of the modalities utilized in energy medicine.

Acupuncture

Acupuncture is one of the one of the key components of traditional Chinese medicine, and is among the oldest healing practices in the world. While a few studies showed some reduction in medication use and improvements in symptoms and quality of life (Tan et al. 2012), at this point, there is insufficient evidence that acupuncture is an effective treatment for asthma.

Manipulative and body-based methods

Manipulative and body-based therapeutic methods include spinal manipulation, mobilization, massage and reflexology. These therapies aim to optimize biomechanical functioning which can ultimately affect somatic, visceral and neurologic processes in the body (Wainapel and Fast 2003). Specifically, when applied to the asthmatic patient, these therapies try to improve rib cage movement to maximize lung functioning and circulation. Additionally, manual techniques like chest tapping, shaking and vibration are thought to facilitate phlegm movement out of the respiratory tract. However, there is not currently enough data to recommend manual therapies for asthma (Hondras et al. 2005).

Alternative medical systems

Alternative medical systems are complete systems of medical theory and practice that developed over time throughout different cultures that are distinct from conventional or western medicine. **Ayurvedic medicine and traditional Chinese medicine are whole medical systems that were developed centuries ago. More contemporary examples of whole medical systems include** homeopathy and naturopathy (Anon. 2017).

Traditional Chinese medicine

In recent years, Traditional Chinese Medicine (TCM), a mainstay in eastern medicine practiced for more than 2,000 years, has been under investigation by the FDA for its efficacy, safety, and role in western medicine as a complementary treatment. TCM integrates herbal therapy, acupuncture, acupressure/massage, mind-body therapy and dietary therapy (Anon. 2017).

The central philosophy of TCM varies significantly from that of western Medicine, as the human being is regarded as a microcosm of the universe and is therefore affected by its forces. Additionally, TCM regards the human body as an integrated system comprised of individual organs and tissues that are all interdependent on one another. Therefore, balance between each component is essential for maintaining a person's health (Anon. 2017).

Chinese herbal medicine is one of the most commonly used therapies from TCM. It is a modality that utilizes extracts of plants, minerals and animal products combined into formulas, teas, capsules, tinctures or powders (Anon. 2017). Studies of specific TCM herbal interventions have yielded exciting results for the treatment of asthma and allergy.

The herbal formula, ASHMI (antiasthma herbal medicine intervention), containing *Ganodermalucidum, Sophoraflavescentis* and *Glycyrrhizauralensis*, is one of the few TCM remedies with reliable evidence in the treatment of asthma. While ASHMI's exact mechanism of action is largely unknown, it has shown to reduce the use of rescue inhalers, suppress IgE and Th2 responses, decrease IFN-γ and cortisol levels, and improve lung functions (FEV_1 and PEV) without causing adrenal suppression when compared to treatment with inhaled steroids All of the trials found therapy with ASHMI to be safe and well tolerated (Kelly-Pieper 2009).

TCM and food allergy herbal formula-2 (FAHF-2) has been investigated in human clinical trials for its safety profile and efficacy in treating food allergies (Wang and Li 2012, Wang et al. 2015) which currently have no conventional treatment.

While TCM offers promising results as complementary and alternative therapies to asthma and allergy management, much data and evidence is still needed to prove its safety and efficacy.

Conclusion

Ultimately, integrative medicine or CAM, provides clinicians and patients with additional options for treatment and control of allergic diseases. Many patients have an interest in utilizing complementary modalities to find relief from their allergic symptoms. It is important for us to know what our patients are using in regard to natural products and patient administered forms can provide a rapid form of that information. Although there remains much in the way of scientific evidence to support CAM modalities as safe and reliable therapeutic options, it is our job to be aware of their effects and proper role in asthma and allergic rhinitis management. In listening to our patients concerns with traditional medications, lack of symptom control and realizing concerns about medication costs or side effects we can have meaningful conversations with our patients and come to mutually agreeable care plans. This can provide a great amount of satisfaction for both patients and health care providers and ultimately lead to better control of our patients allergic disorders.

References

Aggarwal AN, Chaudhry K, Chhabra SK, D'Souza GA, Gupta D, Jindal SK, et al. Prevalence and risk factors for bronchial asthma in Indian adults: a multicentre study. Indian J Chest Dis Allied Sci 2006; 48(1): 13–22.

Allan KM, Prabhu N, Craig LC, McNeill G, Kirby B, McLay JP. Maternal vitamin D and E intakes during pregnancy are associated with asthma in children. Eur Respir J 2015; 45(4): 1027–36.

Anon. nccih. [Online] Available at: www.nccih.nih.gov/health/asthma/facts [Accessed 21 November 2019] 2017.

Anon. n.d. What Is Complementary and Alternative Medicine? [Online] Available at: http://nccam.nih.gov/health/whatiscam#informed [Accessed 29 Jan 2013].

Barnes CS, Kennedy K, Gard L, Forrest E, Johnson L, Pacheco F, et al. The impact of home cleaning on quality of life for homes with asthmatic children. Allergy Asthma Proc 2008; 29(2): 197–204.

Barry AC, Mannino DM, Hopenhayn C, Bush H. Exposure to indoor biomass fuel pollutants and asthma prevalence in Southeastern Kentucky: results from the Burden of Lung Disease (BOLD) study. J Asthma 2010; 47(7): 735–741.

Berdnikovs S, Abdala-Valencia H, McCary C, Somand M, Cole R, Garcia A, et al. Isoforms of vitamin E have opposing immunoregulatory functions during inflammation by regulating leukocyte recruitment. J Immunol 2009; 182(7): 4395–4405.

Bernstein JA, Davis BP, Picard JK, Cooper JP, Zheng S, Levin LS.A randomized, double-blind, parallel trial comparing capsaicin nasal spray with placebo in subjects with a significant component of nonallergic rhinitis. Ann Allergy Asthma Immunol 2011; 107(2): 171–178.

Bontinck A, Maesand T, Joos G. Asthma and air pollution: recent insights in pathogenesis and clinical implications. Curr Opin Pulm Med 2020; 26(1): 10–19.

Burgess J, Ekanayake B, Lowe A, Dunt D, Thien F, Dharmage SC. Systematic review of the effectiveness of breathing retraining in asthma management. Expert Rev Respir Med 2011; 5(6): 789–807.

Bush R. Indoor allergens, environmental avoidance, and allergic respiratory disease. Allergy Asthma Pro 2008; 29(6): 575–579.

Castro-Rodriguez JA, Garcia-Marcos L, Alfonseda Rojas JD, Valverde-Molina J, Sanchez-Solis M. Mediterranean diet as a protective factor for wheezing in preschool children. J Pediat 2008; 152(6): 823–828, e821–822.

Chapman MD, Wood RA. The role and remediation of animal allergens in allergic diseases. J Allergy Clin Immunol 2001; 107(3 Suppl): S414–421.

Chatzi L, Ramirez-Hernandez M, Padilla O, Pacheco-Gonzalez RM, Pérez-Fernández V, Garcia-Marcos L. Mediterranean diet in pregnancy is protective for wheeze and atopy in childhood. Thorax 2008; 63(6): 507–513.

Chatzi L, Kogevinas M. Prenatal and childhood Mediterranean diet and the development of asthma and allergies in children. Public Health Nutr 2009; 12(9A): 1629–1634.

Clapp PW, Jaspers I. Electronic cigarettes: their constituents and potential links to asthma. Curr Allergy Asthma Rep 2017; 17(11): 79.

Clinic M. Mayo Clinic Book of Alternative Medicine 2010. Vol 2 ed. New York, NY: Time Home Entertainment.

Das R. Therapeutic role of probiotics in asthma and allergic rhinitis. Pediatr Pulmonol 2012; 47(2): 206.

Dave ND, Xiang L, Rehm KE, Marshall, Jr GD. Stress and allergic diseases. Immunol Allergy Clin North Am 2011; 31(1): 55–68.

de Marco R, Pesce G, Girardi P, Marchetti P, Rava M, Ricci P, et al. Foetal exposure to maternal stressful events increases the risk of having asthma and atopic diseases in childhood. Pediatr Allergy Immunol 2012; 23(8): 724–729.

Diette GB, McCormack MC, Hansel NN, Breysse PN, Matsui EC. Environmental issues in managing asthma. Respir Care 2008; 53(5): 602–617.

Eggleston P. Methods and effectiveness of indoor environmental control. Ann Allergy Asthma Immunol 2001; 87(6 Suppl 3): 44–47.

Eichenberger PA, Diener SN, Kofmeh R, Spengler CM. Effects of exercise training on airway hyperreactivity in asthma: a systematic review and meta-analysis. Sports Med 2013; 43(11): 1157–70.

Ellwood P, Asher MI, García-Marcos L, Williams H, Keil U, Robertson C, et al. Do fast foods cause asthma, rhinoconjunctivitis and eczema? Global findings from the International Study of Asthma and Allergies in Childhood (ISAAC) Phase Three. Thorax 2013; 68(4): 351–60.

Evans R3. Environmental control and immunotherapy for allergic disease. J Allergy Clin Immunol 1992; 90(3 Pt 2): 462–468.

George M, Avila M, Speranger T, Bailey HK, Silvers WS. Conducting an Integrative Health Interview (Complementary and Alternative Practice in Allergy Committee Workgroup Report). J Allergy Clin Immunol Pract 2018; 6(2): 436–439.

German JA, Harper MB. Environmental control of allergic diseases. Am Fam Physician 2002; 66(3): 421–426.

Giovannini M, Agostoni C, Riva E, Salvini F, Ruscittov, Zuccotti GV, et al. A randomized prospective double blind controlled trial on effects of long-term consumption of fermented milk containing Lactobacillus casei in pre-school children with allergic asthma and/or rhinitis. Pediatri Res 2007; 62(2): 215–220.

Gupta S, Guar S. A placebo controlled trial of two dosages of LPC antagonist—choline in the management of bronchial asthma. Indian J Chest Dis Allied Sci 1997; 39(3): 149–156.

Güvenç IA, Muluk NB, Mutlu FS, Eşki E, Altıntoprak N, Oktemer T, et al. Do probiotics have a role in the treatment of allergic rhinitis? A comprehensive systematic review and meta-analysis. Am J Rhinol Allergy 2016; 30(5): 157–175.

Hodge L, Salome CM, Hugh JM, Liu-Brennan D, Rimmer J, Allman M, et al. Effect of dietary intake of omega-3 and omega-6 fatty acids on severity of asthma in children. Eur Respir J 1998; 11: 361–365.

Holloway E, West R. Integrated breathing and relaxation training (the Papworth method) for adults with asthma in primary care: a randomised controlled trial. Thorax 2007; 62(12): 1039–1042.

Hondras MA, Linde K, Jones AP. Manual therapy for asthma. Cochrane Database Syst Rev2005; Issue 2. Art. No.: CD001002. DOI: 10.1002/14651858.CD001002.

Kalliomaki M, Salminen S, Poussa T, Arvilommi H, Isolauri E. Probiotics and prevention of atopic disease: 4-year follow-up of a randomised placebo-controlled trial. Lancet 2003; 361(9372): 1869–1871.

Kalliomaki M, Salminen S, Poussa T, Isolauri E. Probiotics during the first 7 years of life: a cumulative risk reduction of eczema in a randomized, placebo-controlled trial. J Allergy Clin Immunol 2007; 119(4): 1019–1021.

Kelly-Pieper K, Patil SP, Busse P, Yang N, Sampson H, Li XM, et al. Safety and tolerability of an antiasthma herbal Formula (ASHMI) in adult subjects with asthma: a randomized, double-blinded, placebo-controlled, dose-escalation phase I study. J Altern Complement Med 2009; 15(7): 735–43.

Khianey R, Oppenheimer J. Is nasal saline irrigation all it is cracked up to be? Ann Allergy Asthma Immunol 2012; 109(1): 20–28.

Kiecolt-Glaser JK, Heffner KL, Glaser R, Malarkey WB, Porter K, Atkinson C, Laskowski B, et al. How stress and anxiety can alter immediate and late phase skin test responses in allergic rhinitis. Psychoneuroendocrinology 2009; 34(5): 670–680.

Kozyrskyj AL, Mai XM, McGrath P, Hayglass KT, Becker AB, Macneil B, et al. Continued exposure to maternal distress in early life is associated with an increased risk of childhood asthma. Am J Respir Crit Care Med 2008; 177(2): 142–147.

Lange NE, Rifas-Shiman SL, Camargo Jr CA, Gold DR, Gillman MW, Litonjua AA. Maternal dietary pattern during pregnancy is not associated with recurrent wheeze in children. J Allergy Clin Immunol 2010; 126(2): 250–255, e251–254.

Lau BH, Riesen SK, Truong KP, Lau EW, Rohdewald P, Barreta RA. Pycnogenol as an adjunct in the management of childhood asthma. J Asthma 2004; 41(8): 825–832.

Laumbach R. Outdoor air pollutants and patient health. Am Fam Physician 2010; 81(2): 175–180.

Marshall G. Internal and external environmental influences in allergic diseases. J Am Osteopath Assoc 2004a; 104(5 Suppl 5): S1–6.

Marshall G. Neuroendocrine mechanisms of immune dysregulation: applications to allergy and asthma. Ann Allergy Asthma Immunol 2004b; 93(2 Suppl 1): S11–17.

Marshall GD, J. Agarwal SK. Stress, immune regulation, and immunity: applications for asthma. Allergy Asthma Proc 2000; 21(4): 241–246.

Marshall GD, J. Stress and immune-based diseases. Preface. Immunol Allergy Clin North Am 2011a; 31(1): xiii–xiv.

Marshall GD, J. The adverse effects of psychological stress on immunoregulatory balance: applications to human inflammatory diseases. Immunol Allergy Clin North Am 2011b; 31(1): 133–140.

Mehta A, Singh BP, Arora N, Gaur SN. Choline attenuates immune inflammation and suppresses oxidative stress in patients with asthma. Immunobiology 2010; 215(7): 527–534.

Mickleborough AA, Ionescu, KW Rundell. Omega-3 Fatty acids and airway hyperresponsiveness in asthma. J Altern Complement Med 2004; 10(6): 1067–1075.

Mishra V. Effect of indoor air pollution from biomass combustion on prevalence of asthma in the elderly. Environ Health Perspect 2003; 111(1): 71–78.

Moreira A, Bonini M, Pawankar R, Anderson SD, Carlsen KH, Randolph C, et al. A World Allergy Organization international survey on physical activity as a treatment option for asthma and allergies. World Allergy Organ J 2014; 7(1): 34.

Naik RD, Vaezi MF. Extra-esophageal gastroesophageal reflux disease and asthma: understanding this interplay. Expert Rev Gastroenterol Hepatol 2015; 9(7): 969–82.

Neuman I, Nahum H, Ben-Amotz A. Prevention of exercise-induced asthma by a natural isomer mixture of beta-carotene. Annals Of Allergy, Asthma & Immunology 1999; 82(6): 549–553.

Oddy W. Breastfeeding, Childhood Asthma, and Allergic Disease. Ann Nutr Metab 2017; 70 Suppl: 26–36.

Okamoto M, Mitsunobu F, Ashida K, Mifune T, Hosaki Y, Tsugeno H, et al. Effects of dietary supplementation with n-3 fatty acids compared with n-6 fatty acids on bronchial asthma. Intern Med 2000; 39: 107–111.

Po JY, FitzGerald JM, Carlsten C. Respiratory disease associated with solid biomass fuel exposure in rural women and children: systematic review and meta-analysis. Thorax 2011; 66(3): 232–239.

Powell C. The role of magnesium sulfate in acute asthma: does route of administration make a difference? Curr Opin Pulm Med 2014; 20(1): 103–8.

Protudjer JL, Sevenhuysen GP, Ramsey CD, Kozyrskyj AL, Becker AB. Low vegetable intake is associated with allergic asthma and moderate-to-severe airway hyperresponsiveness. Pediatr Pulmonol 2012; 47(12): 1159–1169.

Quon BS, Goss CH. Maternal stress: a cause of childhood asthma? Am J Respir Crit Care Med 2012; 186(2): 116–117.

Reisman R. Do air cleaners make a difference in treating allergic disease in homes? Ann Allergy Asthma Immunol 2001; 87(6 Suppl 3): 41–43.

Ritz T. Airway responsiveness to psychological processes in asthma and health. Front Physiol 2012; 3: 343.

Schapowal A. Randomised controlled trial of butterbur and cetirizine for treating seasonal allergic rhinitis. BMJ 2002; 324: 144.

Scott M, Roberts G, Kurukulaaratchy RJ, Matthews S, Nove A, Arshad SH. Multifaceted allergen avoidance during infancy reduces asthma during childhood with the effect persisting until age 18 years. Thorax 2012; 67(12): 1046–51.

Shen J, Oraka E. Complementary and alternative medicine (CAM) use among children with current asthma. Preventive Medicine [serial online] 2012; 54(1): 27–31.

Silvers W. Chapter 25: Allergic rhinitis. pp. 271–223. In: Rakel D (ed.). Integrative Medicine. Philadelphia: Saunders 2003.

Sopo SM, Radzik D, Calvani M. Does treatment with proton pump inhibitors for gastroesophageal reflux disease (GERD) improve asthma symptoms in children with asthma and GERD? A systematic review. J Investig Allergol Clin Immunol 2009; 19(1): 1–5.

Sublett J. Effectiveness of air filters and air cleaners in allergic respiratory diseases: a review of the recent literature. Curr Allergy Asthma Rep 2011; 11(5): 395–402.

Sulser C, Schulz G, Wagner P, Sommerfeld C, Keil T, Reich A, et al. Can the use of HEPA cleaners in homes of asthmatic children and adolescents sensitized to cat and dog allergens decrease bronchial hyperresponsiveness and allergen contents in solid dust? Int Arch Allergy Immunol 2009; 148(1): 23–30.

Tan C, Zhang C, Gao D, Bai J, Wang J, Wang P, et al. Impacts on the life quality of patients with bronchial asthma treated with acupuncture in terms of the lung and large intestine theory. Chinese Acupuncture and Moxibustion 2012; 32(8): 673–677.

Thomet OA, Schapowal A, Heinisch IV, Wiesmann UN, Simon HU. Anti-inflammatory activity of an extract of Petasiteshybridus in allergic rhinitis. J Immunopharmacol 2002; 2: 997–1006.

Turyk ME, Hernandez E, Wright RJ, Freels S, Slezak J, Contraras A, et al. Stressful life events and asthma in adolescents. Pediatr Allergy Immunol 2008; 19(3): 255–263.

Valencia M, Randazzo L. Substance P: immuno-allergic implications. AllergoImmunopathol 1992; (Madr) 20(1): 3–8.

Vedanthan PK, Kesavalu LN, Murthy KC, Duvall K, Hall MJ, Baker S, et al. Clinical study of yoga techniques in university students with asthma: a controlled study. Allergy Asthma Proc 1998; 19(1): 3–9.

Wainapel SF, Fast A. Alternative Medicine and Rehabilitation. New York: Demos, 2003. Web. 29 Jan 2013. New York: s.n.

Wang J, Li XM. Chinese herbal therapy for the treatment of food allergy. Curr Allergy Asthma Rep 2012; 12(4): 332–8.

Wang J, Jones SM, Pongracic JA, Song Y, Yang N, Sicherer SH, et al. Safety, clinical, and immunologic efficacy of a Chinese herbal medicine (Food Allergy Herbal Formula-2) for food allergy. J Allergy Clin Immunol 2015; 136(4): 962–970.

Warburton CJ, Niven RM, Pickering CA, Fletcher AM, Hepworth J, Francis HC. Domiciliary air filtration units, symptoms and lung function in atopic asthmatics. Respir Med 1994; 88(10): 771–776.

Welsh EJ, Bara A, Barley E, Cates CJ. Caffeine for asthma. Cochrane Database Syst Rev2010; Issue 1 Art. No.: CD001112. DOI: 10.1002/14651858.CD001112.pub2.

Wood RA, Johnson EF, Van Natta ML, Chen PH, Eggleston PA. A placebo-controlled trial of a HEPA air cleaner in the treatment of cat allergy. Am J Respir Crit Care Med 1998; 158(1): 115–120.

Wood LG, Gibson PG. Reduced circulating antioxidant defences are associated with airway hyper-responsiveness, poor control and severe disease pattern in asthma. Br J Nutr 2010 Mar; 103(5): 735–41.

Wright R. Prenatal maternal stress and early caregiving experiences: implications for childhood asthma risk. Paediatr Perinat Epidemiol 2007; 21(Suppl 3): 8–14.

Wu K, Tantisira, Li L, Fuhlbrigge AL, Weiss ST, Litonjua A. Effect of vitamin D and inhaled corticosteroid treatment on lung function in children. Am. J. Respir. Crit. 2012; 186(6): 508–513.

31

Ayurveda and Yoga Therapy for Allergy and Asthma

Satyam Tripathi, Kashinath G Metri,* Purnandu Sharma, Amit Singh* and Ahalya Sharma*

INTRODUCTION

Chronic Non-Communicable Disorders (NCDs) have become the leading cause of death and disability worldwide. Unhealthy lifestyle is considered to be an important cause of NCDs. Chronic respiratory problems such as asthma has been highly widespread over the last three decades. The underlying pathology in asthma is chronic airway inflammation that substantially contributes to airway hyper-responsiveness, air-flow limitation, respiratory symptoms and disease chronicity (Myers 2011). And there has been an increased prevalence of different kinds of allergies in modern society. Conventional management of asthma and allergies includes administration of anti-inflammatory, bronchodilators and steroids which are often limited to symptomatic management and also have side effects. Despite, the availability of advanced modern medical treatment the prevalence of asthma and different kinds of allergies has been on rise (Alavinezhad and Boskabady 2018).

Recently, Complementary and Alternative Medicines (CAMs) such as Ayurveda and Yoga have drawn the attention of the healthcare system due their health benefiting effects. Ayurveda is among the most ancient health care systems on Earth. Ayurveda provides a guideline for a healthy lifestyle to prevent diseases and promote health. Further, Ayurveda has mentioned the various kinds of lifestyle related disorders including allergies and asthma and their management. Yoga is also an ancient science with its roots in India; yoga helps the growth of physical, mental, spiritual aspects of an individual. Yoga emphasizes the mind which determines our lifestyle as a fundamental factor that leads to a healthy or unhealthy lifestyle. The 'adhi' the negative emotions, ignorance and addictions in the mind provokes the person for an unhealthy lifestyle and yoga helps to eliminate the adhi. Both Ayurveda and Yoga propose that the physical body is governed by three biological forces called vata (responsible for movements), pitta (responsible for metabolism) and kapha (responsible for growth and nourishment) and disease is the result of imbalance in one or more of these energies. Ayurveda recognizes asthma as Tamak shwasa (Rajnik and Varsakiya 2018). According to Ayurveda tamaka swas (asthma) is the result of imbalance in kapha and vata doshas in the respiratory system (pranvaha srotas) (Hemlatha 2006).

Union Yoga Ayurveda, Singapore &SVYASA University, Bengaluru, India.
 Emials: ayur.st@gmail.com; spurnandu@gmail.com
* Corresponding authors: kgmhetre@gmail.com; dramits90@gmail.com; ahalyasharma@yahoo.com

According to Ayurveda, the cause of asthma involves both internal factors like genetic make-up (prakriti), excess of anxiety, anger, grief and external factors like unwholesome food, irregular sleeping habits, exposure to pollutants, etc. (Haslett et al. 2002). Allergies are caused by imbalance in the kapha and pitta dosha in the body (Vidyadhar ravi 2004). Unhealthy lifestyle is the basic cause of imbalance in tridoshas, hence, Ayurveda and Yoga both insist on lifestyle modification as a treatment approach for chronic diseases like asthma and allergies.

Ayurveda and Yoga as complementary and alternative medicines

Both Ayurveda and Yoga are accepted as complementary and alternative medicines in most of the countries across the world. A large number of people suffering from various kinds of chronic diseases, including asthma and allergies, use Ayurveda (herbs/formulation) and Yoga for management and to improve their health condition. Recently, scientific studies have been conducted to test the health benefiting effects of Yoga and Ayurveda and these studies have shown positive effects.

Scientific studies on the role of Ayurveda in management of asthma and allergy

Pippali Rasyana is mentioned as one of the best formulations in the management of respiratory problems and disease of kapha and vata imbalance in Ayurveda texts. A study by Bisthi reported that 2.5 gms of pippalin Rasayana every day for 45 days was effective in the management of respiratory disease as an adjuvant (Bisht et al. 2009). Ethanolic extract of Myrica esculenta, an Ayurvedic herb containing significant anti-allergic and anti-inflammatory activities can be used in the treatment of allergic disorders and allergic rhinitis by decreasing bronchial hyper-responsiveness (Patel et al. 2010). The extract of *S. potatorum* Linn. shows a significant anti-allergic property by stabilizing peritoneal mast cell membranes and inhibiting the release of nitric oxide from mast cells (Biswas et al. 2002). Chyawanprash maintains adequate hydration in the respiratory system. It strengthens the respiratory system by eliminating coughs, inflammation and brochospasm which might be seasonal or non-seasonal. It is helpful in tuberculosis, respiratory infection and the common cold (Ojha et al. 1975). Padmapatradi yoga in the dose of 2 gms per day in two divided doses acts as a brochodilator, anti-inflammatory and antihistaminic and is effective in reducing the severity of attacks and helps in increasing the breath holding time and peak expiratory flow rate Panda and (Panda and Doddangali 2011). Ethyl acetate extract of *Tectona grandis* Linn., at a dose of 100 mg/kg body weight possesses an anti-asthmatic activity. This can be attributed to mast cell stabilizing and adaptogenic activity, suggestive of its potential in treatment and prophylaxis of asthma (Goswami 2010).

Stem bark decoction of the ayurvedic herb Shirish (Albizzia lebbeck) was found to be helpful in bronchospasm. Studies on Shirish showed fall in total leukocyte count, Erythrocyte sedimentation rate, eosinophil count and increase in PEFR (Swamy et al. 1997). The hot aqueous decoction (DO81) and butanolic fraction (FO82) of *Shirish* showed positive results in mast cells stabilizing activities (Brauca et al. 2001). Similarly, a study in a guinea pig model of curcumin demonstrated anti-asthmatic property by improvement in impaired airways features (Ram et al. 2003). In a study of the powdered rhi-zome of SHATI *(Hedychium spicatum)* given for 4 weeks in divided doses of 10 gm to 25 patients with recurrent paroxysmal attacks of dyspnoea (bronchial asthma), patients reported complete relief from dyspnoea, coughs and restlessness (Chaturvedi and Sharma 1975). Coleus forskholii, an Ayurvedic medicine, has been shown to increase intracellular levels of cyclic AMP (Kaik and Witte 1986) alongwith a powerful bronchodilating effect that may have fewer side effects than Formetorol (Bauer et al. 1993).

A literature survey on these studies proves that Ayurveda has a potency to move ahead by matching every step with the main stream of biomedical medicine.

Scientific studies on the role of Yoga in management of asthma and allergies

A study carried on for a period of nine months that was done to compare a group of patients treated by physiotherapy with a group of patients who received yogic training showed the yogic group performed significantly better on objective tests of exercise tolerance (Tendon 1978). Regular yogic practices were found helpful in increasing efficiency and performance of respiratory muscles and movements, which can help in improvement of total pulmonary function (Yadav and Das 2001, Beutler et al. 2016). A control trial in patients with mild as well as moderate COPD showed a statistically significant improvement in transfer factor of the lung for carbon monoxide (TLCO) after two months of yoga training (Soni et al. 2012). Behera studied the effect of yoga on allergic chronic bronchitis in 15 patients and showed that lung function parameters (Forced Vital Capacity (FVC), Forced Expiratory Volume in the first second (FEV$_1$) and Peak Expiratory Flow Rate (PEFR) improved (Bahera 1998). A study of 14 patients with COPD concluded that there was s positive effect of short term yoga practice on oxygen saturation with no increment on dyspnea (Pomidori et al. 2009). A randomized control trial has shown that adding yoga-based life style intervention to the modern treatment improves pulmonary function in patients with mild to moderate bronchial asthma—suggesting a decrease in exercise-induced bronchoconstriction particularly in exercise-sensitive subjects in the yoga group (Vempati et al. 2009). A controlled clinical trial 24 asthmatic patients who received yoga for 4 weeks daily for 50 minutes showed significant improvement in Peak Expiratory Flow Rate (PEFR) and decreased number of day and night attacks and medication (Mekonnen and Andualem 2010). Similarly, a study on the integrated approach of yoga therapy, including asanas, pranayama, relaxation and meditation for 65 minutes a day showed a significant decrease in weekly asthamatic attacks, medication score and increment on peak flow rate (Nagarathna and Nagendra 1985). Yoga training for six weeks was able to reduce the sweating response to a step test and produce a marked increase in respiratory function (Balakrishna et al. 2008). In another study, 12 weeks of yoga practice resulted in a significant increase in maximum expiratory pressure, maximum aspiratory pressure, breath holding time after expiration, breath holding time after inspiration and hand grip strength (Bhavanani 2003). Six weeks of a pranayama breathing course demonstrated improved ventilatory function in the form of a lowered respiratory rate, and increases in the forced vital capacity, forced expiratory volume at the end of one second, maximum voluntary ventilation, peak expiratory flow rate and prolongation of breath holding time (Singh et al. 2011). Similar beneficial effects were demonstrated with 10 weeks of yoga practice (Birkel and Edgren 2000).

Looking into all these studies, one can conclude that Complementary and Alternative Medicines (CAM) including Ayurveda and Yoga can be an adjuvant to biomedical treatments.

Possible mechanism of action of Ayurveda and Yoga in asthma and allergies

Allergic bronchitis/Asthma and yoga therapy

Yogic breathing techniques help to reduce the bronchospasm by decreasing tone bronchial smooth muscle tone. Yogic breathing may help in improving the strength and efficiency of pulmonary muscles, which can help in the development of lung volumes and capacities. Yogic cleansing techniques (kriyas) help by increasing total lung capacities and volumes by removal of infective nasal secretions from the respiratory tract. Goyeche et al. claimed that psychosomatic imbalance is present in many patients with asthma. Suppressed emotion, anxiety, dependence and extreme self consciousness may all be associated with generalized and localized muscle tension, including that of the voluntary respiratory musculature. Yoga helps in reduction of the anxiety score leading to a balance of the Autonomic Nervous System (ANS) and finally subsiding of acute asthmatic attacks and reducing symptoms of bronchitis. A study showed a significant reduction in the level of anxiety after the practice of pranayama, showed increased skin resistance and a decrease in pulse rate, urinary catecholamine concentration, urinary cholinesterase activity and anxiety scores. Yoga brings reduction in psychological hyper-reactivity, decrease in stress and emotional instability which can help to reduce efferent vagal reactivity, which has been proved as the mediator of the psychosomatic factor in reversible allergic bronchitis like-asthma.

Management of allergic bronchitis/Asthma (Shwasa) in Ayurveda

Pippali rasayana is one of the most important herbal formulations prescribed in Ayurveda for Shwasa roga which pacifies vata-kapha (Vata-Kapha hara), breaks the mechanism of manifestation of disease (srotoshodhana) and removes kapha (kapha nisarana) leading to clearing the pathway for proper circulation of vata thus relieving respiratory problems.

Herbal preprations like-Sitopaladi Churna (Sitopala (sugar), Vamasarocana (*Bambusa arundinaceae* Retz.), fruits of Pippali (*Piper longum* Linn.), Seeds of Ela (*Amomum subulatum* Roxb.) and Tvak (bark of *Cinnamomum Zeylanicum* Blume.) have been mentioned in classical texts and proved to be effective in the treatment of immediate allergic conditions because of their ability to stabilize mast cell by decrease in the mediators release and inflammation mediated by them and thus influence the course of disease.

Conclusion

Ayurveda and Yoga are the effective, safe and cost effective. Evidence suggest the promising role of these interventions in the management of various kinds of allergies and asthma. Present conventional management of Asthma and allergies should include Ayurveda and Yoga intervention to have better results.

References

Alavinezhad A, Boskabady MH. The prevalence of asthma and related symptoms in Middle East countries. Clin Respir J. 2018 Mar; 12(3): 865–77.

Balakrishnan S, Gopalakrishnan M, Prakash E. Effect of six weeks yoga training on weight loss following step test, respiratory pressures, handgrip strength and handgrip endurance in young healthy subjects. Indian J Physiol Pharmacol 2008; 52(2).

Baruah CC, Gupta PP, Patnaik GK, Dubey MP, Goel RK, Dhawan BN. Comparative study of the anti-PCA and mast-cell stabilizing activity fractions of Albizzia Lebbeck: a traditional medicinal plant. Journal of Medicinal and Aromatic Plants Sciences (OAJMAX); 22: 42.

Bauer K, Dietersdorfer F, Sertl K, Kaik B, Kaik G. Pharmacodynamic effects of inhaled dry powder formulations of fenoterol and colforsin in asthma. Clin Pharmacol Ther 1993; 53(1): 76–83.

Behera D. Yoga therapy in chronic bronchitis. The Journal of the Association of Physicians of India 1998; 46(2): 207–208.

Beutler E, Beltrami FG, Boutellier U, Spengler CM. Effect of Regular Yoga Practice on Respiratory Regulation and Exercise Performance. PloS one 2016 Apr 7; 11(4): e0153159.

Bhavanani AB. Effect of yoga training on handgrip, respiratory pressures and pulmonary function. Indian J Physiol Pharmacol 2003; 47(4): 387–392.

Birkel DA, Edgren L. Hatha yoga: improved vital capacity of college students. Altern Ther Health Med 2000; 6(6): 55.

Bisht D, Sharma YK, Mehra BL. A clinical study to evaluate the efficacy of Pippali Rasayana in certain respiratory disorders. An international quarterly journal of research in Ayurveda (AYU) 2009; 30(3): 337.

Biswas S, Murugesan T, Sinha S, Maiti K, Gayen JR, Pal M, Saha BP. Antidiarrhoeal activity of Strychnos potatorum seed extract in rats. Fitoterapia 2002; 73(1): 43–47.

Brauca CG, Gupta PP, Patnaik GK, Amarnath, Kulshresthra DK, Dubey MP, et al. Comparative study of Anti PCA and mast cell stabilizing activity of few fractions of Albizzia lekkak, a traditional Medicinal plant for further study. J Med and Aroma Plant Sci 2001; 22(4A): 59–93.

Chaturvedi GN, Sharma BD. Clinical studies on Hedychium spicatum (Shati): An antiasthmatic drug. J Red Indian Med 1975; 10(2): 6.

Goswami DV, Sonawane LL, Nirmal SA, Patil MJ. Evaluation of antiasthmatic activity of Tectona grandis Linn. bark. Int. J. Pharm. Sci. Res. (IJPSR) 2010; 1(1): 10–17.

Goyal HR. A clinical study of Tamaka Shwasa (Bronchial Asthma), 1997. New Delhi: Central Council for Research in Ayurveda and Siddh (CCRAS).

Hari SP. Ashtanga Hridayam with commentaries of sarvanga sundra of arun data & ayurveda rasayana of hemadri. Reprint ed. Varanasi: Chaukhamba Subharati Publication 2000; p. 473.

Haslett C, Haslett C, Davidson SS. Davidson's principles and practice of medicine. Churchill Livingstone 2002; pp. 513–14, 532.

Hemlatha N. A clinical and experimental study on the efficacy of Shunthi Pushkaramooladi yoga in the Management of Tamaka Shwasa W.S.R. to childhood Asthma [MD Thesis]. Jamnagar: Gujarat Ayurved University 2006.

Kaik G, Witte PU. Protective effect of forskolin in acetylcholine provocation in healthy probands. Comparison of 2 doses with fenoterol and placebo. Wiener medizinische Wochenschrift (1946) 1986; 136(23-24): 637–641.

Mekonnen D, Andualem. Clinical effect of yoga on asthma paients: A preliminary clinical trial. Ethiop J Health Sci 2010; 20(2); 107–12.

Meyer KC, Raghu G, Baughman RP, Brown KK, Costabel U, du Bois RM, et al. An official American Thoracic Society clinical practice guideline: the clinical utility of bronchiolar lavage cellular analysis in interstitial lung disease. American Journal of Respiratory and Critical Care Medicine 2012 May 1; 185(9): 1004–14.

Nagarathna R, Nagendra HR. Yoga for bronchial asthma: a controlled study. Br Med J (Clin Res Ed) 1985; 291(6502): 1077–1079.

Ojha JK, Khanna NN, Bajpay HS, Sharma N. A clinical study on Chyawanprash as an adjuvant in the treatment of pulmonary tuberculosis. J Res Ind Med 1975; 10: 11–14.

Panda AK, Doddanagali SR. Clinical efficacy of herbal Padmapatradi yoga in bronchial asthma (Tamaka Swasa). JAIM 2011; 2(2): 85.

Patel KG, Rao NJ, Gajera VG, Bhatt PA, Patel KV, Gandhi TR. Anti-allergic activity of stem bark of Myrica esculenta Buch.-Ham. (Myricaceae). J Young Pharm 2010; 2(1): 74–78.

Pomidori L, Campigotto F, Amatya TM, Bernardi L, Cogo A. Efficacy and tolerability of yoga breathing in patients with chronic obstructive pulmonary disease: a pilot study. J Cardiopulm Rehabil 2009; 29(2): 133–137.

Rajnik Jadav AD, Varsakiya J. A clinical study of Shunthyadi churna in the Management of Tamaka shwasa WSR to Bronchial Asthma. Journal of Ayurvedic and Herbal Medicine 2018; 4(2): 48–52.

Ram A, Das M, Ghosh B. Curcumin attenuates allergen-induced airway hyperresponsiveness in sensitized guinea pigs. Biol Pharm Bull 2003; 26(7): 1021–1024.

Singh S, Gaurav V, Parkash V. Effects of a 6-week nadi-shodhana pranayama training on cardio-pulmonary parameters. J Phys Educ 2011; 2(4): 44–47.

Soni R, Munish K, Singh KP, Singh S. Study of the effect of yoga training on diffusion capacity in chronic obstructive pulmonary disease patients: A controlled trial. IJOY 2012; 5(2): 123.

Swamy GK, Bhattathiri PP, Rao PV, Acharya MV, Bikshapathi T. Clinical evaluation of Shirish twak-kwatha in the management of Tamaka Shwasa (Bronchial Asthma). J of Res in Ayurveda and Siddha 1997; 18: 21–27.

Tandon MK. Adjunct treatment with yoga in chronic severe airways obstruction. Thorax 1978; 33(4): 514–517.

Tripathi S, Sharma P, Singh A, Sharma A. Ayurveda and yoga therapy for allergy and asthma. In Textbook of Allergy for the Clinician 2016; pp. 441–451. CRC Press.

Vempati R, Bijlani RL, Deepak KK. The efficacy of a comprehensive lifestyle modification programme based on yoga in the management of bronchial asthma: a randomized controlled trial. BMC Pulmonary Medicine 2009; 9(1): 37.

Vidyadhar S, Ravi DT. Charaka Samhita by Agnivesha. New Delhi: Chowkhamba Sanskrit Pratisthan 2004.

Vijayalakshmi P, Surendiran A. Effect of slow and fast pranayams on reaction time and cardiorespiratory variables. Indian J Physiol Pharmacol 2005; 49(3): 313–318.

Wilkens JH, Wilkens H, Uffmann J, Bovers J, Fabel H., Frolich JC. Effects of a PAF-antagonist (BN 52063) on bronchoconstriction and platelet activation during exercise induced asthma. British Journal of Clinical Pharmacology 1990; 29(1): 85–91.

Yadav RK, Das S. Effect of yogic practice on pulmonary functions in young females. Indian Journal of Physiology and Pharmacology 2001; 45(4): 493–496.

32

Yoga Breathing Techniques in Asthma

Pudupakkam K Vedanthan[1,*] *and R Nagarathna*[2]

INTRODUCTION

'Yoga' is a popular term around the globe today. Its meaning and usage varies widely based on the location, set up, as well as the instructors and students. Yoga has its origin in India thousands of years ago and has been practiced by a few for self realization through relaxation and meditation. In the recent decades, yoga techniques have been practiced by millions across the world. Due to globalization and socioeconomic factors, Yoga has been highly commercialized and modified accordingly.

Abundant objective data now exists indicating that psychological factors can interact with the asthmatic diathesis to worsen or improve the course of the disease and may affect about half of all asthma patients (Nagarathna and Nagendra 1985). The role of the psychological factors in inducing or prolonging attacks in acute exacerbations varies from patient to patient and from episode to episode in the same individual. It has been shown that suggestion can actually decrease or increase the effects of pharmacological stimuli on the airways.

Yoga techniques are meant to develop mastery over the modifications of the mind as defined by Patanjali. Regular long term practice of one or more of these techniques results in this mastery by reducing the surges of habituated responses to stressful situations of life that triggers the psycho-neuro-immunological excitation. Yoga Breathing Techniques (YBT) along with meditation have been in practice as a therapy for several ailments including asthma.

Yoga techniques for asthma

All yoga techniques are meant to offer deep rest to the body mind complex. Techniques include traditional physical postures maintained for a while with mindfulness for experiencing local rest to the structures in the stretched part (Asanas), mindful slow breathing with or without breath holding to reduce the breathing rate (Pranayama) and different steps of meditation to calm down the mind.

The one hour of standardized module of Integrated Approach of Yoga Therapy (IAYT) program used in our studies (Nagarathna and Nagendra 1985, Murthy et al. 1984, Nagendra and Nagarathna 1986) included: (a) preparatory breathing training (10 minutes): Five types of rhythmic, comfortable, breathing synchronized with simple hand and body movements, (b) exercises to loosen the joints (for 5 minutes), (c) Asanas (5 minutes): physical postures : Tiger posture (Fig. 32.1), Shoulder stand (Fig. 32.2), (d) Four types of specific breathing techniques, 'Pranayama' for 10 minutes (Fig. 32.3), (e) devotional session to

---

[1] University of Colorado, Denver,Colorado USA.
[2] Eknathbhavan, 19, gavipuram circle, Kempegowdanagar, Bengaluru 560019, INDIA, Email: rnagaratna@gmail.com
* Corresponding author: pkv1947@gmail.com

dwell in the mood of blissfully calm love for the divine and finally 'Shavasana' for 5 minutes of deep relaxation to relax the muscles regionally followed by conscious slowing of breathing and calming the mind (Fig. 32.4).

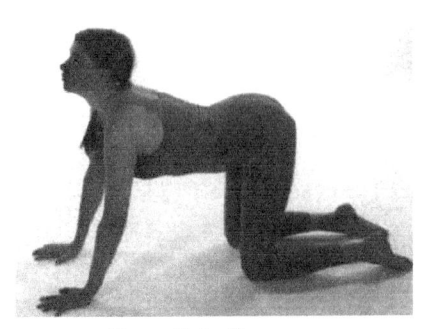

Figure 32.1. Tiger pose.

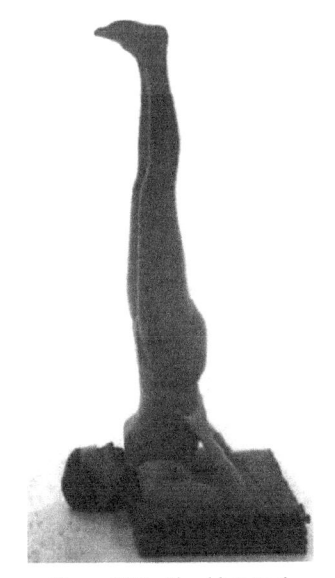

Figure 32.2. Shoulder stand.

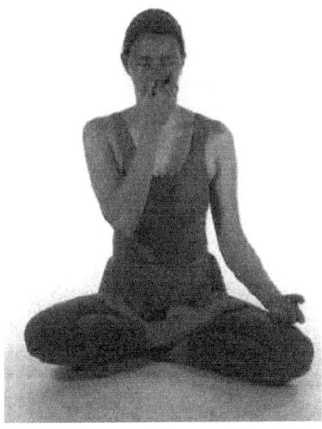

Figure 32.3. Pranayama (Alternate Nostril Breathing).

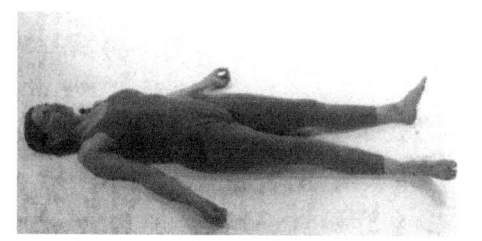

Figure 32.4. Shavasana (Corpse posture).

Discussion

Research evidences on yoga for asthma

Goyeche et al. (Goyeche et al. 1982) used an integrated set of yoga program while Murthy et al. (Murthy et al. 1984) used only the breathing practices documenting the beneficial effects of yoga in patients with asthma. The only long term RCT by Nagarathna and Nagendra (1985) on 53 subjects over a 54-month period that used the integrated module, showed improvement in peak flow rates, medication score and symptom score. The same authors (Nagendra and Nagarathna 1986) demonstrated in a larger study of 570 asthmatics, that regular yoga results in a reduced use of oral, inhaler and parenteral medications for asthma and improves peak expiratory flow rates. Vedanthan et al. (1998) demonstrated that in mild asthmatics practicing yoga 3 times a week for 16 weeks, improved relaxation, positive attitude and exercise tolerance with lesser need for rescue medications. There was no significant improvement in pulmonary functions in this study, which could be due to lack of sufficient power in the study which included only 17 subjects. Sabina et al. (2005) reported that yoga techniques did not exhibit any benefit in a randomized controlled double masked trial of Iyengar Yoga techniques in 62 participants with mild to moderate asthma. Unlike earlier studies, in this study the yoga group practiced only the physical postures followed by a brief session of relaxation and the control group was kept engaged by 'sham yoga' (stretching exercises). In another study (Bhatnager et al. 1991), 46 children with a history of childhood asthma received yoga training that showed improvement in exercise capacity, resting pulmonary functions and exercise-induced bronchial lability index. Raghavendra et al. (2016) performed a randomized, prospective, controlled study to evaluate the immediate effect of 'Kapaalabhaati' (a form of YBT with short rapid inhalations and forceful exhalations) on lung functions of adult patients with mild of moderate asthma using 'Deep slow breathing' technique as a control. Significant increase in lung functions was observed immediately after the practice of Kapaalabhaati for 10-minutes with no change in PFT values in the control group who performed deep slow breathing techniques. Jain (1991) showed that regular yoga increased pulmonary functions and lung capacity in adolescents with asthma . It also decreased frequency and severity of symptoms and drug requirements. Deep breathing exercises and the calm mental state help in ameliorating most of the multiple etiologies of asthma.

Yoga for asthma—review and meta analysis

A review in Cochrane data base in 2000 (Holloway 2000) pointed to some beneficial effects of yoga in asthma, however there was no conclusive evidence. A systematic review in 2011 (Posadzki and Ernst 2011) suggested that yoga leads to a significantly greater reduction in spirometric measures, airway hyper-responsivity, dose of histamine needed to provoke a 20% reduction in forced expiratory volume in the first second, weekly number of asthma attacks and need for drug treatment. Further, three RCTs showed no positive effects compared to various control interventions. Cramer et al. (2014) meta analyzed all available studies with an aim to systematically evaluate the efficacy and safety of yoga. Fourteen randomized controlled trials with 824 patients were included. Evidence for effects of yoga compared with usual care was found for asthma control (Fig. 32.5), asthma symptoms, peak expiratory flow rate, FEV1 (Fig. 32.6) and ratio of FEV1 to FVC; quality of life was better after yoga compared with psychological

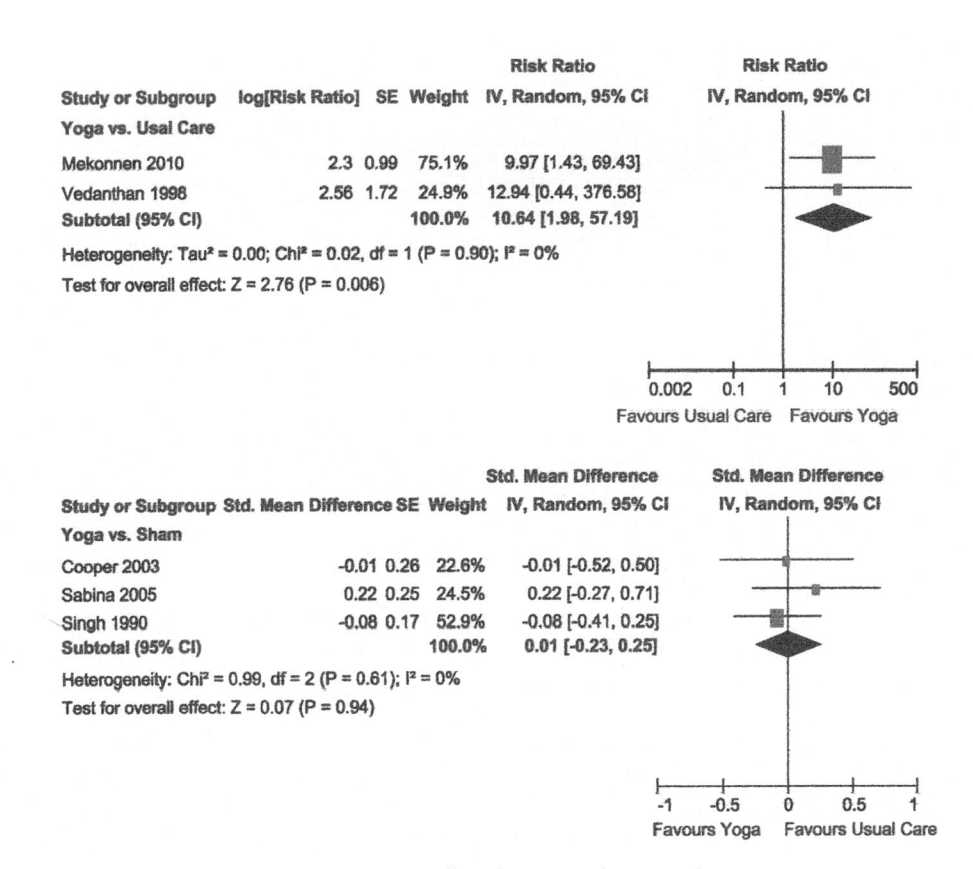

Figure 32.5. Effect of yoga on asthma control.

interventions. No evidence for effects of yoga compared with sham yoga or breathing exercises was revealed in FEV1, FVC, or forced expiratory flow between 25 and 75% values. Yoga was not associated with serious adverse events and concluded that Yoga cannot be considered a routine intervention for asthma patients. Reporting on the safety, the authors recommended that these complex yoga or yoga breathing interventions can be considered ancillary interventions or alternatives to other breathing exercises for asthma patients interested in complementary interventions, as it seems to be a relatively safe in this population. No effect was robust against all potential sources of bias as the studies performed by different groups were difficult to compare as these studies used different techniques and used different outcome measures.

Physiotherapy based breathing for asthma

Several studies on the effect of different types of physiotherapy based breathing exercises have been published. Butyeko breathing was able to reduce symptoms and use of bronchodilators, but there was no significant improvement in lung function tests, bronchial hyper-responsiveness or reduction in inhaled steroid use (Cooper et al. 2003). Fluge et al. (1994) studied the effect of breathing retraining as used in gymnastics with stretching and posture corrections and observed no effect on lung functions or asthma exacerbations. Girodo et al. (1992) used deep diaphragmatic breathing and observed significant reductions in medication use and the intensity of asthma symptoms. The study by Slader et al. demonstrated a substantial and significant improvement in both the breathing exercise group and the control group practicing upper body exercises in patients with mild asthma (Slader et al. 2006).

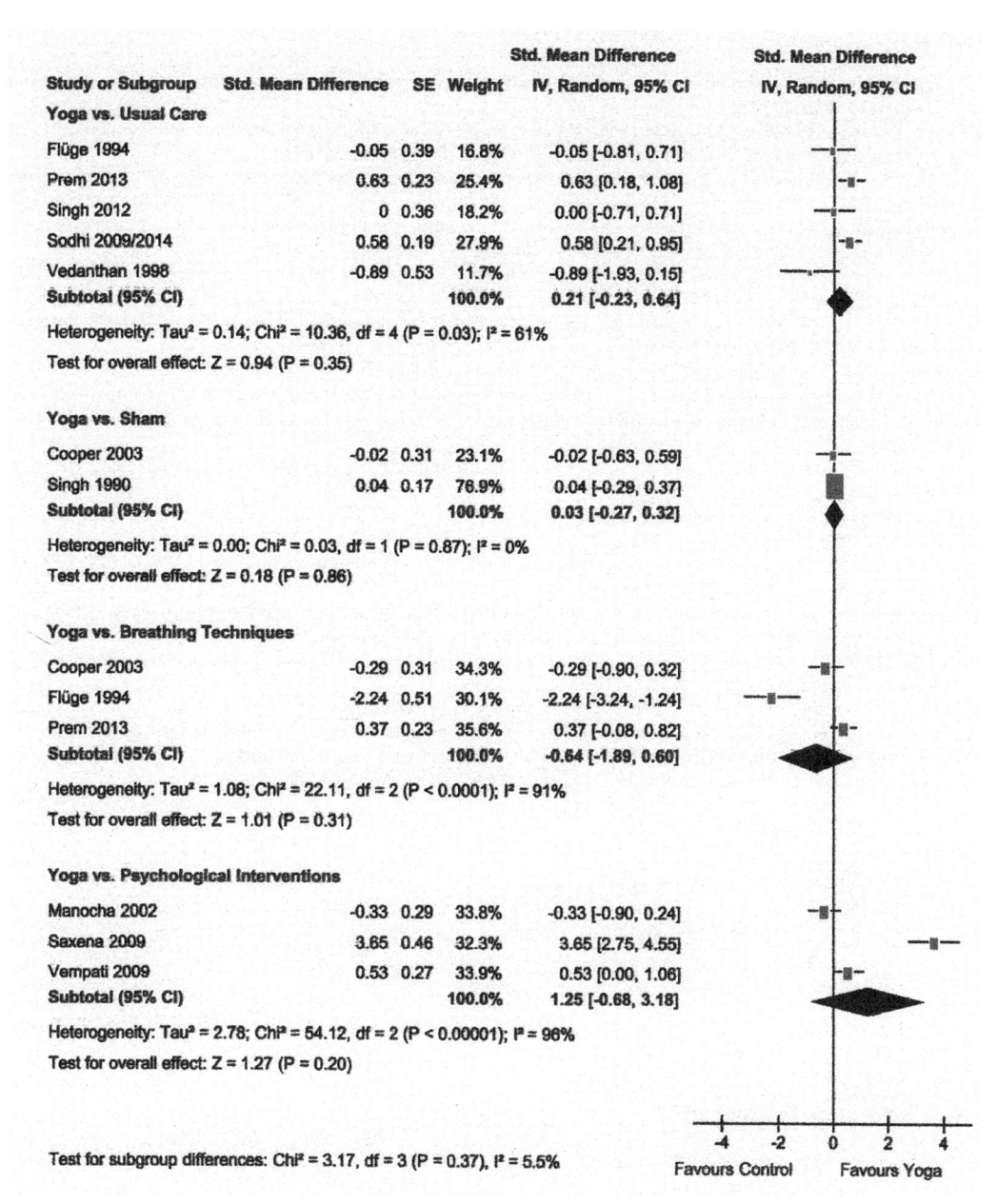

Study or Subgroup	Std. Mean Difference	SE	Weight	Std. Mean Difference IV, Random, 95% CI
Yoga vs. Usual Care				
Flüge 1994	-0.05	0.39	16.8%	-0.05 [-0.81, 0.71]
Prem 2013	0.63	0.23	25.4%	0.63 [0.18, 1.08]
Singh 2012	0	0.36	18.2%	0.00 [-0.71, 0.71]
Sodhi 2009/2014	0.58	0.19	27.9%	0.58 [0.21, 0.95]
Vedanthan 1998	-0.89	0.53	11.7%	-0.89 [-1.93, 0.15]
Subtotal (95% CI)			100.0%	0.21 [-0.23, 0.64]
Heterogeneity: Tau² = 0.14; Chi² = 10.36, df = 4 (P = 0.03); I² = 61%				
Test for overall effect: Z = 0.94 (P = 0.35)				
Yoga vs. Sham				
Cooper 2003	-0.02	0.31	23.1%	-0.02 [-0.63, 0.59]
Singh 1990	0.04	0.17	76.9%	0.04 [-0.29, 0.37]
Subtotal (95% CI)			100.0%	0.03 [-0.27, 0.32]
Heterogeneity: Tau² = 0.00; Chi² = 0.03, df = 1 (P = 0.87); I² = 0%				
Test for overall effect: Z = 0.18 (P = 0.86)				
Yoga vs. Breathing Techniques				
Cooper 2003	-0.29	0.31	34.3%	-0.29 [-0.90, 0.32]
Flüge 1994	-2.24	0.51	30.1%	-2.24 [-3.24, -1.24]
Prem 2013	0.37	0.23	35.6%	0.37 [-0.08, 0.82]
Subtotal (95% CI)			100.0%	-0.64 [-1.89, 0.60]
Heterogeneity: Tau² = 1.08; Chi² = 22.11, df = 2 (P < 0.0001); I² = 91%				
Test for overall effect: Z = 1.01 (P = 0.31)				
Yoga vs. Psychological Interventions				
Manocha 2002	-0.33	0.29	33.8%	-0.33 [-0.90, 0.24]
Saxena 2009	3.65	0.46	32.3%	3.65 [2.75, 4.55]
Vempati 2009	0.53	0.27	33.9%	0.53 [0.00, 1.06]
Subtotal (95% CI)			100.0%	1.25 [-0.68, 3.18]
Heterogeneity: Tau² = 2.78; Chi² = 54.12, df = 2 (P < 0.00001); I² = 96%				
Test for overall effect: Z = 1.27 (P = 0.20)				

Test for subgroup differences: Chi² = 3.17, df = 3 (P = 0.37), I² = 5.5%

Favours Control — Favours Yoga

Figure 32.6. Effect of yoga on forced expiratory volume in 1 second.

Conclusion

Most of the studies done in this context have been short term, with a small number of subjects, no randomization and varying techniques. Due to this variability in the study methods, the modules of yoga intervention used and the duration of follow up, the conclusions that have been drawn are not very consistent. Hence the meta analysis concluded that yoga may be recommended as 'complementary' to the regular management of asthma in motivated patients as it does not cause any adverse effects.

References

Bhatnager S, Jain S, Rai L, Jha U, Ram, K, Valecha A. Effect of yoga training on exercise tolerance in adolescents with childhood asthma. J Asthma 1991; 28(6): 437–42.

Cooper S, Oborne J, Newton S, Harrison V, Thompson coon J, Lewis S, et al. Effect of two breathing exercises (Buteyko and pranayama) in asthma: a randomised controlled trial. Thorax 2003; 58(8): 674–679.

Cramer H, Posadzki P, Dobos G, Langhorst J. Yoga for asthma: a systematic review and meta-analysis. Ann Allergy Asthma Immunol 2014; 112: 503–510.

Fluge T, Richter J, Fabel H, Zysno E, Weller E, Wagner TO. Long-term effects of breathing exercises and yoga in patients with bronchial asthma. Pneumologie 1994; 48(7): 484–490.

Girodo M, Ekstrand KA, Metivier GJ. Deep diaphragmatic breathing: rehabilitation exercises for the asthmatic patient. Arch Phys Med Rehabil. 1992 Aug; 73(8): 717–20.

Goyeche JR, Abo Y, Ikemi Y. Asthma: the yoga perspective. Part II: Yoga therapy in the treatment of asthma. J Asthma 1982; 19(3): 189–201.

Holloway E, Ram FS. Breathing exercises for asthma. Cochrane Database Syst Rev 2000; CD001277.

Jain SC. Effect of Yoga Training on Exercise Tolerance in Adolescents with Childhood Asthma 1991; 28(6): 437–442.

Murthy KJR, Sahay BK, Sitaramaraju P. Effect of pranayama on bronchial asthma. An open study. Lung India 1984; 2: 187–191.

Nagarathna R and Nagendra HR. Yoga for bronchial asthma: a controlled study. Br Med J (Clin Res Ed) 1985; 291(6502): 1077–1079.

Nagendra HR, Nagarathna R. An integrated approach of yoga therapy for bronchial asthma: a 3-54-month prospective study. J Asthma 1986; 23(3): 123–137.

Posadzki P, Ernst E. Yoga for Asthma? A systematic review of randomized clinical trials. J Asthma 2011; 48(6) 632–39. https://doi.org/10.3109/02770903.2011.584358.

Raghavendra P, Shetty P, Shetty S, Manjunath NK, Saoji AA. Effect of high-frequency yoga breathing on pulmonary functions in patients with asthma: A randomized clinical trial. Letters/Ann Allergy Asthma Immunol 2016; 117; 550e572.

Sabina AB, Williams A, Wall Hk, Bansal S, Chupp G, Katz DL. Yoga intervention for adults with mild to moderate asthma, a pilot study. Annals of Allergy 2005; 94: 543–548.

Slader CA, Reddel HK, Spencer LM, Belousova EG, Armour CL, Bosnic-Antecevich SZ, et al. Double blind randomised controlled trial of two different breathing techniques in the management of asthma. Thorax 2006; 61(8): 651–656.

Vedanthan PK, Kesavalu LN, Murthy KC, Duvall K, Hall MJ, Nagarathna S, et al. Clinical study of yoga techniques in University students with asthma: a controlled study. Allergy Asthma Proc 1998; 19(1): 3–9.

33

Drug Allergy

Jay M Portnoy* and Aarti Pandya

INTRODUCTION

Adverse Drug Reactions (ADRs) are common with recent estimates of 2–4 million persons/year suffering disabling or fatal injuries from prescription drugs. Adverse drug reactions (ADRs) are defined by the World Health Organization as a noxious, unintended and undesired effect of a drug, which occurs at doses used in humans for prophylaxis, diagnosis or therapy (WAO 1966). They occur after administration of the medication and present with a wide range of clinical manifestations. When surveyed, 8.3% of respondents reported having a drug allergy. Cutaneous manifestations were reported by 68.2%, and Pseudo allergic, Idiosyncratic, Drug intolerance Beta Lactam ringmethox (SMX-NO) Antibiotics, nonsteroidal anti-inflammatory drugs and anesthetics are the most frequently reported causative drug classes. The frequency of self-reported drug allergy is higher in females and adults and they tend to occur in a medical setting (Sousa-Pinto et al. 2017). Additionally, ADRs should be distinguished from Adverse Drug Events (ADEs), which include medication errors or drug/food interactions (Thong and Tan 2011).

The term adverse drug reaction includes all untoward events related to medications. ADRs can broadly be categorized into predictable (type A) and unpredictable (type B) reactions (Joint Task Force on Practice P 2010). Type A, predictable reactions, constitute 80% of all ADRs. They are usually dose- and duration-dependent, they occur in the general population with no unique susceptibility, and generally are related to the known pharmacologic actions of the drug. Examples of predictable reactions include diarrhea from antibiotics, bleeding with anti-coagulants, sedation with first generation antihistamines and urinary retention with anti-cholinergic medications. Additionally, they can occur in otherwise healthy individuals. Predictable reactions generally are not mediated by immunologic mechanisms.

Unpredictable reactions usually are not dose dependent, they manifest with signs and symptoms that are not expected due to the pharmacologic actions of the drug, and they occur only in susceptible individuals. About 10–15% of ADRs are type B reactions. These can be further divided into immunologically-mediated reactions which often are referred to as drug allergies and non-immunologic reactions including pseudo allergic reactions, idiosyncratic reactions and drug intolerances.

This chapter will focus on immunologically mediated ADRs. It is not intended to be comprehensive, but rather to provide useful information about the most common and important immunologic drug allergies.

Section of Allergy, Asthma & Immunology, Children's Mercy Hospital, Kansas City, MO USA.
* Corresponding author: jportnoy@cmh.edu

Immunologically-mediated adverse drug reactions

Immunologically-mediated ADRs begin with recognition of the drug as an antigen by the immune system. This is followed by an interaction between the previously stimulated immune mechanisms and subsequent exposure to the drug. The process begins with immune recognition.

Immune recognition

Drugs can be recognized by the immune system through a variety of pathways that can lead to immune activation. Immune activation generally requires a coordinated response between T and B cells. Initially, drugs are processed by Antigen-Presenting Cells (APCs) and are recognized as foreign by T cells. Known mechanisms for such immune stimulation are as follows:

Hapten-carrier mechanism

Most medications consist of small molecules that are not able to interact directly with receptors on immune cells to activate the immune system. Many of these small molecules (haptens) can covalently bind to host molecules (carriers) forming a complex that is referred to as a hapten-carrier conjugate. These conjugates can stimulate T cells leading to humoral immune responses. Penicillin is the most common and well-studied hapten. Its beta-lactam ring readily reacts with lysine residues on host proteins to form penicilloyl-protein conjugates that are recognized by the immune system.

Prohapten mechanism

Some small molecules form reactive intermediates during drug metabolism. Before they can be conjugated for detoxification, these drug metabolites can act as haptens which are commonly referred to as prohaptens. The best examples of prohaptens are the sulfonamide antimicrobials, which can form sulfamethoxazole nitroso (SMX-NO) molecules that are highly reactive with host proteins.

Macromolecules

Some medications such as hormones, enzymes, vaccines and monoclonal antibodies, are macromolecules or peptides. These can be processed by APCs and therefore are able to directly activate a T cell response in their native form without binding to a carrier.

Direct B cell stimulation

Some small molecular weight drugs contain repetitive motifs that are sufficiently immunogenic to induce B cell antibody formation without requiring processing by APCs or T cells. Neuromuscular blockers are believed to act in this manner. They contain multivalent quaternary ammonium compounds that are immunoreactive enough to induce drug-specific antibodies in the absence of a coordinated immune response.

Pharmacologic interaction with immune receptors (p-I concept)

Another mechanism is known as the pharmacologic interaction with immune receptors or 'p-i concept'. Here, drugs bind noncovalently with T-cell receptors leading directly to a T cell response without requiring previous sensitization. This mechanism may account for some drug reactions that occur on first exposure to the agent.

Danger hypothesis

In the Danger Hypothesis, co-stimulatory signals to the immune system in the setting of infection or acute inflammation help to activate an immune system in a non-specific manner that contributes to an ADR. An example of this is the development of a drug rash to amoxicillin in the setting of Epstein-Barr virus infection.

Drug allergy

Mechanisms of drug allergy usually are organized by the Gell-Coombs classification of hypersensitivity (Coombs et al. 1975). These types of reaction include: IgE-mediated (type I), cytotoxic (type II), immune complex (type III) and delayed hypersensitivity or cell-mediated (type IV). Type IV reactions can be further subdivided into four categories: activation and recruitment of monocytes (IVa), eosinophils (IVb), CD4+ or CD8+T cells (IVc) and neutrophils (IVd).

Table 33.1. Categories of allergic drug reactions.

Type of reaction	Clinical manifestations	Time of onset	Commonly implicated drugs
Type I: Immediate hypersensitivity (IgE-mediated)	Urticaria, angioedema, bronchospasm, anaphylaxis	minutes to hours	Beta-lactams, antiepileptics, platinum agents, perioperative agents
Type II: Cytotoxic	Hemolytic anemia, thrombocytopenia	5 or more days	penicillin, quinine, sulfonamides, heparin
Type III: Immune complex	Serum sickness	1 to 3 weeks	penicillin, infliximab, anti-thymocyte globulin, sulfonamides
Type IV: Delayed type hypersensitivity	Contact dermatitis, exanthems	Days to weeks initial exposure, faster subsequent exposure	Neomycin, bacitracin, nickel, glucocorticoids, penicillin, sulfonamides
Hypersensitivity vasculitis	cutaneous or visceral vasculitis	Weeks to years	Hydralazine, penicillamine, propylthiouracil
DRESS	Fever, rash, eosinophilia, hepatitis, pneumonitis, nephritis	2–12 weeks	Antieplieptics, dapsone, minocycline, sulfonamides, allopurinol
Pulmonary drug hypersensitivity	Pneumonitis, fibrosis	Days to months	Nitrofurantoin, bleomycin, methotrexate
Drug-induced lupus erythematosus	Arthralgias, myalgias, fever, malaise, erythematous/scaly plaques in photodistribution	Weeks to months	Procainamide, hydralazine, isoniazid, minocycline, anti-TNF, ACE inhibitors, calcium channel blockers, hydrochlorothiazide
Drug-induced granulomatous disease	Granulomatosis with polyangiitis, Eosinophilic Granulomatosis with polyangiitis	Weeks to months	propylthiouracil, leukotriene modifiers
Immunologic hepatitis	Hepatitis, cholestatic jaundice	Weeks to months	para-aminosalicylic acid, sulfonamides, phenothiazines
Blistering disorders	Erythema multiforme, SJS, TEN	Days to weeks	Sulfonamides, cephalosporins, imidazole, anticonvulsants, NSAIDs
Immunologic nephropathy	Rash, fever, eosinophilia, glomerulonephritis	Weeks to months	penicillin, sulfonamides, gold, penicillamine, allopurinol
Aspirin-exacerbated respiratory disease	Rhinorrhea, flushing, bronchospasm	Minutes to hours	Cox-1 inhibitors

Type I: Immediate hypersensitivity

Type I reactions are IgE-mediated. This type of reaction requires a sensitization stage in which a coordinated B cell and T helper cell response leads to class switching which generates drug-specific IgE antibodies. These IgE antibodies attach to the surface of mast cells; a condition referred to as sensitization.

On re-exposure to the drug, cross-linking of the drug-specific IgE occurs leading to activation of mast cells and subsequent release of mediators including histamine, tryptase and arachidonic acid metabolites leading to symptoms. Symptoms can consist of pruritus, flushing, urticaria, GI symptoms (pain, emesis or diarrhea), angioedema, wheezing, laryngeal edema and hypotension possibly leading to anaphylactic shock. Type I reactions usually occur within minutes to hours after exposure and therefore are referred to as immediate type hypersensitivity reactions. The most common causative agents include beta-lactam antibiotics, platinum-based chemotherapeutics and perioperative agents. Type I reactions that are not IgE mediated are believed to be caused by direct mast cell activation by a drug. This type of reaction is referred to as a 'pseudoallergic' reaction. Examples include reactions to opiates, vancomycin or iodinated radiocontrast media. The MRGPRX2 receptor is located on mast cells and has been implicated in pseudoallergic reactions (Subramnaian et al. 2016).

Type II: Cytotoxic

Type II hypersensitivity drug reactions are uncommon. Initially a drug binds to and acts as a hapten, stimulating IgG or IgM production to that foreign hapten-protein complex. Subsequent binding of the drug to preformed IgG or IgM causes cell destruction by macrophage- or complement-mediated lysis. These reactions usually occur with high-dose and prolonged treatment courses. Immune-induced thrombocytopenia may occur following treatment with heparin, quinidine, propylthiouracil, gold salts, beta-lactams sulfonamides, vancomycin and other drugs. Membrane damage occurs due to drug–antibody complexes, which are adsorbed onto cell membranes. Type II reactions are usually associated with a positive direct and indirect Coombs test.

Type III: Immune complex

Type III hypersensitivity reactions generally can present as Arthus reactions, serum sickness or vasculitis reactions. Immune complex reactions originally were described following administration of heterologous antisera, but they also may be caused by small-molecular-weight drugs, protein medications such as anti-thymocyte globulin and monoclonal antibodies such as infliximab, though can also occur with prolonged use of small molecule medications including beta-lactams. This type of reaction occurs when drug-specific IgG antibodies bind to drug antigens forming antigen-antibody immune complexes. These immune complexes can precipitate in various tissues including joints and blood vessels leading to complement activation and inflammation. Symptoms often include fever, rash, urticaria, lymphadenopathy and arthralgias, usually starting 1 to 3 weeks after exposure to the offending agent. The prognosis for recovery is excellent; however, symptoms may last for several weeks. Treatment usually consists of corticosteroids and H1 antihistamines.

Serum sickness–like reactions following exposure to cephalosporins (primarily by cefaclor) usually are caused by antibodies directed to reactive intermediates that are formed by altered metabolism of the drug. In contrast, Arthus reactions are localized type III hypersensitivity reactions that can occur as a result of vaccination and present without systemic manifestations.

Type IV: Delayed type hypersensitivity

Type IV hypersensitivity reactions often are responsible for cutaneous drug eruptions. They occur as a result of activation of T cells and do not involve antibody formation. They often involve the skin due to the large numbers of T cells in the skin. Type IV reactions often are divided into subsets based on T cell recruitment of effector cells, which reflect the laboratory findings or histology of the reactions. These effector cells include monocytes (IVa), eosinophils (IVb), CD8+ T cells (IVc) and neutrophils (IVd). Drug reactions may involve a combination of these subdivisions. An example of a type IV drug reaction is allergic contact dermatitis to a topical agent such as such as bacitracin, neomycin, corticosteroids, local anesthetics and antihistamines. This is similar to reactions that occur following exposure to poison ivy which leads to inflammatory plaque and/or vesicle formation involving cytotoxic T cells.

Type IV reactions cause delayed cutaneous eruptions that are usually seen 24 hours or more after the initial exposure to the medication. The most important reaction is a drug-induced exanthem. This often presents as a morbilliform rash starting about 2 weeks after the initial exposure or 24–72 hours after re-exposure to an offending drug and accounts for about 75% of all cutaneous drug reactions. The rash generally resolves following removal of the drug. Type IV reactions are also responsible delayed maculopapular eruptions caused by oral antibiotics such as amoxicillin and sulfonamides. Patch testing may help to identify contact allergens. After avoidance is instituted, topical and/or systemic corticosteroids may be used to treat a contact dermatitis (Fonacier et al. 2015).

Another type IV reaction is a fixed drug eruption which is characterized by localized erythematous plaques often on a limb, the face or in the mouth, frequently leading to hyperpigmentation. On re-exposure to the drug, a rash will recur in the same location. Such reactions are generally not dangerous and resolve with discontinuation of the offending agent.

Acute Generalized Exanthematous Pustulosis (AGEP) is a rare presumed type IV hypersensitivity that presents with superficial pustules typically 24 hours after administration of a drug. It typically begins on the face or intertriginous areas and spreads over several hours. It generally resolves with discontinuation of the drug but in rare cases can progress and can be life threatening (Henning et al. 2019).

Drug exanthems

Erythema multiforme minor is a cell-mediated hypersensitivity reaction associated with viruses, other infectious agents and drugs (Sokumbi et al. 2012). It manifests as pleomorphic cutaneous eruptions, with target lesions being most characteristic.

Blistering disorders

Stevens-Johnson Syndrome (SJS) and Toxic Epidermal Necrolysis (TEN) are severe blistering reactions characterized by fever and necrosis of skin and mucous membranes leading to sloughing of the epidermis. (9)TEN (i.e., Lyell syndrome), is distinguished from SJS (i.e., erythema multiforme major) by the extent of epidermal detachment. It is termed SJS if less than 10% of the body surface area is involved, and TEN if greater than 30%, with the middle percentage considered an overlap syndrome. These syndromes are known to be in part mediated by stimulated cytotoxic CD8 T cells similar to a type IVc reaction, but the precise mechanism is more complex. Research currently points towards production of a cytolytic protein granulysin as being essential, however the mechanism of this stimulation is unknown. The reaction typically begins between 5 and 21 days after exposure to a drug and presents with a prodrome of fever and malaise followed by erythematous macules, targetoid lesions or diffuse erythema progressing to vesicles, bullae and then necrosis of skin and mucous membranes. Well known causes include allopurinol, sulfonamides, antiepileptics and NSAIDs.

Treatment of SJS with systemic corticosteroids is controversial (Antoon et al. 2019). In addition, treatment of TEN with systemic corticosteroids is associated with increased mortality. Treatment with high-dose intravenous immunoglobulin is controversial. Patients with one of these disorders generally should be managed in a burn unit. Additionally, the use of patch testing in such reactions remains controversial (Joint Task Force on Practice P 2010).

DRESS

Drug Rash with Eosinophilia and Systemic Symptoms (DRESS) is a drug hypersensitivity that can lead to multi organ failure. It typically appears between 2 and 12 weeks after drug initiation and can have a variable clinical presentation. The syndrome involves fever, skin eruption, hematologic derangements (eosinophilia, atypical lymphocytosis, or neutropenia) and internal organ damage (hepatitis, pneumonitis, nephritis, myocarditis, pericarditis, myositis, pancreatitis and/or thyroiditis). DRESS is known to be a potentially life-threatening reaction. The pathophysiology of DRESS is unclear, however there is some evidence that drug induced reactivation of herpes viruses is the first step. Drugs usually implicated include antibiotics (74%) (vancomycin [39%], beta-lactams [23%], fluoroquinolones [4%], tetracyclines [4%], sulfonamides [3%]) and anticonvulsants (20%) (Wolfson et al. 2019). Other drugs associated with DRESS include dapsone and minocycline. Management primarily includes identification and prompt withdrawal of the offending drug (Tas et al. 2003). The use of systemic corticosteroids remains controversial. DRESS has been successfully treated with IVIG, cyclosporine and mepolizumab though the role of these agents for treatment remains to be fully defined (Ange et al. 2018, Galvao et al., Ton et al. 2019).

Drug-Induced Lupus Erythematosus (DILE)

Drug-Induced Lupus Erythematosus (DILE) is a complex syndrome that can present either with systemic manifestations including fever, arthralgias, arthritis, serositis, vasculitis and glomerulonephritis or with cutaneous manifestations. While the reaction mechanism is unclear, the implicated drugs lead to auto antibody formation. Drugs traditionally associated with DIL include procainamide, hydralazine, quinidine and others, but strong associations with newer agents, such as TNF alpha inhibitors, are increasingly being recognized (Vaglio et al. 2018). Antihistone antibodies are present in more than 90% of patients with DILE but occur less commonly with minocycline, propylthiouracil and statins. In contrast, **Anti-Ro/SSA** antibodies are more common in patients with drug-induced subacute cutaneous lupus (drug induced SCLE).

Acute interstitial nephritis

Acute Interstitial Nephritis (AIN) is a drug induced renal disease presenting with rash, fever, eosinophilia and glomerulonephritis. Its mechanism is poorly understood. AIN can occur in over 15% of individuals treated with methicillin, which is the most commonly implicated drug though nafcillin is also frequently implicated. AIN can also present as membranous glomerulonephritis which is often related to treatment with gold, penicillamine and allopurinol.

Pulmonary specific drug hypersensitivity reactions

Most pulmonary specific drug hypersensitivity reactions present as an acute pneumonitis, though pulmonary fibrosis also has been described. The most common causes include bleomycin and methotrexate, though pulmonary toxicity also may occur due to other medications.

Anticonvulsant hypersensitivity Syndrome (AHS)

AHS has been estimated to occur in between 1 and 1000 and 1 in 10,000 exposures (Knowles et al. 2012) and is mainly associated with administration of aromatic anticonvulsant drugs and is related to an inherited deficiency of epoxide hydrolase, an enzyme required for the metabolism of arene oxide intermediates produced during hepatic metabolism (Atanaskovic-Markovich et al. 2019). It is characterized by fever, skin nodules, plaques, lymphadenopathy and internal organ involvement (usually the liver), which occurs 2 to 8 weeks after the initiation of therapy. The most common drugs causing AHS include phenytoin, carbamazepine and phenobarbital which are believed to cross-react with each other. Other common triggers include valproic acid, gabapentin and lamotrigine. In addition to a history, skin patch testing has been used to identify drugs associated with this syndrome (Elzagallaai et al. 2009).

AERD

Aspirin Exacerbated Respiratory Disease (AERD) is a chronic condition with four related symptoms: asthma, nasal polyposis with rhinosinusitis and acute respiratory exacerbations with exposure to aspirin or other NSAIDs (Namazy et al. 2002). AERD is an acquired imbalance of arachidonic acid metabolism and altered sensitivity to the downstream lipid mediators of this pathway. All COX-1 inhibitors, including aspirin and other NSAIDs, lead to increased production of proinflammatory cysteinyl leukotrienes and decreased synthesis of anti-inflammatory prostaglandin E2, exacerbating inflammation of the respiratory tract and causing bronchospasm.

Clinical approach to drug allergy

Risk factors

The most important risk factors for a drug-induced hypersensitivity reaction include the specific chemical property and molecular weight of the suspected drug as well as the dose, route of administration, duration of treatment, repetitive exposure and concurrent illnesses (e.g., Epstein-Barr virus infection and amoxicillin rash). Host risk factors include age, sex, atopy, underlying diseases (such as lupus erythematous and human immunodeficiency virus) and the presence of specific genetic polymorphisms.

Clinical history

The first question in the evaluation of a patient with a suspected adverse drug reaction is whether the reaction is drug-related (Joint Task Force on Practice P 2010). The history should focus on the nature of the reaction and the likelihood that a suspected agent was its cause. In particular:

- Are the clinical signs and symptoms consistent with an unpredictable drug reaction?
- Was there exposure to a drug prior to onset of the reaction, by what route and is the time frame consistent with a drug reaction? Note that a drug reaction can begin after the drug has been discontinued.
- Has the patient been exposed to the suspected drug previously and if so, was there a reaction? While it is possible to have a drug reaction without prior exposure, it is not always clear whether a cross-reacting or hidden source of exposure has taken place.
- How likely is the suspected agent to cause a reaction? Some agents are more likely to cause certain types of adverse reaction than others. Immediate reactions most commonly occur after exposure to penicillin.
- Are there other possible explanations for the observed reaction including exposure to other drugs or to foods to which a patient is allergic? Patients might not consider over-the-counter agents such as aspirin to be a drug, so it helps to get a detailed history of drug and food intake.
- Are there other conditions that would increase the likelihood of a drug reaction such as a viral infection with amoxicillin?

Physical examamination

The most common clinical manifestations of drug reactions are cutaneous. Numerous types of rash can be associated with drug reactions including exanthems, urticaria, angioedema, acne, bullous eruptions, fixed drug eruptions, erythema multiforme, photosensitivity, psoriasis, purpura vasculitis, pruritis, blistering associated with SJS and TEN, exfoliative dermatitis and the rash associated with DRESS. While rashes often are not specific, each of these rashes can provide a clue as to whether it was caused by a drug and if so, which agent likely caused it.

The most common drug-induced rash is a drug exanthem (i.e., maculopapular rash). Exanthems often are pruritic, beginning as macules that can evolve into papules which eventually coalesce into plaques. Drug exanthems typically involve the trunk and spread outward to the limbs. They typically begin several days after taking the offending drug, can last days and may resolve with scaling. Drug-induced exanthems are not associated with anaphylaxis because they are not IgE-mediated. Drug likely to cause exanthems include allopurinol, aminopenicillins, cephalosporins, antiepileptic agents and antibacterial sulfonamides.

Fixed drug eruptions are called that because they recur in the same location on reintroduction of the causative drug. Typical fixed drug eruptions present as round or oval, sharply demarcated, red to livid, slightly elevated plaques, ranging from a few millimeters to several centimeters in diameter. They frequently involve the lips, hands and genitalia. A number of medications are associated with fixed drug eruptions including tetracycline, NSAIDs and carbamazepine (Ben Fadhel et al. 2019).

Urticaria and angioedema are the most common IgE-mediated manifestations though they can occur with non IgE reactions such as serum sickness. Angioedema due to ACE inhibitors is mediated by bradykinin.

Photoallergic reactions often present with eczematous eruptions in a sun exposure distribution on the face, the 'V' area of the neck, dorsa of hands and arms. Such reactions often present with erythroderma beginning minutes to hours after exposure to sunlight and can progress to vesicles in severe reactions. Similar eruptions can occur with drug-induced lupus.

Testing for drug allergy

Once a clinical history consistent with a drug reaction has been obtained and the likely agent identified, it is necessary to confirm that the agent caused the reaction (Solensky et al. 2014). If the reaction is suspected to have been IgE-mediated, tests for specific IgE such as a skin test or *in vitro* test may be helpful. Non IgE-mediated reactions require other types of test such as patch tests. If no validated tests are available, it may be necessary to do an oral challenge with the agent or if the reaction was severe, delayed or unpredictable, no testing should be done and the drug should be avoided.

Skin testing to detect drug-specific IgE

Allergy skin testing is done to document the presence of drug-specific IgE. When testing for sensitization to low molecular weight drugs, it is necessary to test both for the drug and for its metabolites (often referred to as 'minor determinants') since they also can bind to IgE. Since such drugs are too small to stimulate an immune response directly, they serve as haptens by binding to protein carrier molecules. Therefore, in addition to testing with a nonirritating concentration of the native drug, it may be necessary to test for IgE directed at a drug-protein conjugate (e.g., penicilloyl-polylysine which is often referred to as the 'major antigenic determinant' of penicillin). This is responsible for at least 95% of immediate type hypersensitivity reactions and is the key to testing for penicillin allergy. Other metabolites such as penilloate and penicilloate are often referred to as the 'minor antigenic determinants'. Specific IgE directed at these moieties has been implicated in allergic reactions, however such reactions are infrequent. Currently, there is no FDA-approved product to use for testing to penicillin minor determinants. Recently it was shown that penicillin skin tests that include penicillin and its major determinant without the minor determinant can safely identify patients who are likely to tolerate penicillin (Macy et al. 2013).

Penicillins currently are the only low-molecular-weight agents for which validated testing is available. Skin testing for penicillin allergy has a high sensitivity in that it will detect most patients who have IgE-mediated allergy. A negative penicillin skin test is highly predictive of penicillin tolerance. On the other hand, it has a low specificity so false positive tests are very common. An example of a form to use for penicillin skin testing is shown in Table 33.2.

Table 33.2. An example of a form for skin testing to detect amoxicillin allergy.

Antigen	Percutaneous (mm wheal/ mm erythema)	Intracutaneous (mm wheal/ mm erythema)
Penicillin G*		
PenicillylPolylysine**		
Amoxicillin*		
Histamine (1mg/mL)***		
Saline		
Oral Challenge****		

*Used at a non-irritating concentration.
**Available commercially as Prepen™.
***Intracutaneous histamine test is not done if the percutaneous histamine test is reactive.
****Oral challenge is done if the skin tests are negative and histamine is positive.

Table 33.3. Non-irritating Concentrations of selected antibiotics. From Solensky and Khan 2014, Table 18.(4).

Antibiotic	Nonirritating Concentration
Amoxicillin	6mg/mL
Azithromycin	10mcg/mL
Cefotaxime	10mg/mL
Cefuroxime	10mg/mL
Cefazolin	33mg/mL
Ceftazidime	10mg/mL
Ceftriaxone	10mg/mL
Clindamycin	15mg/mL
Cotrimoxazole	800mcg/mL
Erythromycin	50mcg/mL
Gentamicin	4mg/mL
Levofloxacin	25mcg/mL
Nafcillin	25mcg/mL
Ticarcillin	20mg/mL
Tobramycin	4mg/mL
Vancomycin	5mcg/mL

Skin testing with nonirritating concentrations of non-beta-lactam antibiotics is not standardized. Since drug derivatives for non-penicillin drugs are not available for skin testing, it is unclear what the performance characteristics of those tests are. Therefore, a negative skin test result does not rule out the possibility of an immediate-type reaction and a positive skin test result suggests the presence of drug specific IgE antibodies. Native skin testing is usually done with carbapenems and monobactams. Non-irritating concentrations for some antibiotics have been determined (Table 33.3) (Empedrad et al. 2003).

Skin testing is both useful and routinely used for detecting specific IgE to peptide-based medications such as insulin and monoclonal antibodies, as well as for two classes of chemotherapeutic drugs: taxanes and platinum agents. There is no validated use of skin testing for other medications.

Patch testing

Patch testing involves applying a drug directly to the skin surface for 24–72 hours to allow penetration through the epidermis and activation of the immune system. It is highly effective for the diagnosis of type IV hypersensitivity contact dermatitis to numerous topical drugs. Common examples include the antimicrobials neomycin and bacitracin. Patch testing is not validated for the diagnosis of cutaneous drug reactions to systemically administered drugs. There is limited evidence that it may be useful with specific medications such as some beta-lactams, sulfonamide antibiotics and aromatic anticonvulsants. This may be useful in the diagnosis of specific type IV cutaneous reactions including maculopapular exanthams, fixed drug eruptions and AGEP. However, sensitivity and specificity of such testing is generally poor. Notably it is not useful in assessing for the severe cutaneous drug reactions SJS/TEN or DRESS.

Drug challenges

Drug challenges are performed either to document that a patient does not have a drug allergy (graded challenge) or to induce tolerance in a patient who needs a drug for which there is an increased likelihood of an adverse reaction (induction of tolerance). The former is used for diagnostic purposes and the latter for treatment. The primary difference between these two procedures is that with a graded challenge the doses are increased rapidly and frequently enough to elicit a reaction in an allergic patient. Induction of tolerance, on the other hand, starts with doses that are low enough to be tolerated and is done gradually to avoid causing a reaction.

A graded challenge is used to prove tolerance in a patient who is unlikely to be allergic to a drug. It is done in a graded fashion when there is no intention to induce tolerance to the drug so that if a reaction does occur it will be mild. Challenge doses need to be high enough and to be given frequently enough to document that the patient is not allergic to the drug and that tolerance was not induced. Patients who tolerate a graded challenge are considered to not be allergic to the drug and are not at increased risk for future reactions compared with the general population. Such testing should not be done when the probability of a reaction is high or if there is history of SJS/TEN or DRESS as drug exposure could be life threatening in such circumstances.

Drug challenges to NSAIDs pose a additional unique problems (Stevenson et al. 2006). The choice of protocol for NSAID challenge depends upon the nature of the patient's initial reaction. Aspirin challenges are the gold standard for diagnosis of patients with suspected AERD. Aspirin challenge and desensitization are often simultaneously done in these patients. The procedure will likely induce symptoms in patients with AERD, therefore safety must be considered prior to initiating this procedure. Risk factors linked to severe bronchial reactions from this procedure include lack of a leukotriene-modifying drug (LTMD) at the time of procedure, baseline FEV_1 of less than 80% of predicted value and a history of a prior emergency department visit for asthma (Hope et al. 2009). Patients with AERD can undergo a challenge by administering aspirin at 90-minute dose escalations, starting at a dose of 40.5 mg bringing the total cumulative daily dose to 325 mg or more (DeGregorio et al. 2019).

Treatment

Once a patient is confirmed to have a drug allergy, treatment depends on the severity of the likely reaction and the need for the drug. If the likely reaction is relatively mild, such as a mildly pruritic rash with no other systemic symptoms, the drug could be given, and the resulting symptoms treated with an antihistamine. If the likely reaction is more severe, the drug should be avoided and an alternate agent given instead. When there is no alternate agent or if the alternatives are very expensive, difficult to administer or are likely to have significant side effects, then induction of tolerance with the initial agent should be considered.

Induction of tolerance

Drug tolerance is defined as a state in which a patient with a drug allergy will tolerate a drug without experiencing an adverse reaction. Induction of tolerance modifies a patient's response to a drug temporarily which permits it to be given when it is needed. A procedure for inducing drug tolerance is also referred to as drug desensitization. It is done in situations where an alternate non–cross-reacting medication cannot be used and has been used to treat reactions that are IgE-mediated, non-IgE mediated, pharmacologic and undefined (Caimmi et al. 2019) (Der Groot and Mulder 2010). The procedure has proven to be markedly effective, allowing for successful drug administration in almost any patient with drug hypersensitivity when supervised by experienced clinicians.

Numerous protocols have been used for inducing tolerance to various medications. Each of these involved administration of increasing doses, usually over the course of several hours or over several days for certain agents (Liu et al. 2011). The dosing generally starts between 1/1,000 to 1/100,000 of the desired therapeutic dose. This slow exposure to a medication decreases responsiveness of mast cells and allows temporary tolerance to a drug. The mechanism of decreased responsiveness is unclear but may have to do with decreased expression of receptors and drug specific IgE on the surface of mast cells during slowly increased exposure. Induction of tolerance generally is contraindicated for serious non–IgE-mediated reactions such as Stevens-Johnson syndrome or toxic epidermal necrolysis.

Several specific protocols for induction of tolerance to penicillin have been widely published, but the one by Sullivan (Sullivan et al. 1982) is the most commonly used (See Table 33.4). For penicillin-derived antibiotics, the oral route has been found to be safer than parenteral administration. IV protocols and protocols that start with oral and then convert to IV have also been described (JACI 2010). For some delayed non–IgE-mediated cutaneous reactions, induction of drug tolerance may be performed to allow treatment with the drug. This has been reported for mild cutaneous drug reactions to sulfonamide antibiotics, for example (Table 33.5) (Demoly et al. 2000).

Induction of tolerance can also be performed in the setting of Aspirin-Exacerbated Respiratory Disease (AERD). While protocols for this procedure are similar to that of other agents, the mechanism of reaction is different. The mechanism is believed to be due to an alteration in arachidonic acid metabolism and a shift away from generation of proinflammatory cys-leukotrienes. An example of an aspirin protocol is shown in Table 33.6 (Macy et al. 2007).

Table 33.4. Protocol for oral induction of tolerance to penicillin. From Sullivan, et al. 1982, Table 1.(31). Doses are given every 15–20 minutes.

Step	Penicillin (mg/mL)	Amount (mL)	Dose (mg)	Cumulative Dose
1	0.5	0.1	0.1	0.1
2	0.5	0.2	0.1	0.2
3	0.5	0.4	0.2	0.4
4	0.5	0.8	0.4	0.8
5	0.5	1.6	0.8	1.6
6	0.5	3.2	1.6	3.2
7	0.5	6.4	3.2	6.4
8	5.0	1.2	6.0	12.4
9	5.0	2.4	12.0	24.4
10	5.0	5.0	25.0	49.4
11	50.0	1.0	50.0	100.0
12	50.0	2.0	100.0	200.0
13	50.0	4.0	200.0	400.0
14	50.0	8.0	400.0	800.0

Table 33.5. Protocol for induction of tolerance to Trimethoprim-Sulfamethoxazole. From Demoly et al. 2000 (32).

Step	Drug Dosage	Concentration of TMP-SMX	Volume of TMP-SMX solution, mL	Time, min
1	0.2/1 mcg	8/40 mcg/mL	0.025	0
2	0.6/3 mcg	8/40 mcg/mL	75	30
3	1.8/9 mcg	8/40 mcg/mL	0.225	60
4	6/30 mcg	8/40 mcg/mL	0.75	90
5	18/90 mcg	8/40 mcg/mL	2.25	120
6	60/300 mcg	8/40 mcg/mL	7.5	150
7	0.2/1 mg	80/400 mcg/mL	2.5	180
8	0.6/3 mg	80/400 mcg/mL	7.5	210
9	1.8/9 mg	0.8/4 mg/mL	2.25	240
10	6/30 mg	8/40 mg/mL	0.75	270
11	18/90 mg	8/40 mg/mL	2.25	300
12	60/300 mg	8/40 mg/mL	7.5	330

Specific classes of drugs

Drug allergies have been reported to a wide array of medications and most drugs can cause multiple different types of allergic reactions. However most reactions are due to certain drugs leading to specific

Table 33.6. Protocol for Aspirin desensitization. It is recommended that patients should be premedication with a leukotriene modifier such as montelukast prior to the procedure. From Macy et al. 2013 (33).

Time (min)	Aspirin Dose (mg)
0	20.25
90	40.5
180	81
270	162.5
360	325

types of reactions. A solid grasp of these more common drug reactions is important for accurate diagnosis and appropriate evaluation and treatment.

Penicillins

Penicillins are the most frequently reported cause of medication allergy, with between 5 and 10% of people reporting an allergy to this class of drugs. However approximately 90% of these individuals can tolerate penicillin. Both inaccurate previous diagnoses and spontaneous resolution of penicillin allergy may account for this discrepancy. Most type I allergic reactions are caused by specific IgE directed to the core ring structure, which is identical in all penicillin antibiotics. *In vivo* the beta-lactam ring degrades into several reactive metabolites that can covalently bind lysine residues on proteins and act as haptens to elicit an immune response. Alternatively, the side chain or R-group, which distinguishes each synthetic penicillin from another can occasionally be antigenic and lead to a specific allergy to a selective type of penicillin. This mechanism accounts for about 1% of reactions. In the case of a true type I hypersensitivity reaction to a penicillin, unless it can be definitively proven to be due to a side chain, a patient must avoid all penicillin class antibiotics as they are cross reactive. Drug induced exanthems can also be seen with penicillins. A delayed drug induced exanthem is generally idiosyncratic and does not imply a cross reactivity with other drugs in this class.

Over diagnosis of penicillin allergy has led to an initiative to avoid overuse of non-beta-lactam antibiotics in patients with a history of penicillin allergy without an appropriate evaluation. While skin testing is part of an appropriate evaluation, there is increasing evidence that testing may not be necessary when the history consists of a delayed reaction that is cutaneous-only. In a recent study, 96% of patients with this type of history tolerated amoxicillin regardless of skin test results and the other 4% developed mild rash (Li et al. 2019).

Given this information, recommendations for performing an oral challenge without doing a skin test have been proposed (Macy and Vyles 2018). These criteria include any of the following if they have occurred more than 12 months previously:

- Any benign rash
- Gastrointestinal symptoms
- Headaches
- Other benign somatic symptoms
- Unknown history.

The authors recommend skin testing first if:

- The reaction occurred within the past 12 months
- The patient has a history of respiratory symptoms or anaphylaxis associated with penicillin
- The patient is uncomfortable doing a direct oral challenge.

Cephalosporins and other beta-lactam antibiotics

Cephalosporins all share a core ring structure that it is distinct from that of penicillin. This ring structure similarly can degrade to form hapten-protein complexes. These have not been isolated, so penicillin-equivalent skin tests are not available for cephalosporins. Most cephalosporin allergies are believed to be due to IgE directed at specific side chains and not at the core ring structure.

Most reactions to cephalosporins are type I hypersensitivity reactions. Skin testing with native cephalosporins can suggest sensitization if positive, but a negative test is not useful for ruling out an allergy if negative. In the setting of a reaction to a cephalosporin, the entire class may need to be avoided given cross reactivity within the family unless the reaction can be demonstrated to be side chain specific. Cross reactivity between penicillins and cephalosporins appears to be low, and most data support that a patient with a confirmed penicillin allergy has no higher likelihood of reacting to a cephalosporin than to any other class of antibiotics. Nevertheless, patients with penicillin allergy in whom a cephalosporin is indicated should be handled cautiously, particularly if the clinical reaction to penicillin was severe. Skin testing and graded challenges are useful tools for ruling out cephalosporin allergy in these patients.

Monobactams such as Aztreonam are another class of beta-lactam. They generally have no cross reactivity to penicillins or cephalosporins and can therefore be given in patients who are allergic to these agents (Adkinson 1990). Carbapenems appear to have low if any cross reactivity to penicillins but are often used cautiously in a patient with a severe penicillin allergy.

Sulfonamides

Approximately 4% of the general population will develop a hypersensitivity reaction to sulfonamide antimicrobials (Jick 1982). Type I reactions are rare as most reactions consist of delayed cutaneous reactions. These drugs usually cause mild type IV drug induced exanthems, but they are also associated with life-threatening SJS/TEN and DRESS (Cribb et al. 1996). The incidence of these serious reactions is relatively low. In contrast to the general population, approximately 60% of patients with HIV develop adverse reactions to sulfonamide antibiotics. In the case of mild cutaneous drug reactions in HIV positive patients, there has been good success with desensitization protocols. There is no evidence of true cross-reactivity between sulfonamide antibiotics and non-antibiotic medications containing sulfonamide or other sulfa moieties.

Vancomycin allergies are rare, however about half of patients will experience cutaneous erythema, flushing and pruritus (red man syndrome) due to non-IgE mediated mast cell degranulation (Polk et al. 1988). This type of reaction is dependent on the infusion rate so treatment can often resume at a slower rate. Both type I and mild type IV hypersensitivity reactions to clindamycin and fluoroquinolones can occur, but the causative metabolites are not well defined and there are no validated diagnostic tests for these agents. Macrolide allergies are generally rare. Immunologic reactions to several antimycobacterial drugs including isoniazid, ethambutol, pyrazinamide and rifampicin are not rare and include a diverse number of the immunologic drug reactions.

NSAIDS

AERD is a chronic condition manifested by asthma, nasal polyposis, rhinosinusitis and acute respiratory reactions to aspirin and other NSAIDs (Simon 2004). Approximately 10% of adults with asthma and a third of patients with asthma with nasal polyposis have AERD (Jenkins et al. 2004). It is caused by abnormal metabolism of arachidonic acid that is exacerbated by NSAIDs (Kim et al. 2008). This condition can be diagnosed by an aspirin challenge. Aspirin desensitization followed by daily aspirin has been associated with improved outcomes in patients with AERD who are poorly controlled with medical and/or surgical management.

Another common reaction from NSAIDs is exacerbation of urticaria or angioedema in patients with chronic urticaria. In these cases, the cause is presumed to be due to inhibition of COX-1 and therefore the reaction can be caused by any COX-1 inhibitor. Aspirin and NSAIDs that inhibit cyclooxygenase

1 (COX-1) cross-react and cause respiratory reactions in AERD, whereas selective COX-2 inhibitors almost never cause reactions in patients with AERD and can be taken safely.

Aspirin and NSAIDs may on rare occasion cause type I hypersensitivity reactions including urticaria and anaphylaxis (Stevenson et al. 2001). The immunologic basis for these reactions in unknown and there is no useful skin or *in vitro* testing for NSAID-specific IgE. Unlike AERD, there does not seem to be cross reactivity among agents in these patients.

Radiocontrast media

Anaphylactoid reactions occur in 1 to 3% of patients who receive ionic RCM and in less than 0.5% of patients who receive nonionic RCM (Coleman et al. 1964). Many patients who previously reacted to hyperosmotic agents will tolerate isosmotic ones (Katayama et al. 1990). For this reason, patients who need a contrast study should be asked if they have a history of acute urticaria, angioedema, bronchospasm and/or hypotension following the administration of RCM. Use of an isosmotic agent is recommended for such patients and to reduce the risk of an RCM reaction in patients who have not had any previous exposure, has become routine.

Since these reactions are not IgE-mediated, there are no tests that can accurately predict individuals who are at increased risk of having one (Yamaguchi et al. 1991). The mechanism of an RCM reaction is believed to be related to direct mast cell activation in susceptible individuals leading to anaphylaxis. There is no evidence that individuals with 'seafood allergy' are at increased risk of anaphylaxis to RCM when compared those without such a history.

Chemotherapeutics and biologics

Drug allergies have been reported for most chemotherapeutic agents. Taxanes and platinum agents are by far the most frequently implicated in type I hypersensitivity anaphylaxis. Cremophor-EL, a carrier molecule for hydrophobic drugs, has also frequently been implicated in type I hypersensitivity anaphylaxis. This is contained in paclitaxel, but also in tacrolimus, cyclosporine and IV vitamin K. Type III reactions have been seen frequently with methotrexate, thymoglobulin and rituximab. Type IV drug-induced exanthems are common with bortezomib, rituximab, fludarabine, gemcitabine and cytarabine. SJS/TEN is rare with all chemotherapeutics but has been reported with over 30 separate agents. Bleomycin and methotrexate have both frequently been implicated in pneumonitis.

Biologic drugs comprise a quickly growing field of medicine including a diverse number of proteins and monoclonal antibodies. Type I hypersensitivity reactions have been reported with most of these medications leading to urticaria or anaphylaxis. A variety of delayed cutaneous reactions have also been noted with several of these medications. Infusions reactions ranging from fevers and chills to acute respiratory distress syndrome have also been seen with several monoclonal antibodies, which is presumed to be due to cytokine release. Given the novelty of these drugs, the full spectrum of reactions is not yet known.

Clinical cases

(1) A 55-year-old woman with multiple myeloma reports that 10 years ago she received oral amoxicillin for pneumonia and developed immediate hives and throat swelling after the first dose. She was treated with diphenhydramine and steroids and switched to levofloxacin. In the years prior to this she had been treated with penicillin on at least two occasions without adverse events. She has avoided penicillin since that event. Five years ago she was treated with oral cephalexin for cellulitis and after the first dose developed immediate hives and wheezing. She has since been labeled with a penicillin and cephalosporin allergy and has avoided all beta-lactam antibiotics. She will likely need antibiotics during her upcoming therapy and is referred for evaluation and planning for desensitization. Given this history, skin testing is performed with penicillin, penicilloyl-polylysine, amoxicillin and ceftazadime. The only positive reaction is to amoxicillin. It is determined she is allergic to the shared side chain that is in both amoxicillin and cephalexin and not to the core beta-lactam ring of either penicillin or cephalosporin. Her allergies are specific to the aminopenicillin and a small subset

of cephalosporin that share this common side chain. She tolerates all other beta-lactam antibiotics without issue.

(2) A 40-year-old male suffers after a fall a subdural hematoma requiring evacuation (day 0). On day 5, he develops an infection of the surgical site and is treated with ceftriaxone. On day 7 he has a seizure and is treated with phenytoin. The infection persists so on day 21 he is treated with vancomycin. He then undergoes debridement on day 29 and vancomycin is stopped. On day 30 he develops a diffuse maculopapular rash, so the ceftriaxone is switched to amoxicillin-clavulanate. Vancomycin and ceftriaxone are listed as allergies causing a rash. The rash persists so on day 33 laboratories are checked which show an elevated eosinophil count of 500, normal renal function and an ALT of 350 and an AST of 260. Amoxicillin-clavulanate is stopped and added to his allergy list. He is put on levofloxacin and metronidazole. Despite the change, the rash persists, and he develops fevers, rigors and myalgias. He is admitted to the hospital and empirically started on prednisone 40 mg. His symptoms continue and repeat laboratory tests show a normal eosinophil count, an ALT of 1100 and an AST of 700. At this point levofloxacin, metronidazole and phenytoin are stopped and prednisone is continued. Over the course of 3 days his fevers and myalgias were solved and in two weeks his rash resolved and his LFTs trend down. A diagnosis of DRESS is made, and phenytoin is identified as the etiology. His other drug allergies are removed from his record.[1]

Conclusion

The spectrum of drug allergy has evolved overtime. There is a broad range of adverse drug reactions including immunologic and non-immunologic reactions. The exact mechanisms of drug allergy are currently unknown. A detailed clinical history is crucial in the diagnosis of drug allergy.

References

Adkinson NF, Jr. Immunogenicity and cross-allergenicity of aztreonam. Am J Med 1990; 88(3C): 12S–5S; discussion 38S–42S.

Ange N, Alley S, Fernando SL, Coyle L, Yun J. Drug Reaction with Eosinophilia and Systemic Symptoms (DRESS) syndrome successfully treated with mepolizumab. J Allergy Clin Immunol Pract 2018; 6(3): 1059–60.

Antoon JW, Goldman JL, Shah SS, Lee B. A retrospective cohort study of the management and outcomes of children hospitalized with stevens-johnson syndrome or toxic epidermal necrolysis. J Allergy Clin Immunol Pract 2019; 7(1): 244–50 e1.

Atanaskovic-Markovic M, Jankovic J, Tmusic V, Gavrovic-Jankulovic M, Cirkovic Velickovic T, Nikolic D, et al. Hypersensitivity reactions to antiepileptic drugs in children. Pediatr Allergy Immunol 2019; 30(5): 547–52.

Ben Fadhel N, Chaabane A, Ammar H, Ben Romdhane H, Soua Y, Chadli Z, et al. Clinical features, culprit drugs, and allergology workup in 41 cases of fixed drug eruption. Contact Dermatitis 2019; 81(5): 336–40.

Caimmi S, Caffarelli C, Saretta F, Liotti L, Crisafulli G, Cardinale F, et al. Drug desensitization in allergic children. Acta Biomed 2019; 90(3-S): 20–9.

Coleman WP, Ochsner SF, Watson BE. Allergic Reactions in 10,000 Consecutive Intravenous Urographies. South Med J 1964; 57: 1401–4.

Cribb AE, Lee BL, Trepanier LA, Spielberg SP. Adverse reactions to sulphonamide and sulphonamide-trimethoprim antimicrobials: clinical syndromes and pathogenesis. Adverse Drug React Toxicol Rev 1996; 15(1): 9–50.

DeGregorio GA, Singer J, Cahill KN, Laidlaw T. A 1-Day, 90-Minute aspirin challenge and desensitization protocol in aspirin-exacerbated respiratory disease. J Allergy Clin Immunol Pract 2019; 7(4): 1174–80.

De Groot H, Mulder WM. Clinical practice: drug desensitization in children. Eur J Pediatr 2010; 169(11): 1305–9.

Demoly P, Messaad D, Reynes J, Faucherre V, Bousquet J. Trimethoprim-sulfamethoxazole-graded challenge in HIV-infected patients: long-term follow-up regarding efficacy and safety. J Allergy Clin Immunol 2000; 105(3): 588–9.

Elzagallaai AA, Knowles SR, Rieder MJ, Bend JR, Shear NH, Koren G. Patch testing for the diagnosis of anticonvulsant hypersensitivity syndrome: a systematic review. Drug Saf 2009; 32(5): 391–408.

Empedrad R, Darter AL, Earl HS, Gruchalla RS. Nonirritating intradermal skin test concentrations for commonly prescribed antibiotics. J Allergy Clin Immunol 2003; 112(3): 629–30.

Fonacier L, Bernstein DI, Pacheco K, Holness DL, Blessing-Moore J, Khan D, et al. Contact dermatitis: a practice parameter-update 2015. J Allergy Clin Immunol Pract 2015; 3(3 Suppl): S1–39.

---

[1] Disclosure:

Dr. Portnoy has nothing to disclose; Dr. Pandya has nothing to disclose

Galvao VR, Aun MV, Kalil J, Castells M, Giavina-Bianchi P. Clinical and laboratory improvement after intravenous immunoglobulin in drug reaction with eosinophilia and systemic symptoms. J Allergy Clin Immunol Pract 2014; 2(1): 107–10.

Gell, P. G. H., and R. R. A. Coombs. Classification of allergic reactions responsible for clinical hypersensitivity and disease. Clinical Aspects of Immunology 2 (1975).

Henning MA, Opstrup MS, Taudorf EH. Acute generalized exanthematous pustulosis to amoxicillin. Dermatitis 2019; 30(4): 274–5.

Hope AP, Woessner KA, Simon RA, Stevenson DD. Rational approach to aspirin dosing during oral challenges and desensitization of patients with aspirin-exacerbated respiratory disease. J Allergy Clin Immunol 2009; 123(2): 406–10.

Jenkins C, Costello J, Hodge L. Systematic review of prevalence of aspirin induced asthma and its implications for clinical practice. BMJ 2004; 328(7437): 434.

Jick H. Adverse reactions to trimethoprim-sulfamethoxazole in hospitalized patients. Rev Infect Dis 1982; 4(2): 426–8.

Joint Task Force on Practice P, American Academy of Allergy A, Immunology, American College of Allergy A, Immunology, Joint Council of Allergy A, et al. Drug allergy: an updated practice parameter. Ann Allergy Asthma Immunol 2010; 105(4): 259–73.

Katayama H, Yamaguchi K, Kozuka T, Takashima T, Seez P, Matsuura K. Adverse reactions to ionic and nonionic contrast media. A report from the Japanese Committee on the Safety of Contrast Media. Radiology 1990; 175(3): 621–8.

Kim SH, Hur GY, Choi JH, Park HS. Pharmacogenetics of aspirin-intolerant asthma. Pharmacogenomics 2008; 9(1): 85–91.

Knowles SR, Dewhurst N, Shear NH. Anticonvulsant hypersensitivity syndrome: an update. Expert Opin Drug Saf 2012; 11(5): 767–78.

Liu A, Fanning L, Chong H, Fernandez J, Sloane D, Sancho-Serra M, et al. Desensitization regimens for drug allergy: state of the art in the 21st century. Clin Exp Allergy 2011; 41(12): 1679–89.

Li J, Shahabi-Sirjani A, Figtree M, Hoyle P, Fernando SL. Safety of direct drug provocation testing in adults with penicillin allergy and association with health and economic benefits. Ann Allergy Asthma Immunol 2019.

Macy E, Bernstein JA, Castells MC, Gawchik SM, Lee TH, Settipane RA, et al. Aspirin challenge and desensitizatio for aspirin-exacerbated respiratory disease: a practice paper. Ann Allergy Asthma Immunol 2007; 98(2): 172–4.

Macy E, Ngor EW. Safely diagnosing clinically significant penicillin allergy using only penicilloyl-poly-lysine, penicillin, and oral amoxicillin. J Allergy Clin Immunol Pract 2013; 1(3): 258–63.

Macy E, Vyles D. Who needs penicillin allergy testing? Ann Allergy Asthma Immunol 2018; 121(5): 523–9.

Namazy JA, Simon RA. Sensitivity to nonsteroidal anti-inflammatory drugs. Ann Allergy Asthma Immunol 2002; 89(6): 542–50; quiz 50, 605.

Polk RE, Healy DP, Schwartz LB, Rock DT, Garson ML, Roller K. Vancomycin and the red-man syndrome: pharmacodynamics of histamine release. J Infect Dis 1988; 157(3): 502–7.

Simon RA. Adverse respiratory reactions to aspirin and nonsteroidal anti-inflammatory drugs. Curr Allergy Asthma Rep 2004; 4(1): 17–24.

Sokumbi O, Wetter DA. Clinical features, diagnosis, and treatment of erythema multiforme: a review for the practicing dermatologist. Int J Dermatol 2012; 51(8): 889–902.

Solensky R, Khan DA. Evaluation of antibiotic allergy: the role of skin tests and drug challenges. Curr Allergy Asthma Rep 2014; 14(9): 459.

Sousa-Pinto B, Fonseca JA, Gomes ER. Frequency of self-reported drug allergy: A systematic review and meta-analysis with meta-regression. Ann Allergy Asthma Immunol 2017; 119(4): 362–73 e2.

Stevenson DD, Sanchez-Borges M, Szczeklik A. Classification of allergic and pseudoallergic reactions to drugs that inhibit cyclooxygenase enzymes. Ann Allergy Asthma Immunol 2001; 87(3): 177–80.

Stevenson DD, Woessner KM, Simon RA, Namazy JA, Lang DM. Evidence-based protocols for oral NSAID challenges. J Pediatr 2006; 148(5): 704–5; author reply 5–6.

Subramanian H, Gupta K, Ali H. Roles of Mas-related G protein-coupled receptor X2 on mast cell-mediated host defense, pseudoallergic drug reactions, and chronic inflammatory diseases. J Allergy Clin Immunol 2016; 138(3): 700–10.

Sullivan TJ, Yecies LD, Shatz GS, Parker CW, Wedner HJ. Desensitization of patients allergic to penicillin using orally administered beta-lactam antibiotics. J Allergy Clin Immunol 1982; 69(3): 275–82.

Tas S, Simonart T. Management of drug rash with eosinophilia and systemic symptoms (DRESS syndrome): an update. Dermatology 2003; 206(4): 353–6.

Thong BY, Tan TC. Epidemiology and risk factors for drug allergy. Br J Clin Pharmacol 2011; 71(5): 684–700.

Ton A, Kassab L, Patel A, Dawson N. Severe acute hepatitis in drug reaction with eosinophilia and systemicsymptoms (DRESS) syndrome resolved following cyclosporine. J Allergy Clin Immunol Pract 2019.

Vaglio A, Grayson PC, Fenaroli P, Gianfreda D, Boccaletti V, Ghiggeri GM, et al. Drug-induced lupus: Traditional and new concepts. Autoimmun Rev 2018; 17(9): 912–8.

WAO. International Drug Monitoring: The Role of the Hospital. Geneva, Switzerland; 1966. Contract No.: Technical Report Series No. 425.

Wolfson AR, Zhou L, Li Y, Phadke NA, Chow OA, Blumenthal KG. Drug Reaction with Eosinophilia and Systemic Symptoms (DRESS) Syndrome identified in the electronic health record allergy module. J Allergy Clin Immunol Pract 2019; 7(2): 633–40.

Yamaguchi K, Katayama H, Takashima T, Kozuka T, Seez P, Matsuura K. Prediction of severe adverse reactions to ionic and nonionic contrast media in Japan: evaluation of pretesting. A report from the Japanese Committee on the Safety of Contrast Media. Radiology 1991; 178(2): 363–7.

34

Latex Allergy

Ronald D DeGuzman[1] *and Pudupakkam K Vedanthan*[2,*]

INTRODUCTION

Natural Rubber Latex (NRL) is a ubiquitous material found in thousands of consumer and medical products. Nearly all of the world's latex is derived commercially from the milky cytoplasmic fluid of the rubber tree, *Hevea brasiliensis* (Yip and Cacioli 2002). This fluid is composed of small hydrocarbon particles of cis-1,4-polyisprene in a phospholipoprotein envelope dispersed in an aqueous serum containing sugars, nucleic acids, carbohydrates, minerals and proteins (Spina and Levine 1999). The protein content can vary from 1 to 2% with 60% associated with the rubber particle and 40% the serum. Approximately 90% of the harvested rubber is used to manufacture solid dry rubber products such as automobile tires, conveyor belts rubber hoses and balls. IgE-mediated hypersensitivity is rarely seen with this type of rubber, but delayed contact hypersensitivity reactions have been reported (Kelly 2010). The remaining 10% of the harvested rubber is used to manufacture dipped products, which include rubber gloves, condoms and balloons. Dipped rubber products are responsible for the majority of allergic reactions to natural rubber latex (Ahmed et al. 2003).

In the manufacture of dipped latex products, a process of vulcanization occurs where the rubber material is mixed with sulfur and heat treated to enhance elasticity and strength. Accelerators such as thiurams, mercapto compounds, carbamates and thioureas, may be used to decrease the production time in the manufacturing of NRL products (Cohen et al. 1998). These compounds rarely cause IgE-mediated reactions, but commonly are involved in delayed hypersensitivity contact dermatitis (Hamann et al. 2005).

There are two immunological reactions to natural rubber latex, an immediate type I IgE-mediated reaction and a delayed type IV reaction also known as contact dermatitis. The first report of immediate type clinical symptoms to NRL dates back to 1927 with severe generalized urticaria and laryngeal edema caused by an NRL dental prosthesis (G.S. et al. 1927) Contact dermatitis to rubber gloves was first reported in 1933 (Downing 1933). Beginning in the late 1980s and extending into the early 1990s, there was a growth in the numbers of individuals affected by latex allergy. Major factors leading to this rise in latex sensitivity included escalated recognition of the disease as well as the increase of glove use due to the institution of universal precautions by the Center for Disease Control in 1987 in response to the concerns for AIDS and other transmissible diseases (Ownby 2002). The apparent rise in latex sensitivity hit its peak in the mid 1990s and has since been decreasing (Ranta and Ownby 2004) The

---

[1] Allergy/Immunology/Immunization Service, Walter Reed National Military Medical Center, Bethesda, Maryland. USA.
  Email: ron.deguzman@amedd.army.mil
[2] University of Colorado, Denver,Colorado. USA.
* Corresponding author: pkv1947@gmail.com

FDA established regulations concerning the latex protein and powdered content of gloves in 1997 and mandated the labeling of medical devices containing natural rubber latex in 1998 (Farnham et al. 2002). In addition, recognition of the disease has led to health care facilities implementing protocols to decrease latex exposure to patients and staff and glove manufacturers have taken steps to reduce the sensitization potential of NRL gloves (Ranta and Ownby 2004).

In contrast to type I and type IV hypersensitivity, the most common reaction associated with latex is a non-immunologically mediated irritant contact dermatitis that is typically seen with people using gloves (Hepner and Castells 2003). The reaction presents as dry crusted lesions localized to the glove-exposed areas, develops within minutes to hours of exposure and is likely due to the alkaline pH of powdered gloves.

Prevelance

The prevalence of IgE-mediated latex allergy varies with the method for making the diagnosis and the population studied (Sussman et al. 2002). A number of studies using skin pinprick testing estimate the prevalence of IgE-mediated allergy to NRL to be around 1% (Liss and Sussman 1999). In contrast, studies using serum latex specific-IgE show the prevalence to be higher. In 1000 healthy volunteer blood donors, Ownby found the rate of sensitization to be 6.5%, however the clinical relevance of the positive tests is unknown (Ownby et al. 1996).

The prevalence of Type IV hypersensitivity to latex has been reported in studies of patients referred to dermatology clinics for patch testing. In a prospective study of 2738 consecutive patients, 1% were positive to a patch test to NRL and in another series of 822 patients, the prevalence of delayed type hypersensitivity to latex was 1.2% (Sommer et al. 2002, Wilkinson and Beck 1996).

Pathogenesis

Immediate type I hypersensitivity to latex is mediated by an IgE response to these latex proteins. Exposure can occur via the skin, mucous membrane or the respiratory tract. In addition, mucous membranes of the gastrointestinal and urogenital tracts can be exposed by direct contact with NRL catheters and internal exposure can occur during surgical procedures by the use of NRL gloves or internally placed latex materials such as wound drains (Weissman and Lewis 2002). Patients become sensitized with plasma cells producing IgE to latex proteins. The IgE binds to the surfaces of mast cells and upon re-exposure to latex these sensitized cells release mediators leading to the onset of symptoms (Hepner and Castells 2003).

Type IV allergy to latex is a delayed cell-mediated reaction where allergen interacts with Langerhans cells in the skin and is presented to CD4+ T cells inducing the clonal expansion of antigen-specific T lymphocytes (Shah and Chowdhury 2011). Further clonal expansion occurs in the regional lymph nodes and the sensitized T cells are then dispersed throughout the body. Upon subsequent exposure of the skin to sufficient antigen, a local inflammatory response ensues (Ownby 1995). This occurs over 24–48 hours and results in a pruritic, eczematous reaction at the site where allergen has been in contact with the skin (Shah and Chowdhury 2011).

Etiology

Exposure is the single most significant risk factor associated with latex allergy (Slater 1994). Occupations with high latex exposure such as healthcare workers, rubber industry workers, agriculture workers and housekeepers are known to have a higher risk of developing latex allergy (Cohen et al. 1998) (Slater 1994). In health care workers, this prevalence ranges from 2.8 (Turjanmaa et al. 1996) to 17% (Yassin et al. 1994). Patients who have undergone multiple operations have higher sensitization rates to latex. This is especially true for patients with spina bifida with reported prevalence ranging from 17 to 64%, likely due to increased mucosal exposure (Johar et al. 2005, Niggemann 2010). Other reported risk factors for NRL allergy include atopy and pre-existing hand dermatitis (Turjanmaa and Makinen-Kiljunen 2002).

There are 14 latex allergens known to elicit IgE antibody, named Hev b 1 to Hev b 14. Certain allergens have been associated with different clinical entities (Table 34.1). Spina bifida is associated with

Table 34.1. Latex allergens: properties.

Allergen	Biological property	Clinical cross reactivity	Allergenic significance
Hev b 1	Elongation		*Major/Minor*
Hev b 2	Defense		*Major*
Hev b 3	Elongation		*Major/Minor*
Hev b 4	Synthesis		NA
Hev b 5	Structural	Kiwi	*Major*
Hev b 6	Major Protein	Banana Avocado, Chestnut	Major
Hev b 7	Inhibitor Esterase	Potato, Egg Plant	Minor
Hev b 8	Binding	Prolifins	NA
Hev b 9	Enolase		Minor
Hev b 10	Protection		Minor
Hev b 11	Chitinase		Minor
Hev b 12	Lipid Transfer Protein	NA	NA
Hev b 13	Elongation	NA	*Major*

Hev b 1 and Hev b 3 and Hev b 7 (Niggemann 2010, Wagner et al. 2001). The major allergens in health care workers are thought to be Hev b 2, Hev b 5, Hev b 6 and Hev b 13 (Bernstein et al. 2003).

There is a well-reported clinical association between latex allergy and allergies to a number of fruits and vegetables. This latex fruit syndrome has been reported with chestnut, avocado, banana, kiwi, papaya, peach, tomato, potato and bell pepper (Wagner and Breiteneder 2002). A group of defense-related proteins, class I chitinases are the major panallergen responsible for this syndrome and have structural homology with Hev b 6.01, a major NRL allergen (Blanco 2003).

Unlike with type I hypersensitivity, delayed contact reactions to NRL are not due to the latex protein but rather to chemicals used in the manufacturing of NRL products to include accelerators and anti-oxidants. The most common accelerators accounting for type IV hypersensitivity to latex gloves are thiurams, carbamates and mercapto compounds (Cohen et al. 1998).

Diagnosis

The diagnosis of immediate Type I latex allergy begins with a thorough history and physical examination with the clinical conclusions supported by appropriate testing (Kelly 2010). The skin is frequently involved and can begin as local urticaria or angioedema in areas of contact to latex products and later become generalized (Ownby 1995). Symptoms usually start within 15 minutes of exposure and last for 30 to 60 minutes after exposure stops (Pecquet at al. 1990). Airborne exposure or contact with respiratory symptoms can lead to rhinitis with sneezing, congestion and rhinorrhea or lower respiratory symptoms of wheezing and dyspnea (Ownby 1995). Although the cornstarch donning powder in powdered latex gloves is not considered allergenic, it is considered a carrier for some latex allergens (Tomazic et al. 1994). More severe reactions are usually associated with parenteral exposure and include flushing vasodilatation severe bronchospasm and cardiovascular collapse (Laxenaire and Mertes 2001).

Skin testing is considered the most sensitive test for confirming the diagnosis of latex allergy. Skin testing is the primary confirmatory test in Europe and Canada and is available commercially with ammoniated and non-ammoniated latex extracts (Bernadini et al. 2008). In the United States, FDA-approved latex skin tests are not available and thus serologic testing for latex specific IgE has become the most widely accepted confirmatory test (Hamilton 2002). This *in vitro* test, however, has suboptimal diagnostic predictive value with highly variable reported sensitivities between 50 to 100% (Lieberman et al. 2010). Provocative testing methods, to include glove use tests, inhalational challenge and nasal provocation, have been reported by a number of investigators. Due to concerns with safety, reproducibility and interpretation of these testing methods, provocation testing has not been recommended by some experts for routine clinical use (Hamilton 2002).

In contrast to immediate hypersensitivity, delayed-type IV reactions to NRL are limited to areas of contact, typically on the hands of individuals occupationally wearing latex gloves (Cohen et al. 1998). Lesions usually occur 24–48 hours after exposure and can present initially with erythema, pruritus, vesicles or blisters. With continued exposure, chronic lesions may develop dryness, scaling, fissuring and thickness (Ownby 1995). The diagnosis is confirmed by patch testing to rubber additives. The standard patch test series for rubber additives in most countries contains mixes of thiuram, carba, mercapto and black rubber (Shah and Chowdhury 2011).

Treatment

For immediate and delayed type hypersensitivity to latex, the mainstay of management is avoidance of latex products. For the latex allergic individual, the management begins with the awareness of possible exposure in the home and work environment and the use of non-latex alternatives. Pharmacotherapy can provide symptomatic relief of symptoms. Urticaria responds to elimination of antigen and use of antihistamines, asthma symptoms are treated with bronchodilators and contact dermatitis responds to topical steroids (Cohen et al. 1998, Kelly 1995). Patients with systemic reactions to latex should always carry self-injectable epinephrine. Other measures recommended for the latex-allergic individual include wearing a medical alert bracelet indicating the latex allergy, carrying non-latex gloves in the event emergency resuscitation is required and alerting healthcare providers early for medical, dental, surgical and gynecological procedures in order to facilitate latex free protocols and a latex-safe environment (Chua et al. 2005). Studies in the U.S. have shown that primary prevention strategies such as switching to low allergen, non-powdered latex gloves have led to a dramatic decrease in the prevalence of latex allergy (Hunt et al. 2002).

A primary prevention study was conducted in Germany (Allmers et al. 2002) among health care workers in facilities serving a population of nearly 3 million consumers. The intervention included switching to the use of Non Powdered Natural Rubber Latex (NRL) gloves. After a lag period of 2 years, the prevalence of occupational NRL allergy cases started to decline significantly along with the decrease in the use of powdered gloves. This study showed that primary prevention of using low protein, non powdered gloves caused significant reduction of NRL glove allergy.

The newer synthetic rubber glove made from Nitrile Butadeine rubber seems to retain all the unique characteristic of the latex glove, namely elasticity, viral impenetrability, toughness against tears as well as the ability to regain the original shape after stretching.

Latex avoidance from birth in Spina Bifida patients (Slater 1994), prevention of IgE sensitization to latex in health care workers after reduction of antigen exposures (Liss and Sussman 1997). Epidemiological study of hospital workers for Latex Allergy (Kelley et al. 2011), identified the latex examination gloves as the causative agent for the epidemic. Dramatic improvement in lowering the sensitization rates occurred after changing to non powdered gloves as well as the usage of powdered gloves by health care workers (Liss and Sussman 1999). Inspite of these positive interventions, there are still 'unanswered questions' (Table 34.2) regarding latex allergy.

In addition, AAAAI, ACAAI and Association of Operating room nurses as well as NIOSH published alerts which also had an impact in reducing the use of powdered gloves However it was the scientific epidemiological and clinical studies across the globe that led to convincing that latex allergen content of the gloves and its transmission via the corn starch granules in the ambient environment was causing the epidemic. The final banning of the powdered surgeons gloves, powdered examination gloves and absorbable powder for lubrication of the surgeons gloves by the Food and Drug administration in January 2017 in the United States will keep this disease under control.

Case scenarios

Case 1: This is a young boy who apparently blew up a latex balloon at the school party. He also touched his eyes, nose and skin over the face during this time. He developed an immediate allergic reaction with

Table 34.2. Unresolved issues in latex allergy*.

FDA-cleared latex skin test reagent
Improved sensitivity of latex-specific IgE serologic assays
Managing daily lives of patients with persistent latex allergy
How do patients with spina bifida get sensitized?
What is the source of sensitization to latex in the general population?
Can we get all occupational-induced latex-allergic patients back to work?
What happens to the occupational asthma of latex allergy over time?
Can we eliminate type 4 contact dermatitis to additive chemicals in all gloves through better manufacturing?
Educating health care providers about latex allergy with its lower prevalence
What should be done with multiple-dose vials that have NRL tops (e.g., vaccine)?

* Permission sought from Elsiever

dermal and respiratory symptoms within minutes. Latex antigen present on the surgical glove probably adsorbed on the starch powder used on the gloves to keep it pliable. Latex antigen is water soluble. He had absorption of the latex antigen through two routes: Oral mucous membrane as well as skin over the face. Mode of transmission of the latex antigen: Mucous membrane and skin.

Case 2: This case demonstrates the importance of being aware of the ambient latex particles in the hospital working environment. The young desk clerk has history of allergic reaction to ingestion of banana, due to cross reactivity with the latex antigen. The Emergency room is a busy place with health professionals changing gloves quite often. This leads to dispersal of the latex antigen into the ambient air. The desk clerk developed acute allergic respiratory symptoms apparently after inhalation of the ambient latex particles in the Emergency room, without any direct contact with any of the latex products. Mode of transmission of the latex antigen: Inhalation from the ambient air.

Case 3: The pulmonologist had developed latex sensitization over a period of time due to exposure due to his occupation as an intensivist working in the hospital. He also had a history of breaking out with urticarial rash with itching after wearing a swimming cap. Over a period of time his latex sensitization got progressively worse. This is a case of cumulative latex allergy.

Clinical pearls

- There are three reactions to natural rubber latex: irritant contact, Type I immediate hypersensitivity and Type IV delayed hypersensitivity (contact dermatitis).
- There is a clinical association between latex allergy and allergies to certain foods due to cross-reactive proteins. This cross-reactivity is seen more often with chestnut, banana, avocado, kiwi, papaya, peach, tomato, potato and bell pepper.
- Groups at highest risk for development of latex allergy include healthcare workers and patients with spina bifida.
- The diagnosis is established by the clinical history and examination with appropriate testing confirming the diagnosis. In the United States, *in vitro* latex specific IgE is the test of choice for immediate hypersensitivity. For contact dermatitis to latex products, patch testing is used.
- The mainstay of management is avoidance of latex products.

Summary

Despite the decrease in latex hypersensitivity due to increased recognition and primary prevention measures, allergy to natural rubber latex continues to be a significant concern, particularly in the health care setting. Providers need to be aware of the clinical presentation and the diagnostic testing modalities available in order to accurately identify latex-allergic individuals. Patient education and establishing of avoidance measures in the home and work environment is critical in order to prevent further exposures and potential reactions.

Disclaimer

The views expressed in this book chapter are those of the author and do not necessarily reflect the official views of the Walter Reed National Military Medical Center, the U.S. Army, U.S. Navy, U.S. Air Force, Department of Defense, nor the U.S. Government.

References

Ahmed DD, Sobczak SC, Yunginger JW. Occupational allergies caused by latex. Immunol Allergy Clin North Am 2003; 23(2): 205–19.

Allmers H, Schmengler J, Skudlik C. Primary prevention of natural rubber latex allergy in the Germn health care system through education and intervention. J Allergy Clin Immunol 2002; 110(2): 318–23.

Bernardini R, Pucci N, Azzari C, Novembre E, De Martino M, Milani M. Sensitivity and specificity of different skin prick tests with latex extracts in pediatric patients with suspected natural rubber latex allergy—a cohort study. Pediatr Allergy Immunol 2008; 19(4): 315–8.

Bernstein DI, Biagini RE, Karnani R, Hamilton R, Murphy K, Bernstein C, et al. *In vivo* sensitization to purified Hevea brasiliensis proteins in health care workers sensitized to natural rubber latex. J Allergy Clin Immunol 2003; 111(3): 610–6.

Blanco C. Latex-fruit syndrome. Curr Allergy Asthma Rep 2003; 3(1): 47–53.

Chua IC, Owen AJ, Williams PE. Management of latex allergy: allergist's perspective. pp. 249–58. *In*: Chowdhury MMU, Maibach HI (eds.). Latex Intolerance: Basic Science, Epidemiology, and Clinical Management. Boca Raton: CRC Press; 2005.

Cohen DE, Scheman A, Stewart L, Taylor J, Pratt M, Trotter K, et al. American Academy of Dermatology's position paper on latex allergy. J Am Acad Dermatol 1998; 39(1): 98–106.

Downing J. Dermatitis from rubber gloves. N Engl J Med 1933; 208(4): 196–8.

Farnham JJ, Tomazic-Jezic VJ, Stratmeyer ME. Regulatory initiatives for natural latex allergy: US perspectives. Methods 2002; 27(1): 87–92.

G.S. Überempfindlichkeit gegen Kautschuk als ursache von Urticaria und Quinckeschem Ödem. Klin Wochenschr. 1927; 6: 1096–7.

Hamann CP, Rodgers PA, Sullivan K. Chemical additives. pp. 28–56. *In*: Chowdhury MMU, Maibach HI (eds.). Latex Intolerance : Basic Science, Epidemiology, and Clinical Management. Boca Raton: CRC Press; 2005.

Hamilton RG. Diagnosis of natural rubber latex allergy. Methods 2002; 27(1): 22–31.

Hepner DL, Castells MC. Latex allergy: an update. Anesth Analg 2003; 96(4): 1219–29.

Hunt LW, Kelkar P, Reed CE, Yunginger JW. Management of occupational allergy to natural rubber latex in a medical center: the importance of quantitative latex allergen measurement and objective follow-up. J Allergy Clin Immunol 2002; 110(2 Suppl): S96–106.

Johar A, Lim DL, Arif SA, Hawarden D, Toit GD, Weinberg EG, et al. Low prevalence of latex sensitivity in South African spina bifida children in Cape Town. Pediatr Allergy Immunol 2005; 16(2): 165–70.

Kelly KJ. Management of the latex-allergic patient. Immunol Allergy Clin North Am 1995; 15(1): 139–57.

Kelly K. Latex allergy. pp. 631–9. *In*: Leung DYM, Sampson HA, Geha R, Szefler SJ (eds.). Pediatric Allergy: Principles and Practice 2nd ed. Edinburgh: Saunders; 2010.

Kelly K, Wang M, Klancick M, Petsonk E. Prevention of IgE sensitization to latex in health care workers After Reduction of Antigen Exposures. J of Occu Envi Med 2011: 53: 934–940

Laxenaire MC, Mertes PM. Anaphylaxis during anaesthesia. Results of a two-year survey in France. Br J Anaesth 2001; 87(4): 549–58.

Lieberman P, Nicklas RA, Oppenheimer J, Kemp SF, Lang DM, Bernstein DI, et al. The diagnosis and management of anaphylaxis practice parameter: 2010 update. J Allergy Clin Immunol 2010; 126(3): 477–80 e1–42.

Liss GM, Sussman GL. Latex sensitization: occupational versus general population prevalence rates. Am J Ind Med 1999; 35(2): 196–200.

Niggemann B. IgE-mediated latex allergy—an exciting and instructive piece of allergy history. Pediatr Allergy Immunol 2010; 21(7): 997–1001.

Ownby D. Manifestations of latex allergy. Immunol Allergy Clin North Am. 1995; 15(1): 21–9.

Ownby DR, Ownby HE, McCullough J, Shafer AW. The prevalence of anti-latex IgE antibodies in 1000 volunteer blood donors. J Allergy Clin Immunol 1996; 97(6): 1188–92.

Ownby DR. A history of latex allergy. J Allergy Clin Immunol 2002; 110(2 Suppl): S27–32.

Pecquet C, Leynadier F, Dry J. Contact urticaria and anaphylaxis to natural latex. J Am Acad Dermatol 1990; 22(4): 631–3.

Ranta PM, Ownby DR. A review of natural-rubber latex allergy in health care workers. Clin Infect Dis 2004; 38(2): 252–6.

Shah D, Chowdhury MM. Rubber allergy. Clin Dermatol 2011; 29(3): 278–86.
Slater JE. Latex allergy. J Allergy Clin Immunol 1994; 94(2 Pt 1): 139–49; quiz 50.
Sommer S, Wilkinson SM, Beck MH, English JS, Gawkrodger DJ, Green C. Type IV hypersensitivity reactions to natural rubber latex: results of a multicentre study. Br J Dermatol 2002; 146(1): 114–7.
Spina AM, Levine HJ. Latex allergy: a review for the dental professional. Oral Surg Oral Med Oral Pathol Oral Radiol Endod 1999; 87(1): 5–11.
Sussman GL, Beezhold DH, Liss G. Latex allergy: historical perspective. Methods 2002; 27(1): 3–9.
Tomazic VJ, Shampaine EL, Lamanna A, Withrow TJ, Adkinson NF, Jr, Hamilton RG. Cornstarch powder on latex products is an allergen carrier. J Allergy Clin Immunol 1994; 93(4): 751–8.
Turjanmaa K, Alenius H, Makinen-Kiljunen S, Reunala T, Palosuo T. Natural rubber latex allergy. Allergy 1996; 51(9): 593–602.
Turjanmaa K, Makinen-Kiljunen S. Latex allergy: prevalence, risk factors, and cross-reactivity. Methods 2002; 27(1): 10–4.
Wagner B, Buck D, Hafner C, Sowka S, Niggemann B, Scheiner O, et al. Hev b 7 is a Hevea brasiliensis protein associated with latex allergy in children with spina bifida. J Allergy Clin Immunol 2001; 108(4): 621–7.
Wagner S, Breiteneder H. The latex-fruit syndrome. Biochem Soc Trans 2002; 30(Pt 6): 935–40.
Weissman DN, Lewis DM. Allergic and latex-specific sensitization: route, frequency, and amount of exposure that are required to initiate IgE production. J Allergy Clin Immunol 2002; 110(2 Suppl): S57–63.
Wilkinson SM, Beck MH. Allergic contact dermatitis from latex rubber. Br J Dermatol 1996; 134(5): 910–4.
Yassin MS, Sanyurah S, Lierl MB, Fischer TJ, Oppenheimer S, Cross J, et al. Evaluation of latex allergy in patients with meningomyelocele. Ann Allergy 1992; 69(3): 207–11.
Yassin MS, Lierl MB, Fischer TJ, O'Brien K, Cross J, Steinmetz C. Latex allergy in hospital employees. Ann Allergy 1994; 72(3): 245–9.
Yip E, Cacioli P. The manufacture of gloves from natural rubber latex. J Allergy Clin Immunol 2002; 110(2 Suppl): S3–14.

35

Allergy–Asthma Practice
East vs West

Mark Holbreich,[1] *Pudupakkam K Vedanthan,*[2,*] *PA Mahesh*[3] *and Sitesh Roy*[4]

The Current Status of the Practice of Allergy in the United States

Mark Holbreich

Introduction

Allergy and immunology is one of the smaller medical specialties in the United States. There are approximately 5000 board certified allergists in the United States for a population of 325 million. Although there is only 1 allergist per 50,000 population, allergists generally see the most severe patients and therefore although there is some shortage of allergists most individuals in the United States with severe allergies have access to a well-trained allergist. Many primary care physicians care for patients with mild allergies and asthma.

Becoming a board certified allergist requires a long period of training. Generally this path includes 4 years of university studies followed by 4 years of medical school. College generally begins around 18 years of age. Following medical school individuals interested in allergy must first complete 3 years of training in either pediatrics or internal medicine. This is followed by 2 years of allergy fellowship leading to board certification. There are approximately 80 allergy training programs in United States. Each program produces about two new allergists per year.

After completing an allergy fellowship physicians are required to take a national board examination and upon passing are certified as Board Certified Allergists. Certification is not permanent and allergists must complete ongoing continuing medical education to maintain their board certification.

---

[1] Allergy and Asthma Consultants, Indianapolis. Indiana, U S A, Email: mholbreich@comcast.net
[2] University of Colorado, Denver. Colorado USA.
[3] J S S University, Mysore. India, Email: mahesh1971in@yahoo.com
[4] Dr. Roy Health Solutions Clinics, Mumbai, India, Email: siteshroy@gmail.com
* corresponding author: pkv1947@gmail.com

After completing an allergy fellowship most individuals will enter into the clinical practice of allergy. A few individuals stay on at university medical centers to do research as well as patient care. Most often newly trained allergists will join an existing group of allergists who have an established allergy practice. There are many options for the newly trained allergist.

Healthcare in the United States

Most Americans obtain their healthcare through their employment. This is medical insurance. In this model the employer pays a portion of the cost and the patient is responsible for a portion of the cost. Medical insurance is not universal and therefore there is a portion of the population with no or very poor healthcare insurance. Patients over 65 have healthcare through the federal government (Medicare). The poorest families can receive health care at a very reduced or no cost through programs in each state (Medicaid). Healthcare in the United States is very costly for patients and the society. There is need for more affordable healthcare for much of the population.

Allergists in the United States see a variety of medical conditions. The most common are asthma, allergic rhinitis, urticarial, food allergy, eosinophilic esophagitis and immunodeficiency. In the recent past there have been many changes in the clinical practice of allergy.

Asthma

Asthma is a disorder affecting almost 7% of the population. Many patients with asthma have a mild disease which is managed by a primary care physician who does not have specific training in allergy/asthma. However patients with more complex allergies and asthma are seen by allergists. Currently the evaluation generally includes lung function testing, exhaled nitrous oxide and allergy testing. Since the addition in 2001 of ICS/LABA's the management of asthma has been significantly improved. There are currently a number of preparations containing a combination of ICS/LABA for both children and adults. A small percentage of patients are uncontrolled despite these new and better medications. It is now recognized that a certain phenotype often referred to as eosinophilic asthma in which there are high levels of peripheral eosinophils. These patients are benefited by the addition of new biologic medications that interfere with cytokine production particularly anti-IL-4, anti-IL-5 and anti-IL-13. Currently there are four biologics therapies available for allergists to use in the treatment of severe eosinophilic asthma. These agents are expensive and are only used when all other options are not controlling the patient's asthma. Some biologics are now approved for children 6 years of age and older.

Allergic rhinitis

Allergic rhinitis is found throughout the United States. Patients can be affected with year round or perennial allergic rhinitis or they may have seasonal allergic rhinitis which occurs primarily in the spring and fall of each year. The symptoms are quite characteristic and easy to recognize. The majority of these patients are treated with oral antihistamines and intranasal corticosteroids. Patients who do not do well on these medications can be treated with subcutaneous immunotherapy. They gradually receive increasing doses of the allergens to which they are allergic until they reach a maintenance dose at which time the patient receives concentrated injections of a mixture of the items to which they are allergic. There are risks associated with allergen immunotherapy including the risk of anaphylaxis. Treatment is usually undertaken for 3 to 5 years and then discontinued. Three sublingual products are now available including treatment for grass allergy, weed allergy and dust mite allergy.

Chronic idiopathic urticaria and angioedema

Urticaria will affect to 5–10% of the population at some time in their life. Angioedema is often seen in patients with urticarial or may occur in the absence of urticarial. Episodes of urticaria and angioedema may last for days, weeks or years. In patients with a typical presentation, the likelihood of finding a cause is uncertain. In the past 10 years a new agent for chronic urticaria and angioedema which is Omalizumab has been developed. This medication, also used for asthma, is extremely effective in the treatment of chronic idiopathic urticarial and angioedema. Although used sparingly it is certainly helpful with chronic problematic symptoms. Most allergists treat urticarial and angioedema with antihistamines at a high-dose as most symptoms will resolve spontaneously in 2–3 years. Testing for underlying medical conditions including allergy testing is not recommended unless the patient has an unusual medical history.

Food allergies

Food allergies now affect up to 8% of US children and a similar percentage of adults. The most common allergies in children are cow's milk, eggs, peanuts, tree nuts, wheat, soy, fish and shellfish. In adults the most common food allergy is shellfish. The current understanding is that food allergy develops when a food protein touches abnormal skin in an infant as in atopic dermatitis. Most childhood food allergies with the exception of peanuts, tree nuts, fish and shellfish will be outgrown. Following the publication of the Learning Early About Peanut (LEAP) trial in England it is now recommended that infants with atopic dermatitis begin eating peanuts at 6 months of life to induce tolerance. Currently the treatment for children who have a severe food allergy is avoidance of the food and carrying injectable epinephrine. It is expected that over the next few years treatment for food allergies will change dramatically with the introduction of programs for Oral Induction of Tolerance (OIT). The first product AR 101, which is purified peanut protein, will be commercially available in the near future.

Eosinophilic esophagitis

Eosinophilic esophagitis is a disease characterized most commonly by dysphagia in adults and chronic abdominal complaints in children. It was first recognized in 1986 and over the past 10 years the disease has been better defined. Although found throughout the world it is most prevalent in caucasian males living in developed countries. The treatment may consist of a diet or swallowed corticosteroids. It is a chronic and progressive disease.

Immunodeficiency

Immunodeficiency is a complex aspect of the practice of allergy. For more common diseases like common variable immunodeficiency (CVID) allergists may evaluate and treat with replacement gamma globulin therapy although the more complex diseases are seen in university medical centers by immunologists specializing in immunodeficiency.

Allergists practicing in the United States have the good fortune to have a number of organizations that support the allergist and their patients. Two major organizations are the American Academy of Allergy, Asthma and Immunology (aaaai.org) and the American College of Allergy, Asthma and Immunology (acai.org). Both organizations have medical journals devoted to the practice of allergy as well and many opportunities for continuing medical education. They also have robust teaching websites for patients. There are also national organizations that support families in whom there are serious allergic problems.

The future of allergy in the United States is well established. New highly trained allergists are meeting the need created by retiring allergists. The increase in food allergy and new therapies for food allergy will require the allergist to have excellent skills in food allergy management. New biologic therapy for asthma has improved the lives of many patients and there are a number of new biologic therapies under development that will continue to revolutionize the treatment of asthma. Biologics are under development for a variety of allergic problems including food allergy and eosinophilic esophagitis. The United States has many more well trained allergists than most countries in the world and it is fortunate to have this strong specialty to meet the needs of patients with complex allergic and immunological problems.

ALLERGY-ASTHMA PRACTICE: EAST VS WEST

P.K. Vedanthan

Introduction

It is a privilege to be in this specialty due to my involvement globally for the past three decades in providing care, doing research, charitable work as well as academic work both in USA and India. Hence I have been able to analyze the polarized scenarios in developed and Low to Middle Income Countries (LMIC).

The prevalence and incidence of allergic diseases are on the raise both in developed as well as developing countries. The demand for providing care for allergic patients is increasing worldwide. In developed countries like the USA and western Europe the ratio of an allergist for the population (1: 50,000) has been reached (Table 35.1). While the incidence of allergic diseases are steadily on the rise in India and are even reaching levels that would match those found in western countries, there are significant differences in the practice of diagnosing, treating and overall management. The pharmaceutical manufacturers have done remarkably well in providing the effective therapeutic agents both in developed as well as Low to Middle income countries. The major issue in the Low to Middle Income Countries (LMIC) is the lack of trained technical and medical personnel as well as lack of public awareness with regard to allergic diseases. Although there are well established guidelines to follow, these are not observed in the LMIC, resulting in huge morbidity and expense to the economies. There are major differences in the delivery of the care rendered to patients between the eastern and western hemispheres as outlined below.

Table 35.1. Global challenge (WAO White Paper 2010).

Country	Population (in millions)	Prevalence (in%)	Specialists (estimated)	Ratio of specialists
INDIA	1100	20	400	0.36/million
SRI LANKA	20	25	5	0.25/million
PHILLIPPINES	100	10–25	96	0.96/million
MEXICO	103	40	570	5.53/million
TAIWAN	23	30	358	15/million
BRAZIL	78	10–20	200	2.56/million
EGYPT	78	10–20	500	6.41/million
MALAYSIA	28	10–15	2	0.07/million
RUSSIA	141	20	1700	12.05/million
ZIMBABWE	10	15	1	0.1/million
USA	310	15	6000	19/million

Practice of medicine in USA

In general, the practice of medicine in the USA is highly regulated at several levels. Every practitioner has to meet the requirements of the State Board of Medical Examiners, a powerful arm of the respective state governments. Once the practitioner is licensed, he will able to practice medicine in that particular state. There are 50 different states in the USA and each state has its own licensing authority with slightly different requirements. The license in any state of USA has time limitations and has to be renewed along with evidence of Continued Medical Examination (CME) credits. The board has strict codes of moral and ethical conduct and if a physician is in conflict with those rules, he is liable for severe punishment, including revocation of his license in addition to financial penalties. The issue of medical malpractice is another major issue. The medical practitioner needs to have adequate insurance coverage (generally US$ 1–3 million. This aspect of practice of medicine influences the approach towards patient care and quite often defensive medicine is widely practiced. The medical scene in the USA is greatly influenced by insurance companies who determine how much the health professionals get reimbursed for their services. Nearly 80% of the US population is covered by medical insurance. Twenty percent of the population, translating to nearly 40 million people, have issues with access to adequate medical insurance coverage.

The specialty is very well represented by both professional and layman organizations. These organizations include American Academy of Allergy, Asthma and Immunology (AAAAI), American College of Allergy, Asthma & Immunology (ACAAI), Food Allergy Network and the Allergy Asthma Network. These organizations play a major role in offering continued education to healthcare professionals, paramedical personnel the public and patients. They also develop practice parameters in streamlining the essentials in the evaluation and treatment of common allergic diseases.

Most of the graduating fellows in USA will join established practices (either single specialty or multi specialty) on a salaried position with a guarantee of partnership with in 1–3 years. This arrangement has major advantages compared to entering a solo practice. The solo practitioner has major risks of uncertainness, lack of professional coverage, moral support, financial guarantee, imposing bank loans and a very uncertain prospect of future practice growth.

The most important decision a physician makes is to set his practice, either solo or as a member of the group, is **LOCATION**. It is the location of his medical practice that determines his professional and personal growth. The next very important criterion is the **NEED** for an allergy specialist in the community. It is advisable to limit the practice to the scope of specialization or sub specialization. Physician colleagues feel it less threatening to refer patients, if the services rendered are restricted to the area of specialization. Generally physician referrals are needed to help build the initial patient base, especially in the early years in practice. Patient referrals are the best way to build up the practice.

In the USA, there are several well known allergen extract companies that manufacture and supply standardized allergen extracts for testing and treatment. Clinic supplies and medical supplies are all easily available. Several banks also will be willing to finance the purchase of needed equipment, furniture as well as the needed supplies.

The set up of the practice area, meaning the ground plan and furnishings are very important. It is important to plan this with your office staff (manager, nurses and receptionist) to get a practical feedback on the planning process. Typically the layout of the office includes (Fig. 35.1):

1. Office entry with a clear sign
2. Waiting area: well furnished for patient comfort. Reading materials and pure drinking water are available
3. Reception counter from the business office: For registration
4. Allergy Injection room
5. Nurses station: Lung function, Blood drawing area
6. Examination rooms: equipped with basic equipment, x ray viewer, TV monitor for education, table with waiting chairs
7. Allergen extract storage in the refrigerator
8. Doctor's chamber
9. Storage areas for office supplies
10. Rest rooms (separate for staff and patients)

Allergy–Asthma Practice: East vs West 415

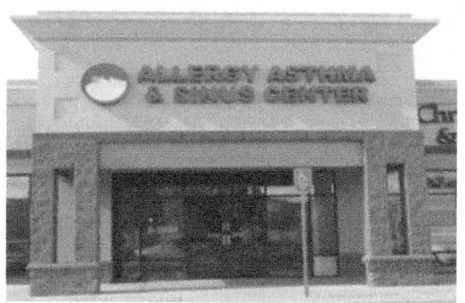

Main office with clear and visible sign
Clean and organized counter in the examination room
Nurse at work
Examination room 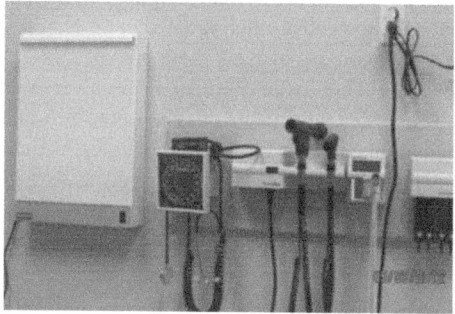
Examination room 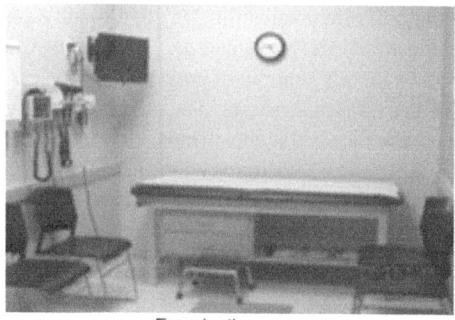
Antigens in the refrigerator 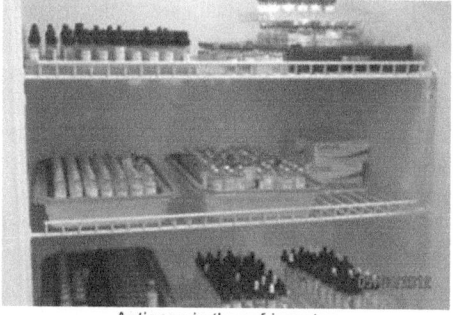
Storage area

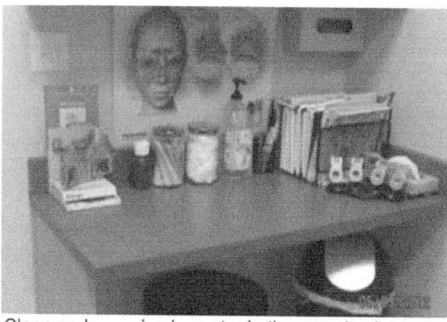

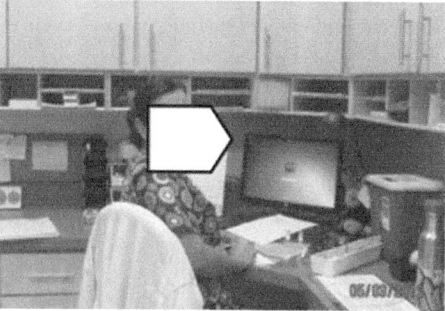

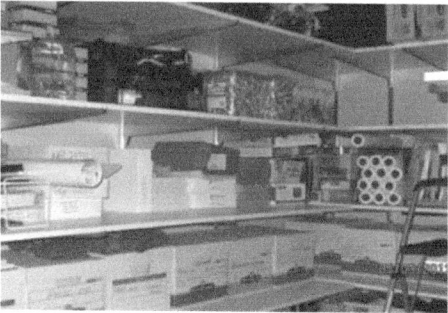

Figure 35.1. Figure 35.1 Allergy asthma office in lakewood, Colorado USA.

Scenario of Allergy–Asthma Practice in India

P.A. Mahesh

Introduction

Compared to the Western world where allergy practice is an established specialty, there are no courses offered in the specialty of allergy by the medical council of India at any medical university. Therefore, it is far more difficult to establish the field of allergy practice in India. There is paucity of recognition from both the colleagues in the medical profession and the patients alike as they are not aware of the progresses in the management of allergies. Except a handful of medical universities in India where, even though there are no courses offered, there are specialty clinics in allergy being run on a regular basis, most of the teaching faculties in other medical universities are not even aware of the field of allergy. Naturally, it is difficult for the students passing out from these universities to be well versed with even the basics of evaluation and management of allergies, which translates to poor management of allergic diseases in their patients. The following paragraphs deals with the SWOT analysis of the allergy practice in India. The key outcome measures used for the SWOT analysis are the four key features of management; patient counseling, pharmacotherapy, allergy avoidance and immunotherapy.

Strengths

One of the key strengths available to the Indian population is the availability of good quality generic drugs related to the management of allergic rhinitis and asthma. Relievers and preventers are available as dry powder or metered dose inhalers at a nominal cost. A month's supply of preventers costs less than US$ 3 dollars. The drugs are available even in most of the rural pharmacies. The other key strength is availability of medical personnel in the urban areas and paramedical personnel in most villages. At present the paramedical personnel are trained to administer vaccines under the national control program, conduct antenatal checkups and administer iron and folic acid tablets, conduct deliveries, malaria, tuberculosis and other infectious diseases, national control programs and referral services to the nearest primary health center where a medical officer is available when required. There is some support from the Government of India, which has established an Asthma Task Force under the aegis of the Indian Council of Medical Research to promote research into the field of allergies and asthma. Over the last decade many of the general practitioners have been trained in the management of asthma and use of inhalers and DPI's and even in the rural areas, practitioners have started prescribing these medications, which is a welcome change, though they are yet to incorporate practices to assess the severity of asthma such as spirometry and prescribe the appropriate dosage. Nebulizers are now available in many primary health care centers in the rural areas. It has been observed that even non-allopathic practitioners such as Ayurveda and other practitioners have started prescribing inhaled medications.

Weakness

For the practice of allergy in most developing countries, including India, the weaknesses outnumber the strengths. To start with, there is a need to have a comprehensive program or at least a formal fellowship in India in the specialty of allergy. A semi-formal diploma in allergies is offered at leading medical universities, but still leaves a lot to be desired. There is a need to introduce allergy in the curriculum of undergraduate and postgraduate courses such as medicine, pediatrics, ENT, skin and ophthalmology since these specialties find allergic diseases an important part of their clinical practice. Though the doctors who graduate are highly skilled in their chosen specialties, unless the subject is introduced in the curriculum and is practiced at medical college hospitals, they will find it difficult to master the subject on their own after they graduate. At present there is very little being taught about allergies to post graduate students in various disciplines, which leaves them ill equipped to manage patients with allergies. Aerobiology data is not available for most parts of the country and where available is quite old. The data is likely to have been changed since there are a lot of changes in the environment over the last few decades with rapid urbanization of most cities in India. There is a need for standardized collection of aerobiological data throughout the country with establishment of national aerobiological monitoring laboratories. Very few botany departments in most universities in India have trained aerobiologists in their teaching faculty and therefore most postgraduate students in botany with MSc or PhD are not aware of aerobiology and do not possess enough skills to run an aerobiology laboratory. There is also a need for greater standardization of allergens available for clinical testing in India. Many allergens are still available as weight by volume rather than in standardized units such as biological units. The most difficult allergens to standardize have been those of the house dust mite, which is also the most important allergen. This translates to poor choices during designing immunotherapy for the patients. Unfortunately, although pharmacotherapy include short and long acting bronchodilators and inhaled steroids alone or in combination are available at a very nominal cost in India, most clinicians still do not prescribe inhaled medications. The most common prescription by the family practitioner for asthma remains oral bronchodilators (Salbutamol or Theophylline or their combination) and for allergic rhinitis remains antihistamines. This greatly reduces the quality of life of most patients and the main reason for this practice behavior is the poor training received by the graduates in the field of allergy, since their teachers in the medical colleges themselves do not prescribe inhaled medications, especially for the graduates of various disciplines other than respiratory medicine. Most medical colleges also do not perform spirometry on a regular basis and this translates to the graduates not being trained to assess asthma appropriately and prescribe evidence-based dosages of inhaled steroids according to the severity of asthma. Most clinicians in India are not aware about the practice of allergy and the tools used for evaluation and when they should refer a case for specialist allergist consultation. Most practitioners also do not understand the basics of allergy and are unable to counsel their patients effectively regarding the need for regular medications, need for ICS, need for assessing the severity of the disease, assessing risk and preventing complications related to allergies. There is also very little research going on in the field of allergy and asthma in India except for few centers either in the field of epidemiology, clinical, basic science or new drug discovery.

Opportunities

If the curriculum of various sub-specialties is appropriately modified to include allergy as an important part in both theory and clinical practice, there is a good chance that there will be a tremendous change in the practice behavior of most clinicians. If a department of allergy is established in all the medical colleges and postings for students of various related sub-specialties is made mandatory for at least 3 months in the department of allergy, the clinicians will practice better evidence-based medicine for the management of various allergies and become more aware when and which case needs specialist care from an allergist. Since the drugs are quite economical, they could be provided at the primary health care centers and medical officers could be trained to administer them, which would make high quality care accessible to most patients in the rural areas. The Asthma Task Force under ICMR can promote more research in the field of allergy and asthma including better standardization of allergens for testing and treatment. Asthma guidelines are available for both adults and pediatric patients from national societies such as the Indian Chest Society (ICS) and Indian association of Pediatrics (IAP), but needs to be better disseminated to improve the quality of standardized care for patients.

Threats

Studies in India have shown an increase in the prevalence and severity of allergies, especially in children in some areas, though nationwide data are lacking. In the year 2020, the global asthma network will have the latest information on the burden of asthma and allergies in 12 cities in India, but more data from other cities are needed. Without the promotion of allergy as an important specialty there is a significant likelihood that most patients in the country would not be receiving appropriate treatment, though they can afford such treatment. There is a need to also conduct good quality epidemiologic and basic research in the field of allergies and retain the protective factors that may be present in the environment that has so far kept the prevalence of allergies low in India, especially related to food allergies, which are among the lowest in the world. Patients respond less well to medicines than they did two decades ago and that is another important cause for concern. India does not have the trained personnel as well as the required manpower to adequately manage the problem of food allergy if the prevalence were to increase to those levels found in the western population.

The Differences and Similarities between India and the USA

Sitesh Roy

If it is estimated that 20–40% of the US population (Pawankar et al. 2011) suffers from allergic disorders which would mean that about 100 million people are suffering from such diseases there. The incidence of asthma one of the classic allergic disorders seems to have plateaued in the US in the recent years (Bousquet et al. 2005). However, it is clearly rising in India and is expected to reach the levels of westernized countries in the next decade or two. Even if one conservatively estimates the number of allergy sufferers of all ages in India, based on regional clinical data from the International Study of Allergies and Asthma in Childhood (ISAAC) study centers as well as other published adult data, at only 20% (Shah and Pawankar 2009) one is left with a staggering number of 260 million allergic individuals in the country.

Patients tend to have much better access to and rapport with their General Practitioners (family physicians) in India and can only connect with physicians who are practicing allergy through referrals or via self-initiated searches on the internet or by word of mouth. Such specialists usually practice allergy out of their own choice and interest and include chest physicians (Pulmonologists), ENT specialists and internists or pediatricians who have taken some special training (certificate/diploma courses) to be allergologists. While there are over 4500 formally trained allergists-immunologists practicing in the US, it has been estimated that there are only about 450–500 physicians with any specialized training in allergy in India. This number has increased by around 150–200 in the past 5 years through certificate courses and the DAA type training programs which are truly trying to bridge the gap in allergy-asthma training and care in India. Fellowship program approval from MCI has been received but programs have not yet formally started. Interestingly, of the 600–650 Indian allergists only about 150–200 of them practice allergy as their primary specialty. The undergraduate curriculum in medical colleges also lacks adequate allergy training and basic management of life-threatening allergic reactions to food and insect stings, which are rising rapidly in India and is also lacking amongst recently trained medical graduates. The one positive trend in the past 4–5 years has been that every national level ENT, pediatrics or pulmonary conference has had sessions or workshops dedicated to allergies and their impact on patient management and disease control.

As would be expected, only few specialist trained allergy nurses and almost no formally trained respiratory therapists focus on asthma (as asthma educators) to support the growing number of patients in India except in select pockets (hospitals/multispecialty centers) where specialists practice.

Most specialists in India utilize the asthma guidelines released by Global initiative for asthma (GINA) or the World allergy organization (WAO) and a very few might even refer to the National Asthma Education and Prevention Program (NAEPP) guidelines. Asthma Awareness Programs within national organizations as well as at the local level have grown in the recent years.

The general awareness amongst the public and treating physicians regarding allergy and asthma symptoms, chronicity and progression of disease as well as its correct/optimal treatment is low. Even if the clinical diagnosis is correctly made, the utilization of the latest best confirmatory tests and treatment options by general physicians and sometimes even internists and pediatricians is sub-optimal in India. The use of simple tests like Peak Expiratory Flow (PEF) readings or slightly more sophisticated measurements with a Spirometer or Exhaled Nitric Oxide for diagnosis or follow up care is extremely low. Only when a patient finds their way to a specialist in a tertiary allergy/asthma center can they expect some semblance of care in keeping with international guidelines.

There are many diagnostic difficulties including access to qualified allergologists, lack of standardized reagents for testing and limited array of testing devices. The price of these allergy tests, also make the improvisation of testing techniques necessary to achieve feasibility. Huge reliance on *in vitro* allergy tests with strong promotion by laboratories for the same, without proper clinical correlation has created a major issue for those with positive results since allergy vs. sensitization is not well understood. False reporting or suboptimal testing with old techniques like (RAST) is also a major issue in these *in vitro* tests.

While house dust mite remains the most common sensitizing allergen all across India (Podder et al. 2010), there is a clear lack of data with regards to clinically relevant pollen producing trees, grasses and weeds as well as regional pollen calendars which would aid specialists and patients better understand how to manage their seasonal symptoms/exacerbations. Most patients tend to be poly-sensitized with environmental and/or food allergens. Regional variation in flora and type of foods consumed, make uniform testing kits harder to gain ready acceptability.

With regards to desensitization (immunotherapy) protocols for allergies once detected, there are significant issues. Once again the lack of standardized allergen extracts is the main concern. There are now Indian allergen immunotherapy practice parameters in place for guiding specialists in performance of effective allergen immunotherapy. Patient choice gravitates towards sublingual immunotherapy due to greater perceived safety as well as access to clinics/centers for weekly injections being an issue. Sublingual immunotherapy is performed with a wide array of non-standardized allergens for which there is little scientific data to guide their optimal dosing and duration of therapy. Without clear research of the reactivity of local allergens, effectiveness of mixes of these allergens for convenience into single vials creates problems. Thus some specialists get disheartened by the lack of clinical efficacy of oral/sublingual immunotherapy and cease to practice it. Similarly with subcutaneous (injectable) immunotherapy the lack of standardization and suboptimal knowledge regarding the dosage and compatibility of allergens that can be mixed with one another safely affects the efficacy of immunotherapy. Allergen immunotherapy is practiced by 'specialists' without knowledge of the exact contents of the major allergens in these mixes. The dosages administered are also sub therapeutic. The majority of specialists practicing allergy rely on local antigen manufacturers to determine the exact concentration of allergens to be included in their patient's immunotherapy mixes. The only standardized allergen extracts for testing and immunotherapy available in India are from Allergopharma, Merck India, but, unfortunately been withdrawn from the country recently. The Central Government intervention with policy changes for ease of quality care access to patients alone can help fix these issues. Hopefully the care of allergic and asthma patients will improve in the coming years as awareness grows universally.

Oral food allergen desensitization using non-standardized commercial extracts, while not recommended or proven safe or effective in clinical trials, is done by some allergy specialists in India. Fortunately most of these are conducted in cases that are non-anaphylactic in nature but serious/fatal reactions likely go unreported and under-diagnosed.

There are a lot more pharmaceutical treatment options available for allergy and asthma in India, but due to the lack of stringent drug control regulations for making existing drug combinations, these had been in use for years before being withdrawn by legislation. There is a greater reliance on Methylxanthines (e.g., Theophylline, Doxifylline, Acebrophylline) in the first- and second-line treatment of asthma in both children and adults in India than in the US. Also the use of oral beta-2 agonists alone or in combination with Methylxanthines is more prevalent in the East due to cost and compliance reasons. There is over use and misuse of antibiotics as well as systemic steroids to treat these common disorders (Prasad et al. 2002). A series of histaglobin injections, a mixture of histamine with gamma globulin is still used by many skin and allergy specialists in India for atopic disease including urticaria, and other skin/respiratory allergies. This drug does not even have a mention in the management guidelines for the above mentioned diseases in the West. These are matters of concern and need to be addressed at different levels with scientific evidence based practice parameters.

There are no local manufacturers or bulk-importers of pre-loaded, self-inject able Epinephrine for use after anaphylactic reactions in India. Actually, the awareness, diagnosis and treatment of anaphylaxis in India is extremely poor. Even at major medical institutions and well known medical centers, epinephrine is still NOT used as the primary drug for anaphylaxis; instead antihistamines and steroids are being widely used. This is a matter of major concern and needs to be addressed towards all practicing physicians in India.

There is still a certain degree of social and cultural taboo in the Indian society with the diagnosis/label of asthma that is not seen in the West. Fear of communicability/transmission remains in the minds of some people leading to the use of many untested alternative therapies to get rid of these diseases. The fear of using inhalers and being viewed as the 'last resort' rather than being the 'first line of treatment' is still widely prevalent in both rural and urban settings.

Most expenses for allergy and asthma care in the USA or European nations is either subsidized by the government or medical insurance carriers, however in India right from the consultation visits and follow-ups to testing and therapy is all paid for by the patient without any medical insurance coverage/support. Actually 70% of the medical expenses are borne directly by the consumers (WHO 2012) and this is reflective of the lack of subsidy by the government as well as poor insurance coverage. Some government run hospitals and clinics do provide urgent and emergency as well as outpatient care including specialty care at very subsidized rates; but their impact is limited by the magnitude of sufferers who cannot reach them either due to distance from such centers or long waiting hours once there. Serious lack of dedicated asthma allergy centers, except in large government or private multi-specialty hospitals, is a glaring problem as the incidence of allergic disorders and asthma continue to rise in India.

Similarities

Patients in India also think of asthma and allergies as episodic diseases that do not require chronic preventive treatment and follow up. Patient adherence/compliance remains as much of an issue if not more just as is seen in the West. Fear of chronic medication usage, fear of dependency on inhalers and concerns about steroid safety remain problems in both the East and the West. *In vitro* diagnostic tests such as Thermofisher-Phadia Immuno-CAP testing are very widely available all over India now. This has helped bring the options for diagnostic testing up to international standards here to some extent. Therapeutic options are excellent and generally of high quality, even at much lower prices than in the West, but some forms of treatment such as Anti-IgE remain out of reach for most patients due to the largely self-pay scenario in India. Steroid phobia is a universal phenomenon in the East and West.

Future needs

1. Greater awareness regarding manifestations of allergies and asthma as well its effective treatment both amongst the general population, as well as grass root level general physicians and specialists is necessary. 2. Better diagnostic options by way of devices and standardized antigens. 3. Regional pollen studies for clinical relevance and pollen calendars. 4. Introduction of safer medium- and high-dose allergen immunotherapy with standardized allergens to alter the natural course of these chronic diseases. 5. More formal training programs for allergy and asthma specialists recognized by the Government of India and local State governments to train the future cadre of specialists who can provide higher standards of care to a growing populace of allergic individuals. 6. Enhancing the medical school curriculum to include the topics related to allergy and immunology. 7. More dedicated asthma and allergy centers manned by trained physicians, nurses and respiratory therapists all over India that can cater to the needs of such patients. 8. More rigorously tested therapeutic choices in keeping with international guidelines. 9. Better

insurance coverage for outpatient allergy and asthma diagnosis and treatment. 10. Establishment of centers of excellence in the field to facilitate research and education.

Conclusions

There are significant differences in disease burden, physician and para-medical personnel manpower, training opportunities, educational outreaches as well as over all care for patients between the East and West. In this chapter, USA and India have been taken as model scenarios to represent the western and eastern hemispheres.

Bibliography

Bousquet J, Bousquet PJ, Godard P, Daures JP. The public health implications of asthma. Bulletin of the WAO 2005 Jul; 83(7): 548–54.
Pawankar R, Canonica GC, Holgate ST, Lockey RF. World Health Organization. White Book on Allergy 2011–2012 Executive Summary.
Podder S, Kumar S, Saha G. Incrimination of *Blomia tropicalis* as a potent allergen in house dust and its role in allergic asthma in Kolkata Metropolis, India. World Allergy Organ J 2010 May; 3(5): 182–187.
Prasad R, Prescribing pattern of GPs for asthma in India. Indian J Allergy Asthma Immunol 2002; 16(2): 89–92.
Shah A, Pawankar R. Allergic Rhinitis and Co-morbid Asthma: Perspective from India- ARIA Asia-Pacific Workshop Report. Asian Pac J Allergy 2009; 27: 71–77.
World health organization: World Health Statistics 2012.

Index

A

AAAAI 412, 414
ACAAI 414
Acute Urticaria 288–291, 294–296
Adaptive immunity 348, 350
adenoids 113
Adverse reaction to foods 322, 330
Aerobiology 49–51, 53, 63
air pollutant 219–221, 223, 224, 226–228
air pollution 70, 75, 219, 221–223, 225–228
Airway inflammation 139, 140, 145
Airway remodeling 140
allergen avoidance 82, 83, 87
allergen immunotherapy 82, 87, 165
allergen immunotherapy administration 185
Allergic conjunctivitis 99–101, 104, 105, 107
Allergic Contact Dermatitis 312
allergic disease 207, 211, 213, 215, 216
allergic reaction 255, 258, 259, 264
allergic rhinitis 78–82, 86, 87, 219, 223, 225
allergies 69, 70, 72, 74
allergy 19–24, 28–30, 242, 245, 366, 368, 369, 372, 373
Allergy diagnosis 417
Allergy Fellowship 410, 411
Allergy Practice US 411
allergy skin tests 40
Alternate nostril breathing 382
anaphylaxis 255–268, 273–277, 279–284, 389, 393, 398, 400
Anemophilous 50, 53, 54, 60, 63
Angioedema 287–291, 293, 296–300
antibody 5, 6
aspirin desensitization 185, 201, 203
aspirin exacerbated respiratory disease 89, 90
aspirin sensitivity 90, 91, 94
Aspirin triad 91
asthma 69–74, 125–136, 219–228, 231–233, 235, 237, 238, 366, 368–373, 381, 383–385
Asthma treatment 153
Atopic dermatitis 303–309
Atopic Kerato-conjunctivitis 100
Atopic march 10, 12, 17
atopy patch testing 185, 196
Autoimmunity 290, 351

B

B cell 1–3, 5
basophil activation test 45, 277
Board certification 410
Bronchial reactivity 10

C

Calcineurin inhibitor 307, 309
CAM 367, 373
Challenge test 335, 394, 396
chemicals 75
child 128, 130, 133, 135, 136
childhood asthma 221, 223
choana 109, 110, 113, 115, 120–123
chronic rhinosinusitis 89, 90, 93, 94
Chronic Spontaneous Urticaria 290, 292, 293
clinical history 19, 22, 24
clinical skill 418
Cobblestone papillae 102
co-factors 258
Complement system 348, 352
complementary and alternative medicine 376–378
component resolved diagnostics 45
concha bullosa 113
Contact dermatitis 306, 403, 404, 406, 407
Continued Medical Education 413
COPD 231–233, 235–238
Corpse posture 383
correlation 34, 35, 40, 41
Cross reactivity 324, 325, 328
cytokine 3–8
Cytokine signaling defects 352

D

decongestants 148, 150–152
diagnosis 332–335, 337–340, 343
diagnostic criteria 255, 257, 268
diagnostic testing 333, 336, 343
diet 70–72
dietary management 366, 369

Diffusion capacity 183
dosing 167, 169, 170, 172, 173
DRESS 389, 391–393, 395, 396, 399, 401
Drug Allergy 387, 389, 394–396, 401
Dupilumab 304, 308, 309

E

Early and late phase reaction 11, 14
Eczema 303–307
emergency management 266–268
endoscopic sinus surgery 90, 92, 93, 95
energy therapies 366, 372
Entomophilous 50
environment 207, 213, 214
environmental control 213
Eosinophilic esophagitis 327, 329
Epicutaneous Skin test 33, 34
epidemiology 246
Epigenetic regulation 226
etiology 255
eucapnic voluntary hyperventlilation 185
exercise challenge 185, 187, 188, 205
exposure 207–211, 213–216

F

factors influencing 37
FEF25–75% 183
FESS 94, 95
FEV$_1$ 179, 182, 183, 250
fluorescent enzyme immunoassay 43
Food allergy 321–324, 326–330
Food intolerance 322
Forced expiratory volume 383, 385
fractional exhaled nitric oxide measurement 185, 188, 189
FVC 179, 180, 182, 183

G

Gene by environment response 11–13
Genetic defects 350
GERD 141
Giant Papillary conjunctivitis 100, 103–105
Global Burden of Disease Study 139
Global initiative on asthma 418
Graded Challenge 395, 396, 399
Graft versus host disease 362

H

Health insurance 411
Hereditary Angioedema (HAE) 296
High affinity receptor 32
high molecular weight 242, 245, 246, 252
High-affinity IgE receptors (FcεRI) 288
Histamine 33, 36–41

Horner-Tranta's dots 103
Hymenoptera 271, 273, 275–279, 283, 284
Hypersensitivity 389–396, 398–400

I

immediate hypersensitivity 406, 407
immune response 4, 8
immunity 10–15
Immunodeficiency 347, 348, 350–352, 354, 356, 358, 360, 363
Immunoglobulin and IgE 10–11, 32, 33
Immunoglobulin replacement therapy 362, 363
Immunologic asthma 127, 144
immunomodulators 151, 153–155, 158, 161
Immunotherapy 271, 273, 279, 281, 282
Impulse Oscillometry 178
in vitro 35, 40
Indian Association of Pediatrics 417
Induction of Tolerance 395–397
inhaled corticosteroids 153, 155, 157, 161
inhaled short-acting beta agonist 153
inhalers 158, 159
Innate immunity 348, 352, 358, 362
innate immunity and hygiene hypothesis 13, 211, 212, 362
innate lymphoid cell 7
Insect sting 273–274, 276, 277, 284
integrative medicine 367, 373
Intradermal skin test 33, 34
intradermal skin testing 33, 34
Intradermal test 276, 277
intradermal testing 185, 193, 195
intranasal corticosteroids 147–152, 161
Irritant Contact Dermatitis 313, 314
irritant-induced asthma 249, 253

L

Laboratory tests for immune defects 358–360
Large local reaction 273, 279, 280
larynx 109, 111–113, 117–121, 124
latex allergy 403–407
latex-fruit syndrome 405
leukotriene pathway modifying 153, 154
lifestyle 207, 211–213, 215, 216
lifestyle therapies 366, 368
Lipid transfer Protein 324
local anesthetic testing 185, 193
long-acting beta agonist 161
low molecular weight 242, 245
Lung Functions 383, 384
Lung Volumes 178, 179, 181, 182
lymphocyte 3, 5, 6
management 332, 340, 342, 343

M

Mast cell 32, 33
Mastocytosi 274, 280, 281, 283, 284
Mediators of allergic reaction 11, 14
Medicaid 411
Medicare 411
meditation 378
methacholine challenge 185, 188, 189
Microbiota and inflammation 15
mind-body interventions 366, 371
mixed rhinitis 80

N

nasal cavity 108–110, 112–114, 116, 119–121
nasal polyps 89–95, 114
nasal septum 110, 114
nasopharynx 108, 109, 111, 113, 115–117, 119–122
natural products 367, 373
nebulizer administration 185
NK cell 1, 6
Non IgE mediated allergy 328, 329
nonallergic rhinitis 78, 80, 82–84, 86
Nummular Eczema 306

O

Obstructive Lung disease 179, 181, 182
occupational asthma 241–253
Omalizumab 295, 299
Oral allergy Syndrome 328
oral antihistamines 148–152, 161
oral food challenge 185, 199, 200
Oral tolerance 324
oropharynx 109, 111, 113, 115–117, 122

P

Palynology 49
Papillary hypertrophy 100, 102
patch testing 185, 195, 196, 312–316, 318, 319
pathophysiology 255, 259, 261, 268
patient selection 167
Pattern recognition receptors 347, 348, 355
Peak Flow measurement 178, 182
Peak flow rate 383
Penicillin 388, 389, 393–400
penicillin testing 185, 194
peptide array 45, 46
perinatal 70, 72
Phagocytic cells 352, 361
pharmacotherapy 84
Photophobia 99, 100, 103
P-K or Prausnitz and Kustner reaction 11
Pollen calendar 49–52
Pollination 49–51, 53–55
post-natal 70

prenatal 70, 71
prevalence 207, 214, 216
prevention 332, 342
prick skin testing 36, 38–40
primary prevention 406, 407
procedures 185, 187, 189, 197, 199, 205
Pulmonary Function testing 178, 179, 183
pulmonary medicine 418

R

radioallergosorbent test 44
reactive airways dysfunction syndrome 242
Recognition of immunodeficiency diseases 350
respiratory disorders 418
Restrictive Lung disease 179, 180, 182
rhinitis 78–84, 86, 87
rhinitis treatment 151
rhinoscopy 110, 185, 204, 205
Risk factors 69–71
Routes of sensitization 211

S

safety 165, 166, 173
Samter's triad 90
SCIT 165–166, 168–170, 173, 174
Seed Storage protein 325
Self injectable Epinephrine 420
Sensitization 32–35, 323–328
Severe Asthma Research Program 144
Shoulder stand 381, 382
sinuses 111, 113–115, 120, 123
skin prick testing 185, 191–193
Skin testing 277
SLIT 165, 173, 174
Specific IgE 43–46
Specific IgE tests 276
sphenoethmoidal recess 108, 111, 114, 119–121, 123
spirometry 185–190
Staph aureus 307
Stem cell transplant 348, 357
Subcutaneous Immunotherapy 166
systemic corticosteroids 153, 156
Systemic reaction 271, 273, 274, 279, 281, 282, 284

T

T and B cells 347, 348, 350, 358
T cell 1–6, 8
tests 185, 188, 190–196, 199, 205
Th2 cells and Cytokines 12
Tiger posture 381
traditional Chinese medicine 372
Traditional medicine 366
treatment 333, 335, 337, 338, 340, 341, 343

Tryptase 33
turbinates 110–114
united airway hypothesis 81

U

Upper Airway cough syndrome 141
US training 410

V

Venom Allergy 271, 273–279, 283, 284
Venom Immunotherapy 273, 279, 281

venom testing 185, 194, 195
Vernal Kerato-conjunctivitis 100
vocal folds 112, 113, 117, 118, 120, 123

W

Wiskott Aldrich syndrome 306
workplace 241, 242, 247, 248, 250
World allergy Organization 418

Y

Yoga breathing Techniques 381

About the Editors

Pudupakkam K Vedanthan

Pudupakkam K Vedanthan (PK) is the lead editor of the Text Book of Allergy for the Clinician, 2nd edition. He is a native of Mysore, India and a graduate of Government Medical College, University of Mysore. He comes from a family of physicians including his father and two of his brothers who were alumni of the same medical college. After his initial training in India, he served as a Straight Medical Intern, Resident in Paediatrics and Fellow in Allergy & Immunology in USA. He is board certified by the American Boards of Paediatrics and Allergy, Asthma and Immunology. He served for 25 years in Consultation practice in Fort Collins, Colorado. At the same time, he maintained academic affiliation with University of Colorado, Denver where he has been a Clinical Professor of Medicine for the past decade. He has published in both national and international journals, and has been active in the academic circle in various capacities. He has contributed to Colorado Medical Society (CMS), Association of American Physicians of Indian origin (AAPI) in several capacities. His major contribution has been in Global medicine, since he established 'International Asthma Services (IAS), (www.globalchestintitiatives.org) in 1992. IAS has been active in several developing countries like India, Sri Lanka, Mauritius, Kenya, Russia, Myanmar, Philippines, Argentina, Nepal conducting CMEs for health professionals and Asthma allergy Awareness camps for patients and their families and public in general. IAS has also partnered with major medical institutions in India, namely Christian Medical College-hospital (www.cmch-vellore.edu), Vellore, Tamilnadu and Sir Gangaram Hospital & Research Centre (www.pace@sgrh.com), Delhi, in establishing formal diploma courses in allergy, asthma and immunology. These courses have been very well received and had made a significant impact of the care provided in several developing countries. Dr. PK has also been involved in providing voluntary medical care to the refugee population from 22 nations in the Denver area through Colorado Alliance for Health education & Promotion (CAHEP) for the past three decades. In recognition of these activities, IAS was recognized in 2015 by the Centre for Global Health, School of Public Health, University of Colorado by the award of 'Excellence in Global health'. He has been the recipient of AMA Leadership award, Distinguished Service award, Rotary 'Service Above Self Award', International Faculty award, Special Innovator award from the department of Medicine, University of Colorado, Denver.

Harold S Nelson

Dr. Nelson received an undergraduate degree in economics from Harvard College and later earned a doctor of medicine degree from Emory University. He then completed a residency in internal medicine at Letterman General Hospital and a fellowship in allergy/immunology at the University of Michigan. Dr. Nelson has published over 400 articles and book chapters. He has served on the Board of Regents of the American College of Allergy, Asthma, and Immunology (ACAAI), as well as on the Board of Directors of both the American Academy of Allergy, Asthma, and Immunology (AAAAI) and the American Board of Allergy and Immunology (ABAI). He was a member of the First, Second and Third Expert Panels of the NIH—NAEPP for developing the Guidelines for the Diagnosis and Management of Asthma. Dr. Nelson has been honored with the 'Fellow Distinguished Award' and 'Gold-Headed Cane Award' by the ACAAI; the 'Distinguished Clinician Award' 'Special Recognition Award' and 'Distinguished Service Award' by the AAAAI; the 'Outstanding Clinician Award' from the World Allergy Organization and the 'Lifetime Achievement Award' by National Jewish Health. He has also been honored with named lectureships at the annual meetings of the ACAAI 2008–2009, the AAAAI 2001–2017 and the Western Society of Allergy and Immunology 2018–2022.

Shripad N Agashe

Professor Shripad N Agashe is a dedicated University teacher and research scientist with vast experience of over three decades in USA and Bangalore, India. During his academic career, he has guided 22 research students for PhD and published more than 75 research papers in National and International scientific journals.

He is the author of the text book 'Palyngology and its Applications' published in 2006. His recent book, 'Pollens and Spores' with special emphasis on Aerobiology and Allergy, jointly authored by Prof. Eric Caulton of U.K. was published in 2009.

Prof. Agashe was the founder president of the Indian Academy of Allergy from 1990–98. He was also the past President of the Indian College of Allergy and applied Immunology with headquarters in Delhi.

His tireless efforts over the years have succeeded in bringing together basic scientists (aerobiologists) and clinicians (allergists) for the common cause of giving relief to allergic patients. He was the pioneer in initiating the daily pollen monitoring and creating awareness among allergy sufferers and clinicians in Bangalore, India.

PA Mahesh

Dr. PA Mahesh, completed his undergraduate medical training at KMC, Mangalore in 1992 and his post graduate training in 1997. He is a Professor of Respiratory Medicine at JSS Medical College, Mysore and is a clinician researcher with over two decades of experience in clinical research. His main interest is in research in airway diseases such as asthma and COPD, allergy and infections. He has 123 publications, an h index of 41 and i10 index of 70 and total citations of 22,124 (google scholar). He has been part of large national and international consortiums such as the Global Burden of Disease (GBD), Europrevall, BOLD study I and II, GLIMP, EMBARC, Global Asthma Network (GAN), APRISE and INSEARCH. As part of the International and National (State level collaborators) for the Global Burden of Disease (GBD) and Local Burden of Disease (LBD) group he has several publications in high impact factor journals. As PI, Co-Investigator or Mentor on several Indian Council of Medical Research (ICMR), Department of Science and Technology (DST), Council of Scientific and Industrial Research (CSIR), European Union (FP6) and GHES (NIH, USA), GID (NIH, USA), MRC (UK), Swedish Heart Lung Foundation grants, He has coordinated large-scale epidemiological studies involving house-to-house surveys and schools of more than 1,00,000 subjects. In addition, he has successfully administered the projects (e.g., staffing, research protections, budget) and has collaborated with other researchers from Imperial College, London, UK, Institute of Food Research, Norwich, UK, Amsterdam Medical Center and Leiden Medical Center in the Netherlands, Chinese University of Hong Kong, Siberian State Medical University in Russia, National Jewish Health, and Yale University, USA and Karolinska Institute, Sweden. He has established three cohorts in urban and rural Mysore; Urban adult (BOLD, 7 years old, 3 follow ups), Rural adult (MUDHRA, 10 years old, 4 follow-ups) and Urban child (Europrevall, 1 follow-up).

He has reviewed several national and international journals and conferences. He reviews for 25 international journals and 5 national journals. He regularly reviews abstracts for American College of Chest Physicians, American Academy of Asthma Allergy and Immunology, Global Health Equity Scholars Program (USA) and the Consortium of Universities for Global Health (CUGH), USA. He is the current Chairman of the Karnataka State Chapter of Indian Chest Society and is a member of the Governing Council of the American College of Chest Physicians. He has received several awards, Young Scientist Award and Raju award for the best clinical research, ShivPuri oration from the Indian College of Allergy Asthma and Immunology, OA Sarma oration from the Indian Chest Society (ICS).

Rohit Katial

Rohit Katial, M.D. is a Professor of Medicine at National Jewish Health and the University of Colorado. He continues in these roles but also is the Respiratory, National Physician Head in US Medical Affairs at AstraZeneca. Dr. Katial received his B.S. from Georgetown University in Physics, a B.E.E. from Catholic University of America and subsequently an M.D. from Georgetown University School of Medicine. He went on to do internal medicine training in the US Army Medical Corps, culminating in specialty training both in Allergy/Immunology (AI) and Clinical Laboratory Immunology. He completed his A/I training at Fitzsimons Army Medical Center/National Jewish Health and clinical immunology at Walter Reed Army Medical Center. He has served in numerous roles, including Associate Vice President of Clinical Research & Industry Relationships, Co-Director of the Asthma Institute at National Jewish Health, Fellowship Director at National Jewish Health and named the Helen Wohlberg & Herman Lambert Chair in Pharmacokinetics. His other roles have included Director of the Allergy/Immunology Clinical Service. Dr. Katial has an international reputation in airway disease and has extensive publications on sinusitis, asthma, particularly on aspirin exacerbated respiratory disease and has especific interest in eosinophilic diseases. He has numerous original publications, as well as has edited and authored many book chapters. He was the Principal Investigator for the American Lung Association Airway Clinical Research Consortium, which is a U.S. based airway research network, and has conducted clinical trials for over 20 years. He also led numerous trials on vaccine immune response, asthma and allergic diseases. Dr. Katial is a fellow of the American Academy of Allergy, Asthma & Immunology, a fellow of the American College of Allergy, Asthma & Immunology, as well as a fellow of the American College of Physicians. He is the Chair of the Accreditation Council on Graduate Medical Education (ACGME) Review Committee for Allergy and Immunology. He is board certified by the American Board of Internal Medicine, American Board of Allergy & Immunology with specialty certification in Clinical Laboratory Immunology. He has received numerous awards for his teaching skills and on six occasions been listed in the Denver 5280 Magazine's Top Doctors, as well as yearly in the US News and World Report's Best Doctors.